Mechanisms, Diagnosis and Treatment of Neurological Disorders

Mechanisms, Diagnosis and Treatment of Neurological Disorders

Editor: Elijah Bowers

AMERICAN
MEDICAL PUBLISHERS
www.americanmedicalpublishers.com

AMERICAN
MEDICAL PUBLISHERS
www.americanmedicalpublishers.com

Cataloging-in-Publication Data

Mechanisms, diagnosis and treatment of neurological disorders / edited by Elijah Bowers.
p. cm.
Includes bibliographical references and index.
ISBN 979-8-88740-313-7
1. Nervous system--Diseases. 2. Nervous system--Diseases--Diagnosis.
3. Nervous system--Diseases--Treatment. 4. Nervous system--Diseases--Pathogenesis.
5. Neurology. I. Bowers, Elijah.
RC346 .M43 2023
616.8--dc23

American Medical Publishers,
41 Flatbush Avenue,
1st Floor, New York,
NY 11217, USA

ISBN 979-8-88740-313-7 (Hardback)

Contents

Preface

Every book is a source of knowledge and this one is no exception. The idea that led to the conceptualization of this book was the fact that the world is advancing rapidly; which makes it crucial to document the progress in every field. I am aware that a lot of data is already available, yet, there is a lot more to learn. Hence, I accepted the responsibility of editing this book and contributing my knowledge to the community.

Neurological diseases are the diseases of the nervous system, which are caused due to electrical, structural and biochemical abnormalities in the brain, spinal cord or other nerves. Neurodegenerative and cerebrovascular diseases are major types of neurological diseases, which are related with high morbidity and mortality. The progressive loss of structure or function of neurons is the primary cause of a neurodegenerative disease and this process is known as neurodegeneration. Cerebrovascular diseases are a range of medical conditions that affect the blood vessels of the brain and cerebral circulation. The diagnosis of neurological disorders is a difficult process since the symptoms generally overlap between multiple disorders. Diagnosing a particular neurological condition involves a study of the medical history of the family, physical examination and imaging tests. Medications, lifestyle changes, surgery, along with supportive and rehabilitative therapies can be used to treat neurological disorders. This book presents researches that have transformed the study of neurological disorders. It is compiled in such a manner, that it will provide in-depth knowledge about the mechanisms, diagnosis and treatment of these disorders. This book will serve as a valuable source of reference for those interested in this field.

While editing this book, I had multiple visions for it. Then I finally narrowed down to make every chapter a sole standing text explaining a particular topic, so that they can be used independently. However, the umbrella subject sinews them into a common theme. This makes the book a unique platform of knowledge.

I would like to give the major credit of this book to the experts from every corner of the world, who took the time to share their expertise with us. Also, I owe the completion of this book to the never-ending support of my family, who supported me throughout the project.

Editor

1

Cerebrovascular Pathology in Hypertriglyceridemic APOB-100 Transgenic Mice

Zsófia Hoyk[1†], Melinda E. Tóth[2†], Nikolett Lénárt[2‡], Dóra Nagy[2], Brigitta Dukay[2], Alexandra Csefová[2], Ágnes Zvara[3], György Seprényi[4], András Kincses[1], Fruzsina R. Walter[1], Szilvia Veszelka[1], Judit Vigh[1], Beáta Barabási[1], András Harazin[1], Ágnes Kittel[5], László G. Puskás[3], Botond Penke[6], László Vígh[2], Mária A. Deli[1] and Miklós Sántha[2*]*

[1] Institute of Biophysics, Biological Research Centre, Hungarian Academy of Sciences, Szeged, Hungary, [2] Institute of Biochemistry, Biological Research Centre, Hungarian Academy of Sciences, Szeged, Hungary, [3] Laboratory of Functional Genomics, Core Facilities, Biological Research Centre, Hungarian Academy of Sciences, Szeged, Hungary, [4] Department of Anatomy, Histology and Embryology, Faculty of Medicine, University of Szeged, Szeged, Hungary, [5] Laboratory of Molecular Pharmacology, Department of Pharmacology, Institute of Experimental Medicine, Hungarian Academy of Sciences, Budapest, Hungary, [6] Department of Medical Chemistry, Faculty of Medicine, University of Szeged, Szeged, Hungary

***Correspondence:**
Mária A. Deli
deli.maria@brc.mta.hu
Miklós Sántha
santha.miklos@brc.mta.hu

† These authors have contributed equally to this work

‡ Present address:
Nikolett Lénárt,
Laboratory of Neuroimmunology, Department of Molecular and Developmental Neuroscience, Institute of Experimental Medicine, Hungarian Academy of Sciences, Budapest, Hungary

Hypertriglyceridemia is not only a serious risk factor in the development of cardiovascular diseases, but it is linked to neurodegeneration, too. Previously, we generated transgenic mice overexpressing the human APOB-100 protein, a mouse model of human atherosclerosis. In this model we observed high plasma levels of triglycerides, oxidative stress, tau hyperphosphorylation, synaptic dysfunction, cognitive impairment, increased neural apoptosis and neurodegeneration. Neurovascular dysfunction is recognized as a key factor in the development of neurodegenerative diseases, but the cellular and molecular events linking cerebrovascular pathology and neurodegeneration are not fully understood. Our aim was to study cerebrovascular changes in APOB-100 transgenic mice. We described the kinetics of the development of chronic hypertriglyceridemia in the transgenic animals. Increased blood-brain barrier permeability was found in the hippocampus of APOB-100 transgenic mice which was accompanied by structural changes. Using transmission electron microscopy, we detected changes in the brain capillary endothelial tight junction structure and edematous swelling of astrocyte endfeet. In brain microvessels isolated from APOB-100 transgenic animals increased *Lox-1, Aqp4*, and decreased *Meox-2, Mfsd2a, Abcb1a, Lrp2, Glut-1, Nos2, Nos3, Vim*, and in transgenic brains reduced *Cdh2* and *Gfap-σ* gene expressions were measured using quantitative real-time PCR. We confirmed the decreased P-glycoprotein (ABCB1) and vimentin expression related to the neurovascular unit by immunostaining in transgenic brain sections using confocal microscopy. We conclude that in chronic hypertriglyceridemic APOB-100 transgenic mice both functional and morphological cerebrovascular pathology can be observed, and this animal model could be a useful tool to study the link between cerebrovascular pathology and neurodegeneration.

Keywords: apolipoprotein B-100, astroglia, blood-brain barrier, brain endothelial cell, cerebrovascular pathology, hypertriglyceridemia, P-glycoprotein, tight junction

INTRODUCTION

There is growing preclinical and clinical evidence that pathological changes at the level of the neurovascular unit (NVU), comprising all the cell types of cerebral microvessels and the surrounding neural tissue, lead to secondary neuronal injury and neurodegenerative diseases, including Alzheimer's disease (AD) (Zhao et al., 2015). The key pathways of vascular dysfunction that are linked to neurodegenerative diseases include blood-brain barrier (BBB) breakdown, hypoperfusion-hypoxia and endothelial metabolic dysfunction (Zlokovic, 2008; Zhao et al., 2015). Morphologically the BBB is formed by the capillary endothelium, the basement membrane and the surrounding pericytes and astrocytic endfeet. The endothelial cells adhere tightly to one another, through junctional structures termed tight junctions (TJs), which restrict paracellular permeability of the BBB [3]. Several families of active influx and efflux transporters and transcytotic receptor systems regulate the exchange of small and large nutrients and metabolites across the BBB (Zlokovic, 2008). Both the structure and functions of the BBB are damaged in AD: the barrier function of TJs is impaired, the energy supply of neural cells is decreased, the entry of neurotoxic agents is elevated and the clearance of Aβ peptides is reduced (Zlokovic, 2008, 2011; Lyros et al., 2014; Di Marco et al., 2015; Zhao et al., 2015). Many studies suggest a direct link of atherosclerosis with not only vascular, but also AD dementia, although the relationship is still unclear (Nelson et al., 2016; Kapasi and Schneider, 2016). NVU and BBB pathologies have been increasingly investigated in genetic and other animal models of AD (Nicolakakis and Hamel, 2011), but there are very few models focusing on the link between atherosclerosis and dementia (Li et al., 2003; Lane-Donovan et al., 2016) or NVU changes.

Previously, we generated a mouse model of human atherosclerosis using transgenic mice overexpressing the human APOB-100 protein in different tissues such as the liver, heart and brain (Bjelik et al., 2006; Csont et al., 2007; Lénárt et al., 2012). Apolipoprotein B-100 (APOB-100) is a large, 512 kDa glycoprotein that circulates in the plasma as the major protein component of low density lipoprotein (LDL) and very low density lipoproteins (VLDL). The higher ratio of LDL and VLDL fractions compared to HDL in the blood of these transgenic animals is similar to the human plasma lipoprotein profile, therefore this mouse strain is more suitable to study the effects of hypercholesterinaemia and hypertriglyceridemia than the wild-type mice (Csont et al., 2007). Several studies have shown that the concentration of APOB is elevated in the serum of AD patients (Caramelli et al., 1999; Sabbagh et al., 2004) which correlates with β-amyloid (Aβ) deposition in AD brains (Kuo et al., 1998). Cholesterol and apolipoprotein accumulates in mature amyloid plaques in brains from both AD patients and animal models of AD (Puglielli et al., 2003). The processing of amyloid precursor protein (APP) is modulated by cholesterol which is enriched in the membrane microdomains of neurons (Ehehalt et al., 2003). The amount of 24S-hydroxycholesterol is increased in the plasma of AD and vascular dementia patients, indicating a change in the metabolism of cholesterol (Lutjohann et al., 2000). High levels of plasma triglyceride preceded the formation of amyloid plaques in transgenic mouse models of AD (Burgess et al., 2006). In our model, APOB-100 transgenic mice showed significantly elevated serum triglyceride and cholesterol level when fed with normal chow and cholesterol rich diet, respectively (Csont et al., 2007), and increased the rigidity of the plasma membrane of brain endothelial cells isolated from these transgenic animals (Lénárt et al., 2015). In the past 10 years we have described in detail the neurodegenerative processes occurring in the brain of hypertriglyceridemic APOB-100 transgenic mice. We detected widespread neuronal cell death and apoptosis of cortical and hippocampal neurons in this model (Lénárt et al., 2012). Synaptic dysfunction in the hippocampal region of APOB-100 transgenic mice using electrophysiolology and hyperphosphorylation of the tau protein (primarily at Ser^{262}, Ser^{396}, $Ser^{199/202}$, Ser^{404}phosphosites) were also shown (Lénárt et al., 2012). As a consequence of the extended neurodegeneration a pronounced enlargement of brain ventricles in transgenic brains was detected using MRI, which was transgene dose-dependent (Bereczki et al., 2008). Moreover, APOB-100 overexpression increased the level of lipid peroxidation in cortical and hippocampal brain regions and impaired cognitive function of the animals (Löffler et al., 2013).

Under cerebral ischemic conditions, decreased cortical microvascular density and increased brain capillary lumen diameter was found in our APOB-100 transgenic atherosclerosis model showing neurodegeneration (Süle et al., 2009). Cerebral ischemia also promoted the swelling of perivascular astrocytes and reduced the ratio of intact capillaries (Süle et al., 2009). Our aim was to further study neurovascular pathology and reveal structural and functional changes in the BBB of APOB-100 transgenic mice that may contribute to the neurodegeneration already described in this model.

MATERIALS AND METHODS

Animals

All animals were handled in accordance with approved procedures as defined by the EU Directive 2010/63/EU and all animal work was approved by the regional Station for Animal Health and Food Control (Csongrád-county, Hungary; project license: XVI/4136/2014). Mice were housed in groups of two to three under standard conditions (24°C, 12 h light–dark cycle) with food and water available *ad libitum*. APOB-100 transgenic mice were produced in our laboratory as described previously (Bjelik et al., 2006). Transgenic mice were backcrossed with C57B/6 strain six times to achieve a homogenous genetic background. Animals were maintained on a regular rodent chow diet. Animal surgeries were performed under sodium pentobarbital (Nembutal) anesthesia and all efforts were made to minimize pain and suffering. For genotyping, tail DNA of 10-day-old pups was purified as described earlier (Bjelik et al., 2006) and integrated transgenes were detected by PCR, using primers from the 5′ promoter region of the human *APOB* gene (Callow et al., 1994).

Materials

All reagents were purchased from Sigma-Aldrich Ltd. (St. Louis, MO, United States) except for those specifically mentioned.

Serum Triglyceride Measurement

Serum triglyceride levels in 7, 9, and 12-month-old APOB-100 transgenic (n = 5) and wild-type mice (n = 5) fed on a normal chow diet were measured using a colorimetric assay (**Supplementary Table S1**). Blood samples were collected through cardiac puncture under terminal anesthesia. After clot formation samples were centrifuged at 4°C, 1000 × g for 10 min, then serum was removed and stored at −80°C until use. Serum triglyceride levels were measured in triplicate using a commercially available enzymatic colorimetric assay kit (Diagnosticum Ltd., Budapest, Hungary) according to the manufacturer's instructions. Test accuracy was monitored using Standard Lipid Controls (Diagnosticum Ltd., Budapest, Hungary). Absorbance of the produced purple color product was measured at 560 nm using a microplate reader (Multiskan FC, Thermo Scientific, United States). Values were expressed in mmol/liter. Experimental groups, (APOB-100 transgenic mice and wild-type littermates) consisted of 5 animals each.

BBB Permeability

Permeability for sodium fluorescein (SF, mw: 376 Da), a marker of paracellular flux, and Evans blue (EB, mw: 67 kDa), a tracer which binds to serum albumin (Patterson et al., 1992), was measured as described in detail earlier (Veszelka et al., 2003). Six-month-old wild-type and transgenic mice (n = 10 animals/group) (**Supplementary Table S1**) were given a solution of both dyes (2%, 5 ml/kg) in an *iv.* injection to the tail vein for 1 h, and at the end of the experiments, the animals were perfused with 25 ml phosphate-buffered saline (PBS) for 15 min. Samples from two brain regions, cerebral cortex and hippocampus, were collected, weighed and stored at −80°C. Tissue pieces were homogenized in 650 μl PBS, then 650 μl of cold, 50% w/v, freshly prepared trichloroacetic acid was added and samples were centrifuged again with 10,000 × g for 12 min at 4°C. Dye concentrations were measured in supernatants by a PTI spectrofluorimeter (T-format, Quanta Master QM-1; Photon Technology International). Five hundred μl of the supernatants were diluted in ethanol (1:3) than emission of Evans blue was measured at 650 nm after excitation at 600 nm wavelength. For SF measurement 500 μl supernatants were diluted in distilled water (1:3) then 100 μl 10N NaOH was added to each sample. Emission of fluorescein was measured at 510 nm after excitation at 492 nm wavelength. BBB permeability was expressed as ng tracer/g brain tissue.

Transmission Electron Microscopy (TEM) and Image Analysis

Seven-month-old wild-type and transgenic mice (n = 4 animals/group) (**Supplementary Table S1**) were anesthetized with sodium pentobarbital (150 μg/g, i.p.), then transcardially perfused with 0.9% NaCl in 0.01 M phosphate buffer (PB), followed by 4% paraformaldehyde containing 2.5% glutaraldehyde in 0.1 M PB. Brains were removed and post-fixed in 4% paraformaldehyde in 0.1 M PB overnight at 4°C. Then, 40-μm-thick coronal sections were cut on an Oxford Vibratome (The Vibratome Company, St. Louis, MO, United States). Sections were washed with PBS and incubated in 1% OsO_4 for 30 min, then rinsed with distilled water and dehydrated in graded ethanol, block-stained with 1% uranyl acetate in 50% ethanol for 30 min and embedded in Taab 812 (Taab; Aldermaston, United Kingdom). Following polymerization at 60°C for 12 h, 60–70 nm ultrathin sections were cut using a Leica UCT ultramicrotome (Leica Microsystems, Milton Keynes, United Kingdom) and examined using a Hitachi 7100 transmission electron microscope (Hitachi Ltd., Tokyo, Japan). Electron micrographs were made by Veleta 2k × 2k MegaPixel side-mounted TEM CCD camera (Olympus, Tokyo, Japan). Contrast/brightness of electron micrographs was edited by Adobe Photoshop CS3 (Adobe Photoshop Inc., San Jose, CA, United States). Altogether 215 non-overlapping images representing 56 capillaries from the frontal cortex and 111 non-overlapping images representing 59 capillaries from the hippocampus were analyzed for morphological changes. All analyzed images were taken at 30,000× magnification. To calculate pericyte coverage on capillary profiles, the circumference of brain endothelial cells at their abluminal side facing the basal membrane was marked manually by a line with one color, and the length of pericytes with another. Only pericyte branches completely embedded in the capillary basement membrane were counted. The length of the lines was determined by Matlab. The background (the original image) was removed and the two colors were seperated to two channels. The pixel number of the two differently labeled lines is a good approximation of the pericyte to brain capillary endothelial circumference in each group. Thus, the ratio of the structures is the ratio of the two cumulative pixel numbers.

Brain Microvessel Isolation

Cortical microvessels were isolated from the brain of 6–7-month-old animals, as described earlier (Veszelka et al., 2007). The forebrains of APOB-100 overexpressing or wild-type mice (n = 6) (**Supplementary Table S1**) were collected in ice-cold sterile phosphate buffered saline (PBS). Meninges were taken off by rolling brains on a sterile wet filter paper. White matter and the choroid plexus were removed and the tissue was minced into 1 mm^3 pieces by scalpels. Samples then were homogenized in ice-cold Ringer-Hepes buffer (4 ml/g of tissue), and the resulting homogenates were centrifuged at 1000 g for 10 min. After centrifugation the microvessel enriched pellets were resuspended in 17.5% dextran (64–76 kDa) in Ringer-Hepes, and centrifuged at 4°C, 1500 × g for 15 min. The resulting pellets were suspended in 2 ml Ringer-Hepes buffer containing 1% BSA, while the supernatants were collected and centrifuged two more times. The resulting pellets were pooled and passed through a 100 μm and a 20 μm nylon mesh. The microvessels retained by the 20 μm mesh were washed off with 10 ml buffer and centrifuged at 4°C, 1000 g for 10 min. Finally, the pellets were resuspended in 1 ml buffer and centrifuged at 4°C, 10,000 g for 2 min, and stored in TRIZOL reagent until use. A small aliquot of the brain microvessel preparation was observed with phase contrast microscopy, and similarly to our previously published data (Veszelka et al., 2007), these fractions only contained brain microvessel endothelial cells and pericytes.

Quantitative Real-Time PCR

Total RNA was extracted from primary cell cultures, cortical microvessel samples, or hippocampal and cortical brain regions using TRIZOL reagent according to the manufacturer's protocol. Hippocampal and cortical brain samples were derived from 6-month-old mice (n = 6 animals/group) (**Supplementary Table S1**). Briefly, samples were homogenized in the appropriate volume of TRIZOL reagent, then 1/5 volume chloroform was added to each mixture and the samples were incubated on ice for 5 min. After centrifugation at 12,000 × g for 15 min at 4°C, the RNA containing aqueous phase was separated from the organic phase. The RNA was precipitated with 100% isopropyl alcohol and incubated for 10 min at −20°C. After centrifugation for 10 min at 12,000 × g at 4°C, RNA was washed with 80% ethanol and samples were centrifuged for 5 min at 12,000 × g at 4°C. RNA pellets were dissolved in RNase free water and then bound to RNA Clean Up column (NucleoSpin RNA clean-up kit, Macherey-Nagel) where they were treated with DNase. RNA was finally eluted from the membrane with RNase-free water, and the concentrations of the samples were measured at 230 nm using a spectrophotometer (NanoDrop ND-1000).

mRNA samples were converted to cDNA by using a reverse transcriptase kit (High Capacity cDNA Reverse Transcription Kit, Applied Biosystems). Each reaction mix consisted of 2 μg RNA (15 μl); 1.5 μl reverse transcriptase; 3 μl primer; 1.2 μl dNTP; 3 μl buffer; 6.3 μl RNase free water. The temperature profile of the reaction was the following: 10 min at 25°C, 2 h at 37°C and 5 min at 85°C (using MJ Mini - Personal Thermal Cycler, BioRad). The cDNA was finally diluted 1:20, and 9 μl of this mix was used as a template in the PCR reaction that follows. Each reaction was performed in a total volume of 20 μl containing 10 μl of 2x Power SYBR Green PCR Master Mix (Applied Biosystems), 1 μl of 5 pmol/μl primer mix (forward + reverse) and 9 μl of cDNA sample. The amplification was carried out on a RotorGene 3000 instrument (Corbett Research) with the following cycling parameters: heat activation at 95°C for 10 min; followed by 45 cycles of denaturation at 95°C for 15 s, annealing at 56°C for 15 s, and extension at 60°C for 40 s in 45 cycles. Fluorescent signals were collected after each extension step at 72°C and at the end the registration of the melting curve was performed between 50 and 95°C. The expression level of target genes was normalized to an endogenous control gene *Gapdh* or *Actb* (ΔCt). Then ΔΔCt was calculated, i.e., the relative expression of the target genes in transgenic animals was compared with the expression levels observed in wild-type animals. Fold-differences were calculated using the $2^{-\Delta\Delta Ct}$ formula and were expressed in percents. Gene expression changes were considered significant if the expression level dropped below 50% or showed a two-fold increase compared with control values. We studied genes involved in different molecular mechanism, such as oxidative stress, transport pathways or endothelial dysfunction. Individual genes were selected based on literature data, especially those identified in BBB transcriptome analysis in mice (Daneman et al., 2010), related to AD pathology (Wu et al., 2005), or selected for our recently published gene expression analysis of different BBB models (Veszelka et al., 2018). Primer sequences used in this study are listed in **Supplementary Table S2.**

Immunohistochemistry and Confocal Microscopy

Standard immunofluorescence protocols were applied. 7–8-months-old mice (**Supplementary Table S1**) were terminally anesthetized with sodium pentobarbital (150 μg/g, i.p.), then transcardially perfused with 0.9% sodium chloride dissolved in 0.01 M PB, pH 7.4, followed by 3% paraformaldehyde in 0.1 M PB, pH 7.4. Brains were removed and postfixed for 4 h in the same fixative. Following fixation the brain samples were washed in 0.1 M PB, pH 7.4, and cryoprotected in 30% sucrose until saturation. Then, 30-μm-thick, hippocampus and frontal cortex containing coronal sections were cut on a cryostat (Floorstanding Cryostat MNT; Slee, Mainz, Germany), collected in 0.1 M PB, pH 7.4 containing 0.01% sodium azide (Fluka) (w/v) and were stored at 4°C.

Antigen retrieving for claudin-5 and occludin immunostainings was performed with 0.5 % Triton X-100 in PBS for 10 min, followed by an incubation in protease type XIV (1 μg/ml) dissolved in $CaCl_2$ (1 mg/ml) for 7 min. Antigen retrieving for the other primary antibodies used included only Triton X-100 treatment at concentrations based on our preliminary experiments [0.1% for Pdgfrβ, 0.2% for vimentin and Gfap, 0.3% for Lox-1, and 0.5% for *P*-glycoprotein (Pgp) for details of Lox-1 immunolabeling see **Supplementary Material**]. Primary antibodies used were rabbit anti-claudin-5, rabbit anti-occludin (Thermo Fisher Scientific, Waltham, MA, United States), goat anti-Gfap (Abcam, Cambridge, United Kingdom), mouse anti-vimentin [Agilent (DAKO), Santa Clara, CA, United States], mouse anti-Pgp (Merck Millipore, Burlington, MA, United States), and rabbit anti Lox-1 (Abcam, Cambridge, United Kingdom), (**Supplementary Table S3**). Appropriate secondary antibodies conjugated with DyLight™ 488 and Alexa Fluor™ 594 (Jackson ImmunoResearch Europe Ltd., Cambridgeshire, United Kingdom) were applied. Sections were counterstained with DAPI, coverslipped with Confocal Matrix® (Micro Tech Lab, Graz, Austria) and examined with a confocal laser scanning microscope (Olympus Fluoview FV1000, Olympus Life Science Europa GmbH, Hamburg, Germany). Images of 512 × 512 px were captured using the following microscope configuration: objective lens: UPLSAPO 60x, numeric aperture 1.35; sampling speed: 8 μs/pixel; scanning mode: sequential unidirectional. In order to obtain high resolution (1024 × 1024 px) images, Yokogawa W1/Olympus IX83-based spinning disk confocal microscope was also used for imaging Gfap, vimentin, and Pdgfrβ immunostainings using excitation and detection parameters optimized for DyLight™ 488, Alexa Fluor™ 594 and DAPI. 405nm (for DAPI), 488 nm (for DyLight™ 488) and 561 nm (for Alexa Fluor™ 594) laser excitation, and 60x objective were used for imaging. The contrast of these images showing Gfap immunostaining was increased by inverting and displaying them as gray scale images using the public domain Fiji software.

Fluorescence Intensity Analysis

Immunostained coronal sections containing the hippocampus and cortical areas (5 animals per group, 3 sections per animal) were selected based on the principle of systematic random sampling (Gundersen and Osterby, 1981; Mayhew, 1991). Three images representing randomly selected parts of the hippocampus and frontal cortex in each section were taken with a laser scanning (for claudin-5, occludin and Pgp immunolabeling) or a spinning disk (for Gfap immunostaining) confocal microscope using a 60× objective lens and the same excitation and detection parameters for each image. Fluorescence intensity of claudin-5, occludin and Pgp immunolabelings was evaluated using the ImageQuant™ software as follows: on every image 10 equally sized small rectangular areas (7 × 7 pixels) were placed randomly on the intensively highlighted immunolabeled structures, and five equal rectangles were placed randomly on areas lacking immunostaining representing the background. Then the average intensity/pixel values of each area were calculated, and the average intensity/pixel values representing the background intensity were subtracted from those of immunolabeled areas. The GFAP immunostained structures represented a more a complex pattern and occupied larger areas, therefore the integrated fluorescence intensity of Gfap immunolabeling was measured using the public domain Fiji software as follows: Grayscale 16-bit images were used. The integrated fluorescence intensity of the whole image and that of a small area lacking immunostained structures were measured, then the background fluorescence intensity of the whole image was calculated and subtracted from the integrated fluorescence intensity value of the whole image. The procedures were performed on each image, and the collected data were statistically analyzed (Farkas et al., 2008).

Statistical Analysis

GraphPad Prism 5.0 software (GraphPad Software Inc. LaJolla, CA, United States) was used for statistical analysis. Gaussian distribution of the data was tested with the Kolmogorov–Smirnov normality test. Data showing Gaussian distribution were analyzed with two-way analysis of variance followed by Bonferroni *post hoc* test. Data showing no Gaussian distribution were analyzed with Kruskal–Wallis and Dunn's multiple comparison tests. The level of statistical significance was taken as $p < 0.05$. Results are presented as means ± SEM.

RESULTS

Chronic Hypertriglyceridemia in APOB-100 Transgenic Mice

A statistically significant difference was detected in transgenic compared to wild-type animals at every time point (7, 9, and 12-month, $n = 5$ animals/group) indicating chronic hypertriglyceridemia in APOB-100 transgenic mice (**Figure 1A**).

Impairment of the BBB Integrity: Permeability Measurements

We measured a significant increase in the BBB permeability ($p < 0.05$) for the small molecular weight marker SF in the hippocampal region of transgenic mice, while alteration in the extravasation of the large serum protein albumin showed a non-significant trend (**Figure 1B**). However, there was no obvious change in the permeability for either of the markers in the cortex of transgenic mice compared to wild-type littermates.

BBB Dysfunction: Changes in Gene and Protein Expression in Brain Microvessels

Reduced expression (16%) of the vascular restricted and mesenchyme homeobox gene 2 (*Meox2*), a key regulator of BBB functions, particularly in AD, was measured in cerebral microvessels of APOB-100 transgenic mice compared to wild-type animals (**Figure 1C**). The gene expression of *Mfsd2a* (44%), the BBB transporter for unsaturated lipid docosahexaenoic acid (DHA), and the primary glucose transporter in brain endothelial cells, *Glut-1* (57%) were also decreased (**Figure 1C**).

Lox-1, a lectin-like protein expressed in endothelial cells in the periphery is considered as the major receptor for oxidized low-density lipoprotein. The level of oxidized LDL (oxLDL) receptor (*Lox-1*) has increased dramatically (297%) in the microvessels of APOB-100 transgenic mice (**Figure 1C**). In contrast to the periphery, where Lox-1 was detected in heart coronal vessels, Lox-1 immunolabeling was observed only in neuronal cell bodies and processes, but not in brain capillaries (**Supplementary Figure S1**). A significant increase in Lox-1 immunoreactive area was detected in the cortex, but no change was seen in the hippocampus of transgenic mice compared to wild-type animals (**Supplementary Figure S2**). While mRNA level of LDL receptor-related protein-1 (*Lrp1*, 70%) slightly decreased, the expression level of *Lrp2* dropped to 56% in transgenic microvessels (**Figure 1C**).

We measured two isoforms of nitric oxide (NO) synthases (NOS), the endothelial (*eNos/Nos3*) and the inducible form (*iNos/Nos2*), and found a significant decrease for both genes in brain microvessels of transgenic animals (**Figure 1C**). Expression of mRNA for caveolin-1 (*Cav-1*), a structural element of brain endothelial caveolae associated with Nos3, was also reduced (**Figure 1C**).

The expression of selected TJ proteins was analyzed at gene expressional level using quantitative real-time PCR, and at protein level using fluorescence immunohistochemistry, too. The mRNA level of transmembrane protein *Ocln*, and TJ cytoplasmic linker *Tjp-1*, was reduced to half in transgenic microvessels, while there was no change in the expression level of *Cldn-5*, the dominant claudin member at the BBB, compared to wild-type animals (100%) (**Figure 1C**). Fluorescence immunohistochemical stainings for claudin-5 (**Figure 2A**) and occludin (**Figure 3A**) showed that both immunolabelings were exclusively localized at endothelial TJs and appeared as continuous lines. There was no statistically significant change

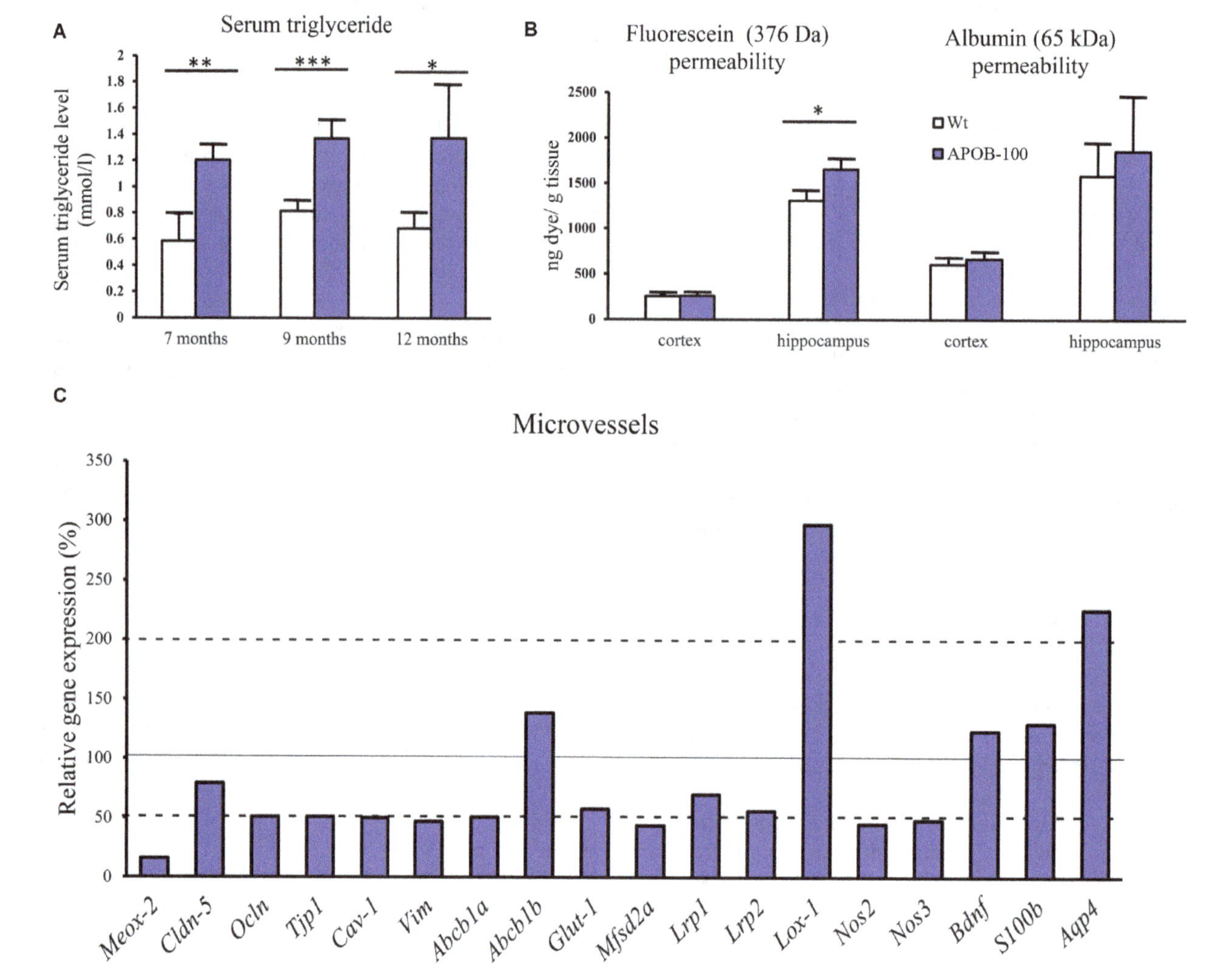

FIGURE 1 | Serum triglyceride levels **(A)**, BBB permeability for fluorescein and albumin in the brain of hypertriglyceridemic APOB-100 transgenic (APOB-100) and wild-type (Wt) mice **(B)**, and gene expression analysis of the microvessel fraction from APOB-100 transgenic mice using QPCR **(C)**. Continuous line indicates the expression level of the corresponding gene in wild-type mice (100%). Dashed lines indicate the levels of significant changes: a 2 fold (200%) increase or an 0.5 fold (50%) reduction in gene expression. $^{***}P < 0.001$, $^{**}P < 0.01$, $^{*}P < 0.05$, compared with Wt mice.

neither in claudin-5 nor in occludin immunostaining intensity in transgenic cortex and hippocampus compared to wild-type animals (**Figures 2B, 3B**).

The gene expression of vimentin, a cytoskeletal protein, which labels reactive astrocytes (Pekny et al., 2007), but can be produced by pericytes (Bandopadhyay et al., 2001) and brain endothelial cells (Deracinois et al., 2013) too, showed a significant reduction in isolated brain microvessels (**Figure 1C**). At protein level, vimentin was localized along capillaries in the frontal cortex of wild-type mice as it can be observed in occludin-vimentin double immunofluorescence stainings (**Figure 3A**), where occludin immunolabeling delineates brain capillaries. Vimentin immunoreactivity was very rarely seen in the frontal cortex of APOB-100 transgenic animals, and it was not detected in the hippocampus of either genotype (**Figure 3A**). The vimentin immunolabeling showed no co-localization with epitopes recognized either by a Gfap antibody (an astroglia marker), or by a Pdgfrβ antibody (a pericyte marker) (**Supplementary Figure S3**). Furthermore, we have established primary pericyte, astrocyte and endothelial cell cultures from wild-type and transgenic mice and vimentin gene expression was measured using QPCR. The vimentin gene expressions normalized to the endogenous mouse actin gene were compared in wild-type animals (ΔCT values). Vimentin was expressed at high level in endothelial cells (ΔCT = 1.3), astrocytes (ΔCT = 2) and pericytes (ΔCT = 2.3) as well. Comparison of the vimentin expression level of wild-type and transgenic animals demonstrates that while the vimentin expression levels were not changed significantly in the transgenic endothelial cells and astrocytes (74 and 124%, respectively) transgenic pericytes showed significantly reduced vimentin level (33%) compared to wild-type cells (**Supplementary Figure S4**). The most widely studied, and AD related ABC transporter at the BBB, *Abcb1* or P-glycoprotein (P-gp) was also examined by QPCR in isolated

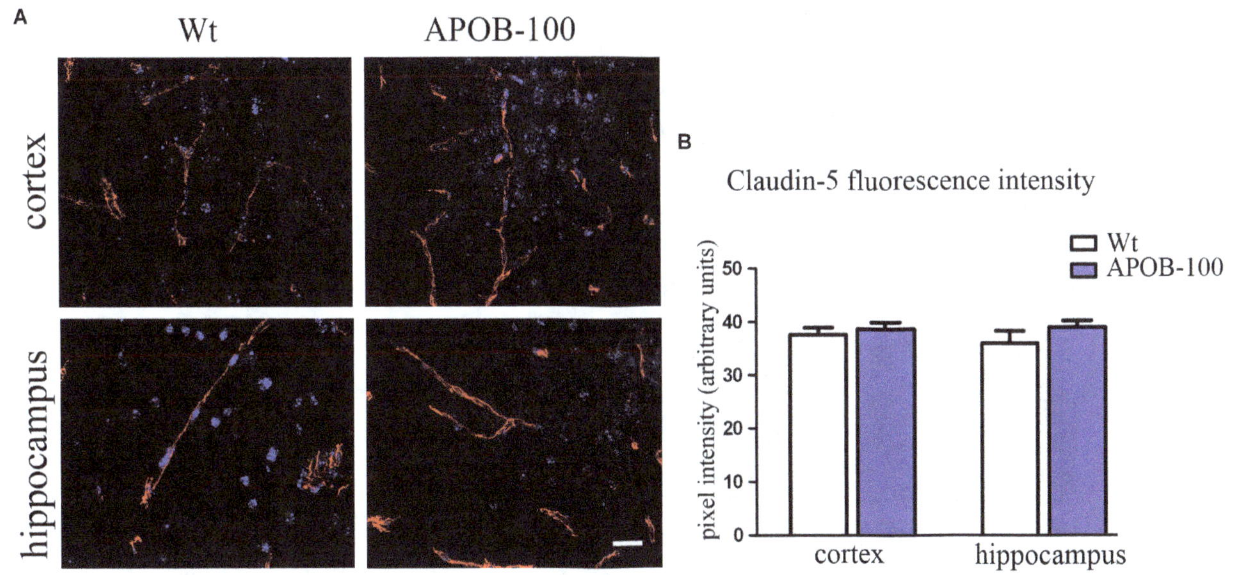

FIGURE 2 | Claudin-5 immunostaining pattern (red) in the cortex and hippocampus of wild-type (Wt) and APOB-100 transgenic mice (APOB-100), counterstained with DAPI (blue) **(A)**. Scale bar: 20 μm. Quantification of fluorescence intensity of claudin-5 immunolabeling in the frontal cortex and hippocampus of Wt and APOB-100 transgenic mice **(B)**.

brain microvessels and by immunohistochemistry in the frontal cortex and hippocampus of wild-type and APOB-100 transgenic mice. From the isoforms of P-gp coding genes, *Abcb1a* mRNA expression was significantly decreased (51%), while *Abcb1b* (138%) showed no significant change (**Figure 1C**). Using a monoclonal antibody recognizing both isoforms of P-gp the immunoreactivity pattern of P-gp was similar to that of TJ proteins delineating a large number of capillaries in the frontal cortex and hippocampus in wild-type animals. However, in the APOB-100 transgenic group, P-gp immunoreactivity could hardly be observed in either brain region examined (**Figure 4A**), which was reflected by a significant drop in P-gp fluorescence intensity in APOB-100 transgenic mice compared to wild-type animals in the cortex and hippocampus, too (**Figure 4B**).

Astroglial endfeet are important structural and functional elements of the BBB. The gene expression level of aquaporin-4 (*Aqp4*), a water channel and a marker of glial endfeet, has increased dramatically (225%) in isolated brain microvessels (**Figure 1C**), while no change was observed in brain samples (**Figure 6**). In the microvessel samples the glial specific calcium-binding cytoplasmic protein *S100b* (129%) and the astrocyte produced brain derived neurotrophic factor (*Bdnf*, 123%) levels showed no change (**Figure 1C**).

Ultrastructural Changes of the BBB in APOB-100 Transgenic Mice

Analysis of the ultrastructure of brain capillaries using TEM revealed several alterations in the NVU of APOB-100 transgenic mice compared to wild-type animals (**Figure 5** and **Table 1**). The most significant changes were observed in the morphology of TJs and astrocytic endfeet. Swollen astrocytic processes around capillaries were predominant in the transgenic group, indicating edema of glial endfeet (**Figure 5A** and **Supplementary Figure S5**). The intercellular junctions of capillary endothelial cells were characterized by a continuous electron dense material in wild-type mice (**Figure 5B**). In the transgenic group, in contrast, nearly half of the endothelial cell contacts displayed a discontinuous electron dense structure (**Figure 5B** and **Table 1**). Further ultrastructural differences include basal membrane alterations, like increased thickness, tortuosity, fragmentation, and alterations in luminal membrane characteristics, like increased number of protrusions in the transgenic group. No significant difference was found in the pericyte coverage of brain capillaries (**Table 1**). The described ultrastructural changes were detected in the frontal cortex and in the hippocampus as well.

Neuroinflammation and Neuron Related Changes in the Cortex and Hippocampus

From the genes of selected cytokines and neuroinflammatory markers the expression of cytokine *Tnfα* (152%) and the inflammation related nuclear factor *NF-κB* (167%) increased in the transgenic cortex but were not substantially changed in the hippocampus. No change was measured for *Il-1β* (**Figure 6**). Similarly, there was no notable change in the expression of other inflammatory markers in the cortex, except for *Tlr4*, the expression of which was dropped down to 60%. Of neuronal synaptic genes, which play an important role in remodeling CNS synapsis, the level of *Nlgn1* (152%) has slightly increased in the hippocampus but was not changed in the cortex. The expression level of *Nmdar* and *Nrxn1* was unchanged both in the hippocampus and in the cortex. However, a significant decrease in the expression level of a cell adhesion molecule, *Cdh2* (*N-cadherin*), (32%) was detected in the hippocampus of

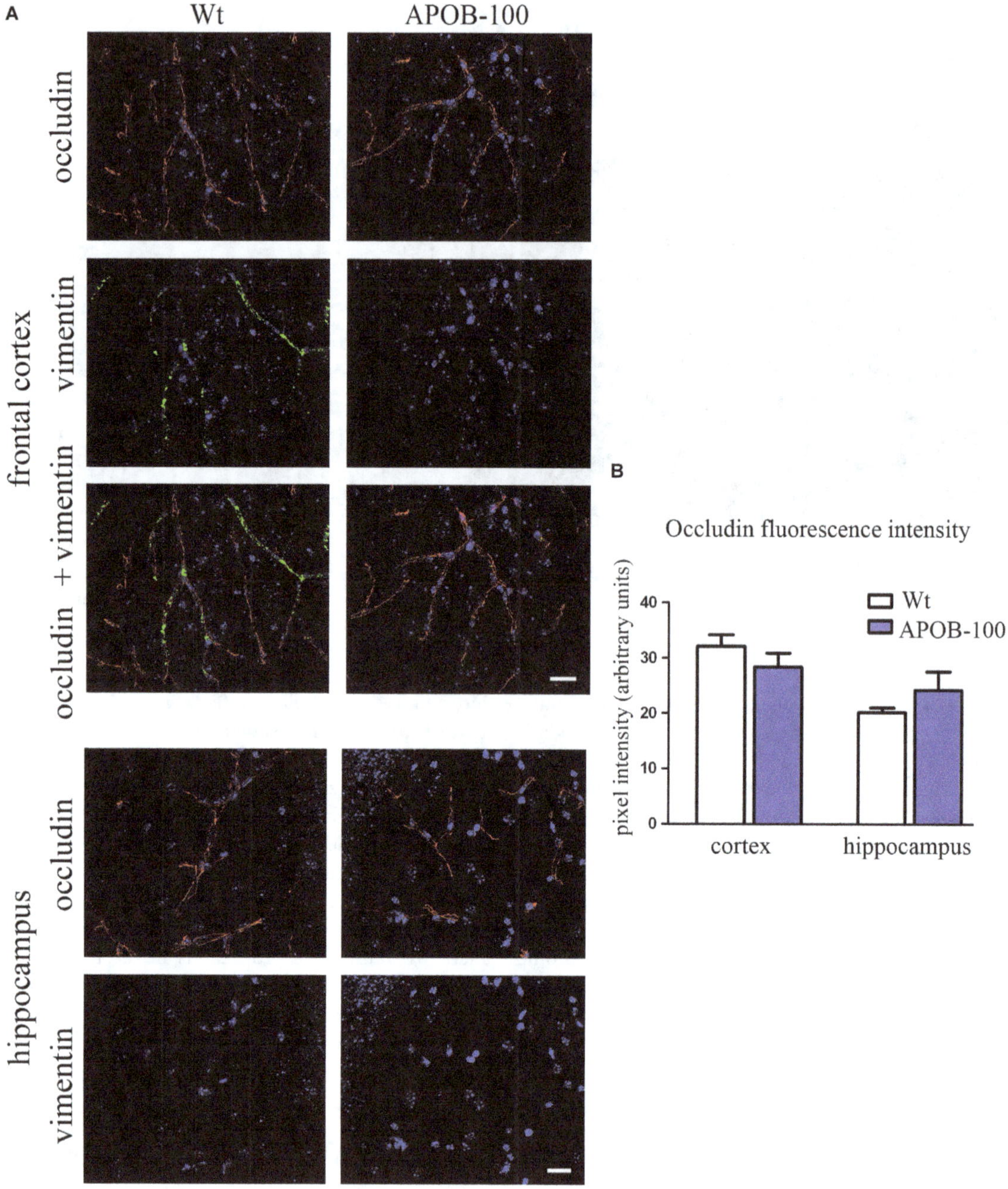

FIGURE 3 | Occludin (red) and vimentin (green) immunostaining pattern in the cortex and hippocampus of wild-type (Wt) and APOB-100 transgenic mice (APOB-100) counterstained with DAPI (blue) **(A)**. Scale bar: 20 μm. Quantification of fluorescence intensity of occludin immunolabeling in the frontal cortex and hippocampus of Wt and APOB-100 transgenic mice **(B)**.

transgenic brains (**Figure 6**). The results of gene expression analysis are summarized in **Table 2**.

Out of 600 miRNAs analyzed, we could detect 10 (1.67%) differentially expressed miRNA genes in APOB100 transgenic cortices (6 upregulated and 4 repressed). List of miRNA genes with altered expression level is shown in **Supplementary Table S4**. Overexpressed miRNAs were mmu-miR-669g, mmu-miR-222, mmu-miR-708, mmu-miR-26a, mmu-miR-1898, and mmu-miR-500, and repressed miRNAs were mmu-miR-7a, mmu-miR-7b, mmu-miR-187, and mmu-miR-1a. Although we found 10 miRNAs showing differential expression, only 4 miRNAs had experimentally validated targets in the IPA database (mmu-miR-1a, mmu-miR-222, mmu-miR-26a, mmu-miR-7b). Some of these target genes (n = 11) were expected to have relevance in neuronal changes. The expression level of these genes was further investigated by QPCR but no significant changes were detected (data not shown) with the exception of *Bdnf*. This gene may be regulated by two differentially expressed

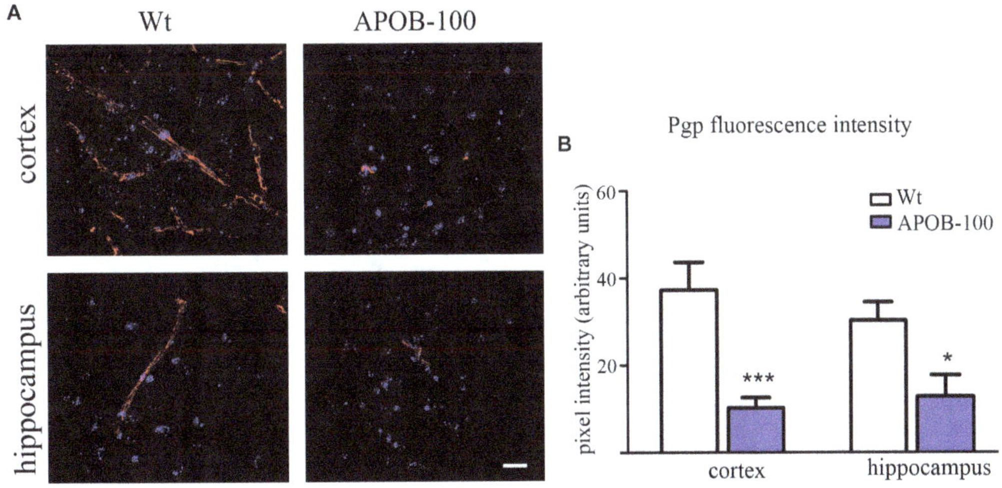

FIGURE 4 | P-gp (ABCB1) transporter immunostaining pattern (red) in cortical and hippocampal areas of wild-type (Wt) and APOB-100 transgenic mice (APOB-100), counterstained with DAPI (blue) **(A)**. Scale bar: 20 μm. Quantification of fluorescence intensity of P-gp immunolabeling in the frontal cortex and hippocampus of Wt and APOB-100 transgenic mice **(B)** $^{***}P < 0.001$, $^{*}P < 0.05$, compared with Wt mice.

miRNAs: mmu-miR-26a (overexpressed), and mmu-miR-1a (repressed). QPCR data showed a two-fold overexpression of *Bdnf* gene in the transgenic cortex (**Supplementary Figure S6**).

Changes in Glial Cell Gene Expression and Morphology

The expression level of the microglial marker (*Iba-1/Aif1*) was slightly increased (145%) in the hippocampus of APOB-100 transgenic mice compared to wild-type animals (**Figure 6**). In contrast, the expression level of glial fibrillary acidic protein (*Gfap*), a cytoskeletal astroglial marker, was dropped down to 38% in transgenic hippocampus (**Figure 6**). The level of two *Gfap* isoforms, *Gfap-α* and *Gfap-σ*, was also reduced to 59 and 41%, respectively, in the hippocampus of APOB-100 transgenic mice compared to wild-type littermates (100%) (**Figure 6**). Gfap immunoreactive cells displayed several processes that were closely associated with microvessels in the cortex and in the hippocampus too, in both experimental groups (**Figure 7A**). The intensity of the fluorescent Gfap immunolabeling showed a significant decrease in the cortex of APOB-100 transgenic mice compared to wild-type animals (**Figure 7B**).

DISCUSSION

Here, we describe, that transgenic mice overexpressing the human APOB-100 protein show chronic hypertriglyceridemia, an increase in permeability for a small molecular marker, and gene expressional, immunohistochemical and ultrastructural alterations at the BBB. Several previous reports have already shown that hypertriglyceridemia is a serious risk factor in the development of neurodegeneration and dementia (Burgess et al., 2006; Raffaitin et al., 2009; Bowman et al., 2012; Klafke et al., 2015) and it was also demonstrated that dyslipidemia is more prevalent in AD subjects with BBB impairment (Bowman et al., 2012). Observations in aging rats, that a decrease in cerebral blood flow is linked to pathologies similar to those found in AD (De La Torre et al., 1992; De la Torre and Mussivand, 1993) and demonstration of brain microvascular injury and BBB leakage in AD patients (Zipser et al., 2007) led to the vascular concept of AD which became generally accepted by today (Zlokovic, 2008; Gosselet et al., 2013; Zhao et al., 2015; Kisler et al., 2017). Lipolysis products generated from triglyceride rich lipoproteins damage endothelial barrier function: perturb the expression of junctional proteins, induce apoptotic cell death *in vitro* in human aortic endothelial cells (Eiselein et al., 2007) and transiently elevate BBB permeability *in vivo* in mice (Lee et al., 2017). Hypertriglyceridemia may contribute to endothelial dysfunction likely through the generation of oxidative stress (Antonios et al., 2008). Indeed, in our recent study (Lénárt et al., 2015) we have shown that oxidized LDL treatment induced barrier dysfunction and increased reactive oxygen species production and membrane rigidity in primary brain endothelial cells.

In the present paper we studied BBB related functional and morphological characteristics as well as gene expression profiling of APOB-100 transgenic mice. We found APOB-100 transgenic mice are characterized by chronic hypertriglyceridemia. Regarding BBB function, a significantly increased extravasation for a small molecule marker, SF, was observed in the hippocampus of transgenic mice, which may suggest an increase in paracellular permeability. Gene expression changes suggesting endothelial dysfunction in APOB-100 transgenic animals include reduced expression of the homeobox regulator *Meox2*, and BBB transporters *Mfsd2a, Glut1, Lrp2, Abcb1a* genes in APOB-100 transgenic brain microvessels may indicate pathomechanisms similar to those observed in conditions of BBB dysfunctions (Zlokovic, 2011; Zhao et al., 2015). Low expression of *MEOX2* was demonstrated in cultured brain endothelial cells isolated from severely affected AD patients (Wu et al., 2005). In the same

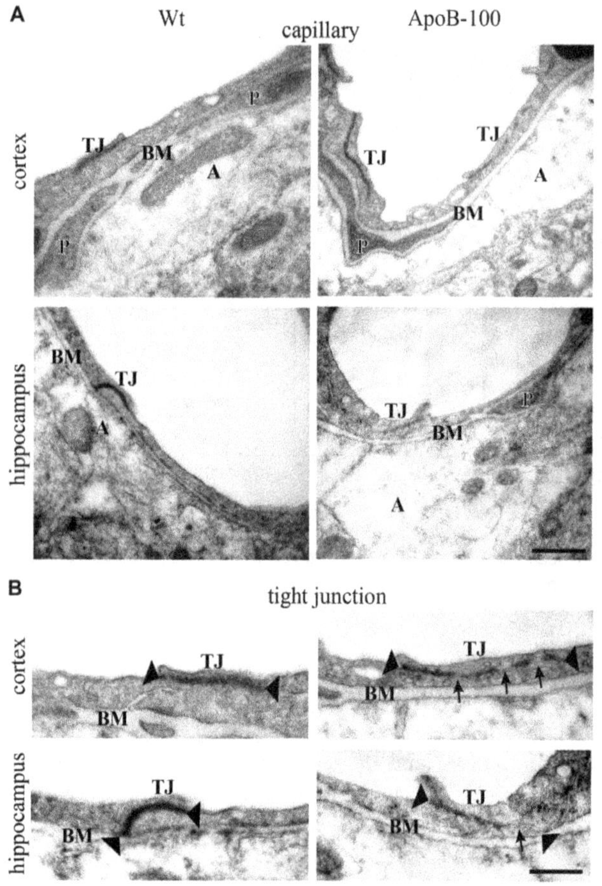

FIGURE 5 | Electron micrographs of brain capillaries **(A)** and tight junctions **(B)** in the frontal cortex and hippocampus of wild-type (Wt) and APOB-100 transgenic (APOB-100) mice. Tight junctions in **(B)** are larger magnifications of tight junctions seen in **(A)**. A, astrocyte; BM, basal membrane; P, pericyte; TJ, tight junction. Scale bars: 500 nm **(A)** and 800 nm **(B)**.

TABLE 1 | Summary of changes in BBB ultrastructure in the frontal cortex and hippocampus of wild-type (Wt) and APOB-100 transgenic (APOB-100) mice.

Frontal cortex		**Wt**	**APOB-100**
Number of capillaries		23	33
Number of images		91	124
Capillary endothelial cell			
Luminal membrane	Smooth	69%	48%
	Protrusions	31%	52%
Tight junctions	Intact	100%	56%
	Discontinuous	0%	44%
Basal membrane	Intact	78%	56%
	Altered	22%	44%
Pericyte			
	Capillary coverage	20%	17%
	Capillary wo pericyte	5%	22%
Astrocyte			
	Intact	77%	12%
	Edema	23%	88%
Hippocampus CA1		**Wt**	**APOB-100**
Number of capillaries		29	30
Number of images		92	129
Capillary endothelial cell			
Luminal membrane	Smooth	78%	46%
	Protrusions	22%	54%
Tight junctions	Intact	100%	29%
	Discontinuous	0%	71%
Basal membrane	Intact	89%	24%
	Altered	11%	76%
Pericyte			
	Capillary coverage	25%	23%
	Capillary wo pericyte	19%	23%
Astrocyte			
	Intact	89%	44%
	Edema	11%	56%

Values are shown as percent of all images analyzed in the group. Pericyte coverage was calculated as written in the Materials and methods section.

study Meox2 deletion in mice resulted in decreased density of brain capillaries, lower levels of cerebral blood flow during rest, a diminished hypoxia-induced angiogenic response in the brain. In addition, in these animals low levels of LRP were observed leading to reduced Aβ efflux. Our observations on the drastically reduced *Meox2* in transgenic brain microvessels might also support the link between Meox2 and neurovascular dysfunction. Beside *Meox2* the other gene for which a dramatic decrease was observed in brain microvessels from transgenic animals was *Mfsd2a,* which might have contributed to the increased BBB permeability in our study and the neurodegeneration in our model described previously (Bereczki et al., 2008). It has been recently discovered, that Mfsd2a is not only a DHA transporter at the BBB, but also a key regulator of BBB integrity and function (Zhao and Zlokovic, 2014). Mutations in *MFSD2A* gene leads to decreased DHA transport into the CNS and severe neurological symptoms (Betsholtz, 2015), and DHA can protect cells of the NVU against amyloid peptide toxicity (Veszelka et al., 2013). At the BBB GLUT1 is the main transporter of glucose, the primary energy source in the CNS. A reduction in Glut1 expression was linked to neurovascular dysfunction and AD in a mouse model (Winkler et al., 2015) emphasizing the importance of the present findings.

Additionally, the receptors Lrp1, Lrp2 and the transporter P-gp responsible for the clearance of Aβ from the brain (Shibata et al., 2000; Deane et al., 2003; Cirrito et al., 2005) are downregulated in AD pathology (Marques et al., 2013). In this study we showed a significant reduction in the expression of the *Abcb1a* gene coding the P-gp isoform predominantly expressed in brain capillary endothelial cells (Croop et al., 1989; Shoshani et al., 1998). In agreement with this finding, the P-gp immunolabeling could hardly be detected in APOB-100 transgenic mouse brains, which may be linked to the previously demonstrated increased accumulation of Aβ in this model (Bereczki et al., 2008).

A significant decrease in inducible *Nos2* and endothelial *Nos3*, and an increase in *Lox-1* expression were detected in microvessels isolated from APOB-100 transgenic animals.

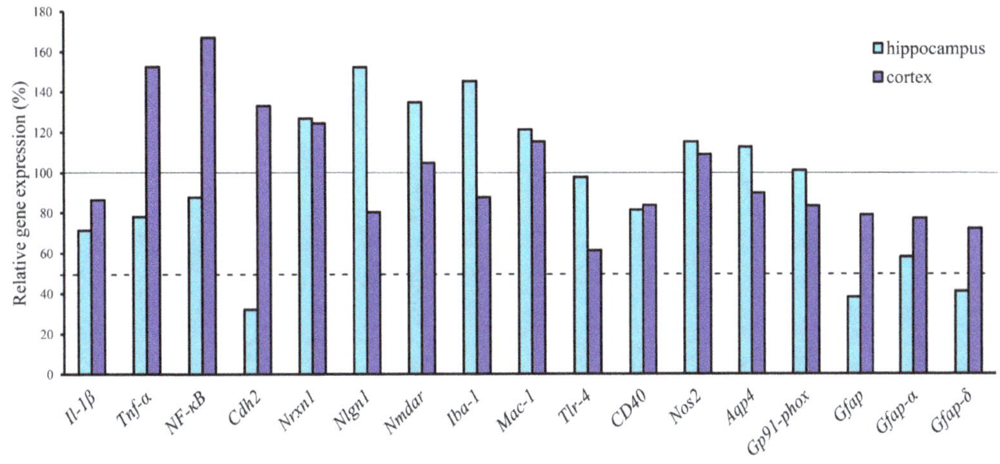

FIGURE 6 | Gene expression analysis of neuroinflammatory markers, transporters and Gfap isoforms in the hippocampus and cortex of APOB-100 transgenic mice. Continuous line indicates the expression level of the corresponding gene in wild-type mice (100%). Dashed line indicates the level of significant changes: a 0.5 fold (50%) reduction in gene expression.

TABLE 2 | Summary of gene expression changes in hypertriglyceridemic APOB-100 transgenic mice.

	mRNA		**Protein**	
	Tissue	**Level**	**Tissue**	**Level**
P-gp (Abcb1a)	Microvessel	Decreased	Hippocampus	Decreased
			Cortex	Decreased
iNOS	Microvessel	Decreased		n.d.
eNOS	Microvessel	Decreased		n.d.
Lox1	Microvessel	Increased	Cortex	Increased
Aqp4	Microvessel	Increased		n.d
Occludin	Microvessel	Decreased	Hippocampus	No change
			Cortex	No change
ZO-1	Microvessel	Decreased		n.d
Caveolin-1	Microvessel	Decreased		n.d
Vimentin	Microvessel	Decreased	Cortex	Decreased
Mfsd2A	Microvessel	Decreased		n.d
Meox-2	Microvessel	Decreased		n.d.
Glut-1	Microvessel	Decreased		n.d
Bdnf	Cortex	Increased		n.d.
Aif-1/Iba-1	Hippocampus	Increased*	Hippocampus	No change
Gfap	Hippocampus	Decreased	Hippocampus	No change
			Cortex	Decreased
Gfap alpha	Hippocampus	Decreased		n.d
Gfap delta	Hippocampus	Decreased		n.d.
IL-β	Hippocampus	Decreased*		n.d
Ncadh	Hippocampus	Decreased		n.d.
TNF-α	Cortex	Increased*		n.d
NF-κB	Cortex	Increased*		n.d.
Tlr4	Cortex	Decreased*		n.d

**Denotes less than two-fold change.*

The area fraction of Lox-1 immunoreactive structures was also significantly increased in the cortex of APOB-100 transgenic mice compared to wild-type animals. The upregulation of *Lox-1* and the downregulation of *Nos2* and *Nos3* mRNA levels confirmed atherosclerotic changes in APOB-100 transgenic mice reported earlier (Chen et al., 2002; Csont et al., 2007) The reduction in *Nos3* gene expression is in line with observations focusing on atherosclerosis-prone regions of the mouse aorta (Won et al., 2007) and on areas of human atherosclerosis (Buttery et al., 1996; Barry et al., 1998). Lox-1 upregulation is observed in atherosclerosis and linked to oxidative stress and inflammatory reactions leading to inhibition of Nos3 enzymatic activity via increased C-reactive protein production (Stapleton et al., 2010; Stancel et al., 2016) and, consequently, microvessel dysfunction in the periphery (Lubrano and Balzan, 2016). Our study suggests for the first time, that there may be a link between neurovascular changes and *Lox-1* upregulation, *Nos2* and *Nos3* downregulation in brain microvessels.

NO or NO donors at low concentrations do not modify the barrier function of BBB culture models, while both the blocking of basal NO production and high levels of NO induce barrier opening (Deli et al., 2005). NO is known to modulate cGMP-pathways which decrease resistance and increase permeability in culture models of the BBB and may mediate the effects of excess NO (Deli et al., 2005), but the exact mechanisms by which NO regulates different BBB permeability pathways are not known.

A significant decrease in *Cav-1* gene expression was detected in microvessels isolated from APOB-100 transgenic brains. Caveolin-1 is a structural protein playing a stabilizing role in caveolae, but it is reported to influence TJ morphology and the expression of junctional proteins occludin and ZO-1, too. Caveolin-1 knock-out mice are characterized by increased paracellular permeability, smaller TJs and defects in the adhesion of endothelial cells to the-basement membrane (Schubert et al., 2002). Knocking down caveolin-1 expression in brain endothelial cells resulted in a decrease in occludin and ZO-1 expression in western blots (Song et al., 2007). However, the effect of caveolin-1 on TJ protein expression is contradictory, since an increase in

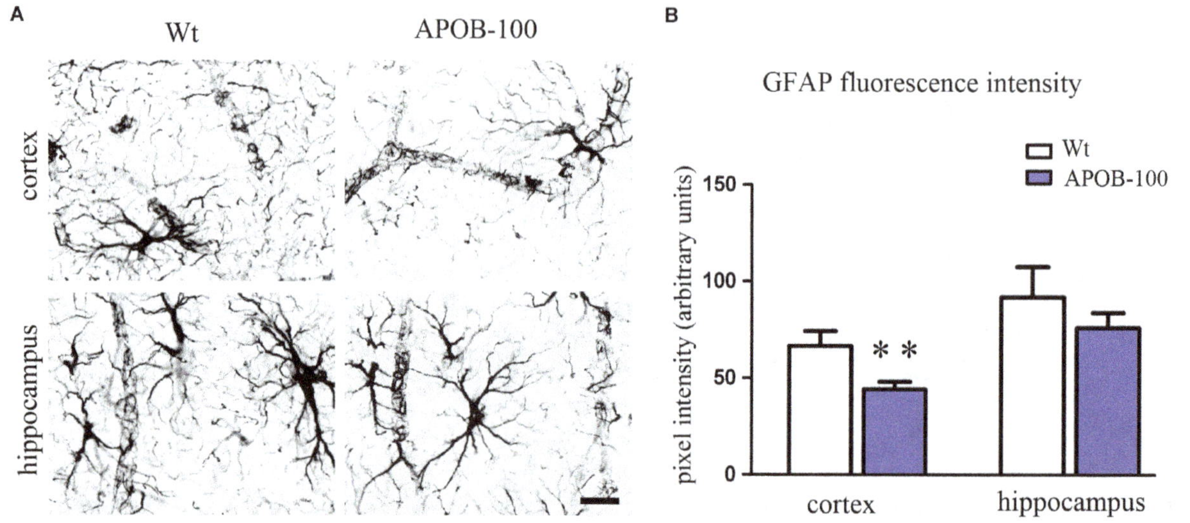

FIGURE 7 | Gfap immunostaining pattern in the cortex and hippocampus of wild-type (Wt) and APOB-100 transgenic mice (APOB-100) **(A).** Scale bar: 25 μm. Quantification of fluorescence intensity of Gfap immunolabeling in the frontal cortex and hippocampus of Wt and APOB-100 transgenic mice **(B).** $^{**}P < 0.01$ compared with Wt mice.

caveolin-1 expression was also linked to a decrease in occludin and or claudin-5 protein expression related to BBB damage (Nag et al., 2007; Beauchesne et al., 2010). In our study a decrease was observed in both caveolin-1 and occludin gene expression using QPCR, which is in concordance with the western blot findings reported by Song et al. (2007).

The increase in BBB permeability in our model may be linked to reduced expression of genes coding important brain endothelial TJ proteins *Cldn-5, Ocln, Tjp-1.* However, the differences detected at mRNA level were not reflected by the immunofluorescent staining pattern of TJ proteins claudin-5 and occludin, suggesting no detectable changes of TJs between the experimental groups at light microscopic level. In contrast, regarding the ultrastructure, a great percentage of discontinuous TJs were observed in TEM images of transgenic brains. Data obtained by PCR and immunohistochemistry do not necessarily show direct positive correlation due to the complex regulation of the gene expression at transcriptional, posttranscriptional, and posttranslational levels resulting in divergences (Vogel and Marcotte, 2012). In addition, during tissue fixation some epitopes may suffer alterations resulting in changes in specific antibody binding. Consequently, both these possibilities may explain the differences between PCR data and the analysis of immunofluorescent TJ signals.

Our findings on functional and gene expressional alterations at the BBB in APOB-100 mice are in agreement with the neurovascular concept of AD. Barrier dysfunction in brain microvessels is well described in AD (Zipser et al., 2007; Nelson et al., 2016), and BBB breakdown was found in the hippocampus in aging human brain which may contribute to cognitive impairment (Montagne et al., 2015).

Due to the observed similarities in gene expression changes present in both AD pathology and in APOB-100 transgenic mice, we examined whether neuroinflammation and neuronal changes were also characteristic features of our model. An increase in the gene expression of *Tnfα*, *NF-κB* and *Aif-1/Iba-1* detected in the brain of APOB-100 transgenic mice suggested inflammation related changes. Among the other inflammatory markers examined, *Tlr4*, which is reported to participate in innate neuroprotective mechanisms (Conte et al., 2017), decreased to 60% in the cortex of APOB-100 transgenic mice. It may indicate a disturbance in neuroprotection. Furthermore, a significant decrease in *Cdh2* expression coding *N*-cadherin was observed in the hippocampus of APOB-100 transgenic animals. *N*-cadherin, as an adhesion molecule, plays an important role in connecting pericytes to endothelial cells, thus maintaining normal BBB integrity (Winkler et al., 2011). Consequently, a loss in *N*-cadherin might lead to the structural and functional disintegration of the BBB.

The miRNA analysis revealed 10 miRNAs showing altered expression in APOB-100 transgenic cortex compared with wild-type ones. Out of these miRNAs mmu-miR-1a, mmu-miR-222, mmu-miR-26a, mmu-miR-7b are correlated with validated target genes. Among the target genes only *Bdnf* can be related to neuronal changes. It is regulated by several miRNAs (Varendi et al., 2014), among others mir-1, miRNA-26a and 26b suppress endogenous BDNF protein levels (Caputo et al., 2011; Varendi et al., 2014) In our study, we measured elevated *Bdnf* mRNA level, while the expression level of two posttranscriptional regulator miRNAs was changed in the opposite direction, miR-1a was downregulated and inversely, miR-26b was upregulated. The reduced expression of miR-1a and the increased expression of miR-26a is in accordance with findings related to high cholesterol levels and AD, respectively. High-cholesterol diet induced a significant decrease of miR-1 expression in ApoE deficient mice (Wang et al., 2013). Blocking miR-1 with antagomir enhanced endothelial permeability, while miR-1 mimics attenuated endothelial barrier dysfunction, strongly

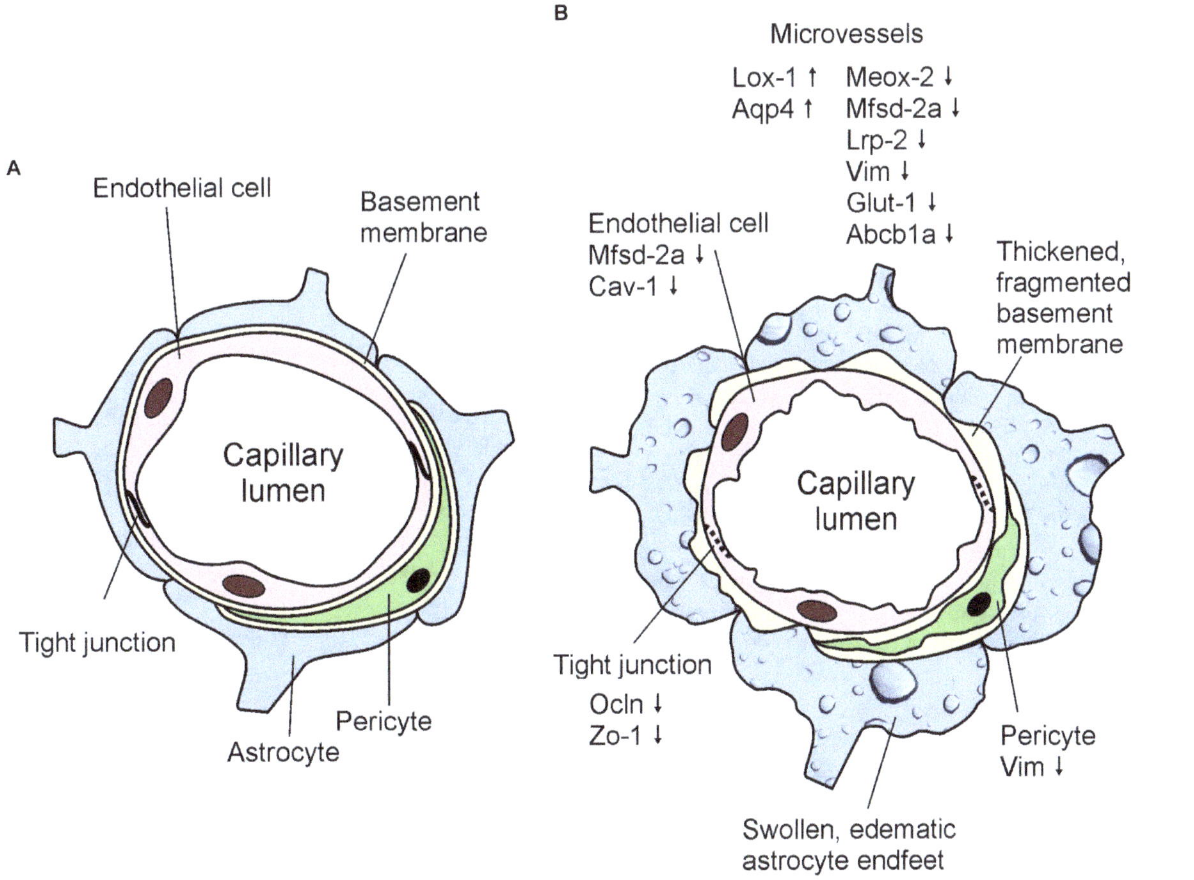

FIGURE 8 | Schematic drawings showing the basic structure of the BBB **(A)** and highlighting the most characteristic morphological and gene expression changes detected in cerebral microvessels of APOB-100 transgenic mice **(B)**.

indicating that miR-1 contributes to the regulation of endothelial barrier function (Wang et al., 2013). Similarly to our result, miR-26a was shown to be upregulated in AD brains (Cogswell et al., 2008) indicating that miR-26a might serve as a therapeutic target for patients with AD (Li and Sun, 2011).

In addition to brain capillary endothelial cells and neurons, alterations in other structural components of the NVU, such as astrocyte endfeet and pericytes may also contribute to BBB dysfunction. Astrocytes participate in the development and maintenance of BBB features, including tightening of TJs, inducing the expression of influx and efflux transporters, as well as specialized enzyme systems (Deli et al., 2005; Abbott et al., 2006; Deracinois et al., 2013). The expression level of Gfap, an astroglia marker, is critical in maintaining BBB integrity. Either an increase or a decrease in Gfap expression results in TJ protein expressional changes and BBB dysfunction (Willis, 2012). The fluorescence intensity of Gfap immunolabeling was significantly decreased in the cortex of APOB-100 transgenic mice compared to their wild-type littermates, which may contribute to the observed decrease in the expression of various TJ protein coding genes. It also may be in line with ultrastructural changes of astrocytes, characterized by edematic swellings around capillaries in the brain of APOB-100 transgenic mice. In a recent study (Ito et al., 2017), an increased sodium fluorescein permeability was reported following electroconvulsive stimulations. Regarding brain capillary ultrastructure, intact TJs were detected in this model of epilepsy, while astrocytic endfeet were swollen. In another paper (Haley and Lawrence, 2017) increased BBB permeability and astrocytic endfeet swelling occurred after cerebral ischaemia, but TJs remained intact and TJ proteins claudin-5 and occludin expression showed no change in western blots. Our study is in concordance with these data on both astroglia morphology and TJ protein expression. The abnormalities in astrocytic endfeet may be linked to the increased expression of *Aqp4* in brain microvessels isolated from APOB-100 transgenic animals. The loss of polarized expression of AQP4 in astrocyte foot processes has an important impact on development of BBB dysfunction and perivascular edema, and also disturbed homeostasis in the brain parenchyma in various pathologies (Wolburg et al., 2009).

S100b, another predominantly glial protein may also indicate BBB disruption. S100B is considered a plasma biomarker in traumatic brain injury (Halstrom et al., 2017), and cerebral small vessel disease, in which it is associated with cognitive impairment in patients (Gao et al., 2015). S100B is also linked to pathological changes observed in early AD (Mattsson et al., 2014).

In our model, no significant difference was found in *S100b* gene expression in the transgenic microvessels. In contrast, the gene expression of vimentin, another intermediate filament protein, dropped to less than 50% in the microvessel fraction of APOB-100 transgenic mice. The decrease in vimentin expression was observed at protein level too, based on immunohistochemical findings. Vimentin is expressed by endothelial cells, fibroblasts and α-smooth muscle actin producing cells in the middle cerebral artery of hyperlipidemic rabbits (Kacem et al., 2006). In an attempt to identify which cell type of the NVU is producing vimentin in our experimental animals, double immunolabeling studies were performed. Vimentin did not colocalize either with Gfap or Pdgfrβ, but a drop of vimentin mRNA expression was only observed in cultured pericytes from transgenic mice. Although cultures do not fully reflect the *in vivo* situation, the immunohistochemistry data together with the vimentin QPCR results on microvessels and cultured cells point to the possibility, that the change in the vimentin staining in brain microvessels of APOB-100 transgenic mice is related to pericytes. The reduction in vimentin immunostaining in the cortical microvessels of APOB-100 transgenic mice reflects that vimentin expression may react very sensitively to hypertriglyceridemic conditions.

Pericytes are embedded between endothelial cells and astrocyte endfeet in brain capillaries and they are crucial components of the NVU. They induce the expression of BBB-specific genes in cerebral endothelial cells and the polarization of glial endfeet which cover brain microvessels (Armulik et al., 2010). Pericyte deficiency leads to accelerated amyloid angiopathy and cerebral β-amyloidosis in a mouse AD model (Sagare et al., 2013). In our TEM analysis we detected an increase in the ratio of capillaries displaying no pericyte branches in the frontal cortex of APOB-100 transgenic mice compared with wild-type animals. It may suggest a decrease in pericyte number, which is in accordance with earlier findings demonstrating a reduction in the number of pericytes during neurodegeneration (Sagare et al., 2013).

CONCLUSION

In conclusion, we demonstrated here, that APOB-100 transgenic mice are characterized by elevated serum triglyceride levels and show functional, morphological, and gene expression alterations suggesting BBB dysfunction (**Figure 8**). Based on our findings we propose APOB-100 transgenic mice as a novel mouse model of vascular neurodegeneration. This model might provide researchers a useful tool to gain deeper insights into the pathomechanism of neurodegenerative diseases of vascular origin, which is fundamental for the development of efficient therapies.

AUTHOR CONTRIBUTIONS

MD, ZH, MT, and MS contributed to the conception and design of the study. DN, NL, and MT performed the BBB penetration study. ÁK, ZH, MT, and MD conducted the ultrastructural studies. ZH, MT, BD, FW, SV, JV, and BB performed the immunohistochemistry. MT, NL, DN, BD, and AZ investigated the QPCR analysis. AZ investigated and LP supervised the miRNA analysis. ZH, AH, GS, AK, BB, AZ, BD, AC, and MT performed the software analysis. MD, LP, LV, BP, and MS supervised the work. MD, LV, BP, and MS were the grant holders. MD, ZH, MT, and MS wrote the manuscript draft. LV, LP, and BP reviewed the manuscript. All authors approved the final manuscript.

FUNDING

This work was supported by funding from National Research, Development and Innovation Office, Hungary (GINOP 2.3.2.-15.2016-00060) and the Hungarian Basic Research Fund (OTKA NN111006).

ACKNOWLEDGMENTS

We thank I. Kis-Sebestyén for her technical assistance, M. Tóth for artwork preparation, T. Márkus-Vadóc and Dr. Marcus Mark Philip for reviewing the manuscript.

REFERENCES

Abbott, N. J., Rönnbäck, L., and Hansson, E. (2006). Astrocyte-endothelial interactions at the blood-brain barrier. *Nat. Rev. Neurosci.* 7, 41–53. doi: 10.1038/nrn1824

Antonios, N., Angiolillo, D. J., and Silliman, S. (2008). Hypertriglyceridemia and ischemic stroke. *Eur. Neurol.* 60, 269–278. doi: 10.1159/000157880

Armulik, A., Genové, G., Mäe, M., Nisancioglu, M. H., Wallgard, E., Niaudet, C., et al. (2010). Pericytes regulate the blood-brain barrier. *Nature* 468, 557–561. doi: 10.1038/nature09522

Bandopadhyay, R., Orte, C., Lawrenson, J. G., Reid, A. R., De Silva, S., Allt, G., et al. (2001). Contractile proteins in pericytes at the blood-brain and blood-retinal barriers. *J. Neurocytol.* 30, 35–44. doi: 10.1023/A:1011965307612

Barry, S. O., Marcel, R. T., Nelson, G., Victor, B., Tadeusz, M., Thomas, F. L., et al. (1998). Reduced endothelial nitric oxide synthase expression and production in human atherosclerosis. *Circulation* 97, 2494–2498. doi: 10.1161/01.CIR.97.25.2494

Beauchesne, E., Desjardins, P., Butterworth, R. F., and Hazell, A. S. (2010). Up-regulation of caveolin-1 and blood-brain barrier breakdown are attenuated by N-acetylcysteine in thiamine deficiency. *Neurochem. Int.* 57, 830–837. doi: 10.1016/j.neuint.2010.08.022

Bereczki, E., Bernát, G., Csont, T., Ferdinandy, P., Scheich, H., Sántha, M., et al. (2008). Overexpression of human apolipoprotein B-100 induces severe neurodegeneration in transgenic mice. *J. Proteome Res.* 7, 2246–2252. doi: 10.1021/pr7006329

Betsholtz, C. (2015). Lipid transport and human brain development. *Nat. Genet.* 47, 699–701. doi: 10.1038/ng.3348

Bjelik, A., Bereczki, E., Gonda, S., Juhasz, A., Rimanoczy, A., Zana, M., et al. (2006). Human apoB overexpression and a high-cholesterol diet differently modify the brain APP metabolism in the transgenic mouse model of atherosclerosis. *Neurochem. Int.* 49, 393–400. doi: 10.1016/j.neuint.2006.01.026

Bowman, G. L., Kaye, J. A., and Quinn, J. F. (2012). Dyslipidemia and blood-brain barrier integrity in Alzheimer's disease. *Curr. Gerontol. Geriatr. Res.* 2012:184042. doi: 10.1155/2012/184042

Burgess, B. L., McIsaac, S. A., Naus, K. E., Chan, J. Y., Tansley, G. H. K., Yang, J., et al. (2006). Elevated plasma triglyceride levels precede amyloid deposition in Alzheimer's disease mouse models with abundant A beta in plasma. *Neurobiol. Dis.* 24, 114–127. doi: 10.1016/j.nbd.2006.06.007

Buttery, L. D., Chester, A. H., Springall, D. R., Borland, J. A., Michel, T., Yacoub, M. H., et al. (1996). Explanted vein grafts with an intact endothelium demonstrate reduced focal expression of endothelial nitric oxide synthase specific to atherosclerotic sites. *J. Pathol.* 179, 197–203. doi: 10.1002/(SICI)1096-9896(199606)179:2<197::AID-PATH587>3.0.CO;2-D

Callow, M. J., Stoltzfus, L. J., Lawn, R. M., and Rubin, E. M. (1994). Expression of human apolipoprotein-B and assembly of lipoprotein (A) in transgenic mice. *Proc. Natl. Acad. Sci. U.S.A.* 91, 2130–2134. doi: 10.1073/pnas.91.6.2130

Caputo, V., Sinibaldi, L., Fiorentino, A., Parisi, C., Catalanotto, C., Pasini, A., et al. (2011). Brain derived neurotrophic factor (BDNF) expression is regulated by microRNAs miR-26a and miR-26b allele-specific binding. *PLoS One* 6:e28656. doi: 10.1371/journal.pone.0028656

Caramelli, P., Nitrini, R., Maranhao, R., Lourenco, A. C., Damasceno, M. C., Vinagre, C., et al. (1999). Increased apolipoprotein B serum concentration in Alzheimer's disease. *Acta Neurol. Scand.* 100, 61–63. doi: 10.1111/j.1600-0404.1999.tb00724.x

Chen, M., Masaki, T., and Sawamura, T. (2002). LOX-1, the receptor for oxidized low-density lipoprotein identified from endothelial cells: implications in endothelial dysfunction and atherosclerosis. *Pharmacol. Ther.* 95, 89–100. doi: 10.1016/S0163-7258(02)00236-X

Cirrito, J. R., Deane, R., Fagan, A. M., Spinner, M. L., Parsadanian, M., Finn, M. B., et al. (2005). P-glycoprotein deficiency at the blood-brain barrier increases amyloid-beta deposition in an Alzheimer disease mouse model. *J. Clin. Invest.* 115, 3285–3290. doi: 10.1172/JCI25247

Cogswell, J. P., Ward, J., Taylor, I. A., Waters, M., Shi, Y., Cannon, B., et al. (2008). Identification of miRNA changes in Alzheimer's disease brain and CSF yields putative biomarkers and insights into disease pathways. *J. Alzheimers Dis.* 14, 27–41. doi: 10.3233/JAD-2008-14103

Conte, C., Roscini, L., Sardella, R., Mariucci, G., Scorzoni, S., Beccari, T., et al. (2017). Toll like receptor 4 affects the cerebral biochemical changes induced by mptp treatment. *Neurochem. Res.* 42, 493–500. doi: 10.1007/s11064-016-2095-6

Croop, J. M., Raymond, M., Haber, D., Devault, A., Arceci, R. J., Gros, P., et al. (1989). The three mouse multidrug resistance (mdr) genes are expressed in a tissue-specific manner in normal mouse tissues. *Mol. Cell. Biol.* 9, 1346–1350. doi: 10.1128/MCB.9.3.1346

Csont, T., Bereczki, E., Bencsik, P., Fodor, G., Görbe, A., Zvara, A., et al. (2007). Hypercholesterolemia increases myocardial oxidative and nitrosative stress thereby leading to cardiac dysfunction in APOB-100 transgenic mice. *Cardiovasc. Res.* 76, 100–109. doi: 10.1016/j.cardiores.2007.06.006

Daneman, R., Zhou, L., Agalliu, D., Cahoy, J. D., Kaushal, A., and Barres, B. A. (2010). The mouse blood-brain barrier transcriptome: a new resource for understanding the development and function of brain endothelial cells. *PLoS One* 5:e13741. doi: 10.1371/journal.pone.0013741

De La Torre, J. C., Fortin, T., Park, G. A. S., Butler, K. S., Kozlowski, B. A., Pappas, B. A., et al. (1992). Chronic cerebrovascular insufficiency induces dementia-like deficits in aged rats. *Brain Res.* 582, 186–195. doi: 10.1016/0006-8993(92)90132-S

De la Torre, J. C., and Mussivand, T. (1993). Can disturbed brain microcirculation cause Alzheimer's disease? *Neurol. Res.* 15, 146–153.

Deane, R., Du Yan, S., Submamaryan, R. K., LaRue, B., Jovanovic, S., Hogg, E., et al. (2003). RAGE mediates amyloid-beta peptide transport across the blood-brain barrier and accumulation in brain. *Nat. Med.* 9, 907–113. doi: 10.1038/nm890

Deli, M. A., Abrahám, C. S., Kataoka, Y., and Niwa, M. (2005). Permeability studies on *in vitro* blood-brain barrier models: physiology, pathology, and pharmacology. *Cell. Mol. Neurobiol.* 25, 59–127. doi: 10.1007/s10571-004-1377-8

Deracinois, B., Pottiez, G., Chafey, P., Teerlink, T., Camoin, L., Davids, M., et al. (2013). Glial-cell-mediated re-induction of the blood-brain barrier phenotype in brain capillary endothelial cells: a differential gel electrophoresis study. *Proteomics* 13, 1185–1199. doi: 10.1002/pmic.201200166

Di Marco, L. Y., Venneri, A., Farkas, E., Evans, P. C., Marzo, A., and Frangi, A. F. (2015). Vascular dysfunction in the pathogenesis of Alzheimer's disease-A review of endothelium-mediated mechanisms and ensuing vicious circles. *Neurobiol. Dis. Rev.* 82, 593–606. doi: 10.1016/j.nbd.2015.08.01

Ehehalt, R., Keller, P., Haass, C., Thiele, C., and Simons, K. (2003). Amyloidogenic processing of the Alzheimer beta-amyloid precursor protein depends on lipid rafts. *J. Cell. Biol.* 160, 113–123. doi: 10.1083/jcb.200207113

Eiselein, L., Wilson, D. W., Lamé, M. W., and Rutledge, J. C. (2007). Lipolysis products from triglyceride-rich lipoproteins increase endothelial permeability, perturb zonula occludens-1 and F-actin, and induce apoptosis. *Am. J. Physiol. Heart Circ. Physiol.* 292, H2745–H2753. doi: 10.1152/ajpheart.00686.2006

Farkas, A. S., Acsai, K., Nagy, N., Tóth, A., Fülöp, F., Seprényi, G., et al. (2008). Na (+)/Ca (2 +) exchanger inhibition exerts a positive inotropic effect in the rat heart, but fails to influence the contractility of the rabbit heart. *Br. J. Pharmacol.* 154, 93–104. doi: 10.1038/bjp.2008.83

Gao, Q., Fan, Y., Mu, L. Y., Ma, L., Song, Z. Q., and Zhang, Y. N. (2015). S100B and ADMA in cerebral small vessel disease and cognitive dysfunction. *J. Neurol. Sci.* 354, 27–32. doi: 10.1016/j.jns.2015.04.031

Gosselet, F., Saint-Pol, J., Candela, P., and Fenart, L. (2013). Amyloid-β peptides, Alzheimer's disease and the blood-brain barrier. *Curr. Alzheimer Res.* 10, 1015–1033. doi: 10.2174/15672050113106660174

Gundersen, H. J., and Osterby, R. (1981). Optimizing sampling efficiency of stereological studies in biology: or 'do more less well!'. *J. Microsc.* 121, 65–73. doi: 10.1111/j.1365-2818.1981.tb01199.x

Haley, M. J., and Lawrence, C. B. (2017). The blood-brain barrier after stroke: structural studies and the role of transcytotic vesicles. *J. Cereb. Blood Flow Metab.* 37, 456–470. doi: 10.1177/0271678X16629976

Halstrom, A., MacDonald, E., Neil, C., Arendts, G., Fatovich, D., and Fitzgerald, M. (2017). Elevation of oxidative stress indicators in a pilot study of plasma following traumatic brain injury. *J. Clin. Neurosci.* 35, 104–108. doi: 10.1016/j.jocn.2016.09.006

Ito, M., Bolati, K., Kinjo, T., Ichimura, K., Furuta, A., McLoughlin, D. M., et al. (2017). Electroconvulsive stimulation transiently enhances the permeability of the rat blood-brain barrier and induces astrocytic changes. *Brain Res. Bull.* 128, 92–97. doi: 10.1016/j.brainresbull.2016.11.011

Kacem, K., Sercombe, C., Hammami, M., Vicaut, E., and Sercombe, R. (2006). Sympathectomy causes aggravated lesions and dedifferentiation in large rabbit atherosclerotic arteries without involving nitric oxide. *J. Vasc. Res.* 43, 289–305. doi: 10.1159/000093010

Kapasi, A., and Schneider, J. A. (2016). Vascular contributions to cognitive impairment, clinical Alzheimer's disease, and dementia in older persons. *Biochim. Biophys. Acta* 1862, 878–886. doi: 10.1016/j.bbadis.2015.12.023

Kisler, K., Nelson, A. R., Rege, S. V., Ramanathan, A., Wang, Y., and Ahuja, A. (2017). Pericyte degeneration leads to neurovascular uncoupling and limits oxygen supply to brain. *Nat. Neurosci.* 20, 406–416. doi: 10.1038/nn.4489

Klafke, J. Z., Porto, F. G., Batista, R., Bochi, G. V., Moresco, R. N., da Luz, P. L., et al. (2015). Association between hypertriglyceridemia and protein oxidation and proinflammatory markers in normocholesterolemic and hypercholesterolemic individuals. *Clin. Chim. Acta* 448, 50–57. doi: 10.1016/j.cca.2015.06.013

Kuo, Y. M., Emmerling, M. R., Bisgaier, C. L., Essenburg, A. D., Lampert, H. C., Drumm, D., et al. (1998). Elevated low-density lipoprotein in Alzheimer's disease correlates with brain A beta 1-42 levels. *Biochem. Biophys. Res. Commun.* 252, 711–715. doi: 10.1006/bbrc.1998.9652

Lane-Donovan, C., Wong, W. M., Durakoglugil, M. S., Wasser, C. R., Jiang, S., Xian, X., et al. (2016). Genetic restoration of plasma ApoE improves cognition and partially restores synaptic defects in ApoE-deficient mice. *J. Neurosci.* 36, 10141–10150. doi: 10.1523/JNEUROSCI.1054-16.2016

Lee, L. L., Aung, H. H., Wilson, D. W., Anderson, S. E., Rutledge, J. C., and Rutkowsky, J. M. (2017). Triglyceride-rich lipoprotein lipolysis products increase blood-brain barrier transfer coefficient and induce astrocyte lipid droplets and cell stress. *Am. J. Physiol. Cell Physiol.* 312, C500–C516. doi: 10.1152/ajpcell.00120.2016

Lénárt, N., Szegedi, V., Juhász, G., Kasztner, A., Horváth, J., Bereczki, E., et al. (2012). Increased tau phosphorylation and impaired presynaptic function in hypertriglyceridemic ApoB-100 transgenic mice. *PLoS One* 7:e46007. doi: 10.1371/journal.pone.0046007

Lénárt, N., Walter, F. R., Bocsik, A., Sántha, P., Tóth, M. E., Harazin, A., et al. (2015). Cultured cells of the blood-brain barrier from apolipoprotein B-100 transgenic mice: effects of oxidized low-density lipoprotein treatment. *Fluids Barriers CNS.* 12:17. doi: 10.1186/s12987-015-0013-y

Li, B., and Sun, H. (2011). MiR-26a promotes neurite outgrowth by repressing PTEN expression. *Physiol. Genomics* 43, 521–528. doi: 10.3892/mmr.2013.1534

Li, L., Cao, D., Garber, D. W., Kim, H., and Fukuchi, K. (2003). Association of aortic atherosclerosis with cerebral beta-amyloidosis and learning deficits in a mouse model of Alzheimer's disease. *Am. J. Pathol.* 163, 2155–2164. doi: 10.1016/S0002-9440(10)63572-9

Löffler, T., Flunkert, S., Havas, D., Sántha, M., Hutter-Paier, B., Steyrer, E., et al. (2013). Impact of APOB-100 expression on cognition and brain pathology in wild-type and hAPPsl mice. *Neurobiol. Aging* 34, 2379–2388. doi: 10.1016/j.neurobiolaging.2013.04.008

Lubrano, V., and Balzan, S. (2016). Roles of LOX-1 in microvascular dysfunction. *Microvasc. Res.* 105, 132–140. doi: 10.1016/j.mvr.2016.02.006

Lutjohann, D., Papassotiropoulos, A., Bjorkhem, I., Locatelli, S., Bagli, M., Oehring, R. D., et al. (2000). Plasma 24S-hydroxycholesterol (cerebrosterol) is increased in Alzheimer and vascular demented patients. *J. Lipid Res.* 41, 195–198.

Lyros, E., Bakogiannis, C., Liu, Y., and Fassbender, K. (2014). Molecular links between endothelial dysfunction and neurodegeneration in Alzheimer's disease. *Curr. Alzheimers. Res.* 11, 18–26. doi: 10.2174/1567205010666131119235254

Marques, F., Sousa, J. C., Sousa, N., and Palha, J. A. (2013). Blood-brain-barriers in aging and in Alzheimer's disease. *Mol. Neurodegener.* 8:38. doi: 10.1186/1750-1326-8-38

Mattsson, N., Insel, P., Nosheny, R., Trojanowski, J. Q., Shaw, L. M., Jack, C. R. Jr., et al. (2014). Effects of cerebrospinal fluid proteins on brain atrophy rates in cognitively healthy older adults. *Neurobiol. Aging* 35, 614–622. doi: 10.1016/j.neurobiolaging.2013.08.027

Mayhew, T. M. (1991). The new stereological methods for interpreting functional morphology from slices of cells and organs. *Exp. Physiol.* 76, 639–665. doi: 10.1113/expphysiol.1991.sp003533

Montagne, A., Barnes, S. R., Sweeney, M. D., Halliday, M. R., Sagare, A. P., Zhao, Z., et al. (2015). Blood-brain barrier breakdown in the aging human hippocampus. *Neuron* 85, 296–302. doi: 10.1016/j.neuron.2014.12.032

Nag, S., Venugopalan, R., and Stewart, D. J. (2007). Increased caveolin-1 expression precedes decreased expression of occludin and claudin-5 during blood-brain barrier breakdown. *Acta Neuropathol.* 114, 459–469. doi: 10.1007/s00401-007-0274-x

Nelson, A. R., Sweeney, M. D., Sagare, A. P., and Zlokovic, B. V. (2016). Neurovascular dysfunction and neurodegeneration in dementia and Alzheimer's disease. *Biochim. Biophys. Acta* 1862, 887–900. doi: 10.1016/j.bbadis.2015.12.016

Nicolakakis, N., and Hamel, E. (2011). Neurovascular function in Alzheimer's disease patients and experimental models. *J. Cereb. Blood Flow Metab.* 31, 1354–1370. doi: 10.1038/jcbfm.2011.43

Patterson, C. E., Rhoades, R. A., and Garcia, J. G. (1992). Evans blue dye as a marker of albumin clearance in cultured endothelial monolayer and isolated lung. *J. Appl. Physiol.* 72, 865–873. doi: 10.1152/jappl.1992.72.3.865

Pekny, M., Wilhelmsson, U., Bogestål, Y. R., and Pekna, M. (2007). The role of astrocytes and complement system in neural plasticity. *Int. Rev. Neurobiol.* 82, 95–111. doi: 10.1016/S0074-7742(07)82005-8

Puglielli, L., Tanzi, R. E., and Kovacs, D. M. (2003). Alzheimer's disease: the cholesterol connection. *Nat. Neurosci.* 6, 345–351. doi: 10.1038/nn0403-345

Raffaitin, C. H., Gin, J. P., Empana, J. P., Helmer, C., Berr, C., Tzourio, C., et al. (2009). Metabolic syndromeand risk for incident Alzheimer's disease or vascular dementia: the Three-City study. *Diabetes Care* 32, 169–174. doi: 10.2337/dc08-0272

Sabbagh, M., Zahiri, H. R., Ceimo, J., Cooper, K., Gaul, W., Connor, D., et al. (2004). Is there a characteristic lipid profile in Alzheimer's disease? *J. Alzheimers Dis.* 6, 585–589. doi: 10.3233/JAD-2004-6602

Sagare, A. P., Bell, R. D., Zhao, Z., Ma, Q., Winkler, E. A., Ramanathan, A., et al. (2013). Pericyte loss influences Alzheimer-like neurodegeneration in mice. *Nat. Commun.* 4:2932. doi: 10.1038/ncomms3932

Schubert, W., Frank, P. G., Woodman, S. E., Hyogo, H., Cohen, D. E., Chow, C. W., et al. (2002). Microvascular hyperpermeability in caveolin-1 (-/-) knock-out mice. Treatment with a specific nitric-oxide synthase inhibitor, L-NAME, restores normal microvascular permeability in Cav-1 null mice. *J. Biol. Chem.* 277, 40091–40098. doi: 10.1074/jbc.M205948200

Shibata, M., Yamada, S., Kumar, S. R., Calero, M., Bading, J., Frangione, B., et al. (2000). Clearance of Alzheimer's amyloid-beta (1-40) peptide from brain by LDL receptor-related protein-1 at the blood-brain barrier. *J. Clin. Invest.* 106, 1489–1499. doi: 10.1172/JCI10498

Shoshani, T., Zhang, S., Dey, S., Pastan, I., and Gottesman, M. M. (1998). Analysis of random recombination between human MDR1 and mouse mdr1a cDNA in a pHaMDR-dihydrofolate reductase bicistronic expression system. *Mol. Pharmacol.* 54, 623–630.

Song, L., Ge, S., and Pachter, J. S. (2007). Caveolin-1 regulates expression of junction-associated proteins in brain microvascular endothelial cells. *Blood* 109, 1515–1523. doi: 10.1182/blood-2006-07-034009

Stancel, N., Chen, C. C., Ke, L. Y., Chu, C. S., Lu, J., Sawamura, T., et al. (2016). Interplay between CRP, atherogenic LDL, and LOX-1 and its potential role in the pathogenesis of atherosclerosis. *Clin. Chem.* 62, 320–327. doi: 10.1373/clinchem.2015.243923

Stapleton, P. A., Goodwill, A. G., James, M. E., Brock, R. W., and Frisbee, J. C. (2010). Hypercholesterolemia and microvascular dysfunction: interventional strategies. *J. Inflamm.* 7:54. doi: 10.1186/1476-9255-7-54

Süle, Z., Mracskó, E., Bereczki, E., Sántha, M., Csont, T., Ferdinandy, P., et al. (2009). Capillary injury in the ischemic brain of hyperlipidemic, apolipoprotein B-100 transgenic mice. *Life Sci.* 84, 935–939. doi: 10.1016/j.lfs.2009.04.011

Varendi, K., Kumar, A., Härma, M. A., and Andressoo, J. O. (2014). miR-1, miR-10b, miR-155, and miR-191 are novel regulators of BDNF. *Cell. Mol. Life Sci.* 71, 4443–4456. doi: 10.1007/s00018-014-1628-x

Veszelka, S., Pásztói, M., Farkas, A. E., Krizbai, I., Ngo, T. K., Niwa, M., et al. (2007). Pentosan polysulfate protects brain endothelial cells against bacterial lipopolysaccharide-induced damages. *Neurochem. Int.* 50, 219–228. doi: 10.1016/j.neuint.2006.08.006

Veszelka, S., Tóth, A., Walter, F. R., Tóth, A. E., Gróf, I., Mészáros, M., et al. (2018). Comparison of a rat primary cell-based blood-brain barrier model with epithelial and brain endothelial cell lines: gene expression and drug transport. *Front. Mol. Neurosci.* 11:166. doi: 10.3389/fnmol.2018.00166

Veszelka, S., Tóth, A. E., Walter, F. R., Datki, Z., Mózes, E., Fülöp, L., et al. (2013). Docosahexaenoic acid reduces amyloid-β induced toxicity in cells of the neurovascular unit. *J. Alzheimers Dis.* 34, 487–501. doi: 10.3233/JAD-120163

Veszelka, S., Urbányi, Z., Pázmány, T., Németh, L., Obál, I., Dung, N. T., et al. (2003). Human serum amyloid P component attenuates the bacterial lipopolysaccharide-induced increase in blood-brain barrier permeability in mice. *Neurosci. Lett.* 352, 57–60. doi: 10.1016/j.neulet.2003.08.028

Vogel, C., and Marcotte, E. M. (2012). Insights into the regulation of protein abundance from proteomic and transcriptomic analyses. *Nat. Rev. Genet.* 13, 227–232. doi: 10.1038/nrg3185

Wang, H., Zhu, H. Q., Wang, F., Zhou, Q., Gui, S. Y., and Wang, Y. (2013). MicroRNA-1 prevents high-fat diet-induced endothelial permeability in apoE knock-out mice. *Mol. Cell. Biochem.* 378, 153–159. doi: 10.1007/s11010-013-1606-x

Willis, C. L. (2012). Imaging *in vivo* astrocyte/endothelial cell interactions at the blood-brain barrier. *Methods Mol. Biol.* 814, 515–529. doi: 10.1007/978-1-61779-452-0_34

Winkler, E. A., Bell, R. D., and Zlokovic, B. V. (2011). Central nervous system pericytes in health and disease. *Nat. Neurosci.* 14, 1398–1405. doi: 10.1038/nn.2946

Winkler, E. A., Nishida, Y., Sagare, A. P., Rege, S. V., Bell, R. D., Perlmutter, D., et al. (2015). GLUT1 reductions exacerbate Alzheimer's disease vasculo-neuronal dysfunction and degeneration. *Nat. Neurosci.* 18, 521–530. doi: 10.1038/nn

Wolburg, H., Noell, S., Wolburg-Buchholz, K., Mack, A., and Fallier-Becker, P. (2009). Agrin, aquaporin-4, and astrocyte polarity as an important feature of the blood-brain barrier. *Neuroscientist* 15, 180–193. doi: 10.1177/1073858408329509

Won, D., Zhu, S. N., Chen, M., Teichert, A. M., Fish, J. E., Matouk, C. C., et al. (2007). Relative reduction of endothelial nitric-oxide synthase expression and transcription in atherosclerosis-prone regions of the mouse aorta and in an *in vitro* model of disturbed flow. *Am. J. Pathol.* 171, 1691–1704. doi: 10.2353/ajpath.2007.060860

Wu, Z., Guo, H., Chow, N., Sallstrom, J., Bell, R. D., Deane, R., et al. (2005). Role of the MEOX2 homeobox gene in neurovascular dysfunction in Alzheimer disease. *Nat. Med.* 11, 959–965. doi: 10.1038/nm1287

Zhao, Z., Nelson, A. R., Betsholtz, C., and Zlokovic, B. V. (2015). Establishment and dysfunction of the blood-brain barrier. *Cell* 163, 1064–1078. doi: 10.1016/j.cell.2015.10.06

Zhao, Z., and Zlokovic, B. V. (2014). Blood-brain barrier: a dual life of MFSD2A? *Neuron* 82, 728–730. doi: 10.1016/j.neuron.2014.05.012

Zipser, B. D., Johanson, C. E., Gonzalez, L., Berzin, T. M., Tavares, R., Hulette, C. M., et al. (2007). Microvascular injury and blood-brain barrier leakage in Alzheimer's disease. *Neurobiol. Aging* 28, 977–986. doi: 10.1016/j.neurobiolaging.2006.05.016

Zlokovic, B. V. (2008). The blood-brain barrier in health and chronic neurodegenerative disorders. *Neuron* 57, 178–201. doi: 10.1016/j.neuron.2008.01.003

Zlokovic, B. V. (2011). Neurovascular pathways to neurodegeneration in Alzheimer's disease and other disorders. *Nat. Rev. Neurosci.* 3, 723–738. doi: 10.1038/nrn3114

2

Homer1a Attenuates Endoplasmic Reticulum Stress-Induced Mitochondrial Stress After Ischemic Reperfusion Injury by Inhibiting the PERK Pathway

Jialiang Wei [1,2†], Xiuquan Wu [1†], Peng Luo [1], Kangyi Yue [1], Yang Yu [1], Jingnan Pu [1], Lei Zhang [1], Shuhui Dai [1], Donghui Han [3] and Zhou Fei [1]*

[1]Department of Neurosurgery, Xijing Hospital, Fourth Military Medical University, Xi'an, China, [2]Department of Health Services, Fourth Military Medical University, Xi'an, China, [3]Department of Urology, Xijing Hospital, Fourth Military Medical University, Xi'an, China

***Correspondence:**
Zhou Fei
feizhou@fmmu.edu.cn

†These authors have contributed equally to this work

Homer1a is the short form of a scaffold protein that plays a protective role in many forms of stress. However, the role of Homer1a in cerebral ischemia/reperfusion (I/R) injury and its potential mechanism is still unknown. In this study, we found that Homer1a was upregulated by oxygen and glucose deprivation (OGD) and that overexpression of Homer1a alleviated OGD-induced lactate dehydrogenase (LDH) release and cell death in cultured cortical neurons. After OGD treatment, the overexpression of Homer1a preserved mitochondrial function, as evidenced by less cytochrome c release, less reactive oxygen species (ROS) production, less ATP and mitochondrial membrane potential (MMP) loss, less caspase-9 activation, and inhibition of endoplasmic reticulum (ER) stress confirmed by the decreased expression of phosphate-PKR-like ER Kinase (p-PERK)/PERK and phosphate- inositol-requiring enzyme 1 (p-IRE1)/IRE1 and immunofluorescence (IF) staining. In addition, mitochondrial protection of Homer1a was blocked by the ER stress activator Tunicamycin (TM) with a re-escalated ROS level, increasing ATP and MMP loss. Furthermore, Homer1a overexpression-induced mitochondrial stress attenuation was significantly reversed by activating the PERK pathway with TM and p-IRE1 inhibitor 3,5-dibromosalicylaldehyde (DBSA), as evidenced by increased cytochrome c release, increased ATP loss and a higher ROS level. However, activating the IRE1 pathway with TM and p-PERK inhibitor GSK2656157 showed little change in cytochrome c release and exhibited a moderate upgrade of ATP loss and ROS production in neurons. In summary, these findings demonstrated that Homer1a protects against OGD-induced injury by preserving mitochondrial function through inhibiting the PERK pathway. Our finding may reveal a promising target of protecting neurons from cerebral I/R injury.

Keywords: ischemic stroke, homer1a, mitochondrial dysfunction, endoplasmic reticulum stress, PERK kinase

INTRODUCTION

Ischemic stroke (IS) is a sudden medical condition in which little or restricted blood flow to the brain results in cell death. IS has high mortality, in which almost half of the patients live less than 1 year, and high morbidity, with up to 75% of patients having physical, mental, and emotional disability (Hankey, 2017; Benjamin et al., 2018). Some mechanisms have been found to be responsible for post-IS neuronal injury, such as excitatory neurotransmitter release, calcium overload and free radical injury. However, few therapies have been discovered to treat IS efficiently (Pandya et al., 2011; Chen et al., 2012). The exact molecular pathways underlying the ischemic reperfusion (I/R) neuronal injury have not been fully illustrated.

Homer proteins are best known as scaffold proteins located at the postsynaptic density and are crucial in regulating neuronal signals (Huang et al., 2008). Homer1a, a short form of Homer protein, contains a conserved EVH1 domain but lacks the CC domain, which enables Homer1a to function as a negative regulator of long forms of Homer protein (Foa and Gasperini, 2009). Several studies have shown that Homer1a plays an important role in sleep management, anti-depression and chronic inflammatory pain (Tappe et al., 2006; Serchov et al., 2016; Diering et al., 2017). Our previous study showed that Homer1a protects neurons against N-Methyl-D-aspartate (NMDA)-induced injury (Wang et al., 2015), and we also found that Homer1a protects retinal ganglion cells against retinal I/R injury (Fei et al., 2015). However, the exact role of Homer1a in cerebral I/R injury and the associated mechanism have not been elucidated.

Mitochondria play pivotal roles in supplying cellular energy, signaling, cellular differentiation, and cell death, as well as maintaining control of the cell cycle and cell growth (Schumacker et al., 2014). As an indispensable energy reservoir, mitochondria control the lifeline of most cells. Dysfunction of mitochondria plays a key role in many nervous system diseases such as stroke and neurodegenerative diseases (Prentice et al., 2015). Studies have revealed the pivotal role of mitochondria in aggravating reperfusion injury *via* producing excessive free radicals (Sanderson et al., 2013). Many studies have focused on therapies such as antioxidants and pro-biogenesis targeting mitochondria, with substantial progress, indicating the importance of mitochondria in I/R injury (Mailloux, 2016; Bhatti et al., 2017). The endoplasmic reticulum (ER) is also an important organelle that is responsible for protein folding and calcium homeostasis. Misfolded protein overload under various stresses results in ER turbulence, which is also known as ER stress (Chen et al., 2017). Previous studies have shown that ER stress is a major mechanism in I/R injury-induced apoptosis in the liver, myocardium and brain (Wang et al., 2016; Imarisio et al., 2017; Wu et al., 2017). Our previous studies showed that Homer1a preserves mitochondrial function in PC12 cells under oxidative stress induced by hydrogen peroxide and regulates the calcium equilibrium in HT22 cells under glutamate-induced injury (Luo et al., 2012a; Rao et al., 2016). However, the underlying mechanism between Homer1a and mitochondria and whether Homer1a influences ER stress after cerebral I/R are still unclear.

In the present study, it is aimed to survey the expression dynamics of Homer1a after neuronal ischemia-reperfusion injury and to determine the effect of Homer1a against IR injury. The effect of Homer1a on mitochondria dysfunction and ERS, as well as the relationship between them are also investigated. Furthermore, drug administration is implemented to inquire the specific mechanism involving PKR-like ER kinase (PERK) and inositolrequiring protein 1 (IRE1) pathways.

MATERIALS AND METHODS

Rat Primary Cultured Cortical Neurons

All procedures and animal manipulations were designed according to the National Institute of Health (NIH) Guide for the Care and Use of Laboratory Animals (No. 85-23) and were approved by the Ethics Committee of the Fourth Military Medical University. Primary cultured neurons were sampled from pregnant C57 mice using specified methods. Briefly, we removed embryos at 15–16 days and subsequently minced the meninges and vessels under a microscope. Then, we separated the cortex from the cerebrum and shredded it. The cortex then was digested in pancreatic enzymes for 20 min at 37°C with gentle shaking every 5 min. The digested neurons were resuspended in NM medium composed of neurobasal medium, 0.5 mM L-glutamine and 2% B27 before being plated onto the Poly-L-Lysine (PLL) pretreated dishes with a density of 1.5×10^6 cells/cm^2. The neurons were cultured in a 5% CO_2 incubator at 37°C, and the culture medium was renewed every 3 days.

Lentivirus Construction and Transfection

The preparation of a Homer1a Lentivirus was described previously (Luo et al., 2012a). The lentivirus overexpression open reading frame was the Pgc-fu-Homer1a cDNA-3FLAG construct (GeneChem Co., Shanghai, China). The primary cultured cortical neurons were cultured 8 days before being transfected with lentivirus for 72 h with an approximate multiplicity of infection (MOI) of 20.

Oxygen and Glucose Deprivation (OGD)

To mimic the I/R injury, the culture medium was renewed with glucose-free Neurobasal after being washed three times with PBS, and the neurons were then cultured in a specific chamber containing 5% CO_2 and 95% N_2 at 37°C for 1 h to simulate ischemic injury. Neurons were then removed from the chamber and washed with PBS three times before being reinfused with NM medium and maintained in a 5% CO_2 incubator at 37°C for a designated time to simulate the reperfusion injury.

Cell Viability Assay

The neurons with or without various interventions were cultured with the Cell Counting Kit-8 (CCK-8; Dojindo, Japan) for 4 h at a concentration of 10 μl/5,000 neurons. The absorbance of each well was determined by a microplate reader (Bio-Rad, Hercules, CA, USA) at 450 nm.

Lactate Dehydrogenase (LDH) Assay

A Cytotoxicity Detection Kit Plus (Roche Applied Bioscience, Indianapolis, IN, USA) was used to measure the release of lactate dehydrogenase (LDH), and all procedures were implemented following the manufacturer's protocol. Each group had its own maximum release group, and the LDH release was calculated in each group as the experimental value/maximum release × 100%.

Antibodies and Reagents

The primary antibodies used are listed as follows: anti-cytochrome c (1:1,000, 10993-1-AP, Proteintech, rosemont, IL, USA), anti-caspase-9 (1:1,000, #9508, Cell Signaling, Danvers, MA, USA), anti-PERK (1:1,000, #3192, Cell Signaling, Danvers, MA, USA), anti-phosphorylated-PERK (anti-p-PERK; Thr982;1:800, DF7576, Affinity Biosciences, Cincinnati, OH, USA), anti-IRE1 (1:500, ab37073, Abcam, Cambridge, MA, USA), anti-p-IRE1 (phosphor S724; 1:1,000, ab48187, Abcam, Cambridge, MA, USA), anti-activating transcription factor 6 (anti-ATF6; 1:1,000, ab203119, Abcam, Cambridge, MA, USA), anti-N'ATF6 (1:800, ab37149, Abcam, Cambridge, MA, USA) and anti-β-actin (1:3,000, GTX109639, GeneTex, Irvine, CA, USA). The ER stress activator Tunicamycin (TM) and the p-PERK inhibitor GSK2656157 were obtained from MedChem Express (Monmouth Junction, NJ, USA). The p-IRE1 inhibitor 3,5-dibromosalicylaldehyde (DBSA) was obtained from Tokyo Chemical Industry (TCI, Tokyo, Japan).

Western Blot Analysis

Neurons were lysed by RIPA with a protease inhibitor cocktail (Roche Applied Bioscience, Indianapolis, IN, USA), and the protein concentration of each sample was measured using a BCA quantification assay (Biosynthesis biotechnology, Beijing, China). Equivalent amounts of protein (30 μg) were separated by 6%–12% SDS-PAGE gels before being transferred onto the methanol pretreated polyvinylidene difluoride (PVDF) membranes. After being soaked in 5% defatted milk dissolved in Tris-phosphate buffer with 0.05% Tween 20 (TBST) for 1 h, the membranes were incubated overnight at 4°C. The membrane was incubated in secondary antibody diluent for 1 h at room temperature before its immunoreactivity was detected using Super Signal West Pico Chemiluminescent Substrate (Thermo Scientific, Rockford, IL, USA). The intensity of the protein bands was calculated *via* ImageJ with normalization to that of β-actin.

Cytoplasmic/Mitochondrial Protein Extraction

This procedure was implemented by using ProteoExtract Cytosol/Mitochondria Fractionation Kit (Calbiochem, Germany) and subjected to the described protocols. Briefly, the neurons were collected with Accutase (Invitrogen, Carlsbad, CA, USA) and centrifuged twice with PBS at 600 *g* for 5 min. Then, the 1× cytoplasmic extraction buffer was used to resuspend the neurons on ice for 10 min before homogenizing the neuron suspension, which was then centrifuged at 700 *g* for 10 min at 4°C. The cytoplasmic protein was obtained by collecting the supernatant after centrifuging the supernatant collected in the last step at 10,000 *g* for 30 min at 4°C. The mitochondrial protein was obtained by resuspending the sediment with mitochondrial extraction buffer and vortexing for 10 s.

Measurement of Reactive Oxygen Species (ROS) Production

The intracellular reactive oxygen species (ROS) was determined using 2,7-dichlorodihydrofluorescein diacetate (H2-DCFDA), an intracellular ROS indicator, as previously reported. Cultured cortical neurons were incubated with 10 nM H2-DCFDA for 1 h at 37°C in a dark place. Then, the neurons were resuspended with PBS before being read by a fluorescence plate reader (excitation wavelength of 480 nm, emission wavelength of 530 nm).

Measurement of Mitochondrial Membrane Potential (MMP)

To monitor the mitochondrial membrane potential (MMP) of each group, the neurons were incubated in 10 mM fluorescent dye rhodamine 123 (RH 123) for 30 min at 37°C. Then, the neurons were washed with PBS three times before reading the fluorescence with a fluorescence plate reader (excitation wavelength of 480 nm, emission wavelength of 530 nm).

Measurement of Intracellular ATP

The ATP level was intraneuronally evaluated using an ATP assay kit (Beyotime, Shanghai, China), and the procedures were performed following the manufacturer's protocol. Briefly, the culture medium in the 96-well plate was removed, and the neurons were resuspended with 100 μl of working solution (ATP detection reagent: diluent = 1:5) for 5 min at room temperature. The ATP indication of each group was obtained *via* a fluorospectrophotometer and modified as a percentage of the control.

Immunofluorescence Staining

Cultured neurons were fixed in 4% paraformaldehyde for 20 min at room temperature in a dark place. Then, the neurons were treated with 0.3% Triton-X-100 for 20 min and blocked by 10% donkey serum for 3 h. After being washed with 1× PBS three times, the neurons were then incubated with rabbit anti-p-PERK (1:200) or rabbit anti-p-IRE1 (1:200) at 4°C overnight. The DAPI nuclei-staining was implemented for 10 min after the incubation of Alexa 594 donkey-anti-rabbit IgG (1:400) for 2 h at room temperature. The neurons were then visualized with a fluorescence microscope. To compare the immunoreactivity between different groups, all images were collected using the identical laser power, exposure time and detector sensitivity. At least five images were acquired by an researcher who was blinded to the experimental details.

Statistical Analysis

All the experimental procedures were performed at least three times. The statistical analysis was conducted using Bonferroni's multiple comparisons or an unpaired *t*-test (two groups) and univariate analyses of variance (ANOVA; more than two groups); the results were plotted with GraphPad Prism Software 6.0.

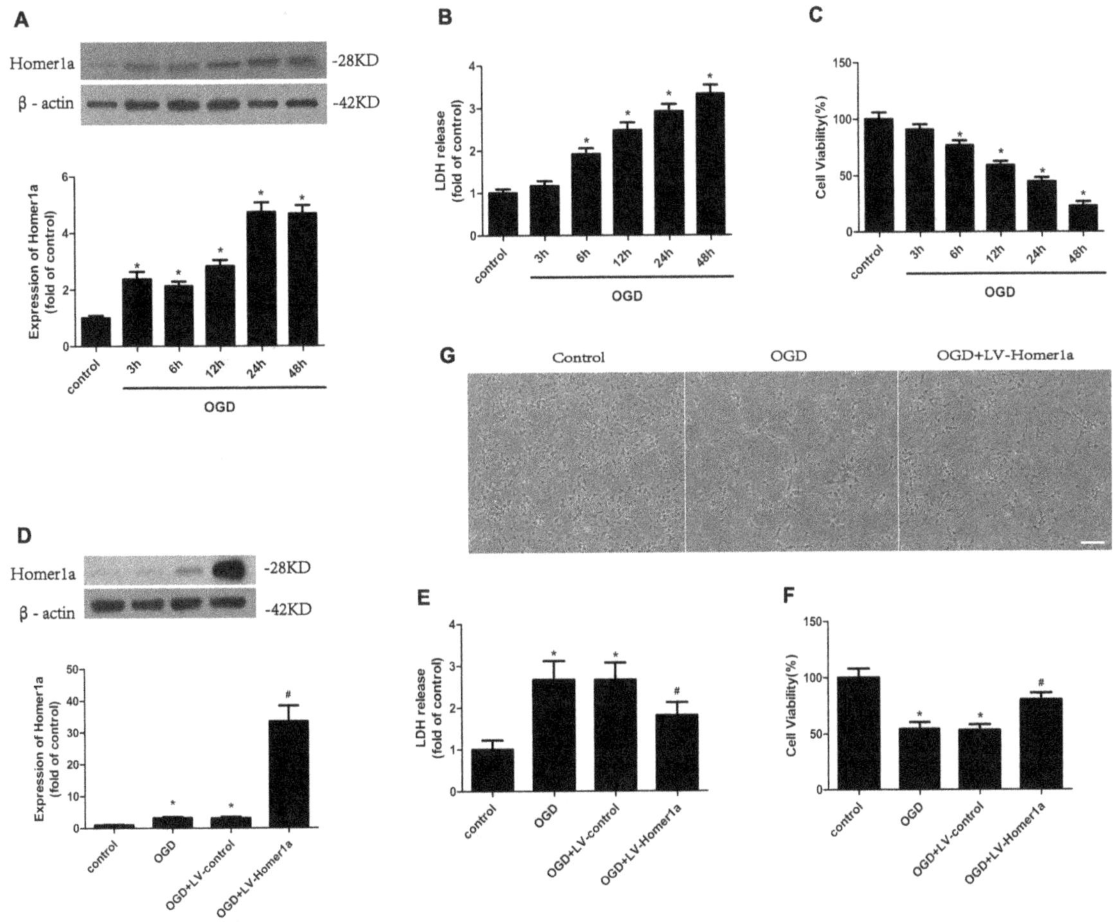

FIGURE 1 | Homer1a protects neurons against ischemia/reperfusion (I/R) injury. Cultured cortical neurons were treated with oxygen and glucose deprivation (OGD) for 1h, and the expression level of Homer1a protein at different reperfusion time points were investigated by Western blot **(A)**. Then the cytotoxicity of neurons was detected by lactate dehydrogenase (LDH) release assay **(B)** and the cell viability was evaluated by CCK-8 test **(C)**. The cortical neurons were then transfected with LV-Homer1a or LV-control for 72 h and exposed to OGD. The Homer1a protein expression was detect by Western blot **(D)**, and cytotoxicity and cell viability were tested in each group **(E,F)**. The cortical neurons were also observed under representative phase photomicrographs **(G)**. The data are represented as means ± SEM. *$p < 0.05$ vs. Control, $^{\#}p < 0.05$ vs. OGD.

RESULTS

Homer1a Protects Neurons Against I/R Injury

To determine the effect of I/R injury on Homerla, the cultured cortical neurons were treated with oxygen and glucose deprivation (OGD) for 1 h, and the expression level of Homerla protein at different reoxygenation time points was investigated using Western blot. The results showed that the Homerla protein levels increased significantly at 6, 12, 24 and 48 h with reperfusion (**Figure 1A**). The I/R injury-induced LDH release (**Figure 1B**) and reduced cell viability of neurons (**Figure 1C**) were elevated in a time-dependent manner. Given that the neuron survival was almost 50%, a 24 h reperfusion after OGD was used in the following experiments. To evaluate the effects of Homerla, the Homerla-targeted lentivirus (LV-Homerla) or the negative control lentivirus (LV-control) was transfected into the neurons for 72 h, and the Western blot results showed that the LV-Homerla protein expression was significantly increased (**Figure 1D**). The overexpression of Homerla clearly decreased LDH release (**Figure 1E**) and promoted cell viability (**Figure 1F**) after I/R injury. Furthermore, representative phase photomicrographs exhibited that the LV-Homerla transfected neurons showed less cell death relative to neurons without LV-Homerla transfection (**Figure 1G**).

Homer1a Conserves Mitochondrial Function in Neurons After I/R Injury

We also evaluated whether Homerla conserves the mitochondrial function following I/R injury. We transfected LV-Homerla 72 h before exposing cultured cortical neurons to the OGD and reperfusion. The results revealed that the overexpression of Homerla clearly decreased the cytochrome c release from the mitochondria to the cytoplasm (**Figure 2A**) and caspase-9 activation (**Figure 2B**). Additionally, Homerla expression alleviated MMP loss (**Figure 2C**), reduced the

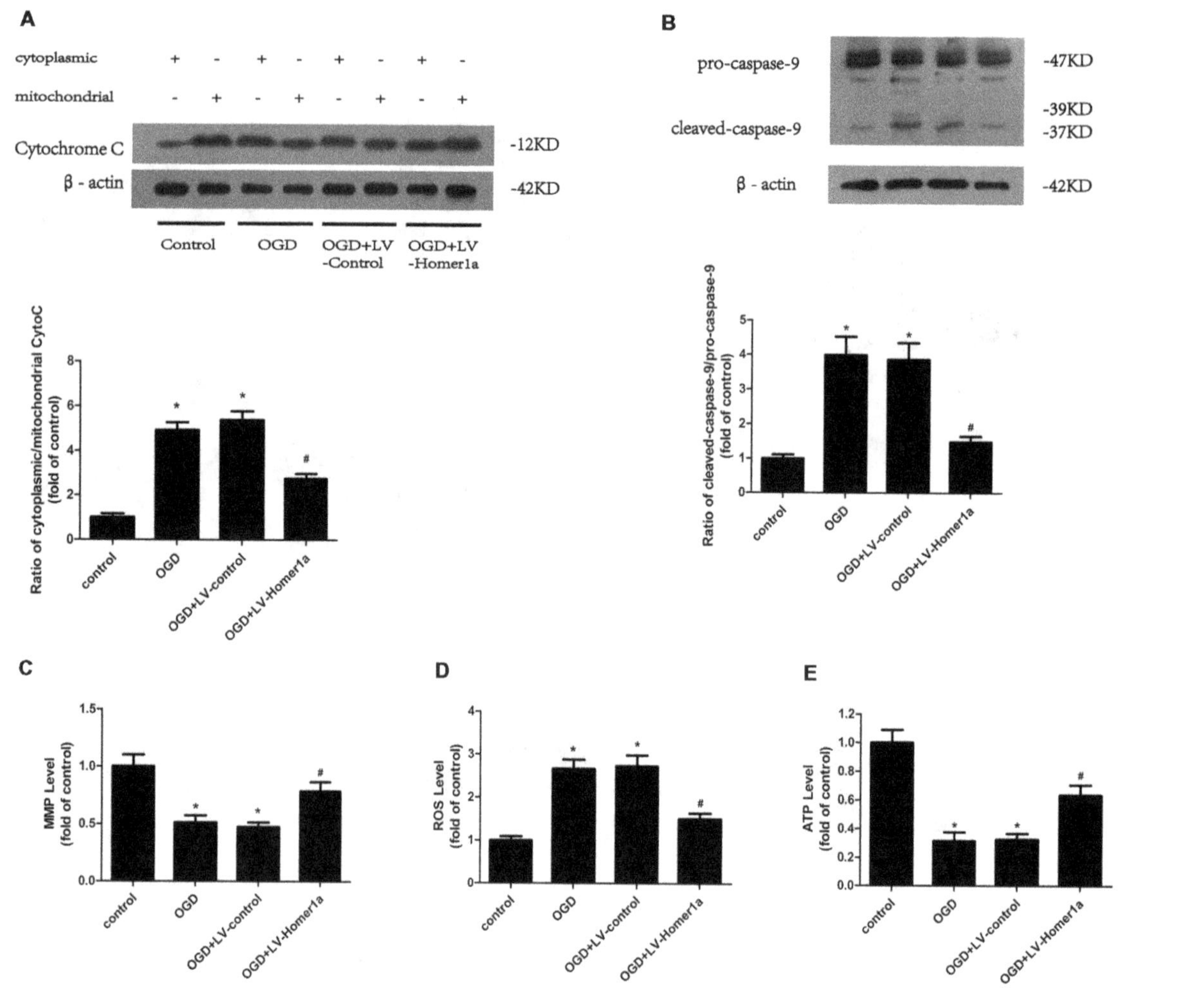

FIGURE 2 | Homer1a conserves mitochondrial function in neurons after I/R injury. Cultured cortical neurons were transfected with LV-Homer1a or LV-control for 72 h and exposed to OGD. The cytochrome c release to cytoplasm and the activation of caspase-9 were detected by Western blot **(A,B)**. The mitochondrial membrane potentials (MMPs) were detected by Rh123 test **(C)**, the intracellular reactive oxygen species (ROS) level was investigated through H_2-DCFDA **(D)** and the intracellular ATP level was measured by ATP assay **(E)**. The data are represented as means ± SEM. $^*p < 0.05$ vs. Control, $^\#p < 0.05$ vs. OGD.

intracellular ROS level (**Figure 2D**) and improved ATP loss (**Figure 2E**) in neurons that underwent I/R injury compared with that in neurons without LV-Homer1a transfection.

Homer1a Reduces ER Stress in Neurons That Underwent I/R Injury

We next examined the effect of Homer1a on ER stress after I/R exposure. The Western blot results showed that under the I/R injury, the ratios of p-PERK/PERK and p-IRE1/IRE1 were both reduced in neurons with Homer1a overexpression compared with neurons without LV-Homer1a lentivirus transfection (**Figure 3A**), whereas the Homer1a overexpression showed little effect on expression of ATF6 and its active form N'ATF6 (**Supplementary Figure S1**). The immunofluorescent results indicated that the effect of I/R injury on neurons significantly increased the fluorescence intensity of p-PERK and p-IRE1. However, neurons with Homer1a overexpression exhibited a significantly decreased fluorescence intensity of p-PERK and p-IRE1 (**Figures 3B,C**). Together, the above data showed that Homer1a overexpression reduced IR-induced ER stress.

Homer1a Alleviates Mitochondria Dysfunction by Reducing ER Stress After I/R Injury

To test whether the Homer1a effect of ER stress reduction is responsible for the conservation of mitochondrial function, we pretreated cortical neurons with 2 μg/L TM, an ER stress activator, 24 h before exposure to the I/R injury to counteract the ER stress reduction of Homer1a overexpression. The Western blot results showed that the TM abolished the reduced p-PERK/PERK and p-IRE1/IRE1 due to Homer1a overexpression (**Figure 4A**). Furthermore, the TM pretreatment of cortical neurons with LV-Homer1a-transfection under I/R injury reversed the ATP loss reduction (**Figure 4B**) and intracellular ROS reduction (**Figure 4C**) achieved by Homer1a

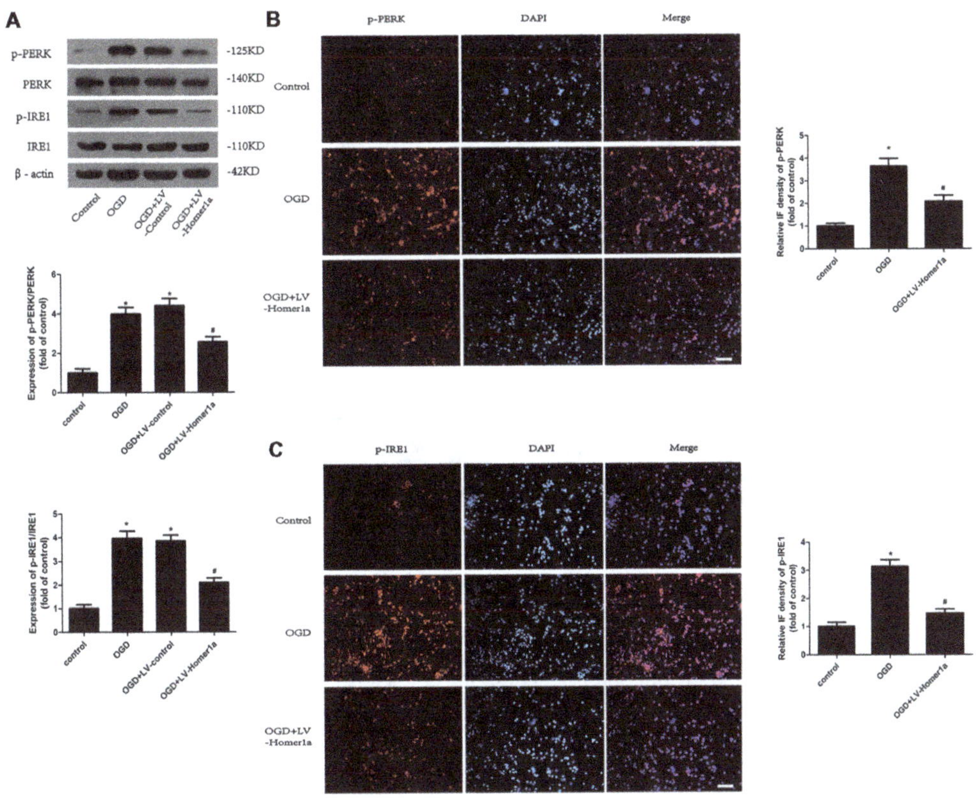

FIGURE 3 | Homer1a reduces endoplasmic reticulum (ER) stress in neurons that underwent I/R injury. Cultured cortical neurons were transfected with LV-Homer1a or LV-control for 72 h and exposed to OGD. Levels of phosphorylated-PKR-like ER kinase (p-PERK), PERK, phosphorylated-IRE1 (p-IRE1) and IRE1 were measured with Western blot **(A)**. The level of p-PERK and p-IRE1 were also determined with immunofluorescence (IF) staining. Images were captured with fluorescence microscope. Red: p-PERK or p-IRE1, blue: nuclei-staining by DAPI. Scale bar = 50 μm. The IF intensity of each group was calculated with ImageJ **(B,C)**. The data are represented as means ± SEM. *$p < 0.05$ vs. Control, #$p < 0.05$ vs. OGD.

overexpression. Additionally, under I/R injury, LDH release was greater in neurons with LV-Homer1a and TM than in neurons with LV-Homer1a alone (**Figure 4D**).

Homer1a Preserves Mitochondrial Function by Reducing ER Stress Mainly *via* the PERK Pathway After I/R Injury

To further elucidate the mechanisms by which Homer1a reduces the ER stress to preserve mitochondrial function, we pretreated cortical neurons 24 h before any intervention with specific inhibitors to separately test each pathway of ER stress. As the Western blot results showed, 20 μM p-IRE1 specific inhibitor DBSA effectively blocked the phosphorylation of IRE1 (**Figure 5A**), and 5 nM GSK2656157, a specific p-PERK inhibitor, was efficient in reducing the phosphorylation of PERK (**Figure 5B**). As the appropriate dosage of each inhibitor was employed, the Western blot results revealed that neurons pretreated with TM and GSK2656157 showed significant reductions in cytochrome c release from mitochondria to the cytoplasm, whereas neurons pretreated with TM and DBSA showed little change under I/R injury (**Figure 5C**). Furthermore, compared with neurons pretreated with TM and DBSA, neurons pretreated with TM and GSK2656157 exhibited less ATP loss and a lower intracellular ROS level (**Figure 5D**).

DISCUSSION

The involvement of Homer1a in some central neuronal stress conditions has been found in our and previous studies (Luo et al., 2014; Schumacker et al., 2014; Wu et al., 2018). In this study, we revealed that Homer1a protects against neuronal I/R injury by preserving mitochondrial function and regulating ERS in primary cortical neurons. First, upregulated expression of Homer1a alleviated the I/R injury with less neuronal death. Second, upregulation of Homer1a helps restore mitochondrial function and mitigates ER stress activation. Third, the anti-ER stress effects of Homer1a were partially responsible for its pro-mitochondrial roles, which was attained mainly through the PERK pathway.

As an immediate early gene (IEG) that regulates the longer form of the homer gene, Homer1a was minimally expressed in the brain and other areas of the nervous system until the physiological conditions were disturbed. Studies have shown that upregulated Homer1a expression evoked by various forms of

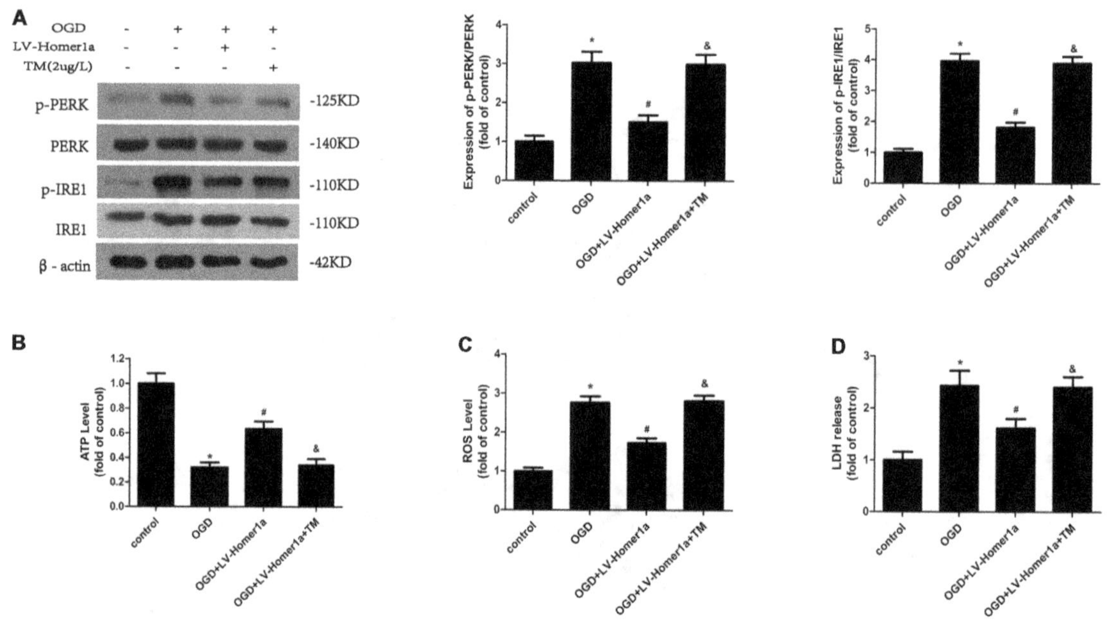

FIGURE 4 | Homer1a alleviates mitochondria dysfunction by reducing ER stress after I/R injury. Cultured cortical neurons were pre-treated with 2 μg/L Tunicamycin (TM) 24 h to activate the ER stress and exposed to I/R injury. The effects of TM were tested by Western blot **(A)**. The intracellular ATP level was measured by ATP assay **(B)** and the intracellular ROS level was investigated through H_2-DCFDA **(C)**. We also investigated the neurons cytotoxicity of each group with LDH release assay **(D)**. The data are represented as means ± SEM. *$p < 0.05$ vs. Control, #$p < 0.05$ vs. OGD, &$p < 0.05$ vs. OGD+LV-Homer1a.

stress could help fight against various pathological processes (Tappe et al., 2006; Diering et al., 2017; Leber et al., 2017). Our previous study has shown that Homerla protects neurons against TNF-a induced injury by interacting with the MAPK pathways (Luo et al., 2012b). Additionally, Wang et al. (2015). found the protective effect of Homerla against NMDA-induced injury (Rao et al., 2016). Recently, Wu et al. (2018) found that Homerla contributed a protective effect in HT22 cells under oxidative stress by inducing autophagy. Similarly, our study demonstrated that Homerla was minimally expressed in rat cortical neurons but rose quickly after the onset of the I/R injury in a time-dependent manner that tended to dynamically stabilize after 24 h of reperfusion. Overexpression of Homerla with a specific lentivirus increased neuronal survival and decreased LDH release after OGD, which indicated that Homerla plays a protective role in the neuronal system in I/R conditions.

Because of the high demand for energy, the nervous system is more susceptible to mitochondrial dysfunction that impaired mitochondria is incapable of producing enough ATP to fill neuronal needs (Shulyakova et al., 2017). ROS production by mitochondria occurs in both physiological and pathological processes, and mitochondria dysfunction leads to the burst of ROS production and hinders oxidative phosphorylation as the mitochondrial membrane breaks down and finally leads to apoptotic cell death (Schieber and Chandel, 2014; Martin et al., 2018). Furthermore, the weakened membrane with higher permeability could lead to apoptotic factor release, such as the release of apoptosis-inducing factor and cytochrome c (Niizuma et al., 2010; Leaw et al., 2017). Cytochrome c includes procaspase-9, which is cleaved into caspase-9 and further triggers neuron apoptosis (Bennetts and Pierce, 2010). Our previous studies showed that Homerla overexpression helps reduce oxidative stress and restore mitochondrial function in PC12 cells and HT-22 cells under oxidative stress (Luo et al., 2012a; Rao et al., 2016). Consistent with these studies, our results showed that Homerla overexpression reduces ROS production and attenuates ATP and MMP loss in cortical neurons. Additionally, the overexpression of Homerla reduces cytochrome c release from mitochondria to the cytoplasm as the ratio of cytoplasmic/mitochondrial cytochrome c decreases, which indicates that the Homerla overexpression prevented the mitochondria from permeabilizing. The apoptic cell death was alleviated as the caspase-9 activation was reduced after Homerla expression. All these results provide evidence that Homerla protects mitochondrial function under I/R injury and thus stops neuronal apoptosis.

Three major transmembrane proteins are involved in the ER stress-activated unfolded protein response (UPR): IRE1, PERK and ATF6. All three proteins are coupled with the chaperone protein Bip and stay inactive under physiological conditions. When the UPR is activated, after the Bip dissociation, the IRE1 and PERK oligomerize and phosphorylate to activate their downstream signals, and ATF6 is cleaved by the Golgi and moves into the nucleus to act as a transcription promoter (Darling and Cook, 2014). ER stress is activated after IS and leads to cell damage (Yu et al., 2017). In our study, the results showed that IR significantly activated ER stress as evidenced by the hyperphosphorylation of PERK and IRE1 and enhanced

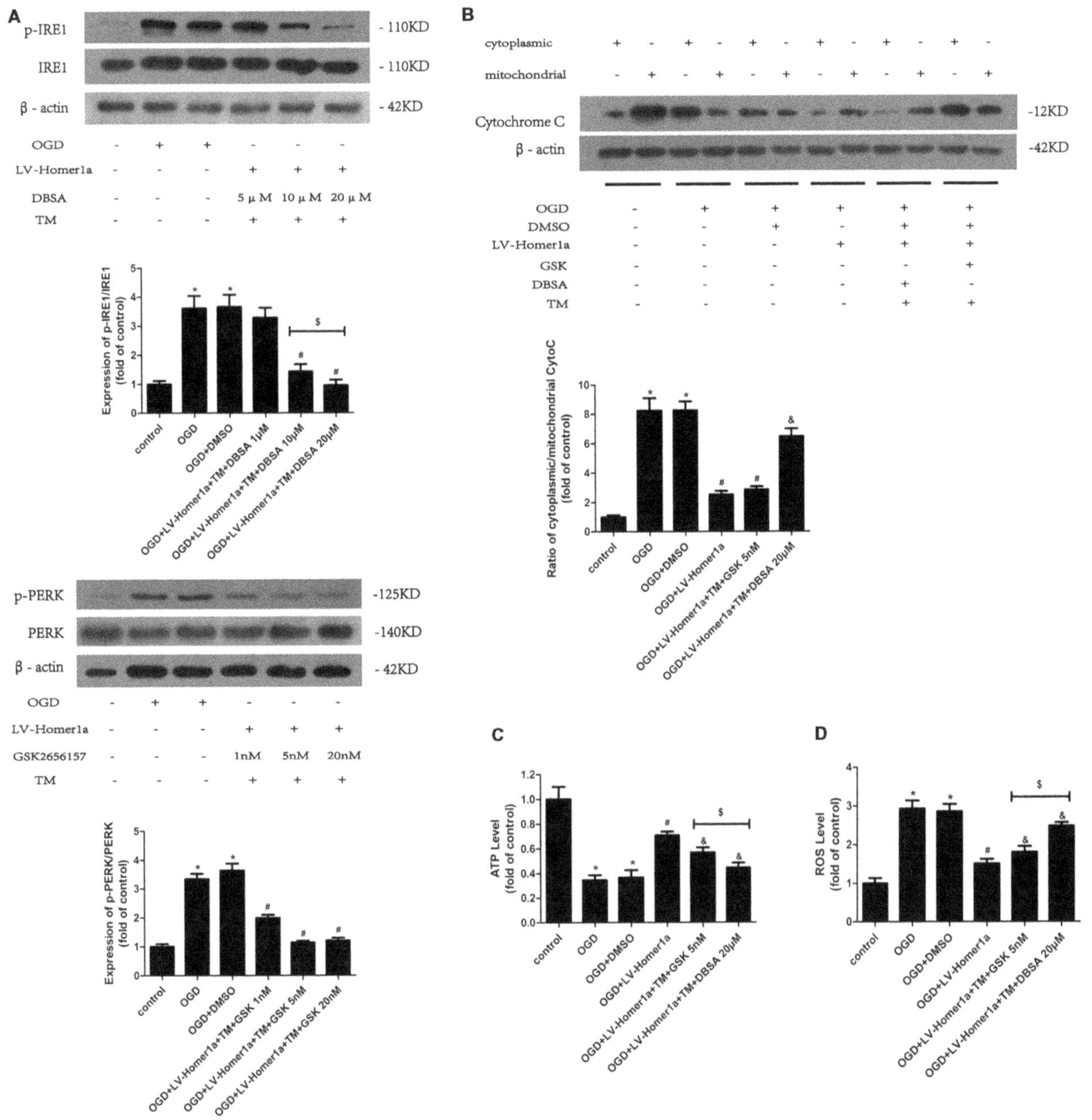

FIGURE 5 | Homer1a preserves mitochondrial function by reducing ER stress mainly *via* the PERK pathway after I/R injury. TM was used to activate the ER stress whereas the GSK2656157 and 3,5-dibromosalicylaldehyde (DBSA) were used to inhibit the PERK and IRE1 respectively. Different DBSA concentrations were tested in cortical neurons and detected by Western blot **(A)** as well as GSK2656157 **(B)**. Then 20 μM DBSA and 5 nM GSK2656157 were chosen to apply to follow experiments. The cytochrome c release to cytoplasm in each group was detected through calculating the ratio of cytoplasmic/mitochondrial cytochrome c by Western blot **(B)**. The intracellular ATP level was measured by ATP assay **(C)** and the intracellular ROS level was investigated through H_2-DCFDA **(D)**. The data are represented as means ± SEM. $^{\$}p < 0.05$, $^{*}p < 0.05$ vs. Control, $^{\#}p < 0.05$ vs. OGD, $^{\&}p < 0.05$ vs. OGD+LV-Homer1a.

fluorescence intensity of p-PERK and p-IRE1. Our previous study showed that downregulation of Homer1b/c, the long form in the homer family that plays an opposite role as Homer1a, inhibited the expression of CHOP, a downstream gene of all three pathways of ER stress, is considered to be a pro-apoptotic protein that mediates ER stress-induced apoptosis (Chen et al., 2012). Similarly, in the present study, our Western blot results showed less phosphorylation of the IRE1 and PERK proteins and reduced fluorescence intensity of phosphorylated IRE1 and PERK. These results demonstrate the anti-ER stress roles of Homer1a. However, our results showed no significant relationship between ATF6 and Homer1a

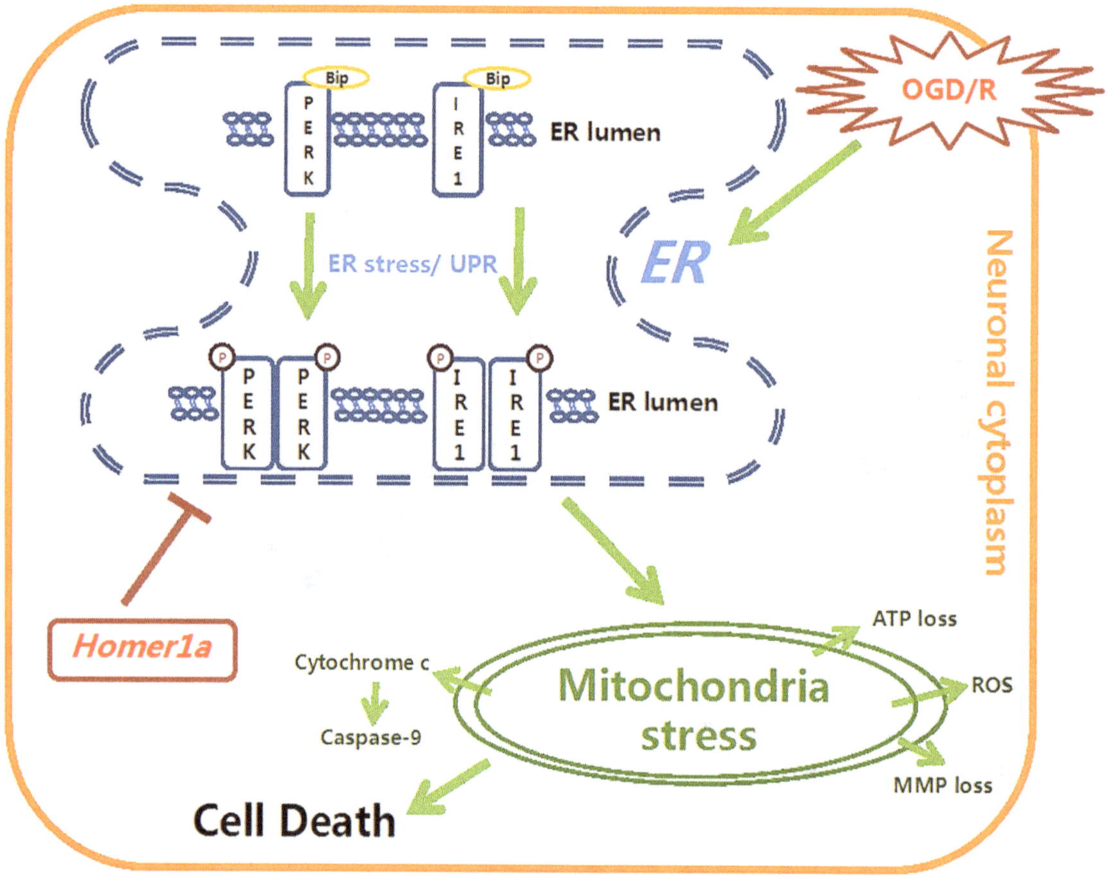

FIGURE 6 | The schematic diagram depicts the molecular mechanisms of homer1a-induced neuron-protection against OGD injury. Homer1a overexpression inhibited the OGD-induced activation of ER stress, which alleviated the secondary mitochondria dysfunction by regulating ATP, MMP, ROS, cytochrome c and caspase-9. In addition, Homer1a-induced preservation of mitochondrial function was achieved mainly *via* inhibiting the PERK pathway.

overexpression which may due to the Homer1a itself, our stroke model, lab environment or other specific details. ATF6 pathway is one of the main branches of ER stress and its activation could upregulates activating transcription factor 4 (ATF4), a cAMP-response element binding protein that could cause retinal and neuronal degeneration (Gully et al., 2016), and CHOP expression (Darling and Cook, 2014). Besides, ATF6 has two isoforms that may be crucial in many scenarios such as embryogenesis (Thuerauf et al., 2007). It is necessary to carry out further experiments to elucidate ATF6's specific roles in brain I/R injury.

ER stress plays different roles in different situations. Under acute or chronic pathologies or stress, ERS elicits UPR, which facilitates the misfolding protein degradation that helps alleviate protein overload that, in turn, helps to avoid cell apoptosis. However, when the cell proteostasis is still not restored, ERS can trigger apoptosis *via* several pathways (Tabas and Ron, 2011). This bifunctional process is essential for maintaining cell homeostasis. Many studies have shown that ERS activation could further aggravate the original pathology, such as pancreatic disease, intestinal inflammation and liver injury (Cunha et al., 2009; Han et al., 2016; Hosomi et al., 2017). In IS, the inhibition of ERS alleviates neuronal injury (Feng et al., 2017). Only a few studies have shown that the activation of ERS protects cells from apoptosis (Tan et al., 2017). In our *in vitro* model, aggravated injury, as demonstrated by increased LDH release, was found in TM-treated neurons. The results indicated that the ERS plays pro-apoptotic roles in cortical neurons under I/R injury.

ER and mitochondria both have dynamic plasticity of their structure in response to cellular requirements, which is the prerequisite for ER-mitochondrial communication functionally and structurally (Bravo-Sagua et al., 2013). The activation of ER stress induced the mitochondrial dysfunction in HT22 cells (Xu et al., 2018), and ER stress sensitized the mitochondria by opening its permeability transition pore in cardiac injury (Chen et al., 2017). Consistent with these studies, our results demonstrate that in cortical neurons under I/R injury, the reactivation of Homer1a overexpression suppressed ER stress *via* TM, which led to increased intracellular calcium load, elevated ROS production and ATP loss. This finding indicated that Homer1a conserves mitochondrial function by inhibiting ER stress under I/R injury in cortical neurons. On the other hand, mitochondria may also have effects on ER stress. Studies showed that the mitochondria and ER stress has crosstalk in many models (Malhotra and Kaufman, 2011; Senft and Ronai, 2015), and the block of respiratory chain complex with rotenone or antimycin A that leads to mitochondrial dysfunction exerts great effects on ER stress (Lee et al., 2010; Jeon et al., 2017; Heo et al., 2019). Further studies are needed to investigate the effects of mitochondria to ER stress regarding Homer1 protein regulation.

Additionally, we further investigated the mechanism by which Homer1a exerts mitochondrial protection *via* ER stress reduction. According to previous studies, the phosphorylated PERK can activate ATF4 transcription, which in turn promotes the expression of bZIP transcription factor C/EBP homologous protein (CHOP) and then influences mitochondrial function by hyperoxidizing the ER lumen structure by activating ER oxidase 1α (ERO1α; Harding et al., 2000; Song et al., 2008). The oxidized ER activates IP3R-induced calcium release and then activates Ca/calmodulin-dependent protein kinase II (CaMKII), which facilitates calcium transfer into the mitochondria. The increasing mitochondrial calcium uptake leads to MMP loss, cytochrome c release and apoptosis (Kashiwase et al., 2005; Li et al., 2009; Timmins et al., 2009). In this study, compared with neurons with Homer1a overexpression, neurons in which the PERK pathway is activated *via* TM and p-IRE1 inhibitor DBSA under I/R injury showed more cytochrome c release, elevated ATP loss and an increased ROS level, which indicated that the PERK pathway is involved in mitochondrial dysfunction. Previous studies also found that in gastric cancer cells, the phosphorylated IRE1 activated Jun N-terminal protein kinase-1 (JNK-1), which in turn activated the transcription of CHOP and influenced mitochondrial related functions (Kim et al., 2018). However, in our study, activating the IRE1 pathway in neurons under I/R injury with TM and the PERK inhibitor GSK2656157 showed less abortion of Homer1a protection with less ATP loss and ROS production than PERK pathway activation. There was no significant difference in cytochrome c release between neurons in which ER stress was inhibited by Homer1a lentivirus transfection and neurons in which IRE1 was activated by TM and GSK2656157. These discrepancies may be attributed to different models, unknown biological traits of the inhibitors and a potential interaction between Homer1a and IRE1-JNK related pathways. All these results indicate that Homer1a preserves mitochondrial function mainly through the PERK pathway and partially through the IRE1 pathway (**Figure 6**).

A limitation of this study was that Homer1a's effect on mitochondria dysfunction and ER stress under I/R injury was only explored in cultured cortical neurons, lacking the interaction with glial cell signaling. Our lab has already built a Homer1a knockout mouse model in which more experiments will be implemented to further evaluate these observations. Additionally, in this study, we investigated molecular mechanisms in pharmacological ways, and future studies with specific gene modulation should elucidate the exact mechanism of Homer1a in mitochondria protection.

In this study, the primary cultured neurons may contain a small portion of astrocytes and may insert mutual or extra efforts on neuron outcome with OGD/R model. Researches revealed that the astrocyte could protect neurons from I/R injury (Liu et al., 2018), while some suggested that the astrocyte plays harmful roles in IS (Yang et al., 2017). Since the ER stress inhibition *via* Homer1a overexpression could inhibit astrocyte activation (Huang et al., 2017), the roles of astrocyte in our present study are still unclear. Further experiments are needed to find the exact roles of astrocyte in IS.

In conclusion, we suggested that Homer1a may protect against I/R neuronal injury by preserving mitochondrial function though suppressing ER stress. Interestingly, Homer1a's protection of mitochondrial function is mainly by inhibiting the PERK pathway. Taken together, our findings provide novel perceptions about the relationship between Homer1a, ER stress and mitochondrial dysfunction in neurons under I/R conditions.

AUTHOR CONTRIBUTIONS

ZF conceived the idea and designed the experiments. JW and XW carried out most of the experiments and composed the manuscript. PL and KY carried out partial experiments. YY and JP helped in analyzing experimental results. LZ and SD assisted with verifying the results. DH helped revising the manuscript.

FUNDING

This work was supported by the National Natural Science Foundation of China (No. 81771239, No. 81430043).

SUPPLEMENTARY MATERIAL

FIGURE S1 | Relationship between Homer1a and ATF6 pathway after I/R injury of neurons. Cultured cortical neurons were transfected with LV-Homer1a or LV-control for 72 h and exposed to OGD. Levels of ATF6 and N'ATF6 were measured with Western blot. The data are represented as means ± SEM. $^{*}p < 0.05$ vs. Control.

REFERENCES

Benjamin, E. J., Virani, S. S., Callaway, C. W., Chamberlain, A. M., Chang, A. R., Cheng, S., et al. (2018). Heart Disease and stroke statistics-2018 update: a report from the american heart association. *Circulation* 137, e67–e492. doi: 10.1161/CIR.0000000000000558

Bennetts, P. S., and Pierce, J. D. (2010). Apoptosis: understanding programmed cell death for the CRNA. *AANA J.* 78, 237–245.

Bhatti, J. S., Bhatti, G. K., and Reddy, P. H. (2017). Mitochondrial dysfunction and oxidative stress in metabolic disorders—a step towards mitochondria based therapeutic strategies. *Biochim. Biophys. Acta Mol. Basis Dis.* 1863, 1066–1077. doi: 10.1016/j.bbadis.2016.11.010

Bravo-Sagua, R., Rodriguez, A. E., Kuzmicic, J., Gutierrez, T., Lopez-Crisosto, C., Quiroga, C., et al. (2013). Cell death and survival through the endoplasmic reticulum-mitochondrial axis. *Curr. Mol. Med.* 13, 317–329. doi: 10.2174/156652413804810781

Chen, T., Fei, F., Jiang, X. F., Zhang, L., Qu, Y., Huo, K., et al. (2012). Down-regulation of Homer1b/c attenuates glutamate-mediated excitotoxicity through endoplasmic reticulum and mitochondria pathways in rat cortical neurons. *Free Radic. Biol. Med.* 52, 208–217. doi: 10.1016/j.freeradbiomed.2011.10.451

Chen, Q., Thompson, J., Hu, Y., Das, A., and Lesnefsky, E. J. (2017). Metformin attenuates ER stress-induced mitochondrial dysfunction. *Transl. Res.* 190, 40–50. doi: 10.1016/j.trsl.2017.09.003

Cunha, D. A., Ladrière, L., Ortis, F., Igoillo-Esteve, M., Gurzov, E. N., Lupi, R., et al. (2009). Glucagon-like peptide-1 agonists protect pancreatic β-cells from lipotoxic endoplasmic reticulum stress through upregulation of BiP and JunB. *Diabetes* 58, 2851–2862. doi: 10.2337/db09-0685

Darling, N. J., and Cook, S. J. (2014). The role of MAPK signalling pathways in the response to endoplasmic reticulum stress. *Biochim. Biophys. Acta* 1843, 2150–2163. doi: 10.1016/j.bbamcr.2014.01.009

Diering, G. H., Nirujogi, R. S., Roth, R. H., Worley, P. F., Pandey, A., and Huganir, R. L. (2017). Homer1a drives homeostatic scaling-down of excitatory synapses during sleep. *Science* 355, 511–515. doi: 10.1126/science.aai8355

Fei, F., Li, J., Rao, W., Liu, W., Chen, X., Su, N., et al. (2015). Upregulation of Homer1a promoted retinal ganglion cell survival after retinal ischemia and reperfusion via interacting with Erk Pathway. *Cell. Mol. Neurobiol.* 35, 1039–1048. doi: 10.1007/s10571-015-0198-2

Feng, D., Wang, B., Wang, L., Abraham, N., Tao, K., Huang, L., et al. (2017). Pre-ischemia melatonin treatment alleviated acute neuronal injury after ischemic stroke by inhibiting endoplasmic reticulum stress-dependent autophagy via PERK and IRE1 signalings. *J. Pineal Res.* 62:3. doi: 10.1111/jpi.12395

Foa, L., and Gasperini, R. (2009). Developmental roles for Homer: more than just a pretty scaffold. *J. Neurochem.* 108, 1–10. doi: 10.1111/j.1471-4159.2008.05726.x

Gully, J. C., Sergeyev, V. G., Bhootada, Y., Mendez-Gomez, H., Meyers, C. A., Zolotukhin, S., et al. (2016). Up-regulation of activating transcription factor 4 induces severe loss of dopamine nigral neurons in a rat model of Parkinson's disease. *Neurosci. Lett.* 627, 36–41. doi: 10.1016/j.neulet.2016.05.039

Han, C. Y., Lim, S. W., Koo, J. H., Kim, W., and Kim, S. G. (2016). PHLDA3 overexpression in hepatocytes by endoplasmic reticulum stress via IRE1-Xbp1s pathway expedites liver injury. *Gut* 65, 1377–1388. doi: 10.1136/gutjnl-2014-308506

Hankey, G. J. (2017). Stroke. *Lancet* 389, 641–654. doi: 10.1016/S0140-6736(16)30962-X

Harding, H. P., Novoa, I., Zhang, Y., Zeng, H., Wek, R., Schapira, M., et al. (2000). Regulated translation initiation controls stress-induced gene expression in mammalian cells. *Mol. Cell* 6, 1099–1108. doi: 10.1016/s1097-2765(00)00108-8

Heo, J. N., Kim, D. Y., Lim, S. G., Lee, K., Suk, K., and Lee, W. H. (2019). ER stress differentially affects pro-inflammatory changes induced by mitochondrial dysfunction in the human monocytic leukemia cell line, THP-1. *Cell Biol. Int.* 43, 313–322. doi: 10.1002/cbin.11103

Hosomi, S., Grootjans, J., Tschurtschenthaler, M., Krupka, N., Matute, J. D., Flak, M. B., et al. (2017). Intestinal epithelial cell endoplasmic reticulum stress promotes MULT1 up-regulation and NKG2D-mediated inflammation. *J. Exp. Med.* 214, 2985–2997. doi: 10.1084/jem.20162041

Huang, G. N., Huso, D. L., Bouyain, S., Tu, J., McCorkell, K. A., May, M. J., et al. (2008). NFAT binding and regulation of T cell activation by the cytoplasmic scaffolding Homer proteins. *Science* 319, 476–481. doi: 10.1126/science.1151227

Huang, R., Zhang, Y., Han, B., Bai, Y., Zhou, R., Gan, G., et al. (2017). Circular RNA *HIPK2* regulates astrocyte activation via cooperation of autophagy and ER stress by targeting *MIR124–2HG*. *Autophagy* 13, 1722–1741. doi: 10.1080/15548627.2017.1356975

Imarisio, C., Alchera, E., Bangalore, R. C., Valente, G., Follenzi, A., Trisolini, E., et al. (2017). Oxidative and ER stress-dependent ASK1 activation in steatotic hepatocytes and Kupffer cells sensitizes mice fatty liver to ischemia/reperfusion injury. *Free Radic. Biol. Med.* 112, 141–148. doi: 10.1016/j.freeradbiomed.2017.07.020

Jeon, Y. M., Lee, S., Kim, S., Kwon, Y., Kim, K., Chung, C. G., et al. (2017). Neuroprotective effects of protein tyrosine phosphatase 1B inhibition against ER stress-induced toxicity. *Mol. Cells* 40, 280–290. doi: 10.14348/molcells.2017.2320

Kashiwase, K., Higuchi, Y., Hirotani, S., Yamaguchi, O., Hikoso, S., Takeda, T., et al. (2005). CaMKII activates ASK1 and NF-κB to induce cardiomyocyte hypertrophy. *Biochem. Biophys. Res. Commun.* 327, 136–142. doi: 10.1016/j.bbrc.2004.12.002

Kim, T. W., Lee, S. Y., Kim, M., Cheon, C., and Ko, S. G. (2018). Kaempferol induces autophagic cell death via IRE1-JNK-CHOP pathway and inhibition of G9a in gastric cancer cells. *Cell Death Dis.* 9:875. doi: 10.1038/s41419-018-0930-1

Leaw, B., Nair, S., Lim, R., Thornton, C., Mallard, C., and Hagberg, H. (2017). Mitochondria, bioenergetics and excitotoxicity: new therapeutic targets in perinatal brain injury. *Front. Cell. Neurosci.* 11:199. doi: 10.3389/fncel.2017.00199

Leber, S. L., Llenos, I. C., Miller, C. L., Dulay, J. R., Haybaeck, J., and Weis, S. (2017). Homer1a protein expression in schizophrenia, bipolar disorder and major depression. *J. Neural Transm.* 124, 1261–1273. doi: 10.1007/s00702-017-1776-x

Lee, J. W., Kim, W. H., Yeo, J., and Jung, M. H. (2010). ER stress is implicated in mitochondrial dysfunction-induced apoptosis of pancreatic β cells. *Mol. Cells* 30, 545–549. doi: 10.1007/s10059-010-0161-5

Li, G., Mongillo, M., Chin, K. T., Harding, H., Ron, D., Marks, A. R., et al. (2009). Role of ERO1-α-mediated stimulation of inositol 1,4,5-triphosphate receptor activity in endoplasmic reticulum stress-induced apoptosis. *J. Cell Biol.* 186, 783–792. doi: 10.1083/jcb.200904060

Liu, X., Tian, F., Wang, S., Wang, F., and Xiong, L. (2018). Astrocyte autophagy flux protects neurons against oxygen-glucose deprivation and ischemic/reperfusion injury. *Rejuvenation Res.* 21, 405–415. doi: 10.1089/rej.2017.1999

Luo, P., Chen, T., Zhao, Y., Xu, H., Huo, K., Zhao, M., et al. (2012a). Protective effect of Homer 1a against hydrogen peroxide-induced oxidative stress in PC12 cells. *Free Radic. Res.* 46, 766–776. doi: 10.3109/10715762.2012.678340

Luo, P., Zhao, Y., Li, D., Chen, T., Li, S., Chao, X., et al. (2012b). Protective effect of Homer 1a on tumor necrosis factor-α with cycloheximide-induced apoptosis is mediated by mitogen-activated protein kinase pathways. *Apoptosis* 17, 975–988. doi: 10.1007/s10495-012-0736-z

Luo, P., Chen, T., Zhao, Y., Zhang, L., Yang, Y., Liu, W., et al. (2014). Postsynaptic scaffold protein Homer 1a protects against traumatic brain injury via regulating group I metabotropic glutamate receptors. *Cell Death Dis.* 5:e1174. doi: 10.1038/cddis.2014.116

Mailloux, R. J. (2016). Application of mitochondria-targeted pharmaceuticals for the treatment of heart disease. *Curr. Pharm. Des.* 22, 4763–4779. doi: 10.2174/1381612822666160629070914

Malhotra, J. D., and Kaufman, R. J. (2011). ER stress and its functional link to mitochondria: role in cell survival and death. *Cold Spring Harb. Perspect. Biol.* 3:a004424. doi: 10.1101/cshperspect.a004424

Martin, J. L., Gruszczyk, A. V., Beach, T. E., Murphy, M. P., and Saeb-Parsy, K. (2018). Mitochondrial mechanisms and therapeutics in ischaemia reperfusion injury. *Pediatr. Nephrol.* doi: 10.1007/s00467-018-3984-5 [Epub ahead of print].

Niizuma, K., Yoshioka, H., Chen, H., Kim, G. S., Jung, J. E., Katsu, M., et al. (2010). Mitochondrial and apoptotic neuronal death signaling pathways in cerebral ischemia. *Biochim. Biophys. Acta* 1802, 92–99. doi: 10.1016/j.bbadis.2009.09.002

Pandya, R. S., Mao, L., Zhou, H., Zhou, S., Zeng, J., Popp, A. J., et al. (2011). Central nervous system agents for ischemic stroke: neuroprotection mechanisms. *Cent. Nerv. Syst. Agents Med. Chem.* 11, 81–97. doi: 10.2174/187152411796011321

Prentice, H., Modi, J. P., and Wu, J. Y. (2015). Mechanisms of neuronal protection against excitotoxicity, endoplasmic reticulum stress and mitochondrial dysfunction in stroke and neurodegenerative diseases. *Oxid. Med. Cell. Longev.* 2015:964518. doi: 10.1155/2015/964518

Rao, W., Peng, C., Zhang, L., Su, N., Wang, K., Hui, H., et al. (2016). Homer1a attenuates glutamate-induced oxidative injury in HT-22 cells through regulation of store-operated calcium entry. *Sci. Rep.* 6:33975. doi: 10.1038/srep33975

Sanderson, T. H., Reynolds, C. A., Kumar, R., Przyklenk, K., and Huttemann, M. (2013). Molecular mechanisms of ischemia-reperfusion injury in brain: pivotal role of the mitochondrial membrane potential in reactive oxygen species generation. *Mol. Neurobiol.* 47, 9–23. doi: 10.1007/s12035-012-8344-z

Schieber, M., and Chandel, N. S. (2014). ROS function in redox signaling and oxidative stress. *Curr. Biol.* 24, R453–R462. doi: 10.1016/j.cub.2014.03.034

Schumacker, P. T., Gillespie, M. N., Nakahira, K., Choi, A. M., Crouser, E. D., Piantadosi, C. A., et al. (2014). Mitochondria in lung biology and pathology: more than just a powerhouse. *Am. J. Physiol. Lung Cell. Mol. Physiol.* 306, L962–L974. doi: 10.1152/ajplung.00073.201

Senft, D., and Ronai, Z. A. (2015). UPR, autophagy, and mitochondria crosstalk underlies the ER stress response. *Trends Biochem. Sci.* 40, 141–148. doi: 10.1016/j.tibs.2015.01.002

Serchov, T., Heumann, R., van Calker, D., and Biber, K. (2016). Signaling pathways regulating Homer1a expression: implications for antidepressant therapy. *Biol. Chem.* 397, 207–214. doi: 10.1515/hsz-2015-0267

Shulyakova, N., Andreazza, A. C., Mills, L. R., and Eubanks, J. H. (2017). Mitochondrial dysfunction in the pathogenesis of rett syndrome: implications for mitochondria-targeted therapies. *Front. Cell. Neurosci.* 11:58. doi: 10.3389/fncel.2017.00058

Song, B., Scheuner, D., Ron, D., Pennathur, S., and Kaufman, R. J. (2008). Chop deletion reduces oxidative stress, improves β cell function, and promotes cell survival in multiple mouse models of diabetes. *J. Clin. Invest.* 118, 3378–3389. doi: 10.1172/JCI34587

Tabas, I., and Ron, D. (2011). Integrating the mechanisms of apoptosis induced by endoplasmic reticulum stress. *Nat. Cell Biol.* 13, 184–190. doi: 10.1038/ncb0311-184

Tan, S. X., Jiang, D. X., Hu, R. C., Dai, A. G., Gan, G. X., Fu, D. Y., et al. (2017). Endoplasmic reticulum stress induces HRD1 to protect alveolar type II epithelial cells from apoptosis induced by cigarette smoke extract. *Cell. Physiol. Biochem.* 43, 1337–1345. doi: 10.1159/000481845

Tappe, A., Klugmann, M., Luo, C., Hirlinger, D., Agarwal, N., Benrath, J., et al. (2006). Synaptic scaffolding protein Homer1a protects against chronic inflammatory pain. *Nat. Med.* 12, 677–681. doi: 10.1038/nm1406

Thuerauf, D. J., Marcinko, M., Belmont, P. J., and Glembotski, C. C. (2007). Effects of the isoform-specific characteristics of ATF6 α and ATF6 β on endoplasmic reticulum stress response gene expression and cell viability. *J. Biol. Chem.* 282, 22865–22878. doi: 10.1074/jbc.m701213200

Timmins, J. M., Ozcan, L., Seimon, T. A., Li, G., Malagelada, C., Backs, J., et al. (2009). Calcium/calmodulin-dependent protein kinase II links ER stress with Fas and mitochondrial apoptosis pathways. *J. Clin. Invest.* 119, 2925–2941. doi: 10.1172/jci38857

Wang, J., Hu, X., and Jiang, H. (2016). ER stress-induced apoptosis: a novel therapeutic target in myocardial ischemia and reperfusion injury. *Int. J. Cardiol.* 214, 233–234. doi: 10.1016/j.ijcard.2016.03.176

Wang, Y., Rao, W., Zhang, C., Zhang, C., Liu, M. D., Han, F., et al. (2015). Scaffolding protein Homer1a protects against NMDA-induced neuronal injury. *Cell Death Dis.* 6:e1843. doi: 10.1038/cddis.2015.216

Wu, X., Luo, P., Rao, W., Dai, S., Zhang, L., Ma, W., et al. (2018). Homer1a attenuates hydrogen peroxide-induced oxidative damage in HT-22 cells through AMPK-dependent autophagy. *Front. Neurosci.* 12:51. doi: 10.3389/fnins.2018.00051

Wu, Y., Wang, X., Zhou, X., Cheng, B., Li, G., and Bai, B. (2017). Temporal expression of apelin/apelin receptor in ischemic stroke and its therapeutic potential. *Front. Mol. Neurosci.* 10:1. doi: 10.3389/fnmol.2017.00001

Xu, Q. H., Song, B. J., Liu, D., Chen, Y. H., Zhou, Y., Liu, W. B., et al. (2018). The MKK7 inhibitor peptide GADD45β-I attenuates ER stress-induced mitochondrial dysfunction in HT22 cells: involvement of JNK-Wnt pathway. *Brain Res.* 1691, 1–8. doi: 10.1016/j.brainres.2018.04.012

Yang, X., Geng, K., Zhang, J., Zhang, Y., Shao, J., and Xia, W. (2017). Sirt3 mediates the inhibitory effect of adjudin on astrocyte activation and glial scar formation following ischemic stroke. *Front. Pharmacol.* 8:943. doi: 10.3389/fphar.2017.00943

Yu, Z., Yi, M., Wei, T., Gao, X., and Chen, H. (2017). KCa3.1 inhibition switches the astrocyte phenotype during astrogliosis associated with ischemic stroke via endoplasmic reticulum stress and MAPK signaling pathways. *Front. Cell. Neurosci.* 11:319. doi: 10.3389/fncel.2017.00319

3

Brain Endothelial Erythrophagocytosis and Hemoglobin Transmigration Across Brain Endothelium: Implications for Pathogenesis of Cerebral Microbleeds

Rudy Chang[1], Juan Castillo[2], Alexander C. Zambon[1], Tatiana B. Krasieva[3], Mark J. Fisher[4] and Rachita K. Sumbria[1,4]*

[1] Department of Biopharmaceutical Sciences, School of Pharmacy and Health Sciences, Keck Graduate Institute, Claremont, CA, United States, [2] Department of Neuroscience, Claremont McKenna College, Claremont, CA, United States, [3] Beckman Laser Institute, University of California, Irvine, Irvine, CA, United States, [4] Departments of Neurology and Pathology & Laboratory Medicine, University of California, Irvine, Irvine, CA, United States

***Correspondence:**
Rachita K. Sumbria
rsumbria@kgi.edu

Peripheral endothelial cells are capable of erythrophagocytosis, but data on brain endothelial erythrophagocytosis are limited. We studied the relationship between brain endothelial erythrophagocytosis and cerebral microhemorrhage, the pathological substrate of MRI-demonstrable cerebral microbleeds. To demonstrate the erythrophagocytic capability of the brain endothelium, we studied the interactions between brain endothelial cells and red blood cells exposed to oxidative stress *in vitro*, and developed a new *in vitro* cerebral microbleeds model to study the subsequent passage of hemoglobin across the brain endothelial monolayer. Using multiple approaches, our results show marked brain endothelial erythrophagocytosis of red blood cells exposed to oxidative stress compared with control red blood cells *in vitro*. This brain endothelial erythrophagocytosis was accompanied by passage of hemoglobin across the brain endothelial monolayer with unaltered monolayer integrity. *In vivo* and confocal fluorescence microscopy studies confirmed the extravasation of RBC exposed to oxidative stress across brain endothelium. These findings, demonstrating erythrophagocytosis mediated by the brain endothelial monolayer and the subsequent passage of iron-rich hemoglobin *in vitro* and RBC *in vivo*, may have implications for elucidating mechanisms involved in the development of cerebral microbleeds that are not dependent on disruption of the microvasculature.

Keywords: erythrophagocytosis, cerebral microbleeds, brain endothelial cells, hemoglobin, red blood cells, transmigration

INTRODUCTION

Cerebral microhemorrhages are tiny deposits of blood degradation products in the brain and are the pathological substrate of cerebral microbleeds (CMB). CMB are associated with increasing age, cerebrovascular diseases, hypertension, and chronic kidney disease (Lau et al., 2017). Mechanistically, it is widely accepted that loss of vascular integrity due to an underlying disruption of the cerebral microvasculature causes CMB development, and these are classified as primary microbleeds (Fisher, 2014). Other mechanisms involved in CMB development include hemorrhagic infarction/microinfarction, and these are classified as secondary microbleeds (Fisher, 2013, 2014). Besides the involvement of hemorrhagic and ischemic processes in the development of CMB, there has been some indication that release of iron from oligodendrocytes during ischemia may result in MRI-demonstrable CMB (Janaway et al., 2014). Further, the existence of *pseudo-microbleeds*, a phenomenon in which iron-rich hemosiderin from red blood cells (RBC) produces signatures of CMB in the absence of vascular disruption, has been proposed (Fisher, 2014).

A recent study showed that brain endothelium have phagocytic properties and that brain vascular endothelial cells are capable of engulfing and translocating intracranial emboli into the brain extravascular space, a process termed angiophagy (Grutzendler et al., 2014). The concept of angiophagy has some similarities to endothelial erythrophagocytosis, a recently described process by which injured or aged erythrocytes are ingested by endothelial cells, undergo hemolysis, and are cleared from the blood circulation (Fens et al., 2010). Endothelial erythrophagocytosis has recently been reported by peripheral endothelial cells using human umbilical vein endothelial (HUVEC) and hepatic sinusoidal endothelial cells *in vitro*, and has further been confirmed *in vivo* (Fens et al., 2010, 2012; Lee et al., 2011).

In the cerebral milieu, macrophage-mediated erythrophagocytosis has been well-documented (Zhao et al., 2009), and the involvement of macrophages in CMB is known (Fisher et al., 2010). Besides macrophages, pericytes are known to have phagocytic function and there is some evidence of pericyte mediated erythrophagocytosis in the brain (Fisher et al., 2010). Phagocytosis of parasitized RBC by brain endothelium within an inflammatory milieu has been reported in *in vitro* studies of cerebral malaria (Jambou et al., 2010). Involvement of brain endothelium in phagocytosis of non-parasitized aged and/or injured RBC and subsequent transmigration of RBC or RBC degradation products (hemoglobin) into the brain has not been reported. It has been proposed that iron-rich extravasated RBC or RBC degradation products may produce MRI signatures of CMB in the absence of vascular disruption (pseudo-microbleeds) (Fisher, 2014).

The above prompted us to investigate the role of the brain endothelium in mediating erythrophagocytosis of aged and/or injured RBC, and subsequent passage of RBC and/or RBC degradation product hemoglobin into the brain. In the current proof-of-concept study to demonstrate brain endothelial erythrophagocytosis, RBC were treated with phosphate buffer saline (PBS) or tert-butylhydroperoxide (t-BHP), an oxidative stressor that results in the exposure of RBC phosphatidylserine (PS) to mimic aged and/or injured RBC marked for phagocytic removal from the circulation (Schroit et al., 1985). Using multiple approaches, our results show robust adhesion and engulfment (erythrophagocytosis) of t-BHP-RBC by brain endothelial cells (bEND3) compared with PBS-RBC. We developed a new CMB *in vitro* model system to study passage of RBC degradation product hemoglobin across bEND3 cells, and show passage of hemoglobin from t-BHP-treated RBC across the bEND3 monolayer with unaltered monolayer integrity. Our *in vitro* results were corroborated by our *in vivo* findings of extrusion of fluorescently-labeled RBC across the mouse brain endothelium. These results may have important implications for elucidating mechanisms involved in the development of CMB demonstrated on brain MRI.

MATERIALS AND METHODS

Red Blood Cell Preparation and Treatment

Purified RBC in Alsevers solution were derived from 2 to 3 month-old male BALB/c mice (BioReclamation IVT, New York, NY). RBC were washed and resuspended in sterile PBS (without $Ca^{2+}$and Mg^{2+}) before experimental treatment with PBS (control; incubation time: 30 min), lipopolysaccharide derived from gram negative bacterium Salmonella Typhimurium (LPS, 10 μg/mL; incubation time: 1 h; an inflammatory stimulus), neuraminidase enzyme from vibrio cholerae (0.125 U or 0.5 U; incubation time: 1 h; for senescence induction) or various concentrations (0.3, 1.0, 3.0 mM) of t-BHP (incubation time: 30 min; an oxidative stressor) at 37°C. LPS, neuraminidase, and t-BHP were selected for the current study based on previous studies using peripheral endothelial cells (Tissot Van Patot et al., 1996; Fens et al., 2012; Yang et al., 2014). After treatment, RBC were washed and resuspended in sterile PBS to desired concentrations described below. All the above materials were purchased from Sigma-Aldrich, St. Louis, MO.

Brain Endothelial Cell Culture

Murine brain microvascular endothelial cells (bEND3 cells; American Type Culture Collection, Manassas, VA) between passages 22 and 31 were grown on T75 flasks in Delbucco's Modified Eagle's Medium (DMEM) containing 0.45% glucose, 0.37% $NaHCO_3$, 4 mM Glutamine, 10% fetal bovine serum, and 100 μg/ml penicillin/streptomycin (Sigma, St. Louis, MO). After reaching 70–80% confluency, cells were subcultured in complete DMEM and seeded onto 6-well plates (5×10^5 bEND3 cells per well), 24 well plates with 0.2% gelatin coated glass cover slips (1×10^5 bEND3 cells per coverslip), or 12-well transwells with 3 μm pore polyester membrane inserts with a surface area of 1.12 cm^2 (Corning, New York, NY) (1×10^5 bEND3 cells per well). For all the experiments, 5×10^6 treated RBC were incubated with the seeded bEND3 cells for up to 24 h at 37°C in 5% CO_2. For initial experiments, 24 h after initial seeding of bEND3 cells grown on 24 well plates with 0.2% gelatin coated cover glass, bEND3 cells were primed with or without 100 ng/mL of LPS for another 24 h before being incubated with treated RBC to determine the effect of endothelial activation on RBC-bEND3 interactions.

Annexin V-FITC Labeling

To quantify the percentage of treated RBC with PS exposure, t-BHP- and PBS-treated RBC were labeled with annexin-V-FITC (BioLegend, San Diego, CA) as per the manufacturer's instructions. Briefly, after wash and resuspension of RBC in sterile PBS, 1×10^6 RBC were incubated in FITC-labeled annexin-V and 1.2 mM Ca^{2+} for 30 min in the dark. After washing and resuspending in sterile PBS, RBC were quantified with a flow cytometer (Accuri C6 Plus, BD, Franklin lakes, NJ) using logarithmic gain for light scatter and fluorescence channels with gating and background settings defined through the PBS/control RBC.

Hematoxylin and Eosin Staining

Twenty-four hours after initial bEND3 seeding on 0.2% gelatin coated glass coverslips in 24 well plates, the cells were incubated with RBC treated either with PBS or t-BHP for 3 h, 18 h and 24 h. Glass cover-slips were then fixed with 4% paraformaldehyde (PFA) for 15 min on ice followed by hematoxylin and eosin (H&E) staining. Briefly, each coverslip was washed with ice cold PBS, stained with hematoxylin for 10 min followed by Scott's Tap Water wash, stained with eosin Y for 8 min, and washed with ethanol and dipped in xylene before mounting. Six fields of view per coverslip were manually quantified by an observer blinded to the treatment using light microscopy at a 20X magnification to estimate: RBC adhesion: RBC to bEND3 ratio (expressed as %) and engulfment: % of bEND3 that were positive for RBC engulfment.

Diaminofluorene Assay

H&E staining results were confirmed using a colorimetric assay which is based on the pseudoperoxidase activity of hemoglobin using 2,7-diaminofluorene (DAF) (Sigma, St. Louis, MO) substrate and hydrogen peroxide (Gebran et al., 1992). For this, bEND3 cells seeded onto 6-well plates at 5×10^5 cells per well for 72 h at 37°C in 5% CO_2 were used. After 72 h, cell media was changed from the FBS-supplemented DMEM to strictly FBS-free DMEM. After media change, RBC treated with PBS or t-BHP were incubated with the bEND3 cells for 24 h. bEND3 cells without RBC served as control (bEND3 only group). After incubation, the supernatant media of the wells was aspirated, wells were washed with distilled water to lyse attached RBC (RBC that are not engulfed by endothelial cells) and incubated with 0.2M Tris-HCl buffer containing 6M urea lysis solution for 30 min, followed by circular scrubbing with cell scrappers to further lyse bEND3 cells to release hemoglobin. DAF dye stock solution (10 mg/mL in 90% acetic acid) was added to 10 mL of 6M urea with 100 μL of hydrogen peroxide to make a DAF working solution which was used to react with 100 μL of supernatant of each well prepared above and immediately read on a SpectraMax 384 microplate reader (Molecular Devices, Sunnyvale, CA) at 620 nm. A hemoglobin standard (Lee Biosolutions, Maryland Heights, MO) was used to estimate the amount of hemoglobin which is an indicator of the extent of erythrophagocytosis. The amount of hemoglobin was expressed as % of hemoglobin detected with the bEND3 only group. Published studies have shown that high concentrations of t-BHP convert hemoglobin to methemoglobin (Murakami and Mawatari, 2003), which is not detected by the DAF assay. This was further confirmed in our lab (data not shown) and as a result, the DAF assay was performed using the lowest dose of t-BHP (0.3 mM).

Red Blood Cell Incubation Viability

The viability of PBS- and t-BHP-treated RBC in cell culture incubation environment was assessed by incubating treated RBC (5×10^6 cells per well) in DMEM or FBS-free DMEM into 24 well plates. After 24 h, 10 μL cells were collected and mixed with trypan blue at 1:1, and manually counted with a hemocytometer for both live and dead RBC based on trypan blue exclusion. Viable RBC were expressed as % of total RBC.

Confocal Microscopy

Brain endothelial cell tight-junctions were imaged and analyzed through Zonula Occludens-1 (ZO-1) staining and confocal microscopy. Twenty-four hours after initial bEND3 seeding on 0.2% gelatin coated glass coverslips in 24 well plates, the cells were incubated with RBC treated either with PBS or t-BHP for 24 h. Glass cover-slips were then fixed with 2% PFA, blocked in 5% bovine serum albumin (BSA) in PBS with 0.1% tritonX-100, incubated with ZO-1 antibody (1:100, ZO-1 Alexa Flour 488, SantaCruz Biotechnology, Dallas, TX; Antibody Registry Accession No. AB_628459) in PBS with 0.75% BSA overnight at 4°C, followed by endothelial nuclear staining with DRAQ5 (BioLegend, San Diego, CA). Cover-slips were mounted with VectaShield Hardset Mounting Medium (Vector Labs, Burlingame, CA) and imaged with a Leica SP5 confocal microscope (Leica, Wetzlar, Germany).

Live Imaging

To visualize the time-lapse of events that occurs between bEND3 cells and RBC, PBS- and t-BHP-treated RBC that were incubated with bEND3 cells on 6-well plates were placed in an incubator (37°C in 5% CO_2) with LumaScope 720 imaging microscope (EtaLuma, Carlsbad, CA) that captured images of each well every 2.5 min over a course of 24 h. The timestamped images were then compiled into an mpeg file that illustrated the time-lapse at 3 frames per second.

Transmigration of Hemoglobin Across the bEND3 Monolayer

To determine the appropriate time to initiate the transmigration experiments, the integrity of the bEND3 monolayer in the transwells was assessed by performing transendothelial electrical resistance (TEER) measurements using the EVOM2 Epithelial Volt/Ohm Meter and an STX-2 electrode system (World Precision Instruments LLC, Sarasota, FL) at various time points (3, 24, 48, and 72 h) in each well.

The experimental setup of the transmigration experiment is shown in **Figure 4A**. To assess whether hemoglobin from treated

RBC migrates through the endothelial monolayer, bEND3 cells were cultured onto the apical wells of the transwells with complete DMEM for 72 h (time at which maximum TEER was obtained; data not shown), followed by replacement of the complete DMEM with FBS-free DMEM. PBS- and t-BHP-treated RBC were then added to the apical wells, incubated undisturbed for 24 h at 37°C in 5% CO_2. Endothelial cells grown on transwell inserts without RBC served as controls (bEND3 only group). After incubation, media in the basolateral well was gently mixed and 200 μL of the media was collected and lysed with 200 μL of 0.2 M Tris-HCl buffer containing 6 M urea for 15 min at RT. The basolateral aliquot was then examined for hemoglobin passage across the bEND3 monolayer using the DAF and hemoglobin standard assay described above. Passage of hemoglobin across bEND3 monolayer-free transwell insert was used to assess spontaneous migration of hemoglobin across the transwell insert. Hemoglobin amount was expressed as % bEND3 only group (control).

TEER measurements were performed in triplicates per insert before addition of RBC to the apical well (0 h) and 24 h after RBC incubation to assess monolayer integrity during the transmigration experiment. All TEER values were corrected for the blank TEER of monolayer-free transwell inserts and represented at % PBS RBC values.

In vivo Passage of RBC Across the Brain Endothelium

All animal procedures were approved by UCI Institutional Animal Care and Use Committee and were carried out in compliance with University Laboratory Animal Resources regulations. Passage of t-BHP-treated RBC across the brain endothelium was visualized using postmortem confocal fluorescence microscopy. Adult male Tie2-GFP mice (10–12 week old, Jackson Laboratory, Bar Harbor, ME) with green fluorescent protein (GFP) labeled endothelial cells were used for imaging. Briefly, autologous blood (200–250 μL) was collected from Tie2-GFP mice ($n = 2$) and RBC were purified using Ficoll-Paque (GE Healthcare, Uppsala, Sweden) gradient. After several washes in PBS, RBC were treated with PBS or 3 mM t-BHP for 30 min at 37°C as described above and stained with PKH-26 Red Fluorescent Cell Linker Kit (Sigma, St. Louis, MO) according to manufacturer's instructions and re-injected into the mice intravenously. Mice were euthanized 24 h after RBC injection using a lethal dose of Euthasol (150 mg/kg, i.p.) and whole brains were harvested for postmortem confocal fluorescence microscopy to visualize passage of RBC across the brain endothelium.

Fluorescence images of whole brains were obtained using Zeiss LSM 510 microscopy system equipped with a longworking distance Zeiss 40x, 0.8 NA water immersion objective. Laser scanning did not induce any visible damage to the tissue or noticeable bleaching of the sample. Stacks of images were acquired with the z-step (distance between consecutive imaging planes) of 2.5 μm. The maximum depth for imaging was up to 80 μm from the brain surface. The probed 3D volume was reconstructed by Zeiss LSM original software.

Measurement of Free Hemoglobin From RBC

bEND3 cells (1×10^5) seeded onto 24 well plates were allowed to grow to confluence and incubated with PBS- or t-BHP-treated RBC in FBS free media for 3 h, 18 h, and 24 h. At the predetermined time intervals, media was collected from each well, and placed in Amicon-100K centrifuge tubes (Fisher Scientific, Hampton, NH). After spinning for 10 min at 14,000 RPM, the filtrate at the bottom containing the free hemoglobin was collected (RBC are retained on top) and processed using the DAF assay described above to determine free hemoglobin present in the media represented as % of hemoglobin from PBS RBC (% control).

Statistical Analysis

All statistical analysis was performed using GraphPad Prism 5 (GraphPad Software Inc., La Jolla, CA). Data are presented as mean ± SEM of at least 3 independent experiments done in duplicates based on power analysis which indicated that at least 3 experiments will be needed to detect a difference of 20% between groups with a power of 80% and significance level of 5%. To compare more than 2 independent groups, one-way ANOVA with Bonferroni's correction was used. For data with more than 2 independent groups and 2 independent variables, two-way ANOVA, with or without repeated measures, was used. A two-tailed $p < 0.05$ for the entire family of comparison was considered statistically significant.

RESULTS

Three-hour incubation of PBS-treated bEND3 cells with PBS-treated RBC resulted in negligible RBC adhesion to bEND3 cells. There was a significant ($p < 0.001$) increase in the adhesion of 3 mM t-BHP-treated RBC to PBS-treated bEND3 cells compared with PBS-treated RBC incubated with PBS-treated bEND3 cells (**Figure 1A**). Treatment of RBC with LPS or neuraminidase (0.125U or 0.5U) did not significantly alter RBC adhesion to PBS-treated bEND3 cells compared with PBS-treated RBC incubated with PBS-treated bEND3 cells (**Figure 1A**). Treatment of the bEND3 cells with LPS did not have a significant effect on RBC adhesion under any condition tested in the current study (**Figure 1A**) or with an increase in incubation time (data not shown).

Phosphatidylserine Exposure

Studies with annexin-V FITC showed that greater than 90% of t-BHP-treated RBC are annexin-V FITC positive confirming PS exposure on the surface of t-BHP-treated RBC compared with PBS-treated RBC (**Figure 1B**).

Concentration and Time Dependent RBC-bEND3 Erythrophagocytosis (Adhesion and Engulfment)

RBC treatment with low and medium concentrations of t-BHP (0.3 and 1 mM) resulted in negligible RBC adhesion to the bEND3 cells following 3 h incubation. RBC treatment with high

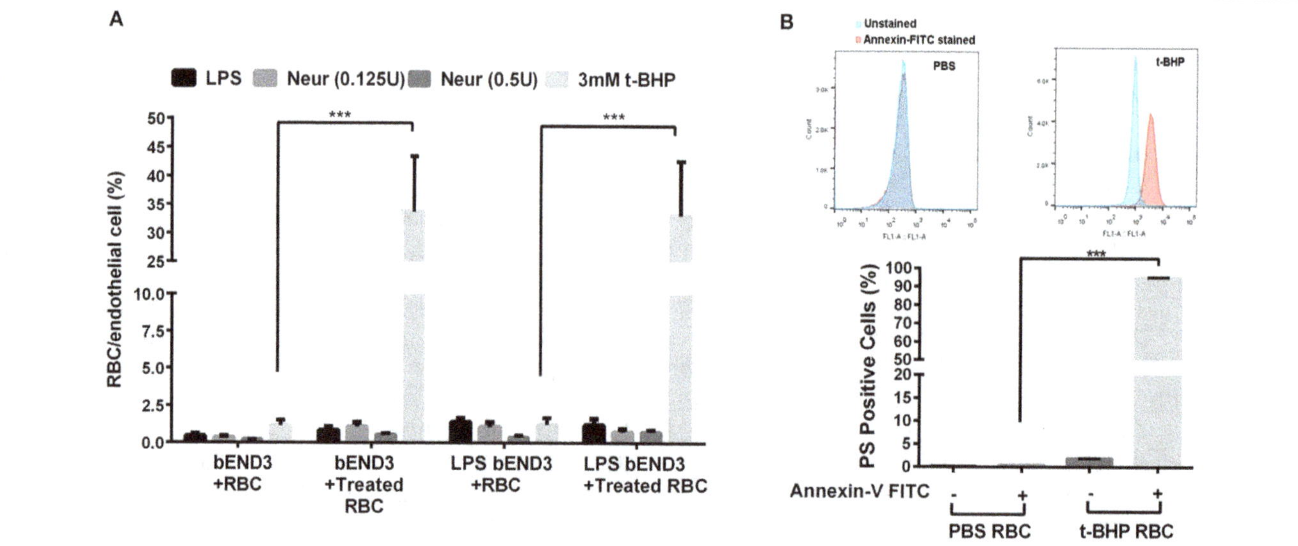

FIGURE 1 | RBC adhesion to brain endothelial (bEND3 cells) under different conditions **(A)** and PS exposure in t-BHP-treated RBC **(B)**. RBC treated with PBS (control), LPS (10 µg/mL) or neuraminidase (0.125 U or 0.5 U) did not significantly alter RBC adhesion to bEND3 cells following 3 h incubation, however, 3 mM t-BHP treatment of RBC resulted in a significant increase in RBC adhesion to bEND3 cells compared with respective PBS-treated RBC. LPS treatment of bEND3 cells did not further enhance RBC adhesion under any treatment conditions. >90% of 0.3 mM t-BHP-treated RBC were PS positive compared with PBS-treated RBC as determined by flow cytometry **(B)**. Data is presented as mean ± SEM of at least 3 independent experiments. $^{***}p < 0.001$.

concentration of t-BHP on the other hand resulted in significant RBC adhesion to the bEND3 cells as early as following 3 h incubation. Overall, adhesion of t-BHP-treated RBC to bEND3 cells, increased in a concentration and time dependent manner. Maximum RBC adhesion for the 0.3 mM t-BHP concentration was observed at 24 h and RBC adhesion plateaued at 18 h for 1 mM and 3 mM t-BHP concentrations (**Figure 2A,B**).

Similarly, low and medium concentrations of t-BHP resulted in no engulfment of RBC by bEND3 cells following 3 h incubation. There was a trend toward an increase in the engulfment of 3 mM t-BHP-treated RBC following 3 h incubation. Engulfment of t-BHP-treated RBC also increased in a concentration and time dependent manner with maximum engulfment of t-BHP-treated RBC occurring following 24 h incubation (**Figure 2C**). Overall, maximum adhesion and engulfment of t-BHP-treated RBC was observed with a concentration of 3 mM. As shown in **Figure 2D**, multiple 3 mM t-BHP-treated RBC are seen engulfed (red arrows) by a single bEND3 cell. The average number of bEND3 cells per field of view remained unchanged with adhesion and engulfment of t-BHP-RBC over the duration of the experiment (**Figure 2E**) for any experimental group and viability of the PBS- and t-BHP-treated RBC in cell culture media was > 90% at 24 h (data not shown).

DAF assay that relies on the pseudoperoxidase activity of hemoglobin was used to confirm erythrophagocytosis (adhesion and engulfment) observed by microscopy. There was no significant difference in the amount of hemoglobin detected in the bEND3 cells incubated with PBS-treated RBC compared with control (bEND3 monolayer only). However, bEND3 cells incubated with t-BHP-treated RBC had a significantly higher amount of hemoglobin, an indicator of erythrophagocytosis, compared with the control and PBS-treated RBC, confirming the light microscopy results (**Figure 2F**).

Adhesion and engulfment of t-BHP-treated RBC by the bEND3 monolayer was further confirmed using live cell time-lapse imaging (see **Supplementary Video 1**), immunofluorescence and confocal microscopy. **Figure 3A** shows a maximum projection of a 6 µm depth z-stack image with a step size of 0.3 µm, and confirms the presence of tight junction protein ZO-1 in the confluent bEND3 monolayer (ZO-1 tight junction protein staining shown in green and bEND3 nuclei stained with DRAQ5 shown in blue). Both PBS- and t-BHP-RBC autofluoresce (green) as shown in the figure. Adhesion and engulfment of t-BHP-treated RBC is further confirmed by orthogonal and single z-stack projections (**Figure 3B**).

Transmigration of Hemoglobin Across the bEND3 Monolayer

We developed a method to determine the passage of hemoglobin across the bEND3 monolayer using an *in vitro* transwell system. Experimental set-up for the transmigration experiment is shown in **Figure 4A**. Migration of hemoglobin across the bEND3 monolayer was determined using the DAF assay as described above. Spontaneous migration reflects the passage of hemoglobin from PBS-RBC across the 3 µm pore size transwell in the absence of a bEND3 monolayer. As expected, hemoglobin passage was observed in the absence of the bEND3 monolayer. However, in the presence of the bEND3 monolayer, the passage of hemoglobin from PBS-RBC across the bEND3 monolayer was the same as control (bEND3 only) indicating no passage of hemoglobin from PBS-RBC across the monolayer. There was a significant increase in the hemoglobin in the basolateral chamber of wells

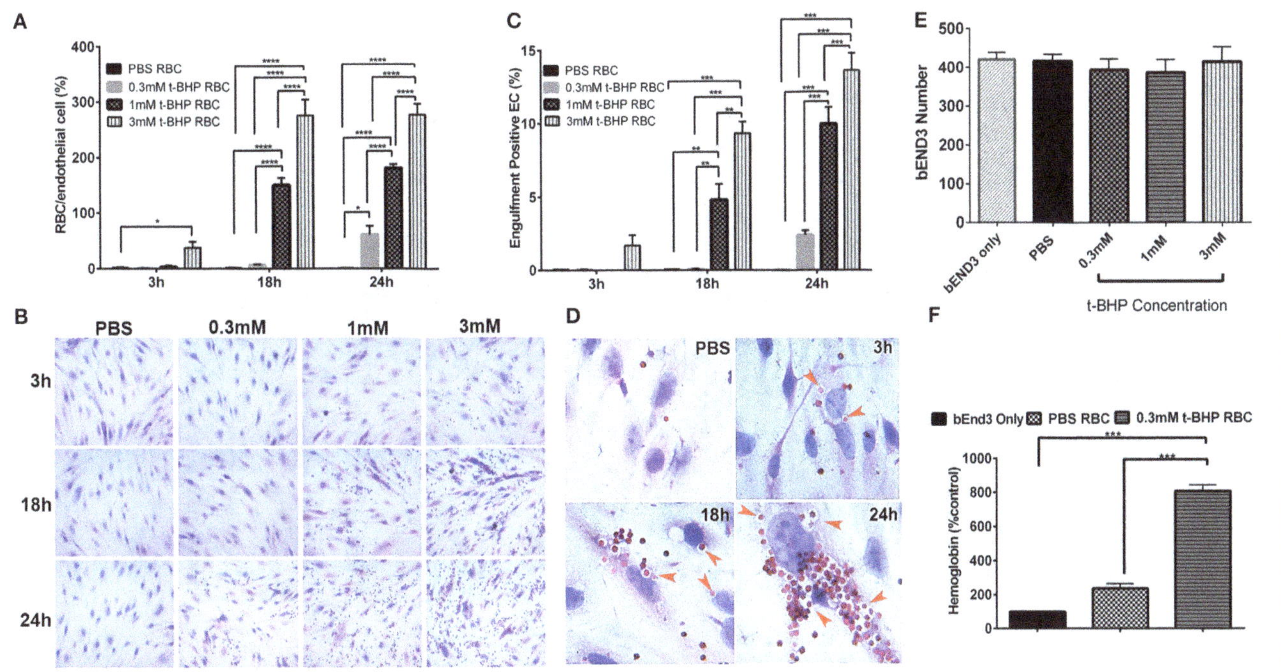

FIGURE 2 | Erythrophagocytosis by brain endothelial cells. Significant time- and concentration-dependent increase in adhesion **(A,B)** and engulfment **(C)** of t-BHP-treated RBC compared with PBS-treated RBC using light microscopy. Marked time dependent increase in engulfment of t-BHP-treated RBC by bEND3 cells indicated by red arrows **(D)**. Brain endothelial erythrophagocytosis at 24 h was not associated with bEND3 degradation or loss **(E)**. Significant increase in the amount of hemoglobin retained by the bEND3 cells incubated with t-BHP-treated RBC compared with PBS-treated RBC following 24 h incubation confirming erythrophagocytosis using the DAF colorimetric method **(F)**. Data is presented as mean ± SEM of at least 3 independent experiments. $^{*}p < 0.05$, $^{**}p < 0.01$, $^{***}p < 0.001$, $^{****}p < 0.0001$. EC, endothelial cells.

incubated with t-BHP-treated RBC compared with PBS-treated RBC confirming passage of hemoglobin from t-BHP-treated RBC across the bEND3 monolayer (**Figure 4B**).

To determine if passage of hemoglobin from the t-BHP-treated RBC was associated with changes in bEND3 monolayer integrity, we measured TEER values, before and 24 h after RBC incubation. No changes in TEER were observed for all concentrations of t-BHP compared with PBS-RBC used as control, confirming that the passage of hemoglobin from t-BHP-RBC was not associated with altered bEND3 monolayer integrity (**Figure 4C**). Further, to rule out the possibility of an increase in hemoglobin release with t-BHP in the apical chamber that may result in higher hemoglobin in the basolateral chamber, we determined the amount of free hemoglobin released by PBS- and t-BHP-treated RBC over the course of 24 h. We found that treating RBC with t-BHP did not increase the free hemoglobin released in the media compared with PBS-treated RBC (**Figure 4D**).

Passage of RBC Across the Brain Endothelium *in vivo*

In vivo studies in Tie2-GFP mice showed that PKH-26 labeled PBS-treated RBC were confined to the cerebral vasculature. However, PKH-26 labeled t-BHP-treated RBC were found inside, outside, partially outside, and partially attached to the cerebral vasculature (**Figure 5**).

DISCUSSION

In this study we demonstrate that RBC exposed to the oxidative stressor t-BHP undergo significant erythrophagocytosis (adhesion and engulfment) by the brain endothelial cells in an *in vitro* cell culture system. Further, this enhanced erythrophagocytosis was associated with an increased passage of RBC degradation product hemoglobin across the brain endothelial cells. No change in brain endothelium monolayer integrity was observed with passage of hemoglobin across the endothelial monolayer in the current study. *In vivo* studies using Tie2-GFP mice further verified the passage of t-BHP-treated RBC across the brain endothelium.

Under normal physiological conditions, the adhesion of RBC to the vascular endothelium is negligible. However, altered RBC-vascular endothelial adhesion has been observed in various pathological conditions including sickle cell disease (SCD), diabetes mellitus, malaria, and retinal vein occlusion (Wautier and Wautier, 2013). Pathological adherence of RBC to the vascular endothelium is associated with vascular complications including vaso-occlusive events observed in SCD (Wautier et al., 1985). Further, cytoadherence of plasmodium falciparum-infected RBC to the brain microvascular endothelium has been demonstrated in cerebral malaria (Jambou et al., 2010; El-Assaad et al., 2013; Howland et al., 2015). Besides abnormal adhesion of RBC to the vascular endothelium, recent studies report endothelial

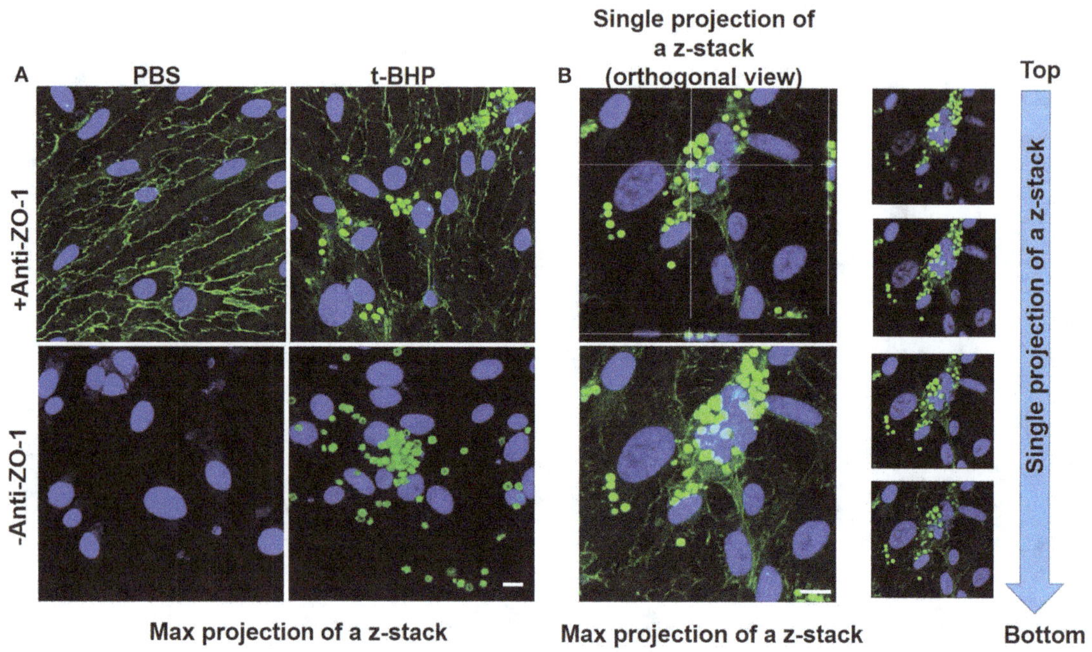

FIGURE 3 | Confocal microscopy of bEND3 cells and RBC to confirm erythrophagocytosis. Maximum projection of z-stack shows adhesion of t-BHP-treated RBC to bEND3 cells and no adhesion of PBS-treated RBC (Blue = DRAQ5 stain for the endothelial nucleus, green = tight junction ZO-1 protein and autofluorescence of RBC) **(A)**. Orthogonal view of a single projection, maximum projection of a z-stack and individual images of a z-stack moving from top to bottom of a cover glass confirm the internalization of t-BHP-treated RBC by bEND3 cells **(B)**. Scale bar = 10 μm.

erythrophagocytosis, a phenomenon by which aged and/or injured RBC adhere to and are engulfed by endothelial cells of peripheral origin including HUVECs and hepatic sinusoidal endothelial cells (Fens et al., 2010, 2012; Lee et al., 2011).

Among the first mechanisms shown to be involved in the phagocytic removal of aged, senescent, or injured RBC from the blood circulation (erythrophagocytosis) is membrane scrambling leading to the exposure of membrane PS to the outer leaflet of the RBC membrane (Bratosin et al., 1998). PS exposure serves as an "eat me" signal that triggers erythrophagocytosis by phagocytes, thereby facilitating erythrocyte clearance from the circulation (Schroit et al., 1985). Some of the seminal studies of RBC erythrophagocytosis showed that RBC with abnormal distribution of PS in the outer cell wall were phagocytized by macrophages more readily than normal or healthy RBC (Bratosin et al., 1998). PS-exposing cells are cleared from the circulation through recognition by receptors, including scavenger receptors, αvβ3 integrins, MerTK, TIM-1 and 4, BAI1, and Stabilin1 and 2, and subsequent attachment, cytoskeleton rearrangement and phagolysosomal processing (Ravichandran and Lorenz, 2007). The role of PS in endothelium-mediated erythrophagocytosis was also recently demonstrated (Lee et al., 2011; Fens et al., 2012). In these studies, PS-mediated endothelial erythrophagocytosis was mediated by the αvβ3 integrins (Fens et al., 2012) or stabilin 1 and 2 (Lee et al., 2011). Apart from endothelial erythrophagocytosis, PS exposure also plays a pivotal role in pathologic RBC adherence to vascular endothelium (Setty et al., 2002; Wautier et al., 2011).

In the current proof-of-concept study, PS exposure to mimic aged and/or injured RBC *in vivo* was triggered by treating RBC with t-BHP **(Figure 1B)** which, although an exogenous agent, is known to result in exposure of PS to the outer-leaflet of RBC (Fens et al., 2010), and is widely used as an external inducer of oxidative stress (Zou et al., 2001). Notably, oxidation of RBC plays an important role in erythrophagocytic clearance of aged and/or injured RBC (Kiefer and Snyder, 2000). As previously demonstrated by others, we found that a large percent of the t-BHP-treated RBC exposed PS (Fens et al., 2012). Consistent with studies using peripheral endothelial cells (Fens et al., 2012), in the current study we found that murine RBC treated with varying concentrations of t-BHP resulted in robust adhesion followed by engulfment of RBC by the murine brain endothelial cells (bEND3) **(Figures 2, 3)**, a well-characterized immortalized brain microvascular cell line known to retain many morphological and biochemical properties similar to *in vivo* conditions (Omidi et al., 2003). Adhesion and engulfment of t-BHP-RBC was confirmed using multiple approaches (H&E, DAF assay, confocal analysis and live imaging). Erythrophagocytosis of t-BHP-RBC was not associated with loss or degradation of brain endothelial cells in the current study and is in agreement with a recent study using HUVEC cells, in which erythrophagocytosis of oxidative stress-exposed RBC did not result in immediate signs of degradation and only a small fraction of HUVEC cells showed signs of apoptosis after 24 h incubation (Fens et al., 2012).

Treatment of RBC with other pathological stimuli such as LPS or neuraminidase did not result in brain endothelial

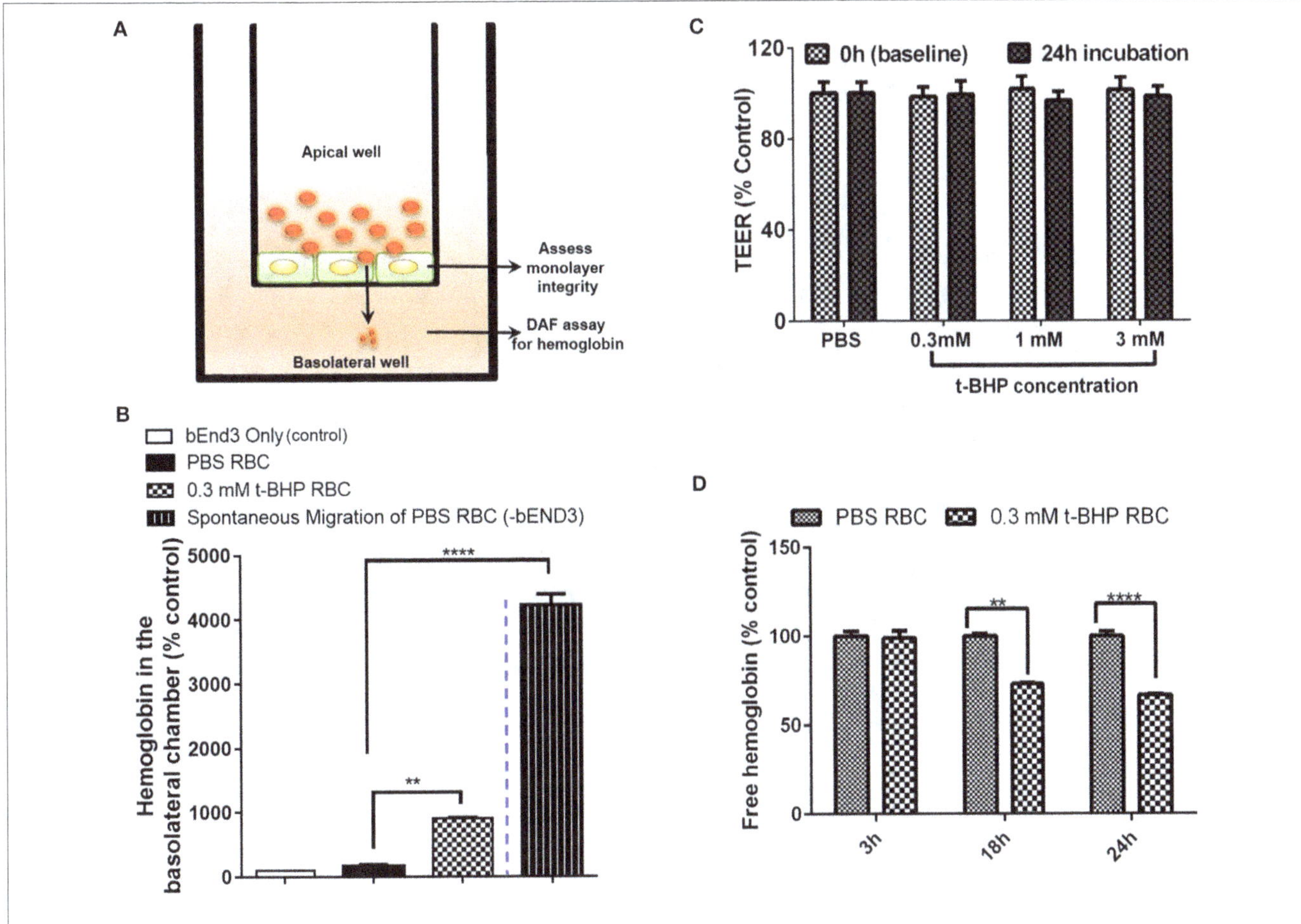

FIGURE 4 | Transmigration of hemoglobin across the bEND3 monolayer. Experimental set up to detect passage of hemoglobin across the bEND3 monolayer **(A)**. Significant increase in the passage of hemoglobin across the bEND3 monolayer incubated with t-BHP-treated RBC compared with PBS-RBC. Spontaneous migration reflects passage of hemoglobin from PBS-RBC across the 3 μm pore size transwell in the absence of a bEND3 monolayer **(B)**. Passage of hemoglobin across the bEND3 monolayer grown on transwells incubated with t-BHP-RBC was not accompanied by a change in TEER; TEER measurements are presented as % of PBS-RBC values **(C)**. Free hemoglobin released by t-BHP-treated RBC is significantly lower compared with PBS-treated RBC. The bEND3 monolayer was grown on standard cell culture wells **(D)**. Data is presented as mean ± SEM of at least 3 independent experiments. $^{**}p < 0.01$, $^{****}p < 0.0001$.

erythrophagocytosis or PS exposure (data not shown) in the current study. Further, activation of the brain endothelial cells with LPS did not augment erythrophagocytosis of t-BHP-treated RBC (**Figure 1**). These results are in contrast to previous studies in which treatment of RBC with LPS or neuraminidase resulted in significant adhesion to vascular endothelium (Tissot Van Patot et al., 1996; Eichelbrönner et al., 2000; Yang et al., 2014), and activation of endothelial cells with LPS further augmented such RBC-endothelial cell interactions *in vitro* (Tissot Van Patot et al., 1996; Eichelbrönner et al., 2000; Setty and Betal, 2008). The use of brain microvascular endothelial cells in the current study, as opposed to peripheral endothelial cells used in all the previous studies, may explain this difference in outcome.

After demonstrating robust erythrophagocytosis of RBC exposed to oxidative stress by the brain microvascular endothelial cells *in vitro*, the main question we wanted to address was whether brain endothelial erythrophagocytosis was associated with the passage of RBC or hemoglobin (RBC degradation product) across the brain endothelium. In the current study, we show significant passage of hemoglobin across the brain endothelial monolayer incubated with t-BHP-treated RBC (**Figure 4**). We further confirmed that the passage of hemoglobin was not associated with a change in the brain endothelial monolayer integrity since the TEER values remained unchanged for the duration of the experiment.

To evaluate the possibility of migration of free apical hemoglobin from t-BHP-treated RBC across the monolayer into the basolateral chamber, we determined the free hemoglobin released by t-BHP-RBC compared with PBS-RBC over 24 h in a separate series of experiments using bEND3 monolayers grown in standard cell culture plates (not transwells). We found that t-BHP-treated RBC did not release more free hemoglobin into the media compared with the PBS-RBC, and there was significantly less free hemoglobin in the media of brain endothelial cells incubated with t-BHP-RBC compared with PBS-RBC (**Figure 4**) following 18 h and 24 h incubation. This suggests that the

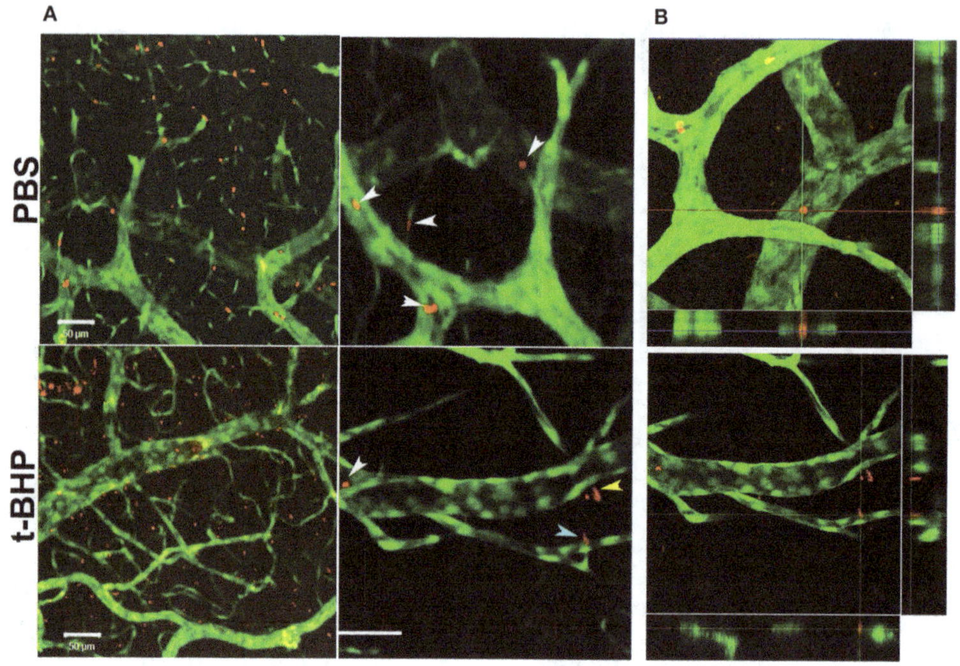

FIGURE 5 | Postmortem confocal microcopy images on mouse brains showing GFP-positive brain endothelium (green) and PKH-26-labeled RBC (red). (**A,** Top): PBS-RBC remain in the blood vessels (white arrows heads). (**A,** Bottom): t-BHP-treated RBC are inside (white arrow head) and outside the blood vessels (yellow arrow head), and also partially extravasated into the brain (blue arrow head). Orthogonal view showing PBS-treated RBC within the blood vessel (**B,** Top) and t-BHP-treated RBC partially and completely outside the blood vessel (**B,** Bottom). Scale bar = 50 μm.

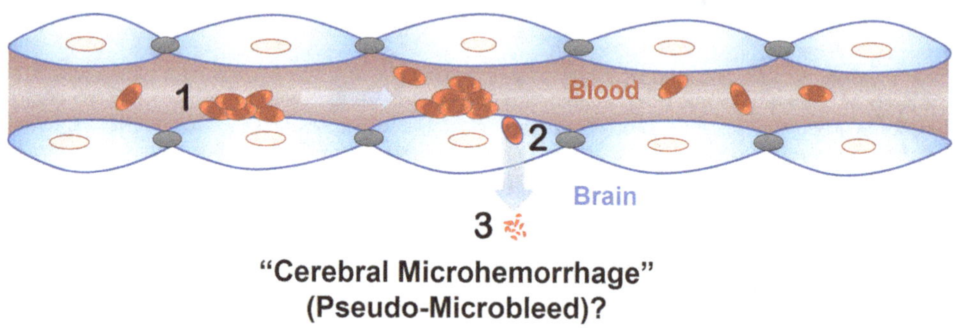

FIGURE 6 | Proposed role of endothelial erythrophagocytosis in cerebral microhemorrhage (pseudo-microbleeds) development. Aged and/or injured RBC adhere to (1) and are engulfed by (2) the brain endothelium. Iron rich RBC or degradation products (e.g., hemoglobin) are translocated across the brain endothelium (3), where they may produce signatures of CMB.

hemoglobin in the basolateral chamber does not represent the migration of free hemoglobin released in the apical chamber. The decrease in free hemoglobin with t-BHP-RBC at 18 h and 24 h is consistent with increased RBC erythrophagocytosis of t-BHP-RBC by brain endothelial cells, and thus lower free RBC available to release hemoglobin at these time points.

A limitation of our *in vitro* findings is the use of an immortalized brain endothelial cell line. Note, however, that passage of RBC degradation product (hemoglobin) across the brain endothelial monolayer were corroborated by our *in vivo* findings of extravasation of fluorescently-labeled t-BHP-treated RBC across the brain endothelium of Tie2-GFP mice using confocal microscopy (**Figure 5**). We reported a similar finding of extravasation of fluorescently-labeled RBC across the brain endothelium of Tie2-GFP mice in an inflammation-induced mouse model of CMB (Sumbria et al., 2016). In the current study, the blood vessel adjacent to the extravasated RBC appeared intact with no visible rupture (**Figure 5**).

Erythrophagocytosis mediated by macrophages involves RBC engulfment, endosomal processing and RBC degradation with subsequent release of hemoglobin and heme. It should be noted that not all engulfed RBC are subjected to phagosomal degradation and that the fate of the engulfed RBC depends on the molecular machinery involved in erythrophagocytosis (Santarino et al., 2017). The intracellular mechanisms involved in the cellular trafficking of engulfed RBC and subsequent RBC processing by endothelial cells are understudied.

In the current study, we report the passage of RBC degradation product hemoglobin *in vitro* and the passage of fluorescently-labeled RBC across the brain endothelium *in vivo*. The possibility of passage of RBC fragments and not intact RBC cannot be ruled-out from the current data. We are unaware of prior reports of extravasation of non-parasitized RBC across the brain endothelium. Our findings are similar to the work done by Grutzendler and co-workers who reported engulfment and subsequent extravasation of emboli into the brain (termed as angiophagy; Grutzendler et al., 2014). Following passage across the brain endothelium, emboli were engulfed and degraded by pericytes and microglial cells. Future *in vitro* studies using co-cultures with pericytes and microglial cells will help elucidate the intracellular trafficking and the fate of the RBC involved in brain endothelial erythrophagocytosis.

The phenomenon of passage of intact RBC or RBC degradation products across an intact endothelial monolayer following endothelial erythrophagocytosis is a novel finding, and brain endothelial erythrophagocytosis is particularly relevant from the standpoint of non-hemorrhagic mechanisms involved in CMB development (**Figure 6**) (Fisher, 2014). This is because CMB are focal deposits of blood degradation products, predominately hemosiderin, which is derived from hemoglobin following hemolysis (Janaway et al., 2014). MRI detection of CMB relies on the paramagnetic properties of hemosiderin and any passage of hemoglobin across the brain endothelium into the perivascular space can thus produce signatures of CMB. Further investigation is required to determine whether brain endothelial erythrophagocytosis and subsequent passage of RBC or RBC degradation products across the brain endothelium occur under physiologically relevant conditions that induce oxidative stress *in vivo* to produce CMB signatures. Notably, PS exposure on erythrocytes and oxidative stress has been reported under several risk factors for CMB, such as chronic kidney disease (Bonomini et al., 1999, 2002; Tucker et al., 2015) and Alzheimer's disease (Nicolay et al., 2007; Gella and Durany, 2009). Further, CMB in the absence of gadolinium extravasation (marker of blood-brain barrier disruption) have been reported in patients with cerebral malaria (Potchen et al., 2018), and recent work showed engulfment of parasitized RBC by human brain endothelial cells in an *in vitro* model of cerebral malaria (Jambou et al., 2010), raising the possibility of erythrophagocytosis-dependent CMB in this disorder.

In conclusion, we show that brain endothelial cells express an erythrophagocytic phenotype for RBC exposed to oxidative stress *in vitro*. Further, brain endothelial erythrophagocytosis is associated with passage of hemoglobin across the brain endothelial monolayer *in vitro*, and passage of RBC exposed to oxidative stress across the brain endothelium *in vivo*. These results may have significant implications for mechanisms of CMB in the absence of frank vascular disruption.

AUTHOR CONTRIBUTIONS

RC performed the experiments, collected and analyzed data, and contributed to manuscript writing. JC performed the experiments and collected data. TK performed confocal microscopy for *in vivo* studies. AZ helped with live imaging. MF helped conceive the study and edited the manuscript. RS conceived the study, designed, analyzed and coordinated the experiments, and drafted and edited the manuscript. All authors read and approved the final manuscript.

FUNDING

This work was partly supported by a grant from the Alzheimer's Association: RG-15-361188 (RS), NIH NS20989 (MF), and intramural support from the Keck Graduate Institute.

ACKNOWLEDGMENTS

Authors thank Russle Benson, Ruaab Patel, Kei-Lwun Yee, Jeffery Woods, and Abrar Al Maghribi for their assistance with the H&E quantification, and Leomar Patam for assistance with the live cell imaging. We also thank Dr. David Cribbs for his assistance with the *in vivo* experimentation. A part of this work was presented at the American Association of Colleges of Pharmacy. (2016).

SUPPLEMENTARY MATERIAL

Supplementary Video 1 | Live cell imaging of brain endothelial erythrophagocytosis. The highlighted region shows attachment and subsequent engulfment of two RBC by brain endothelium.

REFERENCES

American Association of Colleges of Pharmacy. (2016).Correction to 117th annual meeting of the American Association of Colleges of Pharmacy, Anaheim, California, July 23–27. *Am. J. Pharm. Educ.* 80:S22.

Bonomini, M., Sirolli, V., Gizzi, F., Di Stante, S., Grilli, A., and Felaco, M. (2002). Enhanced adherence of human uremic erythrocytes to vascular endothelium: role of phosphatidylserine exposure. *Kidney Int.* 62, 1358–1363. doi: 10.1111/j.1523-1755.2002.kid560.x

Bonomini, M., Sirolli, V., Settefrati, N., Dottori, S., Di Liberato, L., and Arduini, A. (1999). Increased erythrocyte phosphatidylserine exposure in chronic renal failure. *J. Am. Soc. Nephrol.* 10, 1982–1990.

Bratosin, D., Mazurier, J., Tissier, J. P., Estaquier, J., Huart, J. J., Ameisen, J. C., et al. (1998). Cellular and molecular mechanisms of senescent erythrocyte phagocytosis by macrophages. a review. *Biochimie* 80, 173–195. doi: 10.1016/S0300-9084(98)80024-2

Eichelbrönner, O., Sielenkämper, A., Cepinskas, G., Sibbald, W. J., and Chin-Yee, I. H. (2000). Endotoxin promotes adhesion of human erythrocytes to human vascular endothelial cells under conditions of flow. *Crit. Care Med.* 28, 1865–1870. doi: 10.1097/00003246-200006000-00030

El-Assaad, F., Wheway, J., Mitchell, A. J., Lou, J., Hunt, N. H., Combes, V., et al. (2013). Cytoadherence of *Plasmodium berghei*-infected red blood cells to murine brain and lung microvascular endothelial cells *in vitro*. *Infect Immun.*81, 3984–3991. doi: 10.1128/IAI.00428-13

Fens, M. H., Storm, G., Pelgrim, R. C., Ultee, A., Byrne, A. T., Gaillard, C. A., et al. (2010). Erythrophagocytosis by angiogenic endothelial cells is enhanced by loss of erythrocyte deformability. *Exp. Hematol.* 38, 282–291. doi: 10.1016/j.exphem.2010.02.001

Fens, M. H., van Wijk, R., Andringa, G., van Rooijen, K. L., Dijstelbloem, H. M., Rasmussen, J. T., et al. (2012). A role for activated endothelial cells in red blood cell clearance: implications for vasopathology. *Haematologica* 97, 500–508. doi: 10.3324/haematol.2011.048694

Fisher, M. (2014). Cerebral microbleeds: where are we now? *Neurology* 83, 1304–1305. doi: 10.1212/WNL.0000000000000871

Fisher, M., French, S., Ji, P., and Kim, R. C. (2010). Cerebral microbleeds in the elderly: a pathological analysis. *Stroke* 41, 2782–2785. doi: 10.1161/STROKEAHA.110.593657

Fisher, M. J. (2013). Brain regulation of thrombosis and hemostasis: from theory to practice. *Stroke* 44, 3275–3285. doi: 10.1161/STROKEAHA.113.000736

Gebran, S. J., Romano, E. L., Pons, H. A., Cariani, L., and Soyano, A. N. (1992). A modified colorimetric method for the measurement of phagocytosis and antibody-dependent cell cytotoxicity using 2,7-diaminofluorene. *J. Immunol. Methods* 151, 255–260. doi: 10.1016/0022-1759(92)90125-D

Gella, A., and Durany, N. (2009). Oxidative stress in Alzheimer disease. *Cell Adh. Migr.*3, 88–93. doi: 10.4161/cam.3.1.7402

Grutzendler, J., Murikinati, S., Hiner, B., Ji, L., Lam, C. K., Yoo, T., et al. (2014). Angiophagy prevents early embolus washout but recanalizes microvessels through embolus extravasation. *Sci. Transl. Med.* 6:226ra31. doi: 10.1126/scitranslmed.3006585

Howland, S. W., Poh, C. M., and Rénia, L. (2015). Activated brain endothelial cells cross-present malaria antigen. *PLoS Pathog.*11:e1004963. doi: 10.1371/journal.ppat.1004963

Jambou, R., Combes, V., Jambou, M. J., Weksler, B. B., Couraud, P. O., and Grau, G. E. (2010). *Plasmodium falciparum* adhesion on human brain microvascular endothelial cells involves transmigration-like cup formation and induces opening of intercellular junctions. *PLoS Pathog.* 6:e1001021. doi: 10.1371/journal.ppat.1001021

Janaway, B. M., Simpson, J. E., Hoggard, N., Highley, J. R., Forster, G., Drew, D., et al. (2014). Brain haemosiderin in older people: pathological evidence for an ischaemic origin of magnetic resonance imaging (MRI) microbleeds. *Neuropathol. Appl. Neurobiol.*40, 258–269. doi: 10.1111/nan.12062

Kiefer, C. R., and Snyder, L. M. (2000). Oxidation and erythrocyte senescence. *Curr. Opin. Hematol.* 7, 113–116. doi: 10.1097/00062752-200003000-00007

Lau, W. L., Huisa, B. N., and Fisher, M. (2017). The cerebrovascular-chronic kidney disease connection: perspectives and mechanisms. *Transl. Stroke Res.* 8, 67–76. doi: 10.1007/s12975-016-0499-x

Lee, S. J., Park, S. Y., Jung, M. Y., Bae, S. M., and Kim, I. S. (2011). Mechanism for phosphatidylserine-dependent erythrophagocytosis in mouse liver. *Blood* 117, 5215–5223. doi: 10.1182/blood-2010-10-313239

Murakami, K., and Mawatari, S. (2003). Oxidation of hemoglobin to methemoglobin in intact erythrocyte by a hydroperoxide induces formation of glutathionyl hemoglobin and binding of alpha-hemoglobin to membrane. *Arch. Biochem. Biophys.* 417, 244–250. doi: 10.1016/S0003-9861(03)00389-8

Nicolay, J. P., Gatz, S., Liebig, G., Gulbins, E., and Lang, F. (2007). Amyloid induced suicidal erythrocyte death. *Cell Physiol. Biochem.* 19, 175–184. doi: 10.1159/000099205

Omidi, Y., Campbell, L., Barar, J., Connell, D., Akhtar, S., and Gumbleton, M. (2003). Evaluation of the immortalised mouse brain capillary endothelial cell line, b.End3, as an *in vitro* blood-brain barrier model for drug uptake and transport studies. *Brain Res.* 990, 95–112. doi: 10.1016/S0006-8993(03)03443-7

Potchen, M. J., Kampondeni, S. D., Seydel, K. B., Haacke, E. M., Sinyangwe, S. S. Mwenechanya, M., et al. (2018). 1.5 Tesla magnetic resonance imaging to investigate potential etiologies of brain swelling in pediatric cerebral malaria. *Am. J. Trop. Med. Hyg.* 98, 497–504. doi: 10.4269/ajtmh.17-0309

Ravichandran, K. S., and Lorenz, U. (2007). Engulfment of apoptotic cells: signals for a good meal. *Nat. Rev. Immunol.*7, 964–974. doi: 10.1038/nri2214

Santarino, I. B., Viegas, M. S., Domingues, N. S., Ribeiro, A. M., Soares, M. P., and Vieira, O. V. (2017). Involvement of the p62/NRF2 signal transduction pathway on erythrophagocytosis. *Sci. Rep.*7:5812. doi: 10.1038/s41598-017-05687-1

Schroit, A. J., Madsen, J. W., and Tanaka, Y. (1985). *In vivo* recognition and clearance of red blood cells containing phosphatidylserine in their plasma membranes. *J. Biol. Chem.* 260, 5131–5138.

Setty, B. N., and Betal, S. G. (2008). Microvascular endothelial cells express a phosphatidylserine receptor: a functionally active receptor for phosphatidylserine-positive erythrocytes. *Blood* 111, 905–914. doi: 10.1182/blood-2007-07-099465

Setty, B. N., Kulkarni, S., and Stuart, M. J. (2002). Role of erythrocyte phosphatidylserine in sickle red cell-endothelial adhesion. *Blood* 99, 1564–1571. doi: 10.1182/blood.V99.5.1564

Sumbria, R. K., Grigoryan, M. M., Vasilevko, V., Krasieva, T. B., Scadeng, M., Dvornikova, A. K., et al. (2016). A murine model of inflammation-induced cerebral microbleeds. *J. Neuroinflammation* 13:218. doi: 10.1186/s12974-016-0693-5

Tissot Van Patot, M. C., MacKenzie, S., Tucker, A., and Voelkel, N. F. (1996). Endotoxin-induced adhesion of red blood cells to pulmonary artery endothelial cells. *Am. J. Physiol.* 270(1 Pt 1), L28–L36. doi: 10.1152/ajplung.1996.270.1.L28

Tucker, P. S., Scanlan, A. T., and Dalbo, V. J. (2015). Chronic kidney disease influences multiple systems: describing the relationship between oxidative stress, inflammation, kidney damage, and concomitant disease. *Oxid. Med. Cell Longev.* 2015:806358. doi: 10.1155/2015/806358

Wautier, J. L., Galacteros, F., Wautier, M. P., Pintigny, D., Beuzard, Y., Rosa, J., et al. (1985). Clinical manifestations and erythrocyte adhesion to endothelium in sickle cell syndrome. *Am. J. Hematol.* 19, 121–130. doi: 10.1002/ajh.2830190203

Wautier, J. L., and Wautier, M. P. (2013). Molecular basis of erythrocyte adhesion to endothelial cells in diseases. *Clin. Hemorheol. Microcirc.* 53, 11–21. doi: 10.3233/CH-2012-1572

Wautier, M. P., Héron, E., Picot, J., Colin, Y., Hermine, O., and Wautier, J. L. (2011). Red blood cell phosphatidylserine exposure is responsible for increased erythrocyte adhesion to endothelium in central retinal vein occlusion. *J. Thromb. Haemost.* 9, 1049–1055. doi: 10.1111/j.1538-7836.2011.04251.x

Yang, Y., Koo, S., Heng, L. T., Meiselman, H. J., and Neu, B. (2014). Non-adsorbing macromolecules promote endothelial adhesion of erythrocytes with reduced sialic acids. *Biochim. Biophys. Acta* 1840, 288–293. doi: 10.1016/j.bbagen.2013.09.031

Zhao, X., Grotta, J., Gonzales, N., and Aronowski, J. (2009). Hematoma resolution as a therapeutic target: the role of microglia/macrophages. *Stroke* 40 (Suppl. 3), S92–S94. doi: 10.1161/STROKEAHA.108.533158

Zou, C. G., Agar, N. S., and Jone, G. L. (2001). Oxidative insult in sheep red blood cells induced by T-butyl hydroperoxide: the roles of glutathione and glutathione peroxidase. *Free Radic. Res.* 34, 45–56. doi: 10.1080/10715760100300051

4

Role of CXCR1 and Interleukin-8 in Methamphetamine-Induced Neuronal Apoptosis

Si-Hao Du[1†], Wei Zhang[1†], Xia Yue[1], Xiao-Qing Luo[1,2], Xiao-Hui Tan[1], Chao Liu[3], Dong-Fang Qiao[1] and Huijun Wang[1*]*

[1]School of Forensic Medicine, Southern Medical University, Guangzhou, China, [2]Nanfang Hospital, Southern Medical University, Guangzhou, China, [3]Guangzhou Forensic Science Institute, Guangzhou Public Security Bureau, Guangzhou, China

***Correspondence:**
Dong-Fang Qiao
qiaodf@163.com
Huijun Wang
hjwang@smu.edu.cn

†These authors have contributed equally to this work.*

Methamphetamine (METH), an extremely and widely abused illicit drug, can cause serious nervous system damage and social problems. Previous research has shown that METH use causes dopaminergic neuron apoptosis and astrocyte-related neuroinflammation. However, the relationship of astrocytes and neurons in METH-induced neurotoxicity remains unclear. We hypothesized that chemokine interleukin (IL) eight released by astrocytes and C-X-C motif chemokine receptor 1 (CXCR1) in neurons are involved in METH-induced neuronal apoptosis. We tested our hypothesis by examining the changes of CXCR1 in SH-SY5Y cells and in the brain of C57BL/6 mice exposed to METH by western blotting and immunolabeling. We also determined the effects of knocking down CXCR1 expression with small interfering ribonucleic acid (siRNA) on METH-exposed SH-SY5Y cells. Furthermore, we detected the expression levels of IL-8 and the nuclear factor-kappa B (NF-κB) pathway in U87MG cells and then co-cultured the two cell types to determine the role of CXCR1 and IL-8 in neuronal apoptosis. Our results indicated that METH exposure increased CXCR1 expression both *in vitro* and *in vivo*, with the effects obtained *in vitro* being dose-dependent. Silencing of CXCR1 expression with siRNAs reduced the expression of cleaved caspase-3, cleaved poly (ADP-ribose) polymerase (PARP), and other related proteins. In addition, IL-8 expression and release were increased in METH-exposed U87MG cells, which is regulated by NF-κB pathway. Neuronal apoptosis was attenuated by siCXCR1 after METH treatment in the co-cultured cells, which can be reversed after exposure to recombinant IL-8. These results demonstrate that CXCR1 plays an important role in neuronal apoptosis induced by METH and may be a potential target for METH-induced neurotoxicity therapy.

Highlights

- Methamphetamine exposure upregulated the expression of CXCR1.
- Methamphetamine exposure increased the expression of interleukin-8 through nuclear factor-kappa B pathway.

Abbreviations: Bay 11-7082, ((E)3-[(4-methylphenyl)-sulfonyl]-2-propenenitrile; CNS, central nervous system; CXCR1, C-X-C motif chemokine receptor 1; DMEM, Dulbecco's modified Eagle's medium; FBS, Fetal bovine serum; IKK, IκB kinase; IL, Interleukin; METH, Methamphetamine; NF-κB, nuclear factor-kappa B; PARP, poly(ADP-ribose) polymerase; VDF, Polyvinylidenedifluoride; SDS-PAGE, Sodium dodecyl sulfate polyacrylamide gel.

- Activation of CXCR1 by interleukin-8 induces an increase in methamphetamine-related neuronal apoptosis.

Keywords: methamphetamine, CXCR1, IL-8, neurotoxicity, apoptosis, astrocytes

BACKGROUND

Methamphetamine (METH) is a highly addictive psychoactive drug that can have a significant injurious effect on the central nervous system (CNS). The abuse of METH has become more common than that of either heroin or cocaine and has thus placed great pressure on the economy and social order (Dinis-Oliveira et al., 2012).

Clinical and animal model studies of METH have shown that long-term consumption of METH results in significant damage to the dopaminergic system, including direct pharmacological damage of the sensitive brain region (Kita et al., 2009; Zhang et al., 2013), oxidative stress and inflammatory lesions, along with the destruction of dopaminergic neurons (Huang et al., 2015).

Our previous studies and other laboratories' research found that METH can cause neuronal apoptosis through P53 upregulated modulator of apoptosis (PUMA), insulin-like growth factor-binding protein 5 (IGFBP5), and other pathways (Qiao et al., 2014; Carmena et al., 2015; Chen C. et al., 2016; Mendieta et al., 2016). However, the treatment of primary astrocytes with METH showed that the nuclear import of nuclear factor-kappa B (NF-κB) could be increased through Toll-like receptor 4, leading increased release of pro-inflammatory cytokines, such as interleukin (IL)-1β and IL-18 (Du et al., 2017). Our recent study showed that the regulation of chemokines through a NF-κB/IL-8/C-X-C motif chemokine receptor 1 (CXCR1) pathway may play an important role in METH-induced neuronal apoptosis.

The pro-inflammatory IL-8 is a multi-functional CXC chemokine of about 75 amino acids in length (Waugh and Wilson, 2008; Citro et al., 2015). Numerous stresses, including inflammatory signals such as IL-1β and tumor necrosis factor alpha, environmental stresses (including hypoxia and/or reactive oxygen species) or surgical damage can induce IL-8 expression (Hoffmann et al., 2002; Sordillo and Helson, 2015). It turns out that both astrocytes and neurons produce IL-8 *in vitro*, stimulated by pro-inflammatory cytokines (Vlahopoulos et al., 1999; Waugh and Wilson, 2008; Kou et al., 2011). It has also been demonstrated that exposure of the cells to CpG oligodeoxynucleotides and lipopolysaccharides (LPS) increased the expression of IL-8 through mitogen-activated protein kinase (MAPK)-dependent and NF-κB-independent pathways (Kim et al., 2005). Two high-affinity receptors for IL-8 in humans are designated CXCR1 (also called IL-8R-A) and CXCR2 (Lee et al., 1992; Loetscher et al., 1994). The two receptors are expressed not only on leukocytes and tumor cells but also on neutrophils, monocytes, macrophages, basophils, natural killer T-cells and others normal cells; in addition, a lower percentage of T-cells express CXCR1/2 (Flynn et al., 2003; Brat et al., 2005). Additionally, it has been indicated that cells in CNS express chemokine receptors, including CXCR1 and CXCR2 (Dorf et al., 2000).

Chemokine IL-8, also known as CXCL8, exerts its biological effects by binding to the specific G protein-coupled receptors of CXCR1 and CXCR2 (Citro et al., 2015). After their internalization (i.e., via MAPK, phosphoinositide 3-kinase (PI3K), protein kinase c and Src tyrosine kinase, etc.), a wide range of intracellular pathways are activated (Takahashi et al., 2007; Citro et al., 2015). Therefore, in certain pathological conditions, CXCR1 is crucial in inflammatory injury and may be a promising target for neuronal apoptosis (Clunes and Boucher, 2007; Eltzschig and Eckle, 2011). However, the role of CXCR1 in neuronal apoptosis induced by METH remains to be investigated.

We hypothesized that CXCR1 would mediate METH-induced neuronal apoptosis and that the blockade of CXCR1 expression might partially protect against METH-induced neuronal apoptosis. In this study, we examined CXCR1 levels, and they showed elevated expression in METH poisoning models *in vivo* and *in vitro*. We also found that METH treatment of astrocytes resulted in increased expression of IL-8 through the activation of the NF-κB pathway. The apoptosis of neurons increased with the addition of exogenous IL-8, while the apoptosis of neurons was reduced after the silencing of CXCR1. These findings indicated that CXCR1 activation is important in the process of METH-induced neuronal apoptosis. Our study showed that CXCR1 may be a potential target in the mitigation of neuronal damage and apoptosis induced by METH.

MATERIALS AND METHODS

Materials

High Glucose Dulbecco's modified Eagle's medium (DMEM), fetal bovine serum (FBS), opti-MEM, Lipofectamine 3000 and trypsin were purchased from Gibco (Carlsbad, CA, USA). METH (>99% purity) was obtained from the National Institutes for the Control of Pharmaceutical and Biological Products (Beijing, China). Anti-cleaved poly (ADP-ribose) polymerase (PARP), anti-cleaved caspase3, anti-IKK-α, anti-IKK-β, anti-phospho-IKKα/β, anti-phospho-NF-κB, anti-IκB and anti-rabbit and mouse IgG (H + L), F(ab')2 fragment (Alexa Fluor 555 conjugated) were purchased from the Cell Signaling Technology (Boston, MA, USA). Anti-NeuN was purchased from Abcam (Cambridge, UK). Anti-NF-κB, anti-Bax, anti-Bcl-2 and anti-IL-8 were purchased from ABclonal Inc (College Park, MD, USA). Anti-β-actin and goat anti-mouse and rabbit IgG (H + L)-HRP were purchased from Beijing Ray Antibody Biotech (Beijing, China). Anti-CXCR1 was purchased from Bioss (Beijing, China). Fluorescein (FITC)-conjugated goat anti-mouse and rabbit IgG were purchased from DingGuo

(Beijing, China). siRNAs for CXCR1 was purchased from the Shanghai GenePharma Company Limited (Shanghai, China). Human IL-8 ELISA kit was purchased from Cusabio Biotech (Wuhan, China). Super ECL Assay was purchased from KeyGEN Biotech (Nanjing, China). Recombinant IL-8 was purchased from PerproTech (Rocky Hill, NJ, USA). Bay 11-7082 ((E)3-[(4-methylphenyl)-sulfonyl]-2-propenenitrile; a NF-κB inhibitor) was purchased from SelleckChem (Houston, TX, USA). Other reagents, unless specifically mentioned, were purchased from Sigma-Aldrich (St. Louis, MO, USA).

Animal Protocol

Healthy adult male C57BL/6 mice (18–22 g, 6–8 weeks old) were purchased from Southern Medical University Experimental Animal Center (Guangzhou, China) and placed individually in a temperature-controlled tub cage (approximately 22°C) with 12 h of light/dark cycle room. All procedures involving animals were performed in accordance with the ethical standards of Ethics Committee of Nanfang Hospital, Southern Medical University and with the 1964 Helsinki Declaration and its later amendments or comparable ethical standards. This article does not contain any studies with humans performed by any of the authors. Mice were placed in animal facilities for 1 week before use to make them accustomed. Mice were randomly divided into two groups (n = 3/group): saline control group and METH subacute exposure group. METH is dissolved in physiological saline. Mice in the subacute exposure group received an intraperitoneal (i.p.) METH injection (15 mg/kg/injection) every 12 h for a total of eight injections. This pattern of exposure is based on our and other previous studies (Cadet et al., 2003; Krasnova and Cadet, 2009; Qiao et al., 2014; Du et al., 2017). Saline control mice were injected i.p. with a similar volume of saline. Injections were performed at the same time as the subacute exposure group. All animals survived throughout the study. Mice were euthanized 2 h after the last injection (CO_2; followed by decapitation). Brain regions were rapidly isolated, and half hemispheres were cut and placed in 4% paraformaldehyde for 24 h for immunofluorescence experiments. The other half hemispheres were dissected to the prefrontal cortex, hippocampus, midbrain and striatum region on iced glass plates, rapidly frozen and stored at −80°C until analysis.

Cell Culture

SH-SY5Y cells, a human neuroblastoma cell line and U87MG cells, a human primary glioblastoma cell line were purchased from the Cell Bank of Shanghai Institute for Biological Center, Chinese Academy of Science (Shanghai, China). Cells were cultured in DMEM medium containing 10% FBS and placed in a 37°C constant temperature humidification, 5% carbon dioxide cell culture box. The culture medium was changed 1 or 2 days. Cells were passaged to 6-well plate when they reached about 80% to 90%.

Methamphetamine and Inhibitor Treatment

Once cells were reached about 80%, medium was changed to non-serum medium. Then cells were exposed to 0, 0.5, 1.0, 1.5, 2.0 and 2.5 mM METH in U87MG cells or SH-SY5Y cells for 24 h. This concentration range was selected based on our and others previous studies (Cisneros and Ghorpade, 2014; Zhang et al., 2015; Cao et al., 2016) and this concentration covers the non-toxic, sub-toxic and 50% lethal concentrations of METH (Chen C. et al., 2016). In the experiments with inhibitor Bay 11-7082, the cells were pre-cultured for 12 h with 10 μM Bay 11–7082 and then incubated with 2.0 mM METH for 24 h. The concentration of Bay 11–7082 was selected based on earlier studies (Pierce et al., 1997; Zanotto-Filho et al., 2011) and this concentration had optimal inhibition effects in our experiment.

Co-culture of U87MG Cells and SH-SY5Y Cells

U87MG cells and SH-SY5Y cells were cultured to a density of 90% and passaged into transwell dishes (0.4 μM; purchased from Corning (Corning, NY, USA)). SH-SY5Y cells were plated in the upper chamber of the transwell plate and U87MG cells were spread on the bottom of the transwell plate and cultured to a density of 70% to 80% respectively. The upper chamber was then placed above the lower chamber and exposed to 2.0 mM of METH for 24 h.

Western Blot Analysis

We used a Radio Immunoprecipitation Assay (RIPA) cleavage method to extract cell protein. Protein concentration was determined by BCA-100 protein quantification kit, which was purchased from Biosharp (Hefei, China). A sample of 50 μg of protein were taken and separated by 10% to 15% polyacrylamide gel electrophoresis. The protein was transferred to polyvinylidenefluoride (PVDF) membrane (Millipore, Billerica, MA, USA) and then the PVDF membranes were incubated for 1 h at room temperature (RT) in 5% (w/v) skim milk in tris-buffered saline containing 0.1% Tween 20 (TBST), followed by incubated overnight with a primary antibody at 4°C (1:500–1:1,000) in TBST. Next, the PVDF membranes were washed for three times with TBST and then incubated for 1 h at RT with secondary antibody (1:10,000) followed by three times washing with TBST. The membranes were developed with 200 μl of super ECL assay. The band intensities were quantitated by Gel-Pro analyzer (Media Cybernetics Inc., Rockville, MD, USA). We used β-actin as our reference index, and each experiment was repeated three times, with the most representative results presented in the current manuscript.

Small Interfering Ribonucleic Acid and Transient Cell Transfection

Transfection was performed as described previously (Du et al., 2017). The sequences of small interfering ribonucleic acid

TABLE 1 | The sequences of small interfering ribonucleic acids (siRNAs) used in the present study.

Gene	Number	The sequence of siRNA (5′-3′)
CXCR1	1	CCGCCAGGCUUACCAUCCAAACAAU
CXCR1	2	UCGUGCCGCUGUUUGUCAUGCUGUU
Negative control	1	UUCUCCGAACGUGUCACGUTT

(siRNA) are shown in **Table 1**. Twenty-four hours before transfection, 4–5 × 10^5 SH-SY5Y cells were seeded on 6-well culture plates, and 2 ml of DMEM medium containing 10% FBS was added to each well. Then, 20 μMol of CXCRl siRNA or control siRNA (siNC) (GenePharma, Shanghai, China) and 5 μl of lipofectamine 3000 reagent were added to 1 ml opti-MEM medium. The mixed solution was incubated at RT for 20 min, and then added to each well of the culture plate in conjunction with gentle shaking and mixing. The cell culture plates were placed in incubator for 6–12 h and then 1 ml complete medium was added in each well.

Double Immunofluorescence Labeling

Double immunofluorescence labeling was performed as described previously (Du et al., 2017). To determine CXCRl expression levels in SH-SY5Y cells and mice midbrain samples, double immunofluorescence labeling on cells and frozen sections of adult mice midbrains was performed. For immunolabeling, SH-SY5Y cells were seeded on glass bottom cell culture dishes (NEST, Shanghai, China). Cells were fixated in 4% paraformaldehyde. Then cells were incubated with blocking buffer (10% BSA and 0.05% Triton X-100) for 30 min at RT, with the primary antibody (anti-NeuN dilution of 1:200 and anti-CXCR1 dilution of 1:100) overnight at 4°C, and then with the secondary antibody for 1 h at RT (FITC conjugated anti-mouse or rabbit IgG dilution of 1:50, Alexa Fluor 555 conjugated anti-mouse or rabbit IgG dilution of 1:200). All incubation solutions were prepared using PBS supplemented with 10% BSA and 0.05% Triton X-100. 4',6-diamidino-2-phenylindole (DAPI) was used to stain nucleus. The frozen tissue sections were incubated with cold acetone for 15 min to remove the embedding agent. The rest of the steps are the

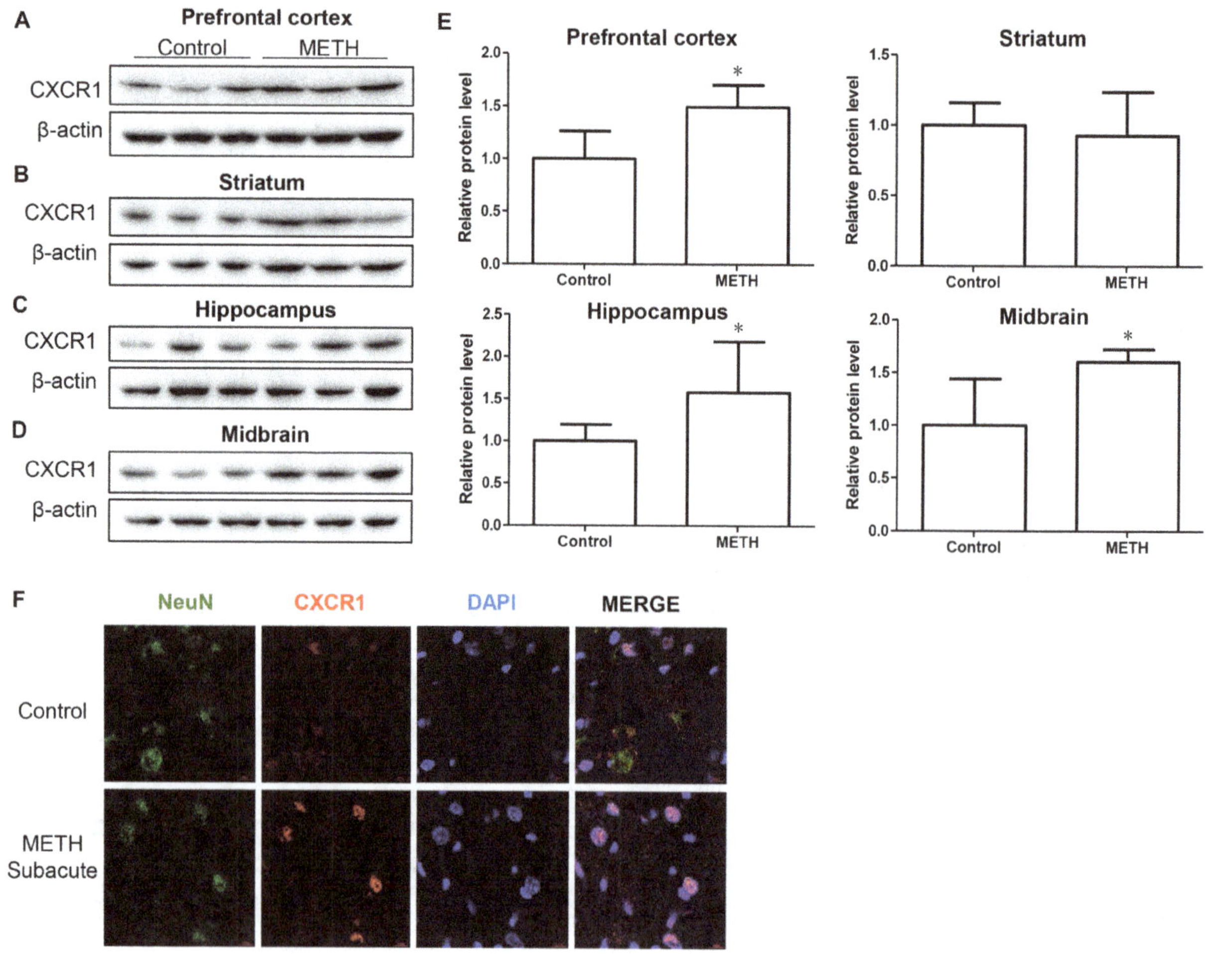

FIGURE 1 | Methamphetamine (METH) increased C-X-C motif chemokine receptor 1 (CXCR1) expression in the brain of male C57BL/6 mice. Male C57BL/6 mice were divided randomly into two groups: experimental group and control group (n = 3/group). Animals were injected intraperitoneally (i.p.) with METH (eight injections, 15 mg/kg/injection, at 12-h intervals) or saline. The prefrontal cortex, hippocampus, midbrain and striatum tissues were separated on ice at 2 h after the last dosing. Western blot **(A–D)** and quantitative analyses **(E)** were performed to determine CXCR1 expression. β-actin was used as a loading control. Fold induction relative to the control group is shown. *Represents a significant difference as compared with the control or vehicle-treated group, *$p < 0.05$. Results are expressed as the mean ± standard deviation (SD) of three experiments. Data were analyzed with Student's t-test. Immunolabeling and confocal imaging analyses **(F)** showed increased CXCR1 expression in the midbrain of METH-exposed mice in comparison with in the controls. Scale bar, 15 μM.

same as for the cells. Microphotographs were taken using fluorescence microscopy (A1+/A1R+; Nikon). All digital images were processed using the same settings to improve the contrast.

Enzyme Linked Immunosorbent Assay (ELISA)

ELISA was performed as Human IL-8 ELISA kit directions described (Cusabio Biotech, China). Briefly, add 100 μl of standard or test sample per well and incubate for 2 h at 37°C. Remove the liquid of each well and add 100 μl of primary antibody and incubate for 1 h at 37°C. Remove the liquid, wash the plate three times with PBS for 2 min each time, add 100 μl horseradish peroxidase labeled avidin secondary antibody, and incubate for 1 h at 37°C. Remove the liquid, wash the plate three times with PBS, add 90 μl of the substrate solution. Incubate for 15–30 min at 37°C to avoid light. Add 50 μl of stop solution to stop the reaction. Determine the optical density of each well within 5 min, using a microplate reader set to 450 nm.

Terminal Deoxynucleotidyl Transferase dUTP Nick End-Labeling (TUNEL) Staining

The DNA fragments of the apoptotic neurons were detected according to the instructions of a terminal deoxynucleotidyl transferase dUTP nick end labeling (TUNEL) fluorescent reagent. First, cells were fixed with 4% paraformaldehyde for 10 min at RT and then incubated for 1 h in cell culture incubator by adding terminal deoxynucleotidyl transferase enzyme conjugated to fluorescein, which was followed by the introduction of DAPI for nuclear count staining. The cross-sectional fragment was observed under a fluorescence microscope. Treatment in the control group was consistent with the addition of terminal deoxynucleotide transferase. TUNEL-positive cells and DAPI-positive cells were counted.

Statistical Analysis

Statistical analysis of data was performed with Student's *t*-test and one-way analysis of variance (ANOVA) followed by Least Significant Difference (LSD) *post hoc* analyses using SPSS 20.0 software (IBM Corporation, Armonk, NY, USA). Data given in the text are expressed as mean ± standard deviation (SD). The value of $P < 0.05$ was considered statistically significant.

RESULTS

Methamphetamine-Induced CXCR1 Expression in Neurons

In order to determine the role of CXCR1 in METH-triggered neurotoxicity, a mouse model treated with METH (eight injections, 15 mg/kg/injection, given at 12-h intervals) was used to detect the expression of CXCR1 *in vivo*. We separated the brain regions of prefrontal cortex, hippocampus,

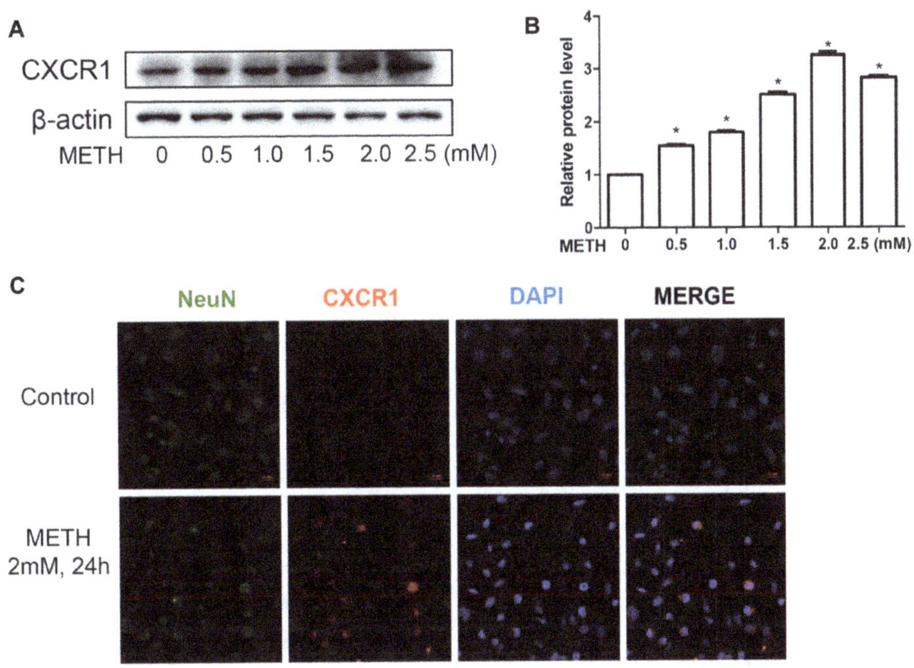

FIGURE 2 | METH increased CXCR1 expression in neurons. SH-SY5Y cells were exposed to 0.5 mM, 1 mM, 1.5 mM, 2 mM and 2.5 mM of METH for 24 h **(A)** or 2 mM of METH for 24 h **(C)**. Western blot **(A)** and quantitative analyses **(B)** were performed to determine CXCR1 protein expression. β-actin was used as a loading control. Fold induction relative to the control group is shown. *Represents a significant difference as compared with the control or vehicle-treated group, *$p < 0.05$. Results are expressed as the mean ± SD of three experiments. Data were analyzed with one-way ANOVA followed by least significant difference (LSD) *post hoc* analyses. Immunolabeling and confocal imaging analyses **(C)** showed elevated CXCR1 expression in the SH-SY5Y cells treated with METH in comparison with in the controls. Scale bar, 50 μM.

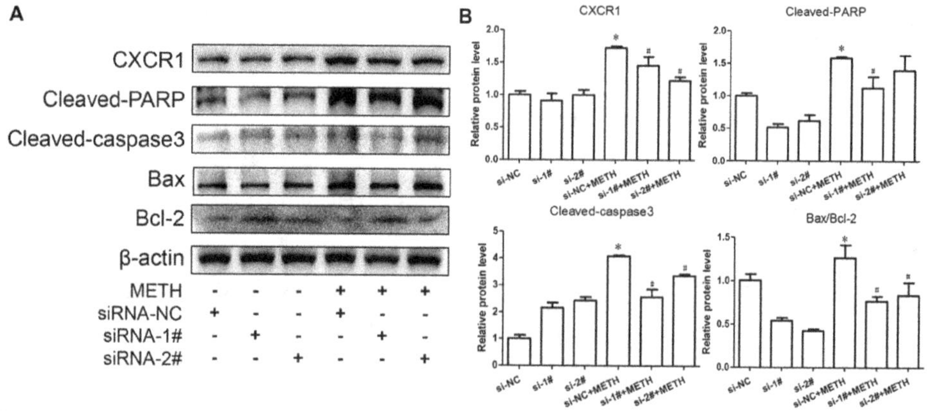

FIGURE 3 | Silencing of CXCR1 expression with small interfering ribonucleic acid (siRNA)-attenuated METH-induced neuronal apoptosis. SH-SY5Y cells were transfected with siRNA targeting CXCR1 or control siRNA for 24 h, followed by 2 mM of METH treatment for 24 h. Western blot **(A)** and quantitative analyses **(B)** were performed to determine CXCR1, cleaved caspase-3, cleaved PARP, Bax and Bcl-2 protein expression. β-actin was used as a loading control. Fold induction relative to the control group is shown. *Represents a significant difference as compared with the non-METH-treated group, $^{*}p < 0.05$. #Represents a significant difference as compared with the scrambled + METH treated group, $^{\#}p < 0.05$. Results are expressed as the mean ± SD of three experiments. Data were analyzed with one-way ANOVA followed by LSD *post hoc* analyses.

midbrain and striatum for further testing. Western blot results showed that CXCR1 protein levels in the prefrontal cortex, hippocampus and midbrain were higher in the subacute exposure group than in the control group (**Figures 1A,C–E**), while the expression of CXCR1 in the striatum showed no obvious effect between the two groups (**Figures 1B,E**). Immunofluorescence staining results also showed that the expression of CXCR1 was increased in the midbrain of METH-treated C57BL/6 mice (**Figure 1F**). In addition, we also observed co-localization of CXCR1 with neurons, indicating that CXCR1 is mainly expressed in the neurons of the midbrain.

To validate this phenomenon *in vitro*, we selected SH-SY5Y cells to determine the expression of CXCR1. SH-SY5Y cells were treated with different concentrations of METH—specifically, 0 mM, 0.5 mM, 1 mM, 1.5 mM, 2 mM, or 2.5 mM—and western blot analysis was performed to detect CXCR1 expression. The results showed that CXCR1 protein expression was increased in a dose-dependent manner in the SH-SY5Y cells (**Figures 2A,B**). CXCR1 protein expression was 3.25-fold higher in the 2.0 mM METH-treated SH-SY5Y cells for 24 h than in the control cells. Immunofluorescence staining results demonstrated the same results (**Figure 2C**). These findings suggest that METH exposure induces CXCR1 protein expression both *in vivo* and *in vitro*.

Importance of CXCR1 Induction in Neuronal Apoptosis Induced by Methamphetamine

To confirm the relationship of CXCR1 and neurotoxicity induced by METH, we designed two siRNA sequences for SH-SY5Y cells to silence CXCR1 expression. The results showed that both of the siRNA sequences could attenuate CXCR1 induction effectively in SH-SY5Y cells (**Figures 3A,B**). After pre-treatment with siRNA#1 or siRNA#2 of CXCR1, the cells were treated with METH (2 mM, 24 h). CXCR1 protein expression decreased respectively, as compared with in the siRNA-NC + METH treatment group (**Figures 3A,B**).

To evaluate the protective effect of CXCR1 silencing from METH-induced neuronal apoptosis, we determined the expression of cleaved caspase-3 and cleaved PARP by western blot analyses. We found that METH increased the level of cleaved caspase-3 and cleaved PARP obviously; this effect was significantly inhibited after CXCR1 silencing (**Figures 3A,B**). We then sought to examine whether Bcl-2/Bax are involved in METH-induced CXCR1-mediated neuronal apoptosis. Western blot analyses were performed to detect changes in Bcl-2 and Bax expression levels with and without CXCR1 knockdown. The results showed that the expression level of Bcl-2, an antiapoptotic factor, was increased following CXCR1 knockdown in comparison with in the si-NC + METH treatment group, while the expression level of Bax, a proapoptotic factor, was decreased (**Figures 3A,B**). Taken together, these results suggest that the silencing of CXCR1 inhibits the Bcl-2/Bax expression and that CXCR1 participates in the mitochondria-mediated apoptosis pathway triggered by METH.

Methamphetamine Increases the Expression of Chemokine IL-8 via Nuclear Translocation of NF-κB in Astrocytes

We have demonstrated that the expression of CXCR1 is upregulated in METH-treated SH-SY5Y cells and may be involved in METH-induced apoptosis. IL-8 is a cytokine secreted mostly by macrophages and epithelial cells. Studies have demonstrated that astrocytes can also secrete IL-8, so we applied METH in human-derived U87MG cells and found that the expression of IL-8 was increased in a dose-dependent manner (**Figures 4A–C**). Specifically, at 2.0 mM, IL-8 protein expression in the U87MG cells was ~1.77-fold higher than in the control cells. Similar effects were observed in the medium of the cells. The concentration of IL-8 in the medium was ~1.38-fold higher than in the control (**Figure 4C**). According to our previous study, the expression of transcription factor NF-κB was upregulated in the METH-treated primary cultured C57BL/6 mouse astrocytes. To verify whether the NF-κB pathway is activated in U87MG cells, cells were exposed to 2.0 mM of METH and then western blot analysis was performed to detect the expressions of NF-κB and phosphor-NF-κB. The results showed that NF-κB protein expression was increased slightly and that phosphor-NF-κB protein expression was significantly increased (**Figures 4D,E**) in the METH-treated U87MG cells as compared with in the control. The expression of IκB kinase (IKK)-α did not change significantly, but the expressions of both IKK-β and phosphor-IKK-α/β were increased, respectively (**Figures 4D,E**). IκB was significantly decreased in the METH-treated U87MG cells. Taken together, these results showed that METH exposure induces the activation of the NF-κB pathway in U87MG cells. To confirm whether the release and expression of IL-8 is associated with NF-κB pathway activation in METH-treated U87MG cells, the inhibitor of NF-κB, Bay 11-7082, was administered to U87MG cells and western blot was performed. Results showed that a blockade of NF-κB reduces METH-induced IL-8 expression in U87MG cells (**Figures 4F,G**). We also detected the concentration of IL-8 in culture medium by ELISA; similar effects were observed (**Figure 4H**).

Co-culture of U87MG Cells and SH-SY5Y Cells Reduced the Apoptosis of SH-SY5Y Cells Induced by Methamphetamine

To explore the effects of METH on neurons in a co-culture mode of astrocytes and neurons, we constructed a cell co-culture model using transwell chambers (**Figure 5A**).

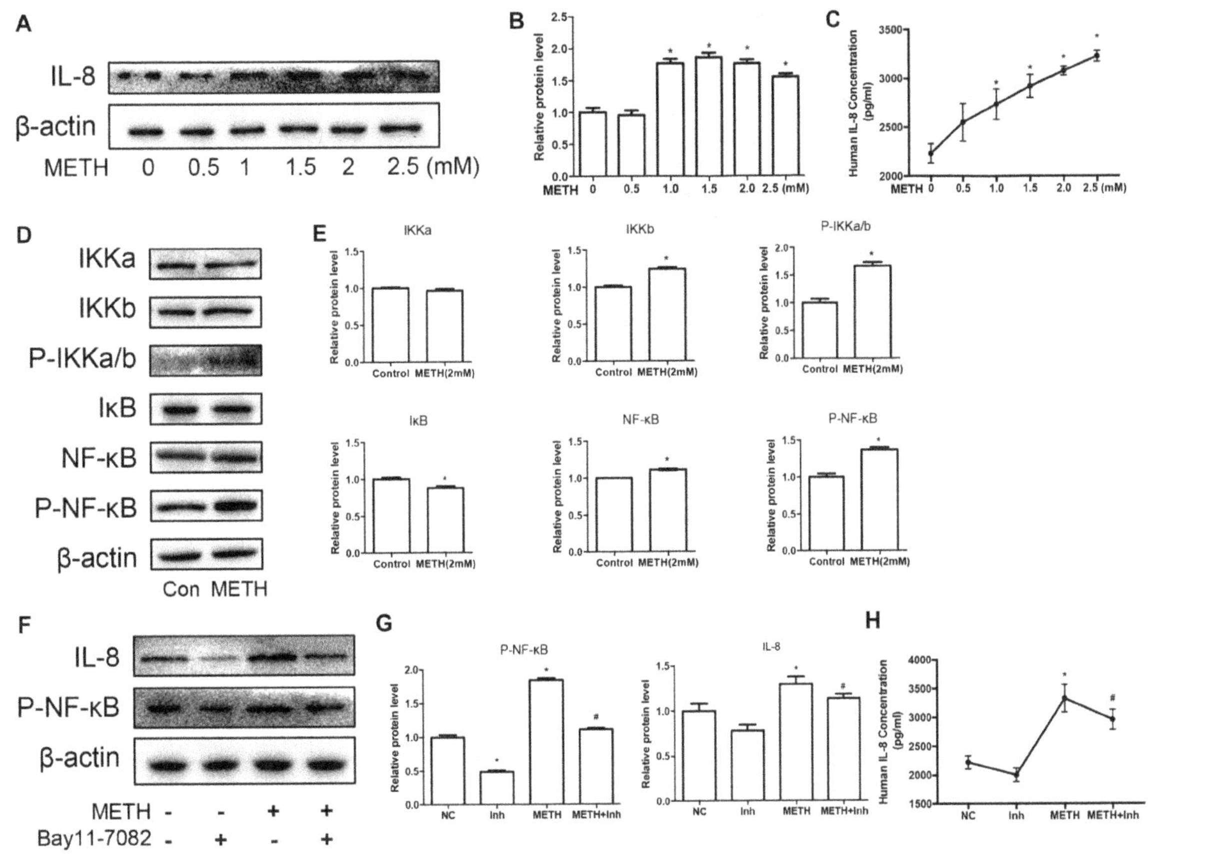

FIGURE 4 | METH increases the expression of chemokine interleukin (IL)-8 via nuclear translocation of NF-κB in astrocytes. U87MG cells were exposed to 0.5 mM, 1 mM, 1.5 mM, 2 mM and 2.5 mM of METH for 24 h **(A)** or 2 mM of METH for 24 h **(D)**. **(F)** U87MG cells were exposed to Bay 11–7082 (10 μM) for 12 h prior to METH (2 mM) treatment as indicated. Western blot **(A,D,F)** and quantitative analyses **(B,E,G)** were performed to determine IL-8, IKK-α, IKK-β, phospho-IKK-α/β, IκB, NF-κB and phospho-NF-κB protein expression. β-actin was used as a loading control. ELISA **(C,H)** was performed to detect the concentration of IL-8 in culture medium supernatant. Fold induction relative to the control group is shown. *Represents a significant difference as compared with the non-METH-treated group, *$p < 0.05$. #Represents a significant difference as compared with the scrambled + METH treated group, #$p < 0.05$. Results are expressed as the mean ± SD of three experiments. Data in **(A,C,F,G)** were analyzed with one-way ANOVA followed by LSD *post hoc* analyses; data in **(D)** were analyzed with Student's *t*-test.

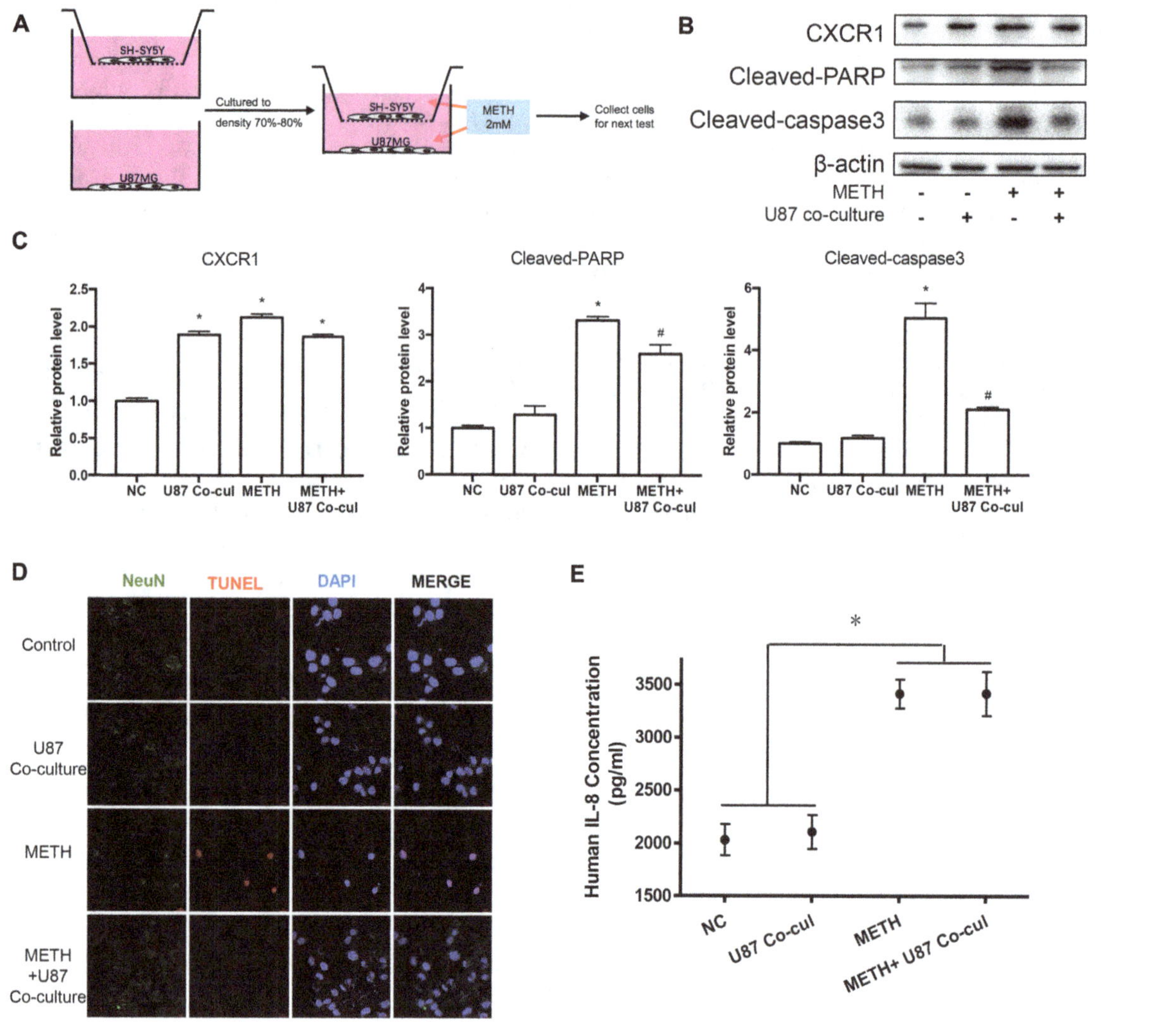

FIGURE 5 | Co-culture of U87MG cells and SH-SY5Y cells reduced the apoptosis of SH-SY5Y cells induced by METH. **(A)** Co-culture pattern diagram. U87MG cells and SH-SY5Y cells were cultured to a density of 90% and passaged into Transwell dishes. SH-SY5Y cells were plated in the upper chamber of the Transwell plate and U87MG cells were spread on the bottom of the Transwell plate and cultured to a density of 70% to 80% respectively. The upper chamber was then placed above the lower chamber and exposed to 2.0 mM of METH for 24 h. Western blot **(B)** and quantitative analyses **(C)** were performed to determine CXCR1, cleaved caspase-3 and cleaved PARP protein expression. β-actin was used as a loading control. Fold induction relative to the control group is shown. *Represents a significant difference as compared with the negative control group, $^{*}p < 0.05$. #Represents a significant difference as compared with the scrambled + METH treated group, $^{\#}p < 0.05$. Results are expressed as the mean ± SD of three experiments. Data were analyzed with one-way ANOVA followed by LSD *post hoc* analyses. terminal deoxynucleotidyl transferase dUTP nick end-labeling (TUNEL) staining and confocal imaging analysis **(D)** was performed to evaluate the SH-SY5Y cells apoptosis. Scale bar, 15 μM. ELISA **(E)** was performed to detect the concentration of IL-8 in culture medium supernatant.

Western blot analysis was performed to detect the expression of neuronal apoptosis-related protein cleaved caspase-3 and cleaved PARP. Our results revealed that cleaved caspase-3 and cleaved PARP expression was significantly attenuated in the co-cultured cells after METH exposure (**Figures 5B,C**). Apoptosis cells were also observed with TUNEL staining (**Figure 5D**). However, the expression of CXCR1 showed no significant difference between in the untreated co-culture group and in the METH-treated co-culture group, which indicated that CXCR1 protein expression is induced by another way in the co-culture model of U87MG cells and SH-SY5Y cells. We also detected the concentration of IL-8 in culture medium by ELISA (**Figure 5E**). Results showed that IL-8 expressions were increased in METH-exposed group, whether co-culture with SH-SY5Y or not.

Silencing of CXCR1 Expression With siRNA Reduced Methamphetamine-Induced Caspase-3 and PARP Activation in Co-cultured Cell Models

To assess the apoptosis levels of co-culture cell models treated by METH with or without CXCR1 siRNA transfection, western blot analysis was conducted. The results are shown

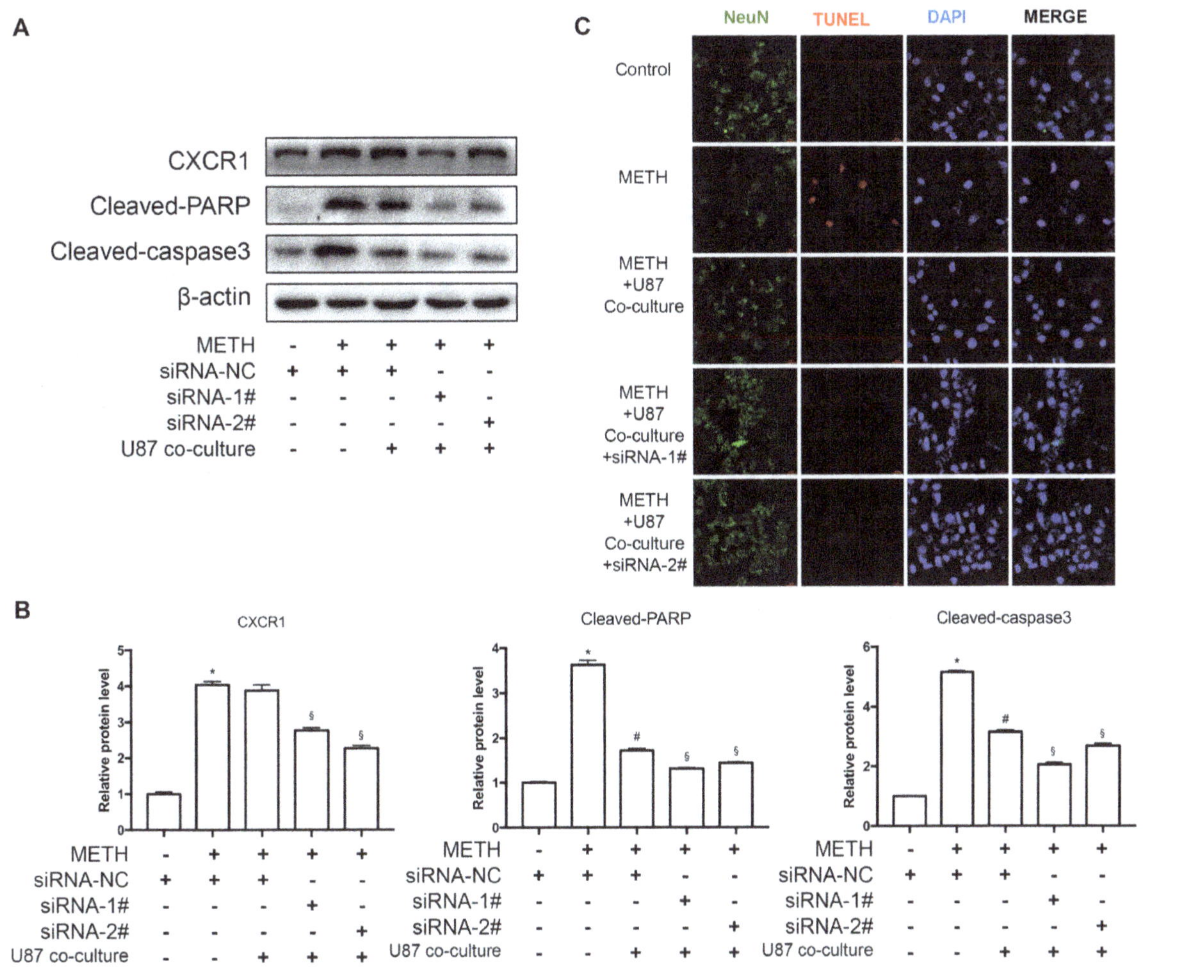

FIGURE 6 | Silencing of CXCR1 expression with siRNA-reduced METH-induced caspase-3 and PARP activation in co-cultured cell models. **(A)** U87MG cells and SH-SY5Y cells were co-cultured in the same manner as before. Before METH treatment, SH-SY5Y cells were transfected with siRNA targeting CXCR1 or control siRNA for 24 h followed by co-cultured with U87MG cells. Simultaneously, 2 mM of METH was added in the medium for 24 h. Western blot **(A)** and quantitative analyses **(B)** were performed to determine CXCR1, cleaved caspase-3 and cleaved PARP protein expression. β-actin was used as a loading control. Fold induction relative to the control group is shown. *Represents a significant difference as compared with the negative control group, $^{*}p < 0.05$. #Represents a significant difference as compared with siRNA NC + METH treated group, $^{\#}p < 0.05$. §Represents a significant difference as compared with siRNA NC + METH treated +U87MG cells co-culture group, $^{\S}p < 0.05$. Results are expressed as the mean ± SD of three experiments. Data were analyzed with one-way ANOVA followed by LSD *post hoc* analyses. TUNEL staining and confocal imaging analysis **(C)** was performed to evaluate the SH-SY5Y cells apoptosis. Scale bar, 15 μM.

in **Figures 6A,B**. The expression of CXCR1 in SH-SY5Y cells was increased in the METH-treated group with or without U87MG cells in the co-culture as compared with in the control group, while both of the siRNA sequences could effectively knockdown the expression of CXCR1. In addition, after the treatment of siRNA of CXCR1, cleaved caspase-3 and cleaved PARP protein expression were significantly decreased in comparison with in the negative control siRNA transfection group. To confirm that silence of CXCR1 protects against METH induced SH-SY5Y cells apoptosis, TUNEL staining was performed (**Figure 6C**). Results suggest that blockade of CXCR1 expression reduces METH-induced apoptosis in SH-SY5Y cells.

Interleukin-8 Increases PARP and Caspase-3 Protein Expression Induced by Methamphetamine *in Vitro*

To verify the effects of IL-8 on neurons in co-culture models treated by METH, exogenous recombinant IL-8 was added to SH-SY5Y cells. We chose two concentrations (10 and 100 ng/ml) to detect the effect of IL-8 on neurons, which were obtained from previous studies (Moriceau et al., 2009; Dwyer et al., 2012; De Buck et al., 2015). In our experiments, these two concentrations of IL-8 had no apparent toxic effects on neurons alone. Then, we checked the expression levels of CXCR1, cleaved caspase-3, and cleaved PARP by use of western blot analysis. Results are shown in **Figures 7A,B**. The expression of CXCR1, cleaved

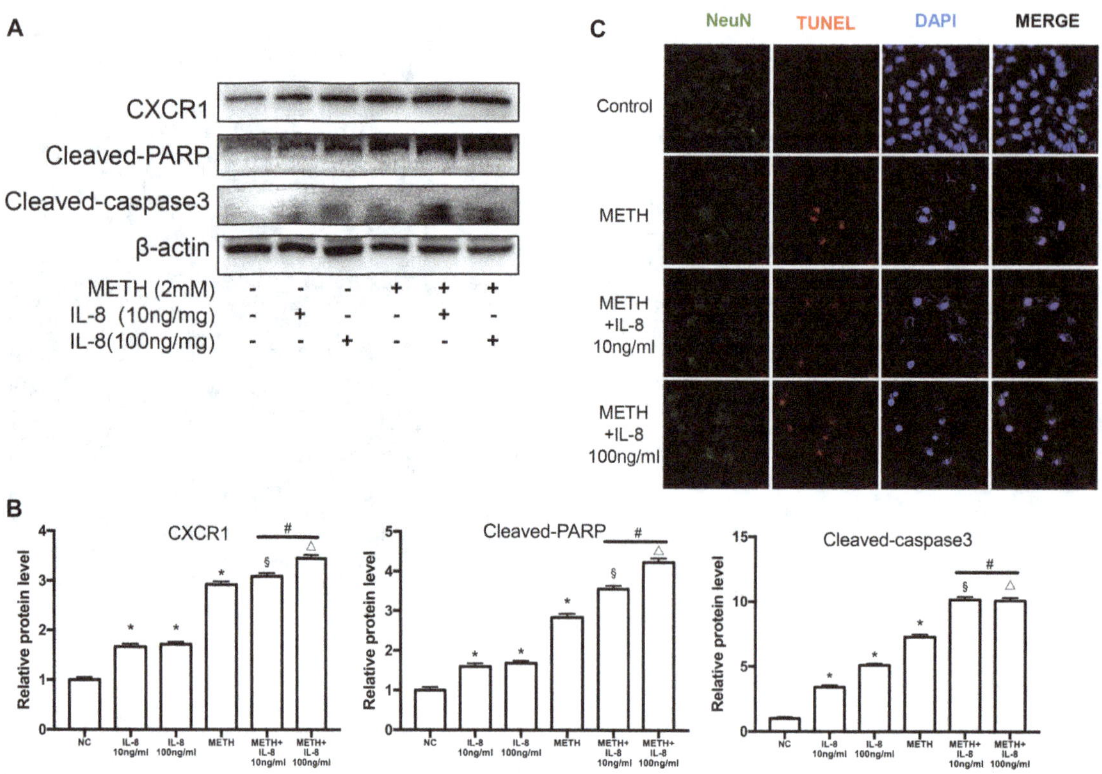

FIGURE 7 | IL-8 increases PARP and caspase-3 protein expression induced by METH *in vitro*. SH-SY5Y cells were treated with 10 ng/ml or 100 ng/ml recombinant human IL-8 for 24 h, given 2 mM of METH simultaneously. Western blot **(A)** and quantitative analyses **(B)** were performed to determine CXCR1, cleaved caspase-3 and cleaved PARP protein expression. β-actin was used as a loading control. Fold induction relative to the control group is shown. *Represents a significant difference as compared with the negative control group, $^*p < 0.05$. #Represents significant difference from METH treated group without IL-8 treatment, $^\#p < 0.05$. §Represents a significant difference as compared with IL-8 (10 ng/mg) treated group, $^\S p < 0.05$. △Represents a significant difference as compared with IL-8 (100 ng/mg) treated group, $^\triangle p < 0.05$. Results are expressed as the mean ± SD of three experiments. Data were analyzed with one-way ANOVA followed by LSD *post hoc* analyses. TUNEL staining and confocal imaging analysis **(C)** was performed to evaluate the SH-SY5Y cells apoptosis. Scale bar, 15 μM.

caspase-3 and cleaved PARP were increased following recombinant IL-8 treatment. Interestingly, METH and two concentrations of recombinant IL-8 exposure together increased the expression of CXCR1, and the expression of cleaved caspase-3 and cleaved PARP was much more increased. We also investigated whether the recombinant IL-8 affects METH-induced neuronal apoptosis using TUNEL staining (**Figure 7C**). These results further demonstrate that IL-8-CXCR1 is involved in METH-induced neuronal apoptosis.

DISCUSSION

In recent years, scholars have studied the direct effects of METH from the classical dopaminergic-related neurotoxicity to more aspects. Researches showed that METH also has direct toxic effects on other cells. The results of our institute and other investigators showed that METH mediates apoptosis of the brain's vascular endothelium through endoplasmic reticulum stress (Cai et al., 2016), mediates the opening of the blood-brain barrier (Xie et al., 2018), activation of astrocytes (Du et al., 2017), and even has some toxic effects to liver and cardiovascular system (Chen R. et al., 2016; Xie et al., 2018). Studies have shown that non-dopaminergic neuron systems play an important role in the development of Parkinson's disease (Guyenet and Crane, 1981; Bonnet, 2000; van der Heeden et al., 2014). METH exposure leads to the loss of neurons in the cerebral cortex and selectively damage pyramidal neurons in the CA3 region of the hippocampus and granule cells with dendritic cells activated by microglia (Kuczenski et al., 2007). In summary, these studies provide more potential targets for METH.

In the present study, we have demonstrated that CXCR1 expression is increased after METH exposure *in vivo* and *in vitro*. We also report that silence of CXCR1 expression using siRNA sequences can protect neuronal apoptosis caused by METH *in vitro* and promote the protective effect of astrocytes. We hypothesized that injury and protection coexist in the effect of astrocytes on METH-induced neuronal apoptosis. IL-8—CXCR1 may play an important role in this dynamic balance.

CXCR1 is a member of the G protein-coupled receptor family that is also a receptor for IL-8. CXCR1 binds IL-8 with high affinity and transduces the signal via the secondary messenger system activated by the G protein (Park et al., 2012; Risnik et al., 2017). Studies have shown that stimulating the neutrophil surface of CXCR1 can lead to neutrophil chemotaxis and activation (Ocana et al., 2017; Tavares et al., 2017), and inhibition of CXCR1 and CXCR2 can reduce the migration of neutrophils to tumor regions (Tavares et al., 2017). Furthermore, oncology research has suggested that blocking CXCR1 can inhibit the differentiation of breast cancer stem cells (Jia et al., 2017), and that CXCR1 is overexpressed in the development of malignant melanoma and involved in cell growth and angiogenesis (Uen et al., 2015; Jacquelot et al., 2016). In the meantime, other study has demonstrated that CX3CR1 can mediate neuronal apoptosis in a cerebral ischemic model, thus potentially playing a role in the pathophysiology of stroke (Wang et al., 2018).

In the current study, we found that the METH exposure increased the expression of CXCR1 *in vivo* and *in vitro*. Immunofluorescence co-localization experiments showed that CXCR1 was mainly expressed on neurons in the midbrain of METH-exposed mice. Besides, the induction of CXCR1 expression by METH occurred in a dose-dependent manner. Inhibition of CXCR1 expression by siRNA sequences also attenuated METH-induced neuronal apoptosis. To verify the role of CXCR1 in METH-induced neuronal apoptosis, we examined two important molecules involved in mitochondrial apoptosis, Bax and Bcl-2. Bax, a water-soluble protein homologous to Bcl-2, is an apoptosis-promoting gene in the Bcl-2 gene family. Bax overexpression can antagonize the protective effect of Bcl-2 and cause cell death (Kuwana et al., 2005; Chen C. et al., 2016). In our previous study, we found that METH exposure can result in the overexpression of Bax and the silencing of Bcl-2 through PUMA, which leads to the mitochondrial apoptotic pathway by releasing cytochrome (Chen C. et al., 2016). The present results showed that, after CXCR1 was inhibited, the expression of Bax was downregulated and the expression of Bcl-2 was upregulated. Meanwhile, the expression of cleaved caspase-3 and cleaved PARP were downregulated, indicating that CXCR1 can mediate METH-induced neuronal apoptosis through the mitochondrial apoptosis pathway.

IL-8 is also known as neutrophil chemokine. It induces target cell chemotaxis, primarily in neutrophils and other granulocytes, causing them to migrate toward the site of infection. IL-8 also induces phagocytosis and is considered to be a potent promoter of angiogenesis (Han et al., 2018; Paulitti et al., 2018). IL-8 can be secreted by any cell that has a Toll-like receptor that is associated with an innate immune response. In our previous study, it was found that Toll-like receptor four mediates METH-induced activation of astrocytes through the NF-κB and caspase-11 signaling pathways (Du et al., 2017). Thus, we detected the expression of IL-8 in U87MG cells and in the culture medium. Results showed that METH application caused the production and secretion of IL-8 in U87MG cells. Furthermore, we also demonstrated that METH exposure induced activation of the NF-κB pathway in U87MG cells, which regulated the expression of IL-8. These findings are consistent with previous studies that suggested that the NF-κB pathway was activated in primary cultured astrocytes exposed to 2.0 mM of METH.

Previous studies have focused on the role of METH in the context of one type of cell, through PUMA, IGFBP5 and other ways to induce neuronal apoptosis (Qiao et al., 2014; Chen C. et al., 2016); METH through NF-κB, caspase-11 and other ways to the induce activation of astrocytes was also evaluated (Du et al., 2017). However, under the stimulation of METH, one question that has not been answered is regarding what happens to neurons when astrocytes and neurons are co-cultured. Studies have found that glial cells involved in the dopaminergic neurons damage (Krencik et al., 2017; Ugbode et al., 2017; Facci et al., 2018). Astrocytes may affect neuronal conditions through diverse molecules such as a-syn or glutamate, with the effect possibly being either protection or damage (Gustafsson et al., 2017; Lee et al., 2017; Madji Hounoum et al., 2017; Yu et al., 2018). In the present study, we used a noncontact, sandwich-type neuron-astrocyte co-culture to study the effects of astrocytes on neurons under the action of METH. Results showed that the neuronal apoptosis was significant reduced in the co-culture group with 2.0 mM of METH for 24 h. This effect is similar to the research of PD, astrocytes rapidly engulf α-syn oligomers resulting in impaired mitochondria, thereby protecting neurons (Gustafsson et al., 2017). According to current research and previous studies (Du et al., 2017), METH treatment of astrocytes alone can cause activation of the TLR4—NF-kB pathway and increased expression of IL 1, 8 and 18. But according to the results of co-culture, astrocytes in the co-culture system protected the damaged neurons. Therefore, we speculate that astrocytes present different states under different processing conditions, and their neuroprotective and injury effects are dynamically balanced. In the present study, the overall performance of astrocytes is the protection state. However, the specific mechanism needs further research.

Other novel findings are that knockdown CXCR1 expression can reduce neuronal apoptosis in an increased fashion. To test whether IL-8 plays a role in this process, we administered exogenous recombinant IL-8 to SH-SY5Y cells in combination with METH. As a result, IL-8 was found to enhance METH-induced apoptosis and to significantly up-regulate CXCR1 expression. These data demonstrated that CXCR1 plays an important role in METH-induced neuronal apoptosis and that the IL-8 secreted by astrocytes is involved in activating CXCR1. The role of astrocytes in neuronal repair may be a double-sided and dynamically balanced process, with damage and protection existing simultaneously. Further studies are needed to illustrate the role of astrocytes.

CONCLUSION

In summary, this study demonstrated that CXCR1 plays an important role in neuronal apoptosis induced by METH. The blockade of CXCR1 expression significantly attenuated METH-induced neuronal apoptosis and enhanced the protective effect of astrocytes on neurons. Moreover, we provide evidence that IL-8 plays a role in neuronal injury. The underlying mechanisms about how astrocytes play a neuroprotective role in the fact of METH exposure and whether other effects could occur requires further research.

AUTHOR CONTRIBUTIONS

S-HD and WZ conducted all the experiments with the help of X-QL and X-HT. D-FQ and HW designed the research. S-HD, CL and XY analyzed and interpreted the results. D-FQ and S-HD wrote the manuscript.

FUNDING

This study was supported by the National Natural Science Foundation of China (Grant No. 81430045 to HW and Grant No.81172907 to D-FQ).

ACKNOWLEDGMENTS

We thank LetPub for its linguistic assistance during the preparation of this manuscript.

REFERENCES

Ashutosh, Kou, W., Cotter, R., Borgmann, K., Wu, L., Persidsky, R., et al. (2011). CXCL8 protects human neurons from amyloid-β-induced neurotoxicity: relevance to Alzheimer's disease. *Biochem. Biophys. Res. Commun.* 412, 565–571. doi: 10.1016/j.bbrc.2011.07.127

Bonnet, A.-M. (2000). Involvement of non-dopaminergic pathways in Parkinson's disease: pathophysiology and therapeutic implications. *CNS Drugs* 13, 351–364. doi: 10.2165/00023210-200013050-00005

Brat, D. J., Bellail, A. C., and Van Meir, E. G. (2005). The role of interleukin-8 and its receptors in gliomagenesis and tumoral angiogenesis. *Neuro Oncol.* 7, 122–133. doi: 10.1215/s1152851704001061

Cadet, J. L., Jayanthi, S., and Deng, X. (2003). Speed kills: cellular and molecular bases of methamphetamine-induced nerve terminal degeneration and neuronal apoptosis. *FASEB J.* 17, 1775–1788. doi: 10.1096/fj.03-0073rev

Cai, D., Huang, E., Luo, B., Yang, Y., Zhang, F., Liu, C., et al. (2016). Nuprl/Chop signal axis is involved in mitochondrion-related endothelial cell apoptosis induced by methamphetamine. *Cell Death Dis.* 7:e2161. doi: 10.1038/cddis.2016.67

Cao, L., Fu, M., Kumar, S., and Kumar, A. (2016). Methamphetamine potentiates HIV-1 gp120-mediated autophagy via Beclin-1 and Atg5/7 as a pro-survival response in astrocytes. *Cell Death Dis.* 7:e2425. doi: 10.1038/cddis.2016.317

Carmena, A., Granado, N., Ares-Santos, S., Alberquilla, S., Tizabi, Y., and Moratalla, R. (2015). Methamphetamine-induced toxicity in indusium griseum of mice is associated with astro- and microgliosis. *Neurotox. Res.* 27, 209–216. doi: 10.1007/s12640-014-9505-9

Chen, C., Qincao, L., Xu, J., Du, S., Huang, E., Liu, C., et al. (2016). Role of PUMA in methamphetamine-induced neuronal apoptosis. *Toxicol. Lett.* 240, 149–160. doi: 10.1016/j.toxlet.2015.10.020

Chen, R., Wang, B., Chen, L., Cai, D., Li, B., Chen, C., et al. (2016). DNA damage-inducible transcript 4 (DDIT4) mediates methamphetamine-induced autophagy and apoptosis through mTOR signaling pathway in cardiomyocytes. *Toxicol. Appl. Pharmacol.* 295, 1–11. doi: 10.1016/j.taap.2016.01.017

Cisneros, I. E., and Ghorpade, A. (2014). Methamphetamine and HIV-1-induced neurotoxicity: role of trace amine associated receptor 1 cAMP signaling in astrocytes. *Neuropharmacology* 85, 499–507. doi: 10.1016/j.neuropharm.2014.06.011

Citro, A., Cantarelli, E., and Piemonti, L. (2015). The CXCR1/2 pathway: involvement in diabetes pathophysiology and potential target for T1D interventions. *Curr. Diab. Rep.* 15:68. doi: 10.1007/s11892-015-0638-x

Clunes, M. T., and Boucher, R. C. (2007). Cystic fibrosis: the mechanisms of pathogenesis of an inherited lung disorder. *Drug Discov. Today Dis. Mech.* 4, 63–72. doi: 10.1016/j.ddmec.2007.09.001

De Buck, M., Berghmans, N., Pörtner, N., Vanbrabant, L., Cockx, M., Struyf, S., et al. (2015). Serum amyloid A1α induces paracrine IL-8/CXCL8 via TLR2 and directly synergizes with this chemokine via CXCR2 and formyl peptide receptor 2 to recruit neutrophils. *J. Leukoc. Biol.* 98, 1049–1060. doi: 10.1189/jlb.3A0315-085R

Dinis-Oliveira, R. J., Carvalho, F., Moreira, R., Duarte, J. A., Proenca, J. B., Santos, A., et al. (2012). Clinical and forensic signs related to opioids abuse. *Curr. Drug Abuse Rev.* 5, 273–290. doi: 10.2174/1874473711205040003

Dorf, M. E., Berman, M. A., Tanabe, S., Heesen, M., and Luo, Y. (2000). Astrocytes express functional chemokine receptors. *J. Neuroimmunol.* 111, 109–121. doi: 10.1016/s0165-5728(00)00371-4

Du, S., Qiao, D., Chen, C., Chen, S., Liu, C., Lin, Z., et al. (2017). Toll-like receptor 4 mediates methamphetamine-induced neuroinflammation through caspase-11 signaling pathway in astrocytes. *Front. Mol. Neurosci.* 10:409. doi: 10.3389/fnmol.2017.00409

Dwyer, J., Hebda, J. K., Le Guelte, A., Galan-Moya, E. M., Smith, S. S., Azzi, S., et al. (2012). Glioblastoma cell-secreted interleukin-8 induces brain endothelial cell permeability via CXCR2. *PLoS One* 7:e45562. doi: 10.1371/journal.pone.0045562

Eltzschig, H. K., and Eckle, T. (2011). Ischemia and reperfusion—from mechanism to translation. *Nat. Med.* 17, 1391–1401. doi: 10.1038/nm.2507

Facci, L., Barbierato, M., and Skaper, S. D. (2018). Astrocyte/microglia cocultures as a model to study neuroinflammation. *Methods Mol. Biol.* 1727, 127–137. doi: 10.1007/978-1-4939-7571-6_10

Flynn, G., Maru, S., Loughlin, J., Romero, I. A., and Male, D. (2003). Regulation of chemokine receptor expression in human microglia and astrocytes. *J. Neuroimmunol.* 136, 84–93. doi: 10.1016/s0165-5728(03)00009-2

Gustafsson, G., Lindstrom, V., Rostami, J., Nordstrom, E., Lannfelt, L., Bergstrom, J., et al. (2017). α-synuclein oligomer-selective antibodies reduce intracellular accumulation and mitochondrial impairment in α-synuclein exposed astrocytes. *J. Neuroinflammation* 14:241. doi: 10.1186/s12974-017-1018-z

Guyenet, P. G., and Crane, J. K. (1981). Non-dopaminergic nigrostriatal pathway. *Brain Res.* 213, 291–305. doi: 10.1016/0006-8993(81)90235-3

Han, J., Li, Y., Liu, X., Zhou, T., Sun, H., Edwards, P., et al. (2018). Metformin suppresses retinal angiogenesis and inflammation *in vitro* and *in vivo*. *PLoS One* 13:e0193031. doi: 10.1371/journal.pone.0193031

Hoffmann, E., Dittrich-Breiholz, O., Holtmann, H., and Kracht, M. (2002). Multiple control of interleukin-8 gene expression. *J. Leukoc. Biol.* 72, 847–855. doi: 10.1189/jlb.72.5.847

Huang, W., Xie, W. B., Qiao, D., Qiu, P., Huang, E., Li, B., et al. (2015). Caspase-11 plays an essential role in methamphetamine-induced dopaminergic neuron apoptosis. *Toxicol. Sci.* 145, 68–79. doi: 10.1093/toxsci/kfv014

Jacquelot, N., Enot, D. P., Flament, C., Vimond, N., Blattner, C., Pitt, J. M., et al. (2016). Chemokine receptor patterns in lymphocytes mirror metastatic spreading in melanoma. *J. Clin. Invest.* 126, 921–937. doi: 10.1172/jci80071

Jia, D., Li, L., Andrew, S., Allan, D., Li, X., Lee, J., et al. (2017). An autocrine inflammatory forward-feedback loop after chemotherapy withdrawal facilitates the repopulation of drug-resistant breast cancer cells. *Cell Death Dis.* 8:e2932. doi: 10.1038/cddis.2017.319

Kim, J. M., Kim, N. I., Oh, Y. K., Kim, Y. J., Youn, J., and Ahn, M. J. (2005). CpG oligodeoxynucleotides induce IL-8 expression in CD34+ cells via mitogen-activated protein kinase-dependent and NF-κB-independent pathways. *Int. Immunol.* 17, 1525–1531. doi: 10.1093/intimm/dxh345

Kita, T., Miyazaki, I., Asanuma, M., Takeshima, M., and Wagner, G. C. (2009). Dopamine-induced behavioral changes and oxidative stress in methamphetamine-induced neurotoxicity. *Int. Rev. Neurobiol.* 88, 43–64. doi: 10.1016/s0074-7742(09)88003-3

Krasnova, I. N., and Cadet, J. L. (2009). Methamphetamine toxicity and messengers of death. *Brain Res. Rev.* 60, 379–407. doi: 10.1016/j.brainresrev.2009.03.002

Krencik, R., Seo, K., van Asperen, J. V., Basu, N., Cvetkovic, C., Barlas, S., et al. (2017). Systematic three-dimensional coculture rapidly recapitulates interactions between human neurons and astrocytes. *Stem Cell Reports* 9, 1745–1753. doi: 10.1016/j.stemcr.2017.10.026

Kuczenski, R., Everall, I., Crews, L., Adame, A., Grant, I., and Masliah, E. (2007). Escalating dose-multiple binge methamphetamine exposure results in degeneration of the neocortex and limbic system in the rat. *Exp. Neurol.* 207, 42–51. doi: 10.1016/j.expneurol.2007.05.023

Kuwana, T., Bouchier-Hayes, L., Chipuk, J. E., Bonzon, C., Sullivan, B. A., Green, D. R., et al. (2005). BH3 domains of BH3-only proteins differentially regulate Bax-mediated mitochondrial membrane permeabilization both directly and indirectly. *Mol. Cell* 17, 525–535. doi: 10.1016/j.molcel.2005.02.003

Lee, J., Horuk, R., Rice, G. C., Bennett, G. L., Camerato, T., and Wood, W. I. (1992). Characterization of two high affinity human interleukin-8 receptors. *J. Biol. Chem.* 267, 16283–16287.

Lee, M. L., Martinez Lozada, Z., Krizman, E. N., and Robinson, M. B. (2017). Brain endothelial cells induce astrocytic expression of the glutamate transporter GLT-1 by a Notch-dependent mechanism. *J. Neurochem.* 143, 489–506. doi: 10.1111/jnc.14135

Loetscher, P., Seitz, M., Clark-Lewis, I., Baggiolini, M., and Moser, B. (1994). Both interleukin-8 receptors independently mediate chemotaxis. Jurkat cells transfected with IL-8R1 or IL-8R2 migrate in response to IL-8, GRO α and NAP-2. *FEBS Lett.* 341, 187–192. doi: 10.1016/0014-5793(94)80454-0

Madji Hounoum, B., Mavel, S., Coque, E., Patin, F., Vourc'H, P., Marouillat, S., et al. (2017). Wildtype motoneurons, ALS-Linked SOD1 mutation and glutamate profoundly modify astrocyte metabolism and lactate shuttling. *Glia* 65, 592–605. doi: 10.1002/glia.23114

Mendieta, L., Granado, N., Aguilera, J., Tizabi, Y., and Moratalla, R. (2016). Fragment C domain of tetanus toxin mitigates methamphetamine neurotoxicity and its motor consequences in mice. *Int. J. Neuropsychopharmacol.* 19:pyw021. doi: 10.1093/ijnp/pyw021

Moriceau, S., Kantari, C., Mocek, J., Davezac, N., Gabillet, J., Guerrera, I. C., et al. (2009). Coronin-1 is associated with neutrophil survival and is cleaved during apoptosis: potential implication in neutrophils from cystic fibrosis patients. *J. Immunol.* 182, 7254–7263. doi: 10.4049/jimmunol.0803312

Ocana, A., Nieto-Jiménez, C., Pandiella, A., and Templeton, A. J. (2017). Neutrophils in cancer: prognostic role and therapeutic strategies. *Mol. Cancer* 16:137. doi: 10.1186/s12943-017-0707-7

Park, S. H., Das, B. B., Casagrande, F., Tian, Y., Nothnagel, H. J., Chu, M., et al. (2012). Structure of the chemokine receptor CXCR1 in phospholipid bilayers. *Nature* 491, 779–783. doi: 10.1038/nature11580

Paulitti, A., Andreuzzi, E., Bizzotto, D., Pellicani, R., Tarticchio, G., Marastoni, S., et al. (2018). The ablation of the matricellular protein EMILIN2 causes defective vascularization due to impaired EGFR-dependent IL-8 production affecting tumor growth. *Oncogene* 37, 3399–3414. doi: 10.1038/s41388-017-0107-x

Pierce, J. W., Schoenleber, R., Jesmok, G., Best, J., Moore, S. A., Collins, T., et al. (1997). Novel inhibitors of cytokine-induced IκBα phosphorylation and endothelial cell adhesion molecule expression show anti-inflammatory effects *in vivo*. *J. Biol. Chem.* 272, 21096–21103. doi: 10.1074/jbc.272.34.21096

Qiao, D., Xu, J., Le, C., Huang, E., Liu, C., Qiu, P., et al. (2014). Insulin-like growth factor binding protein 5 (IGFBP5) mediates methamphetamine-induced dopaminergic neuron apoptosis. *Toxicol. Lett.* 230, 444–453. doi: 10.1016/j.toxlet.2014.08.010

Risnik, D., Podaza, E., Almejún, M. B., Colado, A., Elías, E. E., Bezares, R. F., et al. (2017). Revisiting the role of interleukin-8 in chronic lymphocytic leukemia. *Sci. Rep.* 7:15714. doi: 10.1038/s41598-017-15953-x

Sordillo, P. P., and Helson, L. (2015). Curcumin and cancer stem cells: curcumin has asymmetrical effects on cancer and normal stem cells. *Anticancer Res.* 35, 599–614.

Takahashi, M., Ishiko, T., Kamohara, H., Hidaka, H., Ikeda, O., Ogawa, M., et al. (2007). Curcumin (1,7-bis(4-hydroxy-3-methoxyphenyl)-1,6-heptadiene-3,5-dione) blocks the chemotaxis of neutrophils by inhibiting signal transduction through IL-8 receptors. *Mediators Inflamm.* 2007:10767. doi: 10.1155/2007/10767

Tavares, L. P., Garcia, C. C., Machado, M. G., Queiroz-Junior, C. M., Barthelemy, A., Trottein, F., et al. (2017). CXCR1/2 antagonism is protective during influenza and post-influenza pneumococcal infection. *Front. Immunol.* 8:1799. doi: 10.3389/fimmu.2017.01799

Uen, W. C., Hsieh, C. H., Tseng, T. T., Jiang, S. S., Tseng, J. C., and Lee, S. C. (2015). Anchorage independency promoted tumor malignancy of melanoma cells under reattachment through elevated interleukin-8 and CXC chemokine receptor 1 expression. *Melanoma Res.* 25, 35–46. doi: 10.1097/cmr.0000000000000134

Ugbode, C. I., Smith, I., Whalley, B. J., Hirst, W. D., and Rattray, M. (2017). Sonic hedgehog signalling mediates astrocyte crosstalk with neurons to confer neuroprotection. *J. Neurochem.* 142, 429–443. doi: 10.1111/jnc.14064

van der Heeden, J. F., Marinus, J., Martinez-Martin, P., and van Hilten, J. J. (2014). Importance of nondopaminergic features in evaluating disease severity of Parkinson disease. *Neurology* 82, 412–418. doi: 10.1212/wnl.0000000000000087

Vlahopoulos, S., Boldogh, I., Casola, A., and Brasier, A. R. (1999). Nuclear factor-κB-dependent induction of interleukin-8 gene expression by tumor necrosis factor α: evidence for an antioxidant sensitive activating pathway distinct from nuclear translocation. *Blood* 94, 1878–1889.

Wang, J., Gan, Y., Han, P., Yin, J., Liu, Q., Ghanian, S., et al. (2018). Ischemia-induced neuronal cell death is mediated by chemokine receptor CX3CR1. *Sci. Rep.* 8:556. doi: 10.1038/s41598-017-18774-0

Waugh, D. J. J., and Wilson, C. (2008). The interleukin-8 pathway in cancer. *Clin. Cancer Res.* 14, 6735–6741. doi: 10.1158/1078-0432.ccr-07-4843

Xie, X. L., He, J. T., Wang, Z. T., Xiao, H. Q., Zhou, W. T., Du, S. H., et al. (2018). Lactulose attenuates METH-induced neurotoxicity by alleviating the impaired autophagy, stabilizing the perturbed antioxidant system and suppressing apoptosis in rat striatum. *Toxicol. Lett.* 289, 107–113. doi: 10.1016/j.toxlet.2018.03.015

Yu, W. W., Cao, S. N., Zang, C. X., Wang, L., Yang, H. Y., Bao, X. Q., et al. (2018). Heat shock protein 70 suppresses neuroinflammation induced by α-synuclein in astrocytes. *Mol. Cell. Neurosci.* 86, 58–64. doi: 10.1016/j.mcn.2017.11.013

Zanotto-Filho, A., Braganhol, E., Schröder, R., de Souza, L. H., Dalmolin, R. J., Pasquali, M. A., et al. (2011). NFκB inhibitors induce cell death in glioblastomas. *Biochem. Pharmacol.* 81, 412–424. doi: 10.1016/j.bcp.2010.10.014

Zhang, F., Chen, L., Liu, C., Qiu, P., Wang, A., Li, L., et al. (2013). Up-regulation of protein tyrosine nitration in methamphetamine-induced neurotoxicity through DDAH/ADMA/NOS pathway. *Neurochem. Int.* 62, 1055–1064. doi: 10.1016/j.neuint.2013.03.016

Zhang, Y., Lv, X., Bai, Y., Zhu, X., Wu, X., Chao, J., et al. (2015). Involvement of sigma-1 receptor in astrocyte activation induced by methamphetamine via up-regulation of its own expression. *J. Neuroinflammation* 12:29. doi: 10.1186/s12974-015-0250-7

5

The Effect of Myosin Light Chain Kinase on the Occurrence and Development of Intracranial Aneurysm

Yaying Song[1†], Peixi Liu[2†], Zongwei Li[3], Yuan Shi[2], Jun Huang[4], Sichen Li[2], Yingjun Liu[2], Zhijun Zhang[3], Yongting Wang[3], Wei Zhu[2] and Guo-Yuan Yang[1,3*]*

[1] *Department of Neurology, Ruijin Hospital, Shanghai Jiao Tong University School of Medicine, Shanghai, China,* [2] *Department of Neurosurgery, Huashan Hospital of Fudan University, Shanghai, China,* [3] *Neuroscience and Neuroengineering Research Center, School of Biomedical Engineering, Med-X Research Institute, Shanghai Jiao Tong University, Shanghai, China,* [4] *Shanghai Key Laboratory of Hypertension, Department of Hypertension, Shanghai Institute of Hypertension, Ruijin Hospital, Shanghai Jiao Tong University School of Medicine, Shanghai, China*

***Correspondence:**
Wei Zhu
drzhuwei@fudan.edu.cn
Guo-Yuan Yang
gyyang@sjtu.edu.cn

† These authors have contributed equally to this work

Myosin light chain kinase is a key enzyme in smooth muscle cell contraction. However, whether myosin light chain kinase plays a role in the occurrence or development of intracranial aneurysms is not clear. The present study explored the function of myosin light chain kinase in human intracranial aneurysm tissues. Five aneurysm samples and five control samples were collected, and smooth muscle cells (SMCs) were dissociated and cultured. A label-free proteomic analysis was performed to screen the differentially expressed proteins between aneurysm and control samples. The expression and function of myosin light chain kinase in aneurysms were examined. We found that 180 proteins were differentially expressed between the aneurysm and control samples, among which 88 were increased and 92 (including myosin light chain kinase) were decreased in aneurysms compared to control tissues. In a model of the inflammatory environment, contractility was weakened and apoptosis was increased in aneurysm SMCs compared to human brain SMCs ($p < 0.05$). The knock down of myosin light chain kinase in human brain SMCs caused effects similar to those observed in aneurysm SMCs. These results indicated that myosin light chain kinase plays an important role in maintaining smooth muscle contractility, cell survival and inflammation tolerance.

Keywords: aneurysm, myosin light chain kinase, phenotype switch, proteomic, smooth muscle cell

INTRODUCTION

Intracranial aneurysm (IA), as a cerebrovascular disease, has an annual incidence of approximately 1–2% and is characterized by the ballooning of the intracerebral artery with high mortality due to vascular rupture (Rinkel, 2008; Brown and Broderick, 2014). Ongoing studies characterize the process of IA formation as hemodynamic stress, thrombus formation, extracellular matrix degradation, inflammatory responses and structural changes, including SMC phenotypic modulation and consequently apoptosis (Frosen et al., 2012; Frosen, 2014). The current treatment for IA mainly involves clipping for surgical intervention and endovascular coiling based on its

---

Abbreviations: HBVSMC, human brain vascular smooth muscle cell; IA, intracranial aneurysm; IASMCs, intracranial aneurysm smooth muscle cells; MLCK, myosin light chain kinase; SMA, anti-SM-α actin; SMCs, smooth muscle cells; STA, superficial temporal artery.

special characteristics. Experimental aneurysm studies have mainly focused on endothelial cells, such as the autologous endothelial cell-seed stent (Zhu et al., 2008) and enhanced aneurysm neck endothelialization by erythropoietin-induced endothelial progenitor cell stimulation (Liu et al., 2016). In addition, endothelial injury may result from the reaction and migration of SMCs to the tunica intima (Etminan and Rinkel, 2016). Evidence has also indicated that SMCs might be involved in neo-intima formation in a ligation model (Yuan et al., 2017). Moreover, the dysfunction of endothelial cells and the apoptosis or phenotypic modulation of SMCs could accelerate the progression of aneurysms.

The phenotypic modulation or dedifferentiation of SMCs could be caused by genetic defects or stimulated by stress, which are involved in many vascular diseases (Frosen, 2014; Liu et al., 2015). SMCs alter the synthetic phenotype in the medial layer, thereby weakening the vessel wall, disturbing hemostasis and finally collapsing the vascular structure. Previous studies using microarray (Yu et al., 2014), mRNA sequencing analysis (Kleinloog et al., 2016), and proteomics (Wang et al., 2016) have implicated a group of reported genes, mRNAs and related proteins involved in the proliferation, migration, and apoptosis of SMCs. Previous studies have demonstrated that the injury or death of SMCs by inflammation results in the occurrence and development of aneurysms. Furthermore, SMCs are the main components of the walls of brain vessels and aneurysms (Kondo et al., 1998; Owens, 2007). Because IASMCs were isolated from aneurysm walls, these cells have been considered as a cell model to understand the phenotype and function of SMCs in the formation, progress and rupture of aneurysms (Dai et al., 2006; Bygglin et al., 2011).

The aim of the present study was to explore the role of SMC phenotypic modulation in IA pathogenesis. We used proteomic analysis to explore the specific protein functions in IA pathology. IASMCs were isolated to further explain the results of clinical samples and investigate the role of aneurysm SMCs in IA progression.

MATERIALS AND METHODS

Ethics Statement

This study was approved by the Institutional Review Board (IRB) and the Ethics Committee of Huashan Hospital, Fudan University, China. Each participant provided written informed consent to participate in this study.

Tissue Collection and Label-Free Proteomic

Ten patients with IA who underwent microsurgical clipping were enrolled, and the samples were collected. The control group included patients who underwent STA surgery, followed by unavoidable clipping. Among the 10 samples, 5 were used for label-free proteomics, 2 were used for immunostaining, and 3 were used for western blotting. These 10 samples were frozen immediately at −80°C for further experiments. In addition to these 10 samples, another 4 samples were used for IASMC isolation, of which 3 samples were successful. These 10 samples were all frozen immediately at −80°C for further experiments. Label-free proteomics was commissioned by the Shanghai Branch of the Chinese Academy of Sciences.

IASMC Isolation and Culture

Intracranial aneurysm tissues were obtained from the brain tissues of 3 IA patients during microsurgery. The modified isolation protocol was based on a previously described study (Bygglin et al., 2011; Huang et al., 2017). After clipping, the samples were immediately collected into DMEM supplemented with 5% penicillin/streptomycin. The tissue segments were washed three times with phosphate-buffered saline (PBS) supplemented with 1% penicillin/streptomycin. The surrounding connective tissue was separated, and the endothelial cell layer was scratched gently. Then, the tissues were dissected into 1 mm × 1 mm fragments that were evenly arranged on a dish and incubated in a humidified atmosphere of 5% CO_2 and 95% air at 37°C in a medium comprising DMEM supplemented with 20% fetal bovine serum and 1% penicillin/streptomycin. After 1–2 weeks, the cells grown from the IA explants reached semiconfluence and were subcultured in smooth muscle cell medium (Lonza, Basel, Switzerland) after trypsinization. Control human brain vascular SMCs were obtained from ScienCell Research Laboratories (Carlsbad, CA, United States) and cultured in smooth muscle cell medium. We used the markers anti-myosin-11 and SMA to identify the SMCs.

Immunostaining of Human Tissue Samples

The samples were fixed in 4% paraformaldehyde and embedded in paraffin. Following antigen retrieval by microwaving in pH 6.0 citrate buffer, the sections were incubated with anti-myosin-11 (1:50 dilution; Santa Cruz Biotechnology, Santa Cruz, CA, United States), anti-MLCK (1:200 dilution; Abcam, Cambridge, MA, United States), and anti-SMA (1:100 dilution; Abcam), followed by an immunofluorescent secondary antibody. The brain sections were then stained with DAPI and mounted. Images were taken at different magnifications with a microscope (Leica, Solms, Germany).

MLCK siRNA Interference

Human brain vascular smooth muscle cells (HBVSMCs, Zhongqiao Xinzhou Company, Shanghai, China) were seeded onto six-well plates. Then, 100 nmol/L siRNA was diluted with 250 μl of Opti-MEM (Gibco, Carlsbad, CA, United States) and incubated for 5 min. Next, 10 μl of Lipofectamine® 2000 (Invitrogen, Carlsbad, CA, United States) was diluted with 250 μl of Opti-MEM and incubated for 5 min. The above samples were mixed, generating a final 500 μl Opti-MEM solution, and incubated for 20 min. This medium was added to 2 ml of SMCM (ScienCell, Carlsbad, CA, United States) and incubated with the cells for 6 h. After changing to normal medium, the cells were cultured for 72 h. The interference was detected by real-time PCR and Western blot analysis. The following siRNA sequences were used: si-*mlck*: 5′-3′ CCTGCTTTCATTTTGCCCCC, TCACAAGGCTGAAAGTCCCC.

Cell Viability Assay

Smooth muscle cells were plated in triplicate in 96-well plates at 4×10^3 cells per well. After 24 h, the cells were treated with TNF-α at different doses, including 0, 0.5, 5, 10, 20, and 40 ng/ml for 2 h. The cck-8 assay kit was prepared according to the manufacturer's instructions and then 100 μl was added to each well and incubated for 2 h at 37°C. The absorbance was measured at 450 nm with a spectrometer.

RNA Extraction and Real-Time PCR

Total RNA was isolated from the cells using TRIzol reagent (Invitrogen) according to the manufacturer's instructions. The integrity of the RNA was quantified by using the NanoDrop 1000 spectrophotometer (Thermo Fisher Scientific, UT, United States). The reverse transcription reaction and real-time PCR were performed according to the manufacturer's instructions for the ABScript II cDNA Synthesis Kit (ABclonal, Wuhan, China) and the SYBR Premix ExTaq II Kit (Takara, Dalian, China) by a real-time PCR system (7900HT, ABI). No non-specific amplification was observed based on the dissociation curve. Glyceraldehyde 3-phosphate dehydrogenase (GAPDH) was used as an internal control. The data were analyzed using the comparison Ct ($2^{-\Delta\Delta C_t}$) method and expressed as a fold change relative to the respective control. The following sequences were used for qPCR primers: ACTA2: 5′-3′ TTGAGAAGAGTTACGAGTTG, AGG ACATTGTTAGCATAGAG; MYL9: 5′-3′ CGGGCCACATCCA ATGTCTT, CCATGTTTGAGGATGCGGGT; MLCK: 5′-3′ GGGGACTTTCAGCCTTGTGA, CTGCTTCGCAAAACTTCC TTCT; and CNN1 5′-3′ GGCCCAGAAGTATGACCACC, CCGTCCATGAAGTTGTTGCC.

Western Blotting Analysis

Equal amounts of protein per lane (30 μg) were subjected to electrophoresis on a 12% SDS-PAGE gel. The proteins were electrotransferred onto a polyvinylidene difluoride membrane (PVDF, Millipore, Billerica, MA, United States). The membrane was blocked with 5% non-fat dry milk/0.1% Tween-20 in Tris-buffered saline for 1 h at room temperature. Thereafter, the membrane was incubated with different primary antibodies, including rabbit anti-MLCK (1:5000 dilution, Abcam), rabbit anti-SMA (1:200 dilution, Abcam) and rabbit anti-cleaved caspase-3 (1:1000 dilution, Cell Signaling Technology). Subsequently, the membrane was treated with secondary antibody for 2 h at room temperature. Immunoblots were probed using enhanced ECL substrate (Thermo, Rockford, IL, United States). The chemiluminescence level was recorded using an imaging system (Bio-Rad, Hercules, CA, United States). The results were normalized to β-actin.

Calcium Fluo-4 AM Assay and Contraction Study

Smooth muscle cells were preloaded with the calcium-sensitive fluorophore Fluo-4 AM in extracellular solution for 40 min at room temperature as described in a previous study (Granata et al., 2017). Then, the cells were washed for 30 min at room temperature. Intracellular calcium flux was monitored as a time series, and the acquisition rates were 1 frame every 0.1 ms over 1 min using a Leica confocal microscope before and after the addition of pilocarpine. To detect intracellular calcium release, the SMCs were incubated with calcein. A concentration of 20 mM calcein was used for stimulation. Calcium flux was detected in HBVSMCs (Zhongqiao Xinzhou Company, Shanghai, China), si-*mlck*SMCs, and IASMCs before and after TNF-α stimulation. Five cells were randomly selected from a field of view, and the fluorescent trace was analyzed using ImageJ pro plus software (Media Cybernetics, Bethesda, MD, United States).

Statistical Analysis

All data were expressed as the means ± SE. ANOVA with Student–Newman–Keuls multiple comparisons posttest was used for gene expression. Comparisons between two groups were made by Student's *t*-test. A $p < 0.05$ was considered significantly different. Statistical analysis was carried out with Prism GraphPad 6. Each *in vitro* experimental group was repeated three times, and the experiments were performed separately three times. These outcomes are from data averaged statistically.

RESULTS

Sample Collection and Label-Free Proteomic Analysis

Intracranial aneurysm ($n = 5$) and STA ($n = 5$) groups without significant differences in sex, age, or risk factors were compared. More information is shown in **Supplementary Table 1**. The location of sample collection was shown by HE and Masson staining (**Figure 1A**). The aneurysm wall showed less muscle and collagen compared with the STA wall. Among all 1908 proteins identified from 15426 peptides, 180 significantly differentially expressed proteins between IA and STA were identified, among which 88 were upregulated and 92 were downregulated in IA (**Figure 1B**). GO ontology analysis classified the proteins into "Molecular function," "Cellular component," and "Biological process" subcategories. Further protein expression data were obtained from the KEGG Mapper Pathway to illustrate changes in biological processes (**Figure 1C**). MLCK encodes a regulatory light chain of myosin II, known as myosin light-chain kinase, which was downregulated in IAs. In the vascular smooth muscle contraction pathway, MLCK was involved in the mechanism of smooth muscle contraction (**Figure 1D**).

MLCK Is Downregulated in Both Tissue Samples and Primary IASMCs

Tissue samples from STA and IA were double stained for SMA and MLCK. MLCK showed higher expression in the IA group, and SMA showed weaker expression in the STA group compared with the IA group. Myosin-11 is a marker of mature SMCs, and co-staining with SMA showed a reduction in contractile

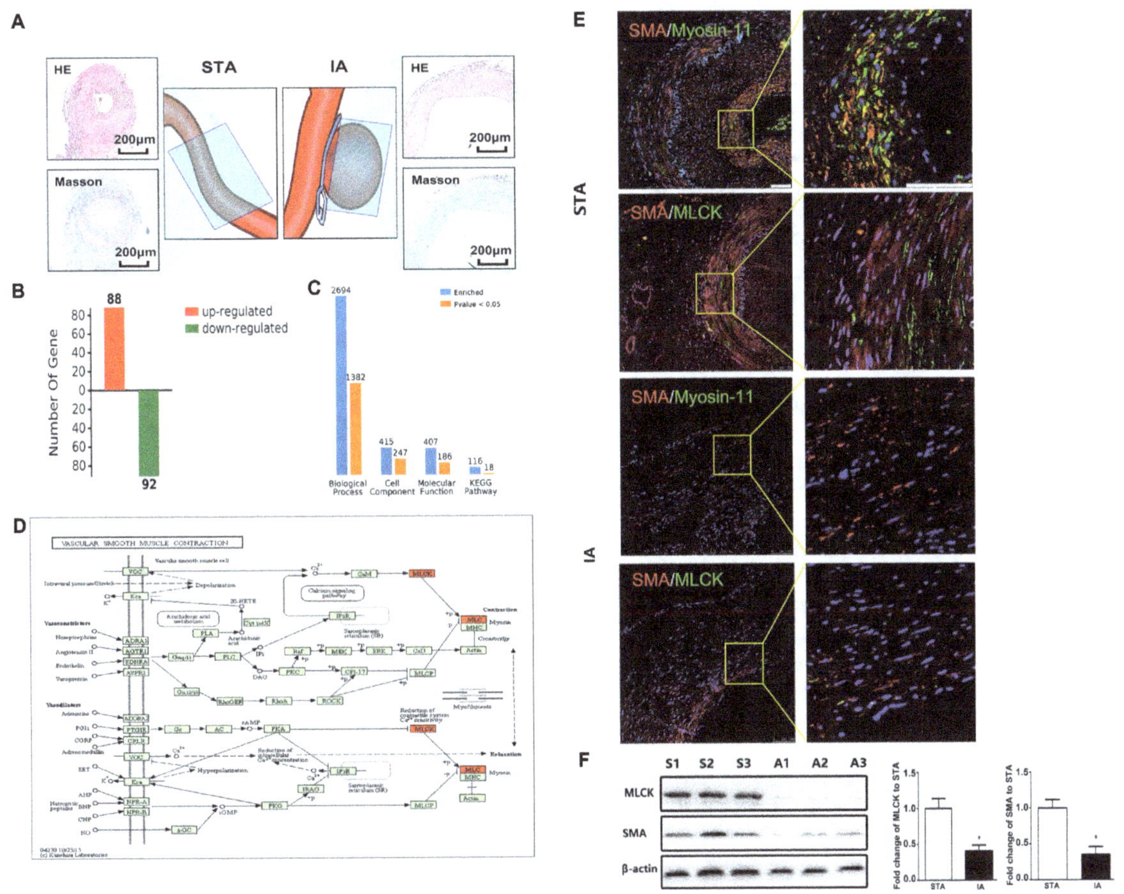

FIGURE 1 | Basic information from label-free proteomics and verification in tissue samples. **(A)** IA and STA illustration with HE and Masson staining show the specimen location for label-free proteomics. **(B)** Significant differences in protein levels between IA and STA. **(C)** GO ontology analysis between IA and STA. **(D)** KEGG pathway mapping of smooth muscle cells (SMCs). **(E)** Double staining for SMA/myosin-11 and SMA/MLCK in STA and IA, with 2× magnification for a closer view. **(F)** Western blot and quantification studies of MLCK and SMA in the tissue sample. S1–S3 represents proteins from three different STA samples, and A1–A3 represents IA samples. STA, superficial temporal artery; IA, intracranial aneurysm.

SMCs. Magnification also showed low SMA expression, which indicated the loss of SMCs in IA tissues. The SMC density showed a significant decrease in the IA sample, indicating that degeneration occurred in the aneurysm wall (**Figure 1E**). The IA samples showed a more significant downregulation of MLCK than STA, consistent with findings in proteomics. SMA was also downregulated, which suggested that functionally mature SMCs were lost in the aneurysm wall (**Figure 1F**). To examine whether the downregulation of MLCK in IA tissue has a similar effect in SMCs, we further isolated primary SMCs from IA walls (IASMCs). IASMCs were morphologically modulated and appeared as spider-like cells with the loss of mature SMC markers. These morphologic changes demonstrated that ductility decreased when stress suddenly increased. Cell viability was also weakened throughout the culture process. IASMCs appeared irregularly shaped and showed weak positivity for SMA, MLCK and myosin-11 compared with HBVSMCs. The results of immunostaining indicated that the IASMCs were in an immature state (**Figure 2**).

MLCK Downregulation in Primary IASMCs and Its Impact on SMC Function

To investigate the function of SMCs, we used siRNA to interfere with *mlck* in HBVSMCs to mimic the genetic defects in IASMCs. The level of *mlck* showed 50% interference, with no significant difference compared with IASMCs (**Figure 3A**). Western blot results showed that the expression of the mature SMC markers MLCK and SMA was decreased in both IASMCs and si-*mlck*SMCs compared with HBVSMCs. We then used cleaved caspase-3 to detect apoptosis. The results indicated that with the loss of mature SMC markers, SMCs probably progressed to apoptosis (**Figure 3B**).

We detected cell contractility in these three groups to further investigate the role of MLCK during SMC contraction. Pilocarpine is a cholinergic agent that can activate the cholinergic receptor. SMCs can respond to the stimulus and contract. When the SMCs were incubated with calcine, intracellular calcium release was detected. The influx of calcium is not the same as "contraction," but the cyclic calcium wave in response to

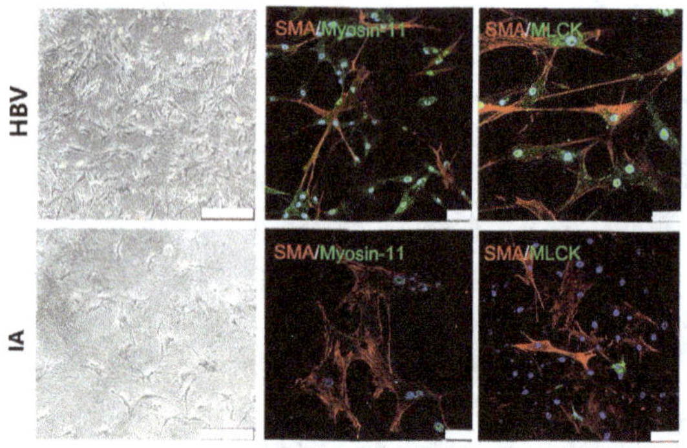

FIGURE 2 | Myosin light chain kinase primary SMCs. Bright field images show IASMCs with more irregular morphology than HBVSMCs. Double staining for SMA/myosin-11 and SMA/MLCK showed that IASMCs were less or weakly positive compared with HBVSMCs. Data are presented as the means ± SD, *$p < 0.05$, bar = 100 μm. HBVSMC, human brain vascular smooth muscle cell; IASMC, intracranial aneurysm smooth muscle cell.

an agonist may reflect cell contractility. SMCs with lower MLCK expression showed reduced contractility in response to stimulation with the cholinergic agent pilocarpine. The local cell morphology of these three groups was also different when simulated by pilocarpine. HBVSMCs showed a spindle shape, and cells with low expression of MLCK showed a more stellate pattern (**Figure 3C**). The intracellular calcium responses of HBVSMCs were different from those of both si-*mlck*SMCs and IASMCs. HBVSMCs generated cyclic calcium waves, whereas si-*mlck*SMCs and especially IASMCs did not generate propagating calcium waves and returned abruptly to basal levels (**Figure 3D**).

Genetic Loss of MLCK Impacts the Inflammatory Responses of SMCs

To mimic the IA environment, we administered TNF-α to explore the proliferation and contractility of SMCs. The mRNA levels of four mature SMC genes, *mlck*, *acta2*, *myl9*, and *cnn1*, were detected after treatment with different doses of TNF-α (**Figure 4A**). We found that mature SMC marker expression was reduced by stimulation with higher doses of TNF-α. The expression of mature SMC markers, such as ACTA2, MYL9, CNN1, and MLCK, was largely decreased after treatment with 40 ng/ml of TNF-α compared with that after treatment with other TNF-α concentrations in cultured SMCs. Therefore, we used a concentration of 40 ng/ml to treat HBVSMCs,

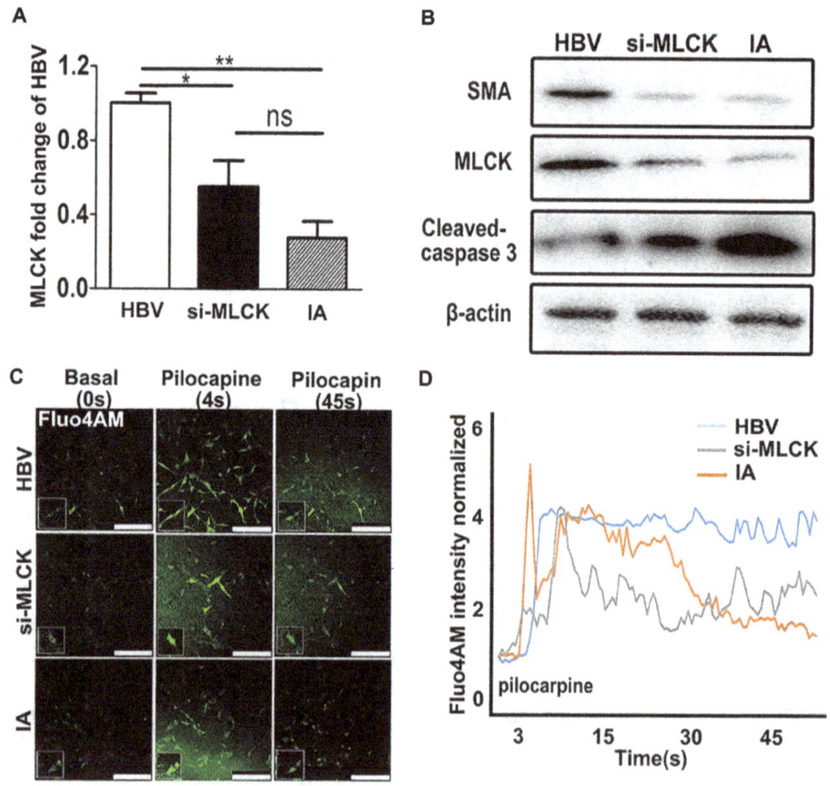

FIGURE 3 | Both si-*mlck*HBVSMCs and IASMCs show weak proliferation and contraction. **(A,B)** MLCK expression in HBVSMCs, si-*mlck*HBVSMCs and primary IASMCs was detected at the mRNA and protein levels. **(C)** Ca^{2+} flux measured by Fluo-4 AM loading and the intensity in HBVSMCs, si-*mlck*HBVSMCs, and IASMCs at a basal level (0 s), upon stimulation with pilocarpine (4 s) and at 45 s after stimulation. **(D)** Quantification of contractility measured as the fluorescence change in the cell surface area of HBVSMCs, si-*mlck*HBVSMCs, and IASMCs. The relative mRNA level was normalized to GAPDH. Data are presented as the means ± SD, *$p < 0.05$, **$p < 0.01$. HBVSMC, human brain vascular smooth muscle cell; IASMC, intracranial aneurysm smooth muscle cell; si-*mlck*SMC, HBVSMCs with interfered *mlck*.

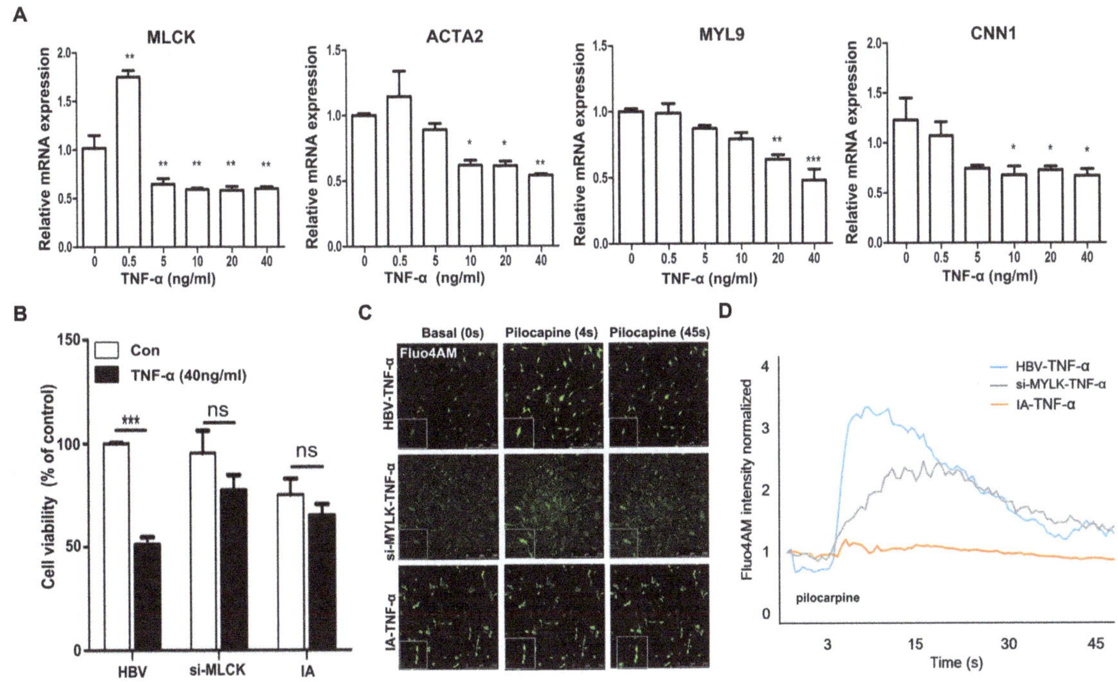

FIGURE 4 | Genetically downregulated MLCK affects cell function more with the stimulation of TNF-α. **(A)** HBVSMCs were treated with a gradient dose of TNF-α and the levels of the mature SMC markers MLCK, ACTA2, MYL9, and CNN1 were detected. **(B)** All three kinds of cells were detected for cell viability by cck-8. **(C)** Ca^{2+} flux measured by loading Fluo-4 AM. **(D)** Quantification of contractility measured as the fluorescence change in the cell surface area of HBVSMCs, si-*mlck*SMCs, and IASMCs. The relative mRNA level was normalized to the control. Data are presented as the means ± SD, *$p < 0.05$, **$p < 0.01$, ***$p < 0.001$. HBVSMC, human brain vascular smooth muscle cell; IASMC, intracranial aneurysm smooth muscle cell; si-*mlck*SMC, HBVSMCs with interfered *mlck*.

si-*mlck*SMC, and IASMCs. Interestingly, HBVSMCs stimulated with TNF-α showed lower cell viability than IASMCs and si-*mlck*SMCs. Thus, the effect of *mlck* deficiency at the genetic level on cell viability may differ from that on inflammation (**Figure 4B**). We redetected cell contractility to further investigate the impact on cell viability. All of the cells showed reduced contractility in response to pilocarpine stimulation, with altered cell morphology. However, HBVSMCs appeared as slim fusiform but still responded to pilocarpine. For IASMCs, the cell morphology was not clear and showed little response to stimulation. The si-*mlck*SMCs appeared as short rod shapes but with a weaker response to calcium stimulation (**Figure 4C**). It was clearly observed that with the reduction of MLCK, the contractility was reduced in all three groups, and IASMCs could hardly generate calcium waves, and cells that genetically lacked MLCK seemed more vulnerable to inflammatory attacks (**Figure 4D**).

DISCUSSION

This study observed the effects of MLCK downregulation in IA samples using a label-free proteomic analysis. SMCs with downregulated MLCK underwent phenotypic modulation and were vulnerable to apoptosis when stimulated with TNF-α. MLCK expression was also decreased in SMCs isolated from IA walls (**Figure 5**). Normal SMCs with downregulated MLCK showed disturbed contractile function and were vulnerable to inflammation. In the label-free proteomic analysis, proteins that play a role in IA pathology were found, which mirrored the results found in previous studies using iTRAQ (Wang et al., 2016). Using a DNA microarray, Chen et al. (2014) found that *myh11, acta2, mlck, and myl9* were differentially expressed genes associated with VSMC contraction (Chen et al., 2014). Our study focused on SMCs and highlighted the impact of losing MLCK on IA formation.

After MLCK was downregulated, the contraction of SMCs was disturbed. SMCs undergo phenotypic modulation with less contractile gene expression and show a pro-inflammatory, dedifferentiated phenotype (Owens, 1998; Owens et al., 2004; Yoshida and Owens, 2005). Phenotypic modulation and eventual degeneration have been considered to promote the formation and progression of IA. IASMCs were first isolated by Bygglin et al. (2011), and the present study was the first to detect the functions of IASMCs and the contractile gene *mlck*. IASMCs were morphologically modulated and appeared as spider-like cells with the loss of mature SMC features. A study of rabbit aneurysm models showed large and stellate cells with long cytoplasmic extensions (Dai et al., 2006). The IASMCs no longer displayed tightly arranged spindle-like cells, and the morphology was replaced by a sparse disordered form whereby the cells dissociated from each other (Merei and Gallyas, 1980). This morphological change suggests a decrease in ductility when placed under sudden stress.

Smooth muscle cell contraction and relaxation are affected not only by how much Ca^{2+} is infused but also by oxidative stress and inflammation directly or indirectly (Carvalho-de-Souza et al., 2013). Previous studies have demonstrated that the myosin light chain phosphatase regulatory light chains were associated with myosin, whose contractions were dictated by the stimulation of myosin ATPase activity (Murthy, 2006). Calcium increased and bound to calmodulin, and the calcium/calmodulin complexes then combined with MLCK, leading to MLC phosphorylation. We also showed the morphological changes and detected the contractility of IASMCs and HBVSMCs with downregulated *mlck* in **Figures 3**, **4**. With increasing Ca^{2+} levels, calcium could bind to calmodulin and lead to MLC phosphorylation. In an aneurysm environment, the intracellular concentration of Ca^{2+}, as a second messenger, decreased. Therefore, the phosphorylation induced by calcium was also downregulated. Ca^{2+}/calmodulin-dependent MLCK phosphorylated MLC is essential for the initiation of smooth muscle contractions. Sustained MLC phosphorylation could be induced by Ca-independent MLCK. Thus, with downregulated MLCK, MLC phosphatase activity may also be downregulated. MLCK and MLC phosphatase activity can coregulate the relaxation of cells (Murthy, 2006). SMC relaxation can result from the activation of TGR5 by the inhibition of the RhoA/Rho kinase pathway. MLC phosphorylation via Ca^{2+}-independent MLCK can sustain G protein activation and regulate the inhibition of MLC phosphatase (Rajagopal et al., 2013).

The *mlck* gene is prominently differentially expressed in IA compared with control arteries. In our experiment, MLCK expression could also be decreased by inflammatory stimulation, and SMCs showed lower viability with a higher dose of TNF-α. During intracranial inflammation, MLCK expression was decreased in SMCs. Additionally, MLC phosphatase activity might also be downregulated (Murthy, 2006). It is largely unknown whether MLCK causes or results from the phenotypic and functional modulation of SMCs. Our results suggested that MLCK might promote SMC dysfunction; however, this is the first study to support this hypothesis. Although TNF-α could suppress the expression of mature SMC genes, normal SMCs could retain the ability of contraction under certain inflammatory conditions (Ali et al., 2013). When inflammation occurred in SMCs lacking MLCK, the contractions were profoundly suppressed, thus explaining why some IA failed to maintain stability throughout the lifetime of an individual.

Intracranial aneurysm pathology also involves apoptosis, which leads to the weakening intima and media of aneurysm walls. Inflammatory factors, such as TNF-α, could trigger an inductive signal in the initiation of apoptosis (Jamous et al., 2007; Sprague and Khalil, 2009; Ait-Oufella et al., 2011). TNF-α and IL-1 are the most important pro-inflammatory factors, which are often used to induce a focal inflammatory response. Numerous studies have demonstrated that TNF-α increases and plays a critical role in the occurrence and development of aneurysms. Therefore, we used TNF-α to mimic the environment of an aneurysm (Ali et al., 2013; Aoki et al., 2014; Starke et al., 2014). Under an inflammatory environment, smooth muscle relaxation was inhibited, which was caused by soluble guanylyl activity (Rajagopal et al., 2015). SMC dysfunction or apoptosis were considered the destructive events in a ruptured IA. Our results indicated that the loss of MLCK in SMCs could lead to apoptotic progression and promote injury in a pro-inflammatory environment. The continuous loss of SMCs and functional synthesis of collagen and matrix components resulted in aneurysm enlargement and rupture (Frosen, 2014). We found that there was a significant decrease in the expression of MLCK in IA by proteomic analysis. After interfering with MLCK RNA silencing, we found that SMC contractility decreased and apoptosis increased. In addition, SMA expression was downregulated. Therefore, we speculated that decreased MLCK could promote aneurysm development. Many other decreased proteins in IA and STA tissues, such as filamin-C, desmin, and aldehyde dehydrogenase, were found through proteomic analysis. We demonstrated that MLCK was less expressed in IASMCs and that other proteins were usually not expressed in SMCs. Therefore, we chose MLCK as a target in the current study.

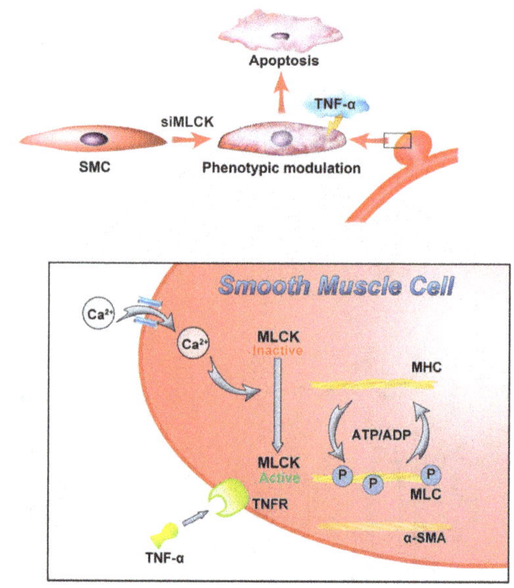

FIGURE 5 | Down-regulation of MLCK weaken the contractile function and with vulnerably reaction to inflammation. The loss of MLCK expressed as phenotypic modulation and calcium dependent phosphorylation was further disturbed. In the TNF environment, the morphologically altered smooth muscle is weaker and more susceptible to apoptosis.

There were also some limitations that need further improvement. IASMCs were isolated from IA tissues and cultured using SMCM. We isolated SMCs from the IA wall directly by cutting small pieces of IA tissues and only used cells within three passages to avoid the effects of *in vitro* culture conditions. The cells were derived with an apoptotic nature and could not be passed for several generations, thus limiting experiments *in vitro*. Whether the *mlck* gene plays a key role in IASMC dysfunction and whether *mlck* mutations exist still needs further exploration.

In summary, the present study provided novel evidence showing that the downregulation of MLCK in SMCs impacted the organization of mature and functional arteries. The lower expression of MLCK further led to increased apoptosis during the inflammatory response, which resulted in the loss of SMCs and contractile dysfunction. This study is the first to use primary IASMCs to detect SMC function. Our results provide further support that MLCK is involved in SMC contraction, proliferation and apoptosis. Our results also showed that the homeostasis of SMCs is crucial to the normal function of intracranial arteries.

AUTHOR CONTRIBUTIONS

YaS and PL designed and performed the experiments, analyzed the data, and drafted the manuscript and figures. G-YY and WZ conceived the project, designed the experiments, and edited the final manuscript. ZL and YuS participated in the study design. JH, SL, and YL contributed to specimen collection. ZZ and YW helped to design the experiments and interpreted the data.

FUNDING

This study was supported by the Shanghai Sailing Program, project no. 16YF1401200 (PL), the NSF of China, no. 81571102 (WZ), the National Key Research and Development Program of China (2016YFC1300600), the National Natural Science Foundation of China (81771251, G-YY; 81771244, ZZ; 81471178, G-YY; and 81522015, YW), the K. C. Wong Education Foundation (G-YY), and the Science and Technology Commission of Shanghai Municipality (17ZR141 3600, ZZ).

ACKNOWLEDGMENTS

The authors would like to thank Yanye Feng for the proteomic analysis and the staff of the Neuroscience and Neuroengineering Center for collaborative support.

REFERENCES

Ait-Oufella, H., Taleb, S., Mallat, Z., and Tedgui, A. (2011). Recent advances on the role of cytokines in atherosclerosis. *Arterioscler. Thromb. Vasc. Biol.* 31, 969–979. doi: 10.1161/ATVBAHA.110.207415

Ali, M. S., Starke, R. M., Jabbour, P. M., Tjoumakaris, S. I., Gonzalez, L. F., Rosenwasser, R. H., et al. (2013). TNF-alpha induces phenotypic modulation in cerebral vascular smooth muscle cells: implications for cerebral aneurysm pathology. *J. Cereb. Blood Flow Metab.* 33, 1564–1573. doi: 10.1038/jcbfm.2013.109

Aoki, T., Fukuda, M., Nishimura, M., Nozaki, K., and Narumiya, S. (2014). Critical role of TNF-alpha-TNFR1 signaling in intracranial aneurysm formation. *Acta Neuropathol. Commun.* 2:34. doi: 10.1186/2051-5960-2-34

Brown, R. D. Jr., and Broderick, J. P. (2014). Unruptured intracranial aneurysms: epidemiology, natural history, management options, and familial screening. *Lancet Neurol.* 13, 393–404. doi: 10.1016/S1474-4422(14)70015-8

Bygglin, H., Laaksamo, E., Myllarniemi, M., Tulamo, R., Hernesniemi, J., Niemela, M., et al. (2011). Isolation, culture, and characterization of smooth muscle cells from human intracranial aneurysms. *Acta Neurochir.* 153, 311–318. doi: 10.1007/s00701-010-0836-x

Carvalho-de-Souza, J. L., Varanda, W. A., Tostes, R. C., and Chignalia, A. Z. (2013). BK channels in cardiovascular diseases and aging. *Aging Dis.* 4, 38–49.

Chen, L., Fan, Y., and Wan, J. (2014). Screening of key genes of unruptured intracranial aneurysms by using DNA microarray data analysis techniques. *Genet. Mol. Res.* 13, 758–767. doi: 10.4238/2014.January.31.2

Dai, D., Ding, Y. H., Kadirvel, R., Danielson, M. A., Lewis, D. A., Cloft, H. J., et al. (2006). A longitudinal immunohistochemical study of the healing of experimental aneurysms after embolization with platinum coils. *AJNR Am. J. Neuroradiol.* 27, 736–741.

Etminan, N., and Rinkel, G. J. (2016). Unruptured intracranial aneurysms: development, rupture and preventive management. *Nat. Rev. Neurol.* 12, 699–713. doi: 10.1038/nrneurol.2016.150

Frosen, J. (2014). Smooth muscle cells and the formation, degeneration, and rupture of saccular intracranial aneurysm wall–a review of current pathophysiological knowledge. *Transl. Stroke Res.* 5, 347–356. doi: 10.1007/s12975-014-0340-3

Frosen, J., Tulamo, R., Paetau, A., Laaksamo, E., Korja, M., Laakso, A., et al. (2012). Saccular intracranial aneurysm: pathology and mechanisms. *Acta Neuropathol.* 123, 773–786. doi: 10.1007/s00401-011-0939-3

Granata, A., Serrano, F., Bernard, W. G., Mcnamara, M., Low, L., Sastry, P., et al. (2017). An iPSC-derived vascular model of marfan syndrome identifies key mediators of smooth muscle cell death. *Nat. Genet.* 49, 97–109. doi: 10.1038/ng.3723

Huang, J., Song, J., Qu, M., Wang, Y., An, Q., Song, Y., et al. (2017). MicroRNA-137 and microRNA-195* inhibit vasculogenesis in brain arteriovenous malformations. *Ann. Neurol.* 82, 371–384. doi: 10.1002/ana.25015

Jamous, M. A., Nagahiro, S., Kitazato, K. T., Tamura, T., Aziz, H. A., Shono, M., et al. (2007). Endothelial injury and inflammatory response induced by hemodynamic changes preceding intracranial aneurysm formation: experimental study in rats. *J. Neurosurg.* 107, 405–411. doi: 10.3171/JNS-07/08/0405

Kleinloog, R., Verweij, B. H., Van Der Vlies, P., Deelen, P., Swertz, M. A., De Muynck, L., et al. (2016). RNA sequencing analysis of intracranial aneurysm walls reveals involvement of lysosomes and immunoglobulins in rupture. *Stroke* 47, 1286–1293. doi: 10.1161/STROKEAHA.116.012541

Kondo, S., Hashimoto, N., Kikuchi, H., Hazama, F., Nagata, I., and Kataoka, H. (1998). Apoptosis of medial smooth muscle cells in the development of saccular cerebral aneurysms in rats. *Stroke* 29, 181–188; discussion 189. doi: 10.1161/01.STR.29.1.181

Liu, P., Zhou, Y., An, Q., Song, Y., Chen, X., Yang, G. Y., et al. (2016). Erythropoietin stimulates endothelial progenitor cells to induce endothelialization in an aneurysm neck after coil embolization by modulating vascular endothelial growth factor. *Stem Cells Transl. Med.* 5, 1182–1189. doi: 10.5966/sctm.2015-0264

Liu, R., Leslie, K. L., and Martin, K. A. (2015). Epigenetic regulation of smooth muscle cell plasticity. *Biochim. Biophys. Acta* 1849, 448–453. doi: 10.1016/j.bbagrm.2014.06.004

Merei, F. T., and Gallyas, F. (1980). Role of the structural elements of the arterial wall in the formation and growth of intracranial saccular aneurysms. *Neurol. Res.* 2, 283–303. doi: 10.1080/01616412.1980.11739584

Murthy, K. S. (2006). Signaling for contraction and relaxation in smooth muscle of the gut. *Annu. Rev. Physiol.* 68, 345–374. doi: 10.1146/annurev.physiol.68.040504.094707

Owens, G. K. (1998). Molecular control of vascular smooth muscle cell differentiation. *Acta Physiol. Scand.* 164, 623–635. doi: 10.1111/j.1365-201X.1998.tb10706.x

Owens, G. K. (2007). Molecular control of vascular smooth muscle cell differentiation and phenotypic plasticity. *Novartis Found. Symp.* 283, 174–191; discussion 191–193, 238–241. doi: 10.1002/9780470319413.ch14

Owens, G. K., Kumar, M. S., and Wamhoff, B. R. (2004). Molecular regulation of vascular smooth muscle cell differentiation in development and disease. *Physiol. Rev.* 84, 767–801. doi: 10.1152/physrev.00041.2003

Rajagopal, S., Kumar, D. P., Mahavadi, S., Bhattacharya, S., Zhou, R., Corvera, C. U., et al. (2013). Activation of G protein-coupled bile acid receptor, TGR5, induces smooth muscle relaxation via both Epac- and PKA-mediated inhibition of RhoA/Rho kinase pathway. *Am. J. Physiol. Gastrointest. Liver Physiol.* 304, G527–G535. doi: 10.1152/ajpgi.00388.2012

Rajagopal, S., Nalli, A. D., Kumar, D. P., Bhattacharya, S., Hu, W., Mahavadi, S., et al. (2015). Cytokine-induced S-nitrosylation of soluble guanylyl cyclase and expression of phosphodiesterase 1A contribute to dysfunction of longitudinal smooth muscle relaxation. *J. Pharmacol. Exp. Ther.* 352, 509–518. doi: 10.1124/jpet.114.221929

Rinkel, G. J. (2008). Natural history, epidemiology and screening of unruptured intracranial aneurysms. *Rev. Neurol.* 164, 781–786. doi: 10.1016/j.neurol.2008.07.012

Sprague, A. H., and Khalil, R. A. (2009). Inflammatory cytokines in vascular dysfunction and vascular disease. *Biochem. Pharmacol.* 78, 539–552. doi: 10.1016/j.bcp.2009.04.029

Starke, R. M., Chalouhi, N., Jabbour, P. M., Tjoumakaris, S. I., Gonzalez, L. F., Rosenwasser, R. H., et al. (2014). Critical role of TNF-alpha in cerebral aneurysm formation and progression to rupture. *J. Neuroinflammation* 11:77. doi: 10.1186/1742-2094-11-77

Wang, J., Yu, L., Huang, X., Wang, Y., and Zhao, J. (2016). Comparative proteome analysis of saccular intracranial aneurysms with iTRAQ quantitative proteomics. *J. Proteomics* 130, 120–128. doi: 10.1016/j.jprot.2015.09.014

Yoshida, T., and Owens, G. K. (2005). Molecular determinants of vascular smooth muscle cell diversity. *Circ. Res.* 96, 280–291. doi: 10.1161/01.RES.0000155951.62152.2e

Yu, L., Fan, J., Wang, S., Zhang, D., Wang, R., Zhao, Y., et al. (2014). Gene expression profiles in intracranial aneurysms. *Neurosci. Bull.* 30, 99–106. doi: 10.1007/s12264-013-1398-8

Yuan, F., Wang, D., Xu, K., Wang, J., Zhang, Z., Yang, L., et al. (2017). Contribution of vascular cells to neointimal formation. *PLoS One* 12:e0168914. doi: 10.1371/journal.pone.0168914

Zhu, W., Tian, Y., Zhou, L. F., Wang, Y., Song, D., Mao, Y., et al. (2008). Development of a novel endothelial cell-seeded endovascular stent for intracranial aneurysm therapy. *J. Biomed. Mater. Res. A* 85, 715–721. doi: 10.1002/jbm.a.31592

6

A Novel Tetramethylpyrazine Derivative Protects Against Glutamate-Induced Cytotoxicity Through PGC1α/Nrf2 and PI3K/Akt Signaling Pathways

Haiyun Chen[1,2], Jie Cao[2], Zeyu Zhu[2], Gaoxiao Zhang[2], Luchen Shan[2], Pei Yu[2], Yuqiang Wang[2], Yewei Sun[2] and Zaijun Zhang[2]**

[1] Institute of Biomedical and Pharmaceutical Sciences, Guangdong University of Technology, Guangzhou, China, [2] Institute of New Drug Research and Guangzhou Key Laboratory of Innovative Chemical Drug Research in Cardio-Cerebrovascular Diseases, Jinan University College of Pharmacy, Guangzhou, China

***Correspondence:**
Yewei Sun
yxy0723@163.com
Zaijun Zhang
zaijunzhang@163.com

Glutamate-induced excitotoxicity is one of the main causes of neuronal cell death in stroke. Compound **22a** has been previously reported as a promising neuroprotective compound derived from tetramethylpyrazine, which is a widely used active ingredient of traditional Chinese medicine Chuanxiong (Ligusticum wallichii Franchat). Compound **22a** can protect neurons from oxidative stress-induced PC12 cell death and alleviates the infarct areas and brain edema in a rat permanent middle cerebral artery occlusion model. In the current work, we further investigated the neuroprotective effects and underlying mechanisms of compound **22a** against glutamate-induced excitotoxicity in primary culture of rat cerebellar granule neurons (CGNs). We found that pretreatment with compound **22a** prevented glutamate-induced neuronal damage by maintaining mitochondrial membrane potential and attenuating cellular apoptosis. Compound **22a** could also enhance peroxisome proliferator-activated receptor gamma coactivator 1-alpha (PGC1α) transcriptional activity and induce nuclear accumulation of Nrf2 in PC12 cells. Accordingly, pretreatment with compound **22a** reversed the glutamate-induced down-regulation of expression of the proteins PGC1α, transcriptional factor NF-E2-related factor 2 (Nrf2), and hemooxygenase 1 (HO-1). In addition, compound **22a** increased the phosphorylation of phosphoinositide 3-kinase (p-PI3K), phosphorylated protein kinase B (p-Akt), and glycogen synthase kinase 3β (p-GSK3β). Meanwhile, the small interfering RNA-mediated silencing of PGC1α expression and selective inhibitors targeting PI3K/Akt (LY294002 and Akt-iv) could significantly attenuate the neuroprotective effect of compound **22a**. Taken together, compound **22a** protected against glutamate-induced CGN injury possibly in part through regulation of PGC1α/Nrf2 and PI3K/Akt pathways.

Keywords: ischemic stroke, tetramethylpyrazine derivative 22a, excitotoxicity, neuroprotection, peroxisome proliferator-activated receptor gamma coactivator 1-alpha

---

Abbreviations: Akt, protein kinase B; CGN, cerebellar granule neurons; Cyt C, cytochrome c; GSK3β, glycogen synthase kinase 3β; HO-1, hemooxygenase 1; MMP, mitochondria membrane potential; Nrf2, transcriptional factor NF-E2-related factor 2; PGC1α, peroxisome proliferator-activated receptor gamma coactivator 1-alpha; PI3K, phosphatidylinositol 3-kinase; ROS, reactive oxygen species; TMP, tetramethylpyrazine.

INTRODUCTION

Ischemic stroke is one of the major causes of human death and disability worldwide (Donnan et al., 2008). Glutamate-induced excitotoxicity has been demonstrated to be involved in neuronal cell death in stroke (Lai et al., 2014). Physiologically, glutamate acts as one of the main excitatory neurotransmitters in the central nervous system (CNS), contributing to normal neural transmission, development, differentiation, and plasticity. Under pathological conditions, however, overproduction of extracellular glutamate leads to uncontrolled, continuous depolarization of neurons in a toxic process called excitotoxicity. Glutamate-induced excitotoxicity is associated with the over-stimulation of glutamate receptors, inducing the impairment of intracellular Ca^{2+} homeostasis and subsequently leading to overproduction of free radicals, overactivation of proteases and kinases, etc. (Wang and Qin, 2010; Lai et al., 2014). Particularly, the overloading intracellular Ca^{2+} and overproduction of free radicals have been shown to induce mitochondrial dysfunction by down-regulating PGC1α, which plays a protective role against neurodegenerative conditions (Sano and Fukuda, 2008; Wareski et al., 2009). Although great progress has been made, the exact mechanism underlying glutamate-induced cytotoxicity is still not clear. Nonetheless, it has been reported that dysregulation of PI3K/Akt and Nrf2 signaling pathways contributes to glutamate-induced excitotoxicity (Jing et al., 2012; Pang et al., 2016). Stimulation of the PI3K/Akt pathway is neuroprotective against hypoxic and excitotoxic neuronal death *in vitro* and ischemic neuronal death *in vivo*, and there is increasingly evidence to indicate cross talk between the Nrf2 and PI3K/Akt pathways in response to glutamate caused cell injury (Jo et al., 2012; Lee et al., 2015).

Since the exact causes of ischemic stroke have yet to be elucidated, currently there are no pharmacological treatments to ameliorate glutamate excitotoxicity and provide neuroprotection for brain ischemic stroke (Lau and Tymianski, 2010). Thrombolysis via the intravenous (i.v.) administration of recombinant tissue plasminogen activator remains the only treatment currently available for acute ischemic stroke. In addition, it is of great concern that clinical trials investigating neuroprotective agents for the development of new stroke therapies have generally been unsuccessful (Grupke et al., 2014). As a result, numerous researchers have been exploring potentially active plant-derived agents, hoping to meet this unmet need and discover a disease-modifying drug (Zhang et al., 2014). Traditional Chinese medicine focuses on the overall regulation of the pathophysiological condition of the entire body, a trait that makes these compounds particularly promising in the treatment of complex diseases (Ghosh et al., 2014). TMP is one of the mainly biologically active constituents derived from the traditional Chinese medicine Chuanxiong (Ligusticum wallichii Franchat) and has been widely used to treat cardio- and cerebro-vascular diseases in clinic (Liu et al., 2003; Xue et al., 2011). In our previous study, a TMP-derived compound **22a** was designed to combine caffeic acid (Touaibia et al., 2011) (another natural compound with versatile pharmacological activities) and a nitrone group (Floyd et al., 2013) (a strong free radical-trapping agent) with TMP. We found that compound **22a** exhibited strong ROS scavenging activity and exerted protective effects in models of ischemic stroke *in vivo* (Chen et al., 2017). In the present study, the neuroprotective effects of compound **22a** against glutamate-induced excitotoxicity on primary culture of rat CGNs, and the underlying mechanisms of action, were further investigated.

MATERIALS AND METHODS

Chemicals and Reagents

All media and supplements used for cell cultures were purchased from Gibco (Carlsbad, CA, United States), unless otherwise noted. ATP assay kit was obtained from Beyotime (Beyotime, China). LY294002 and Akt-iv was obtained from Sigma-Aldrich (St. Louis, MO, United States). PGC1α siRNA, scrambled siRNA and transfection reagent were purchased from Santa Cruz Biotechnology (Santa Cruz, CA, United States). RIPA lysis buffer, phenylmethanesulfonyl fluoride (PMSF), and halt phosphatase inhibitor cocktail were purchased from Pierce Biotechnology (Rockford, IL, United States). Antibodies against phospho-Ser473 Akt, phospho-Ser9 GSK3β, Bcl-2 and Bax were obtained from Cell Signaling Technology (Beverly, MA, United States). Antibodies against β-actin, PGC1α, Nrf2 and HO-1 were obtained from Santa Cruz Biotechnology (Santa Cruz, CA, United States). All other reagents were from Sigma-Aldrich (St. Louis, MO, United States) except where stated otherwise.

Primary Cell Cultures

Eight-day-old Sprague-Dawley rats were obtained from the Experimental Animal Center of Sun Yat-sen University. The detailed methodology used to separate the CGNs is described in our previous publication (Chen H.Y. et al., 2015). Briefly, neurons were seeded at a density of 1.0–1.5 × 10^5 cells/well in basal modified Eagle's medium supplemented with 10% fetal bovine serum, 25 mM KCl, 2 mM glutaMax and penicillin (100 U/mL)/streptomycin (100 μg/mL). The cultures were grown at 37°C for 24 h. The growth of non-neuronal cells was limited by adding cytosine arabinoside (10 μM). Using this protocol, 95–99% of the cultured cells were granule neurons. All experiments were performed in CGNs at 8 days *in vitro* (DIV).

All experiments were conducted in accordance with the guidelines of the Experimental Animal Care and Use Committee of Jinan University. The experimental protocols were approved by the Ethics Committee for Animal Experiments of Jinan University.

MTT Reduction Assay

The tetrazolium salt 3-(4,5-dimethylthiazol-2-yl)-2,5-diphenyltetrazolium bromide dye (MTT) assay was used to assess neurotoxicity. The assay was performed according to the procedure described in our previous work (Chen H.Y. et al., 2015). Briefly, neurons were cultured in 96-well plates for 8 DIV. Treatments of compound **22a** (0.1, 1, 10, 100 μM), TMP (100 μM) and memantine (5 μM) were used as controls for 2 h before 200 μM glutamate was added to the media. To determine the possible pathways involved in the effect of compound **22a**, CGNs were pretreated with 1 μM LY294002 (a PI3K inhibitor) or 1 μM Akt-iv (an Akt inhibitor) for 30 min before administration of compound **22a** (10 μM), and were then challenged by glutamate. After 24 h, the media of each well was supplemented with 10 μL of 5 mg/mL MTT, and the plate was put in an incubator at 37°C for 4 h under humidified conditions. A microplate reader was used to measure the absorbance of the samples at 570 nm wavelength.

Lactate Dehydrogenase (LDH) Release

The activity of LDH released into the incubation medium was used as an indicator to determine cellular injury. CGNs were pretreated with compound **22a** (0.1, 1, 10, 100 μM) or TMP (100 μM) and memantine (5 μM) for 2 h, then 200 μM glutamate was added to incubated for 24 h. The cytotoxicity detection kit (Roche Applied Science, Germany) was used to determine LDH activity. LDH release was calculated according to the manufacturer's instructions. A microplate reader was used to measure the absorbance at 490 nm wavelength. Cytotoxicity (%) was calculated with the following equation:

$$\text{Cytotoxicity (\%)} = (\text{experimental LDH release} - \text{spontaneous LDH release})/(\text{Maximum LDH release} - \text{spontaneous LDH release})^{*}100$$

Experimental LDH release represents the activity of released LDH in cells pretreated with test compounds and glutamate, Spontaneous LDH release represents the activity of released-LDH in untreated normal cells, and Maximum LDH release represents maximum LDH activity determined by lysing the cells (100% dead cells) with Triton X-100 (final concentration 2% for 4 h at 37°C). All assays were performed in six-replicates and repeated three times.

Hoechst Staining

Chromatin condensation was detected by nucleus staining with Hoechst 33342 (Beyotime, China) as previously described (Chen H.Y. et al., 2015). CGNs of 4–5 × 10^5 cells/well were cultured in a 24-well plate for 8 DIV. Pretreatment of compound **22a** (100 μM) and memantine (5 μM) as the positive control at the indicated concentrations for 2 h before 200 μM glutamate was added into the media. After 24 h, cells were washed with ice-cold phosphate-buffered saline (PBS) and fixed with 4% formaldehyde in PBS. Hoechst 33342 (5 mg/mL) was added to the media for 5 min at 4°C. Samples were observed and photos were taken under a fluorescence microscope. The fluorescence images were photo-taken from three different fields of each experiment with a total of three independent experiments. The number of apoptotic nuclei was counted and expressed as a percentage of total 100 nuclei counted/field.

Measurement of Intracellular Reactive Oxygen Species (ROS)

Cerebellar granule neurons were cultured in 96-well plates at a density of 1.0–1.5 × 10^5 cells/well for 8 DIV. After pretreatment with compound **22a** (0.1, 1, 10, 100 μM) or memantine (5 μM) for 2 h, they were then exposed to 200 μM glutamate for 24 h. The total intracellular ROS were detected using H_2DCF-DA (10 μM), and a microplate reader was used to measure the fluorescence intensity. The fluorescence intensity/per well was normalized against the MTT absorption value of the same well. The fluorescence values of the treated group were calculated as a percentage of the fluorescence of the control cells.

Measurement of Mitochondrial Membrane Potential

Cerebellar granule neurons were placed in a 96-well plate at a density of 1.0–1.5 × 10^5 cells/well. After 8 DIV, compound **22a** or memantine was added to pretreat cells at the indicated concentrations for 2 h. After exposure to 200 μM glutamate for 24 h, the cells were washed three times and then stained with 2 μM JC-1 (Beyotime, China), a molecular probe to measure mitochondrial membrane potential (MMP), for 10 min. The microplate reader was used to measure the fluorescence intensity using 490 nm/530 nm excitation and 525 nm/590 nm dual emissions. The mitochondrial accumulation of JC-1 is dependent upon MMP, which is calculated as a decrease in the ratio of 590 nm to 525 nm emissions.

Measurement of Intracellular ATP Levels

Cerebellar granule neurons were placed in a 96-well plate at a density of 1.0–1.5 × 10^5 cells/well. After 8 DIV, **22a** or memantine was added to pretreat at the indicated concentrations for 2 h. After the following incubation with 200 μM glutamate for 24 h, a ATP Assay Kit was used to detect the intracellular ATP levels by using the (Beyotime, China) according to the manufacturer's protocol. The intracellular ATP levels of the treated group were normalized to the control cells'.

Western Blot Assay

Cerebellar granule neurons were cultured in a 6-well plate at a density of 2 × 10^6 per well in 1.5 mL. At 8 DIV, cells were pretreated with **22a** for 2 h before incubation with 200 μM glutamate for another 12 h. Cells were harvested in a cell lysis buffer supplemented with 1% PMSF (phenylmethanesulfonyl fluoride) as well as 1% protease inhibitor cocktail (Roche Applied Science). The cellular protein concentrations were determined by the BCA assay (Pierce, Rockford, IL, United States) after incubation for 15 min on ice and centrifugation (14,000 *g*) for 10 min at 4°C. SDS sample buffer was added to dilute the cell lysates, and the mixture was heated for 5 min at 100°C. The protein (30 μg) was separated on a 10% SDS–polyacrylamide gel. After transferring protein to polyvinyldifluoride membranes, 5% BSA was used as a blocking buffer to block the membranes. After incubation with the primary antibodies at 4°C overnight, signals were attained by binding a secondary antibody conjugated to horseradish peroxidase. Blots were detected using the chemiluminescence enhancer detection ECL plus kit (Fude Biological Technology Co., Ltd., China) and images captured using a detecting system (Carestream Health, United States). Quantitation of the digitalized images was analyzed based on their mean pixel density by using Carestream software system, and described as an expression ratio of target protein to β-actin (a loading control protein).

Silencing of PGC1α by Small Interfering RNA (siRNA)

Cerebellar granule neurons at 8 DIV were transfected with siRNA using transfection reagent Opti-MEM I (Invitrogen, Carlsbad, CA, United States) and Lipofectamine2000 (Invitrogen) according to the manufacturer's instructions and the previous studies' (Kim et al., 2014). Experiments were carried out 24 h after the cells were transfected with PGC1α siRNA or scrambled siRNA.

PGC1α Transcriptional Activity

PC12 cells were plated in 24-well plates and transfected with a PGC1α luciferase reporter plasmid along with Renilla luciferase control vector by using the Amaxa Nucleofector II, which can be used for transfection of any DNA vectors (expression plasmids, shRNA vectors) into difficult-to-transfect cell lines and primary cells. Then 12 h after transfection, the cells were treated with compound **22a** at the indicated concentrations for 24 h. Cells were harvested and analyzed using a Dual-Glo luciferase assay kit (Promega, Madison, WI, United States) following the manufacturer's instructions. Firefly luciferase activity was normalized to Renilla luciferase activity.

Immunofluorescence

Cerebellar granule neurons of 4–5 × 10^5 cells/well were cultured in a 24-well plate for 8 DIV, and were treated with compound **22a** (100 μM). After 12 h, cells were washed with ice-cold phosphate-buffered saline (PBS) and fixed with 4% formaldehyde in PBS for 30 min at room temperature. The cells were washed with ice-cold PBS containing 5% BSA acting as a blocking buffer for 1 h at room temperature before being incubated with anti-Nrf2 antibody (1:500) overnight at 4°C. The cells were then washed with ice-cold PBS and incubated with FITC antibody (1:200) (Sigma-Aldrich, St. Louis, MO, United States) containing 200 nM DAPI for 2 h at room temperature. Samples were observed and photos were taken under a fluorescence microscope.

Statistical Analysis

All experiments were carried out at least three times with different neuronal preparations, data from which was presented as means ± SEM. Analysis of variance (ANOVA) and Bonferroni's

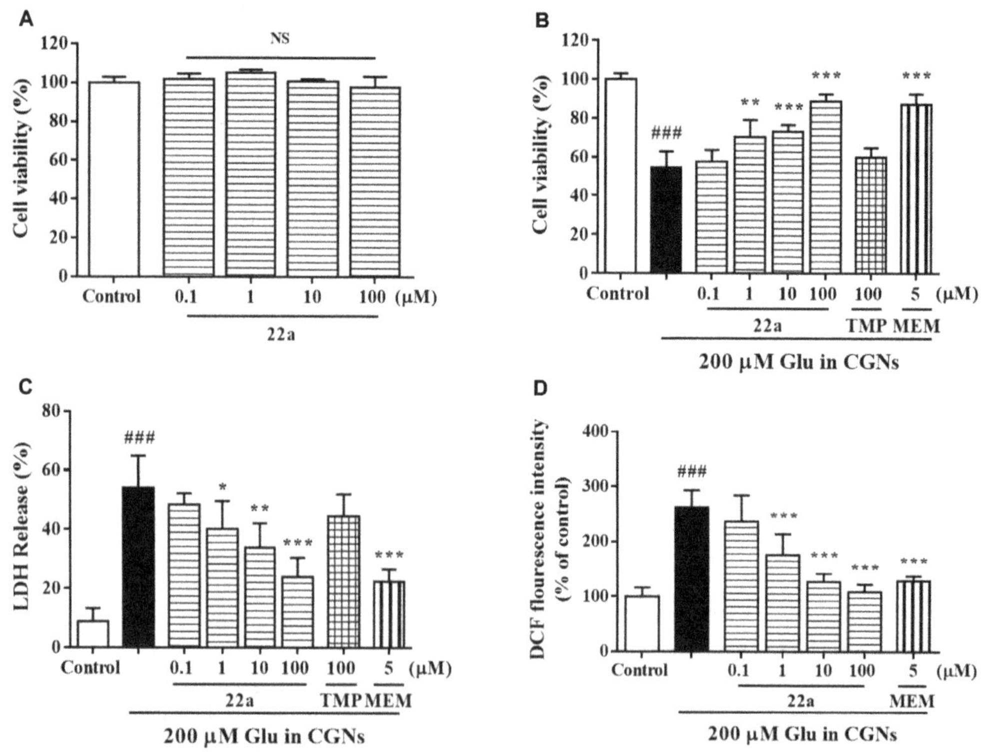

FIGURE 1 | Compound **22a** prevents glutamate-induced neurotoxicity. **(A)** Toxicity of compound **22a** on CGNs. CGNs were pre-incubated with compound **22a** for 24 h. Cell viability was measured using the MTT assay. **(B)** Compound **22a** prevents glutamate-induced neuronal death in CGNs. CGNs were pre-incubated with various agents for 2 h, then exposed to 200 μM glutamate. Cell viability was measured at 24 h post glutamate challenge using the MTT assay. **(C)** Compound **22a** prevents glutamate-induced increase of LDH in CGNs (% of control). CGNs were pre-incubated with various agents for 2 h, then exposed to 200 μM glutamate. LDH release was measured at 24 h after glutamate challenge. **(D)** Compound **22a** attenuates glutamate-induced increase of ROS in CGNs. CGNs were pre-incubated with various compounds for 2 h, then exposed to 200 μM glutamate for another 24 h. Intracellular hydrogen peroxide was measured by DCF-DA. Data were expressed as the mean ± SEM of three separate experiments; $^{###}p < 0.001$ versus control group; $^{*}p < 0.05$, $^{**}p < 0.01$, and $^{***}p < 0.001$ versus glutamate group. Ctrl means control. Glu, glutamate. MEM, memantine.

post-test were used for statistical comparisons, with $P < 0.05$ being considered as statistical significance.

RESULTS

Compound 22a Effectively Prevents Glutamate-Induced Neurotoxicity

At 8 DIV, CGNs were exposed to increasing concentrations of glutamate, which induced a concentration-dependent neuronal death from 50 to 1000 μM (data not shown). Since low doses of glutamate induced apoptosis instead of necrosis in primary CGNs (Du et al., 1997), a 200 μM glutamate concentration that produced approximately 54% neuronal loss was used for the subsequent experiments. Treatment with compound **22a** up to 100 μM for 24 h didn't cause any cytotoxicity to CGNs (**Figure 1A**). Pretreatment with serial concentrations of compound **22a** (1–100 μM) could prevent glutamate-induced toxicity and the maximum cell viability reached 88.7% at 100 μM, similar to that of positive control memantine (87.1%) and higher than that of TMP (60.0%) (**Figure 1B**). The neuroprotection of compound **22a** against glutamate triggered cytotoxicity was more potent than that of TMP.

To further confirm the protection of compound **22a** against glutamate-induced neurotoxicity, we measured the LDH release and intracellular ROS production in CGNs. Compound **22a** and memantine significantly prevented glutamate-induced LDH release. TMP (100 μM) had a marginal effect in this model (**Figure 1C**). Furthermore, pretreatment with compound **22a** from 1 to 100 μM and memantine significantly decreased the intracellular ROS overproduction caused by glutamate in CGNs (**Figure 1D**).

Compound 22a Inhibits Glutamate-Induced Cellular Apoptosis in CGNs

It has been reported that a 200 μM glutamate concentration induced neuronal damage via apoptosis (Du et al., 1997). Compound **22a** and memantine significantly reversed the cell counts of nuclear condensation induced by glutamate (**Figures 2A,B**). In **Figure 2C**, two apoptosis related proteins, Bcl-2 and Bax, were determined by Western blot analysis. It was found that pretreatment with compound **22a** reversed the Bcl-2 down-regulation and Bax up-regulation induced by glutamate. The Bcl-2/Bax ratio was increased by pretreatment with compound **22a** in a concentration-dependent manner (**Figure 2D**).

Compound 22a Improves the Mitochondrial Dysfunction Induced by Glutamate

To examine whether the neuroprotective effects of compound **22a** was due to preservation of mitochondrial function, we

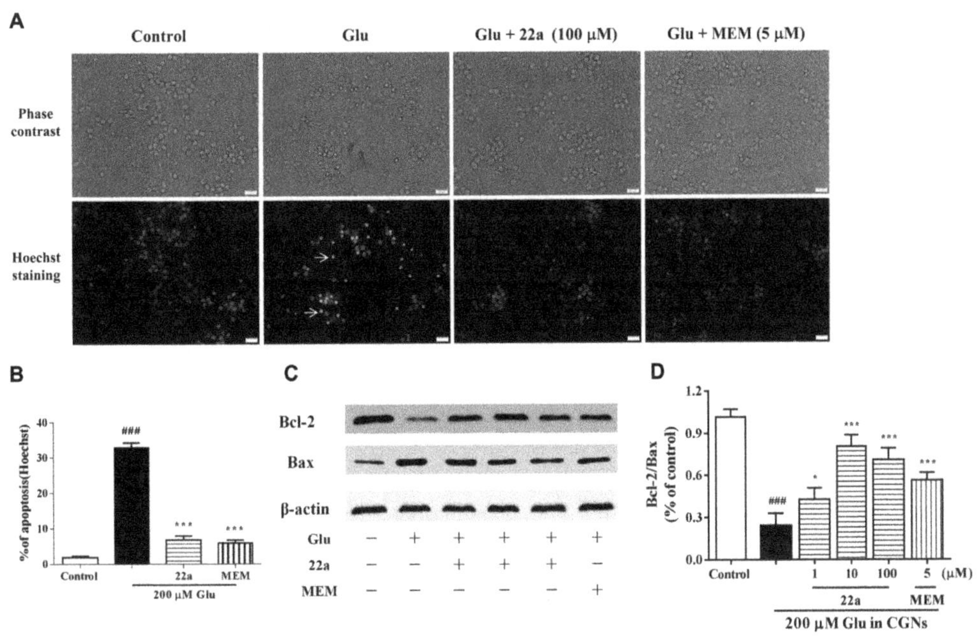

FIGURE 2 | 22a inhibits glutamate-induced cell apoptosis in CGNs. **(A)** Compound **22a** prevents glutamate-induced increase of pyknotic nuclei in CGNs. CGNs were pre-incubated with various agents for 2 h, then exposed to 200 μM glutamate. CGNs were stained with Hoechst 24 h after the glutamate challenge. Photographs were from a representative experiment; experiments were repeated three times (original magnification 400×). **(B)** Statistical analysis of the number of pyknotic nuclei. The number of pyknotic nuclei with condensed chromatin was counted from representative Hoechst staining photomicrographs and is represented as a percentage of the total number of nuclei counted. **(C)** Western blot of apoptosis related proteins Bcl-2 and Bax. **(D)** Densitometry analysis of protein expression ratios of Bcl-2 and Bax. Data were expressed as the mean ± SEM of three separate experiments; $^{###}p < 0.001$ versus control group; $^{*}p < 0.05$ and $^{***}p < 0.001$ versus glutamate group.

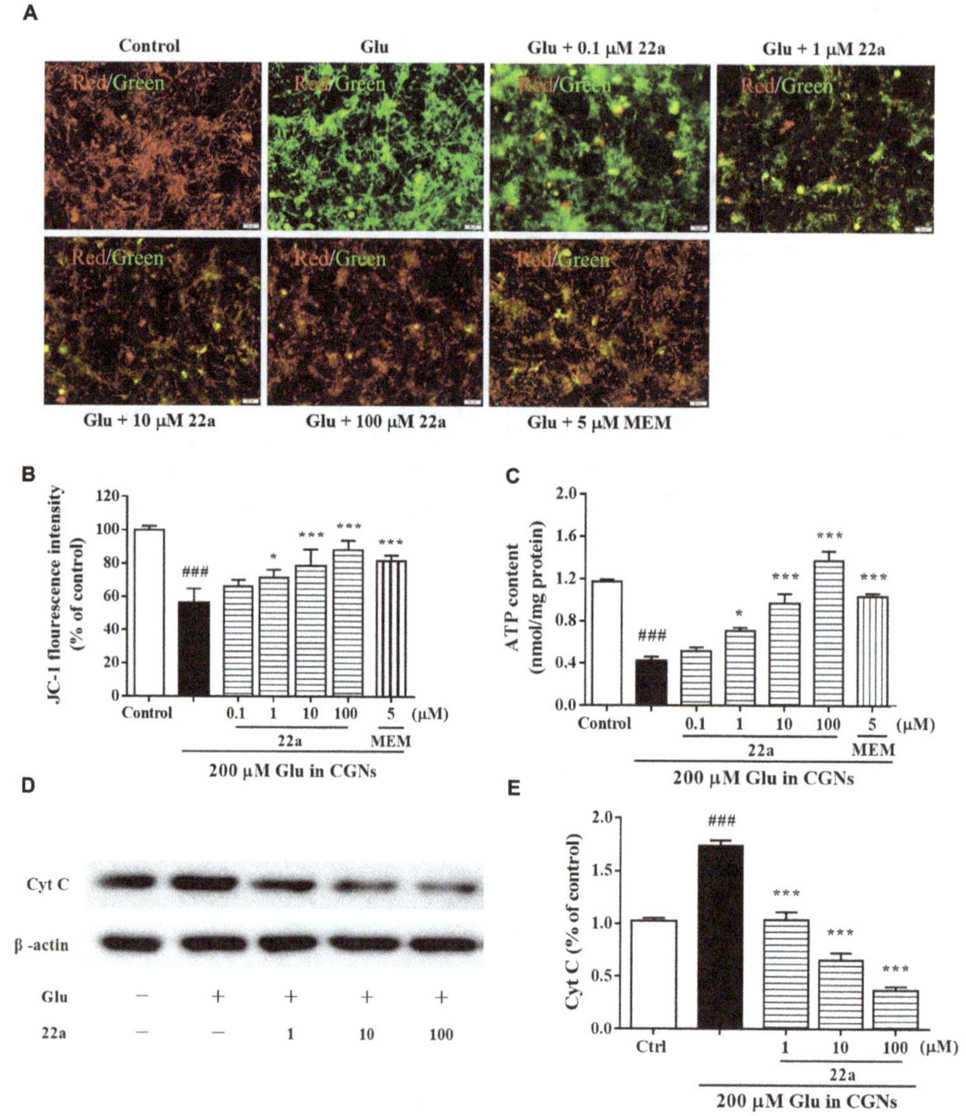

FIGURE 3 | Compound 22a improves mitochondrial dysfunction induced by glutamate. **(A)** Compound **22a** prevents glutamate-induced changes of MMP in CGNs. CGNs were pre-incubated with various agents for 2 h, then exposed to 200 μM glutamate. The MMP was evaluated by staining with the potential sensor JC-1. The fluorescence shift from red to green was detected by a microplate reader. **(B)** Quantitative analysis of the red fluorescence to green fluorescence (590 nm/529 nm) ratio in **(A)**. **(C)** Compound **22a** attenuates glutamate-induced ATP depletion in CGNs. **(D)** Immunoblot assay was performed with antibodies against Cyt C. **(E)** Densitometric analysis of **(D)**. Data were expressed as the mean ± SEM of three separate experiments; $^{###}p < 0.001$ versus control group; $^{*}p < 0.05$, $^{**}p < 0.01$, and $^{***}p < 0.001$ versus glutamate group.

measured the MMP collapse and mitochondrial ATP release. Changes of MMP were monitored by a JC-1 molecular probe, and the fluorescence shift from red to green reflected the depolarization of MMP (Chaoui et al., 2006). It was found that pretreatment with compound **22a** concentration-dependently and strongly restored MMP decrease (red fluorescence/green fluorescence) in glutamate-treated CGNs (**Figures 3A,B**). We also found that glutamate induced a significant decrease in mitochondrial ATP production, whereas pretreatment with compound **22a** significantly prevented glutamate-induced decreases in ATP levels (**Figure 3C**). Memantine was also effective ameliorating the decrease of MMP and ATP in glutamate-treated CGNs. In addition, when Cyt C release was measured by Western blot as shown in **Figures 3D,E**, it was found that **22a** concentration-dependently prevented glutamate-induced Cyt C release.

Compound 22a Up-Regulates PGC1α/Nrf2 Pathway Through Activation of PI3K/Akt

PGC1α was considered to be a major regulator of mitochondrial biogenesis. It is thought to regulate the expression of Nrf2 (Wareski et al., 2009; Robinson et al., 2014), a major transcription

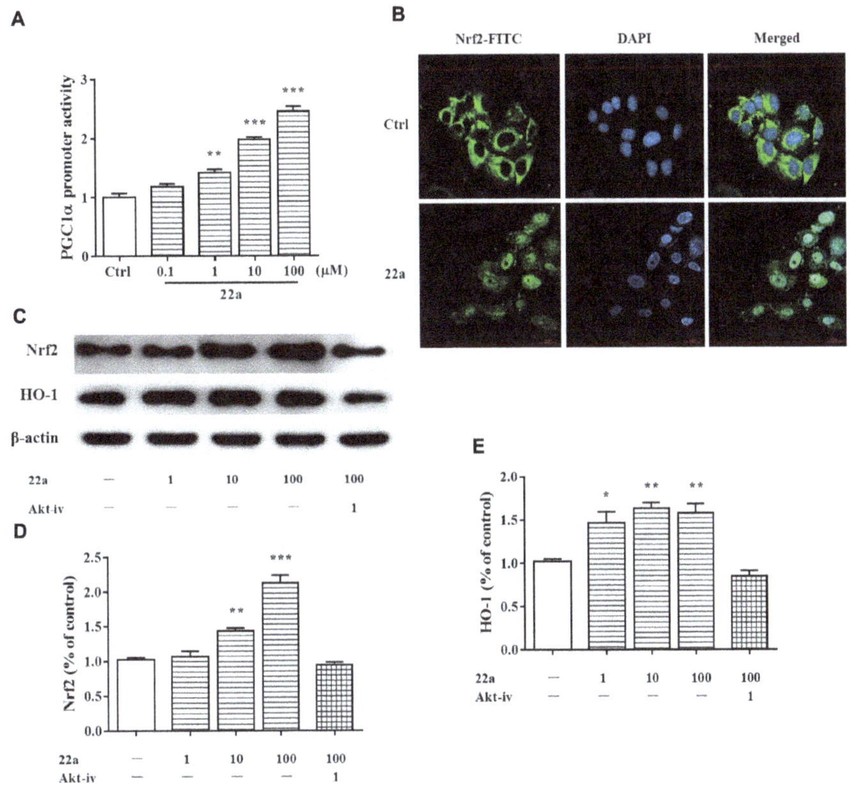

FIGURE 4 | Compound **22a** activates of PGC1α/Nrf2 signaling pathway. **(A)** Compound **22a** (0.1, 1, 10, 100 μM) increased the transcriptional activity of PGC1α determined by the luciferase reporter assay. **(B)** Compound **22a** (100 μM) induced the nuclear translocation of Nrf2 determined by immunofluorescence staining. Left panel: green fluorescence showing Nrf2 localization. Middle panel: stained nucleus with DAPI. Right panel: merged images from green and blue filters. Scale bar: 20 μm. **(C)** Immunoblot assay was performed with antibodies against Nrf2 and HO-1. **(D,E)** Densitometric analysis of the protein expression in **(C)**. CGNs were treated with compound **22a** (1, 10, 100 μM) for 12 h. Data were expressed as the mean ± SEM of three separate experiments; $^{*}p < 0.05$, $^{**}p < 0.01$, and $^{***}p < 0.001$ versus control group.

factor against oxidative stress (Nguyen et al., 2009). As shown in **Figure 4A**, Compound **22a** increased the transcriptional activity of PGC1α in a concentration-dependent manner. Nrf2 nuclear translocation was further investigated with PC12 cells after treatment with 100 μM compound **22a** for 12 h. As shown in **Figure 4B**, **22a** pretreatment increased Nrf2 accumulation in the nucleus. Nrf2 is a crucial regulator against oxidative stress and it is of interest to investigate the involvement of HO-1 protein expression. As shown in **Figures 4C–E**, CGNs treated with compound **22a** concentration-dependently increased Nrf2 and HO-1 expression. PI3K/Akt activation was reported to contribute to the up-regulation of the Nrf2 signal (Lee et al., 2015). We assessed if compound **22a**-induced Nrf2 and HO-1 expression was affected by Akt inhibitor Akt-iv. As shown in **Figures 4C–E**, compound **22a**-induced up-regulation of Nrf2 and HO-1 was completely abolished by Akt-iv.

Compound 22a Activates PGC1α/Nrf2 Signaling Pathway in CGNs Treated With Glutamate

To further elucidate whether the PGC1α/Nrf2 signaling pathways were involved in the protective effect of compound **22a** against glutamate-induced neuron injury, the two protein's expression levels were examined with Western blotting. We found that glutamate significantly decreased PGC1α, Nrf2, and HO-1 protein expression (**Figures 5A,B**); however, compound **22a** pretreatment reversed these decreases. To confirm the role of PGC1α activation in the neuroprotective effects of compound **22a**, we tested the blocking effect of PGC1α siRNA transfection. We found that PGC1α siRNA transfection dramatically decreased PGC1α protein expression (**Figures 5C,D**). In cell viability tests, PGC1α siRNA transfection considerably attenuated the neuroprotection of compound **22a**; however, a scrambled RNA transfection that was used as a negative control did not yield any significant effects on PGC1α expression or on cell viability (**Figure 5E**).

Compound 22a Reversed the Inhibition of PI3K/Akt/GSK3β Pathway Caused by Glutamate

To investigate the signaling pathways involved in the protective effects of compound **22a** against glutamate-caused excitotoxicity, we evaluated the correlation between cell viability and PI3K/Akt activation. The levels of p-PI3K, p-Ser473-Akt and p-Ser9-GSK3β

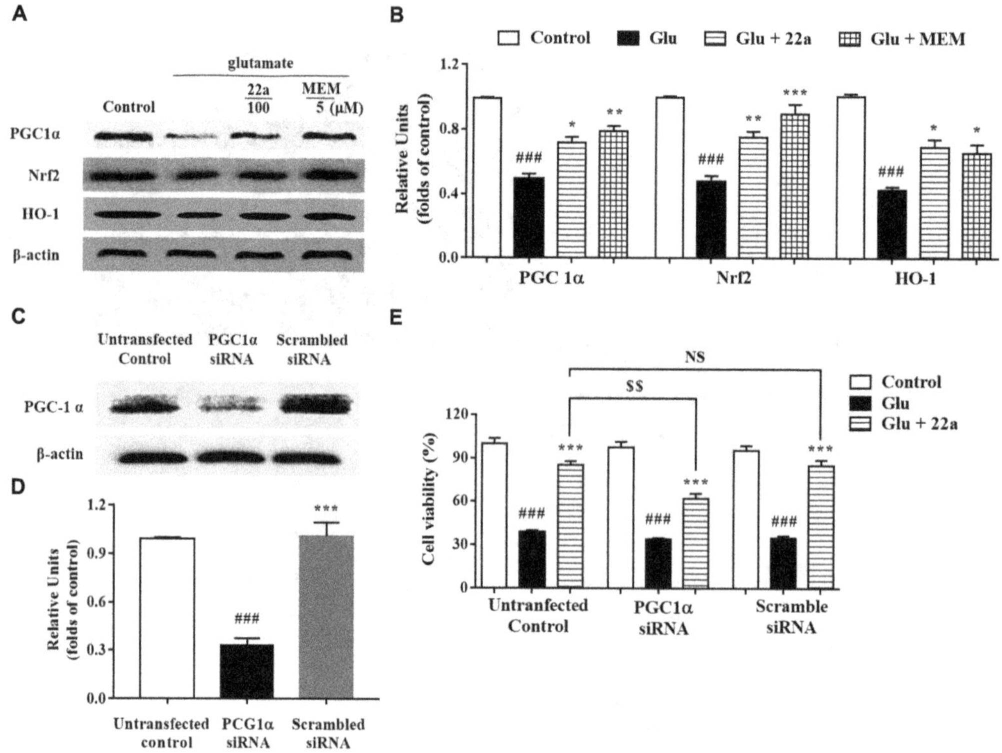

FIGURE 5 | Involvement of the PGC1α/Nrf2 pathway in neuroprotection exerted by compound **22a** in CGNs. **(A)** Representative blots showed the expression of proteins PGC1α, Nrf2 and HO-1 in CGNs after different treatments. **(B)** Densitometric analysis of the protein expression in **(A)**. **(C)** Representative blots showed the protein expression of PGC1α was silenced in CGNs pretreated with PGC1α siRNA, but not when pretreated with scrambled siRNA. **(D)** Densitometric analysis of **(C)**. **(E)** PGC1α siRNA significantly attenuated the neuroprotective effects of compound **22a** against glutamate-induced neuronal cell death in CGNs. CGNs were transfected with either PGC1α siRNA or scrambled siRNA for 24 h and then pretreated with compound **22a** (10 mM) for 2 h before exposure to 200 μM glutamate. Cell viability was measured at 24 h post glutamate exposure using the MTT assay. Data were expressed as the mean ± SEM of three experiments; $^{###}p < 0.01$ versus control group; $^{*}p < 0.05$, $^{**}p < 0.01$, and$^{***}p < 0.001$ versus glutamate group; NS means no significance; $^{\$\$}p < 0.01$ versus **22a** in the not-transfected control group.

were analyzed by Western blot. As shown in **Figures 6A–D**, glutamate down-regulated the phosphorylation of PI3K and Akt, while pretreatment with both compound **22a** and memantine reversed the suppressed phosphorylation of PI3K and Akt. GSK-3β is the molecule downstream of PI3K/Akt and is phosphorylated by the PI3K/Akt pathway. As shown in **Figures 6E,F**, there was a significant increase in the phosphorylation of GSK-3β after treatment with compound **22a** in the presence of glutamate.

PI3K and Akt Inhibitors Attenuate the Neuroprotective Effects of Compound 22a

Activation of the pro-survival PI3K/Akt signaling pathway has been shown to be important for neuroprotection (Cantrell, 2001). Consistent with our previous study (Xu et al., 2016), when exposing the cells to a PI3K inhibitor, LY294002 (1 μM), 30 min prior to the addition of compound **22a**, phosphorylation of Akt and GSK3β was nearly completely blocked by LY294002 as shown in **Figures 7A–D**. Pretreatment with LY294002 reversed compound **22a**-prompted Bcl-2 up-regulation and Bax down-regulation; the Bcl-2/Bax ratio was decreased by LY294002 (**Figures 7E,F**). In line with previous reports that PI3K/Akt is involved in Nrf2 mediated HO-1 expression (Lee et al., 2015), when cells were exposed to an Akt inhibitor, Akt-iv (1 μM), 30 min prior to **22a** treatment, the up-regulation of PGC1α, Nrf2 and HO-1 proteins' expression by compound **22a** was almost completely suppressed by Akt-iv, as shown in **Figures 7G,H**.

To further confirm the involvement of the PI3K/Akt pathway in the neuroprotection exerted by compound **22a** in CGNs damaged by glutamate, a specific PI3K inhibitor LY294002 and an Akt inhibitor Akt-iv were applied in a cell viability assay. LY294002 and Akt-iv significantly attenuated the neuroprotection of compound **22a** against glutamate toxicity (**Figure 7I**).

DISCUSSION

Glutamate is the principal excitatory amino acid neurotransmitter with complex biological activities (Pita-Almenar et al., 2006; Paoletti, 2011). However, a high concentration of extracellular glutamate is toxic to nerve cells

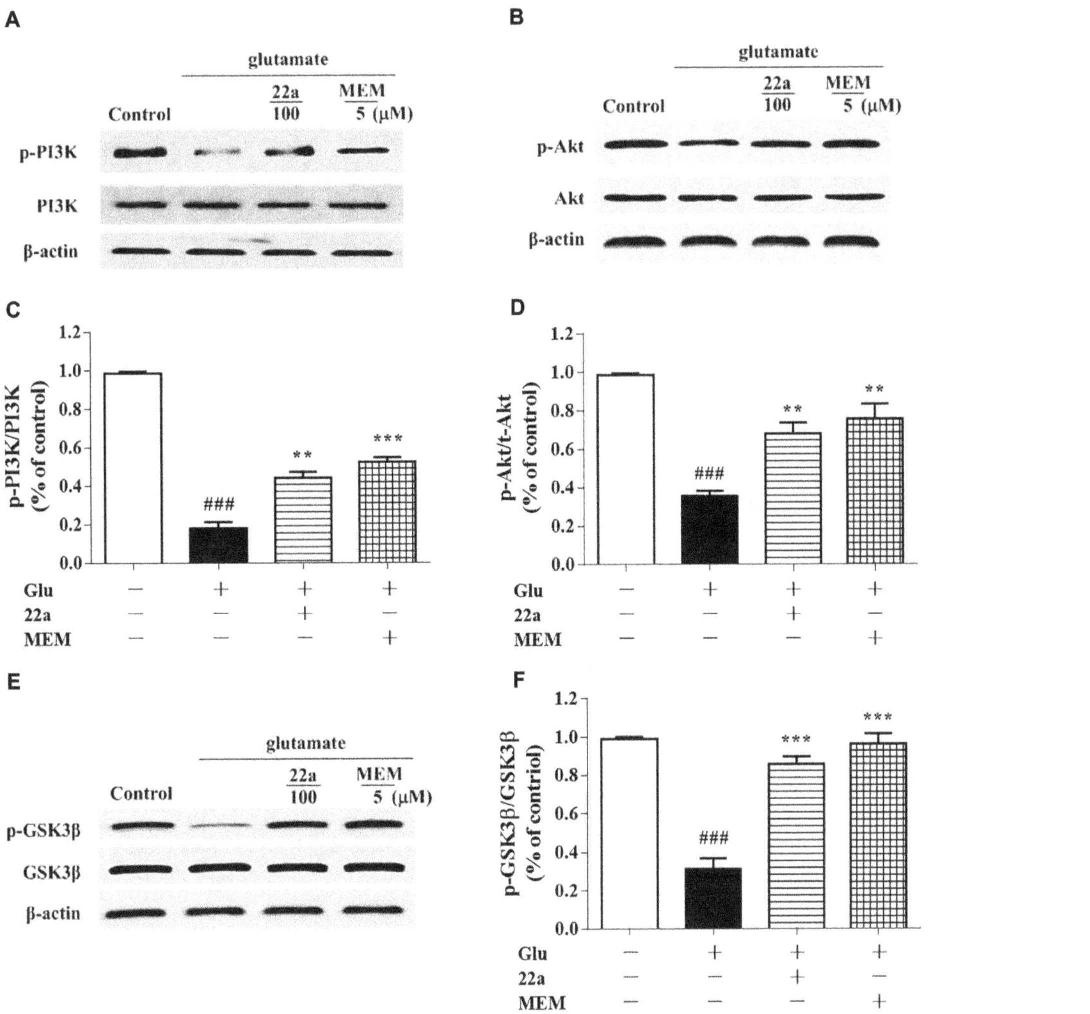

FIGURE 6 | Compound **22a** activates PI3K/Akt pathway in glutamate treated CGNs. **(A,C,E)** Representative blots showed the protein expression of p-PI3K/PI3K **(A)**, p-Akt/Akt **(C)**, and p-GSK3β/GSK3β **(E)** in CGNs. CGNs were pretreated with compound **22a** and memantine for 2 h before exposure to glutamate. **(B,D,F)** Densitometric analysis of the protein expression in **(A,C,E)**. Data were expressed as the mean ± SEM of three experiments; $^{###}p < 0.001$ versus control group; $^{**}p < 0.01$ and $^{***}p < 0.001$ versus glutamate treatment group.

and is considered to be a key contributor in the pathogenesis of neurodegenerative diseases such as ischemic stroke (Wahl et al., 1994). In our previous study, we reported that compound **22a** exhibited neuroprotective effects against oxidative stress-induced neuronal loss *in vitro* and protected against ischemic stroke *in vivo* (Chen et al., 2017). However, the exact mechanisms underlying the neuroprotection of compound **22a** is still unknown. Therefore, the neuroprotective effects of compound **22a** against glutamate-induced excitotoxicity were investigated in the current study. We demonstrated that compound **22a** protected against glutamate-induced neurotoxicity in CGNs. Meanwhile, we found that compound **22a** reversed the MMP collapse and alternation of Bcl-2 and Bax expression to attenuate glutamate-induced cellular apoptosis. Our research further demonstrated that the neuroprotective effects of compound **22a** were intermediated by the stimulation of PI3K/Akt and PGC1α/Nrf2 pathways.

Glutamate is one of the pathological factors in cerebral ischemic disease, and can cause cell apoptosis and MPP reduction, both of which are initiated by the interaction between pro- and anti-apoptotic Bcl-2 family members (Chen Q. et al., 2015). In addition, glutamate toxicity induces mitochondrial dysfunction. Mitochondria are recognized as a center of intracellular energy metabolism, and mitochondrial Ca^{2+} is a positive effector of ATP synthesis (Feissner et al., 2009). Ca^{2+} overload, however, results in free radical generation and mPTP opening, which in turn causes mitochondrial depolarization, matrix solute loss, and Cyt C release (Bernardi and Rasola, 2007). Moreover, the overproduction of ROS is also reported to be related to mPTP opening (Christophe and Nicolas, 2006). In our study, compound **22a** pretreatment significantly prevented intracellular ATP reduction and ROS aggregation, and mitigated MMP dissipation and Cyt C release. Our data further uncovered that compound **22a**

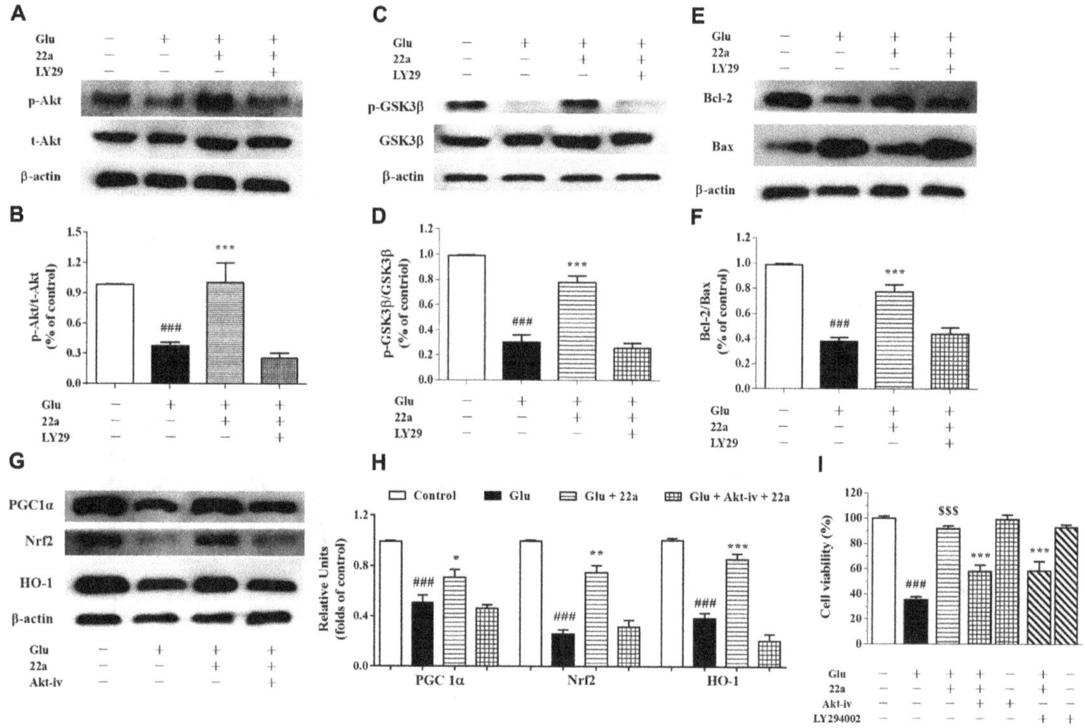

FIGURE 7 | Involvement of the PI3K/Akt pathway in neuroprotection exerted by compound **22a** in CGNs. **(A,C,E)** Representative blots showed the protein expression of p-Akt/Akt **(A)**, p-GSK3β/GSK3β **(C)**, Bcl-2 and Bax **(E)**. CGNs were pretreated with 1 μM LY294002 for 30 min before administration of compound **22a** (10 mM), followed by glutamate challenge. **(B,D,F)** Densitometric analysis of the protein expression in **(A,C,E)**. **(G)** Representative blots showed the protein expression of PGC-1α, Nrf2 and HO-1. **(H)** Densitometric analysis of the protein expression in **(G)**. **(I)** Pretreatment with an Akt inhibitor (Akt-iv) and a PI3K inhibitor (LY294002) attenuated the protective effects of compound **22a** on glutamate-treated CGNs. Data were expressed as the mean ± SEM of three experiments; $^{###}p < 0.001$ versus control group; $^{*}p < 0.05$, $^{**}p < 0.01$, and$^{***}p < 0.001$ versus glutamate treatment group; $^{\$\$\$}p < 0.001$ versus "**22a**+glutamate" treatment group. LY29 refers to PI3K inhibitor LY294002.

reversed the up-regulation of Bax and down-regulation of Bcl-2 expression induced by glutamate. Furthermore, the expression of Bcl-2, an integral membrane protein, is recognized as a hallmark of cell death associated with mitochondria dysfunction (Wallgren et al., 2013). Altogether, these results imply that increased Bcl-2 expression may represent an endogenous repair mechanism against apoptotic pathway, indicating that **22a** may block the Bax-mediated decrease of MMP or promote mitochondrial homeostasis against glutamate-caused CGNs damage.

As described above, mitochondria play a vital role in many fundamental cellular processes, ranging from energy production and metabolism to apoptosis (Robinson et al., 2014). PGC1α is a transcriptional co-activator that regulates the transcription of numerous genes involved in cellular metabolism, including mitochondrial biogenesis and respiration and ROS metabolism (Shin et al., 2011). PGC1α is also a potent stimulator of mitochondrial respiration and gene transcription that acts by activating nuclear respiratory factors Nrfl and Nrf2, which in turn regulate expression of mitochondrial transcription factor A (Tfam) and other nuclear-encoded mitochondrial proteins (Wareski et al., 2009). Numerous studies indicate that Nrf2 combines with the promoter of ARE to create general antioxidant responses, which is recognized as a promising method to therapeutically reestablish the CNS redox balance in neurodegenerative disorders (Lim et al., 2014). Among the enzymes that are redox-sensitive inducible is HO-1, which can protect neurons from acute insults under stress conditions thanks to its antioxidant and anti-inflammatory properties (Chen, 2014). In line with previous studies, we found that compound **22a** could enhance PGC1α transcriptional activity and induce nuclear accumulation of Nrf2 in PC12 cells (**Figures 4A,B**). In addition, we found that glutamate treatment significantly down-regulated the protein expression of PGC1α and pretreatment with compound **22a** significantly reversed the down-regulated expressions of PGC1α, Nrf2 and HO-1 induced by glutamate in CGNs (**Figures 5A,B**). Several investigations present that Nrf2 is tightly regulated in neurons through signaling pathways such as PI3K/Akt, which is reported to have a Nrf2-dependent role in activating HO-1 expression (Wang et al., 2008; Zhang et al., 2012; Yin et al., 2015). In this sense, the present study was designed to investigate whether the PI3K/Akt pathway is involved in regulating the PGC1α and Nrf2/HO-1 activation resultant from compound **22a**'s presence, and what effect that has on compound **22a**'s subsequent protective against glutamate-induced neurotoxicity. Our results demonstrated that a specific Akt inhibitor significantly suppressed the enhanced expression of PGC1α, Nrf2 and HO-1 induced by compound **22a** (**Figures 7G,H**). Moreover, to some extent, knockdown of PGC1α was found to reverse the neuro-protective effect of compound **22a** against toxic stress (**Figures 5C–E**). As such, compound **22a** may pave an effective and practical way to modulate PGC1α activity in neurons.

The PI3K/Akt pathway plays a critical role in preventing the neuronal cell death seen in hypoxic and excitotoxic conditions *in vitro*. Inhibiting the PI3K/Akt pathway exacerbates ischemic neuronal death (Lai et al., 2014). Previous reports indicate that neuroprotective strategies against glutamate-induced excitotoxicity in the cortex and hippocampus of postnatal brains can trigger the activation of PI3K/Akt (Shah et al., 2014). Additionally, Akt activation is capable of suppressing several pro-apoptotic proteins, including members of the Bcl-2 family and some signaling molecules such as GSK-3β (Maurer et al., 2014). In our study, phosphorylation of PI3K, Akt and GSK3β in CGNs was significantly down-regulated when cells were exposed to glutamate; however, compound **22a** pretreatment reversed these changes (**Figures 6A–F**). In addition, PI3K inhibitor LY29004 significantly inhibited the up-regulation of phosphorylated Akt and GSK3β expression while reversing compound **22a**-induced up-regulation of Bcl-2 and down-regulation of Bax expression (**Figures 7A–F**). Importantly, PI3K and Akt inhibitors completely abolished the neuroprotection conferred by compound **22a** pretreatment (**Figure 7I**). Summarily, our results indicate that PI3K/Akt pathway activation is involved in the neuro-protection of compound **22a** against CGNs injury induced by glutamate.

In summary, compound **22a** effectively prevented glutamate-induced excitotoxicity of CGNs via involvement of the PI3K/Akt and PGC1α/Nrf2 pathways. Our results suggest that compound **22a** might be of benefit in preventing neuronal death from ischemic stroke.

AUTHOR CONTRIBUTIONS

HC conceptualized and designed the experiments, performed the research, analyzed and interpreted the results, and wrote the manuscript. JC and ZyZ helped design and performed the experiments. YW, ZjZ, YS, GZ, LS, and PY conceptualized and designed the experiments, analyzed and interpreted the results, and revised the manuscript.

FUNDING

This work was partially supported by the Natural Science Fund of China (81502908), the China Postdoctoral Science Foundation (2017M622646), the Science and Technology Project of Guangdong Province (2013A022100030, 2014A030310174, 2015A020211019, 2015B020232011, 2016A020217013, and 2016A030313107), GD-HK Cooperative Project (2016A050503030), the Key Laboratory Project of Guangzhou (151800010), the Science and Technology Program of Guangzhou (201704020181); as well as the Fundamental Research Funds for the Central Universities (21617469).

ACKNOWLEDGMENTS

We thank Ms. Linda Wang for proof-reading the manuscript.

REFERENCES

Bernardi, P., and Rasola, A. (2007). Calcium and cell death: the mitochondrial connection. *Subcell. Biochem.* 45, 481–506. doi: 10.1007/978-1-4020-6191-2_18

Cantrell, D. (2001). Phosphoinositide 3-kinase signalling pathways. *J. Cell Sci.* 114, 1439–1445.

Chaoui, D., Faussat, A. M., Majdak, P., Tang, R., Perrot, J. Y., Pasco, S., et al. (2006). JC-1, a sensitive probe for a simultaneous detection of P-glycoprotein activity and apoptosis in leukemic cells. *Cytometry B Clin. Cytom.* 70, 189–196. doi: 10.1002/cyto.b.20100

Chen, H., Tan, G., Cao, J., Zhang, G., Yi, P., Yu, P., et al. (2017). Design, synthesis, and biological evaluation of novel tetramethylpyrazine derivatives as potential neuroprotective agents. *Chem. Pharm. Bull.* 65, 56–65. doi: 10.1248/cpb.c16-00699

Chen, H. Y., Xu, D. P., Tan, G. L., Cai, W., Zhang, G. X., Cui, W., et al. (2015). A potent multi-functional neuroprotective derivative of tetramethylpyrazine. *J. Mol. Neurosci.* 56, 977–987. doi: 10.1007/s12031-015-0566-x

Chen, Q., Xu, H., Xu, A., Ross, T., Bowler, E., Hu, Y., et al. (2015). Inhibition of Bcl-2 sensitizes mitochondrial permeability transition pore (MPTP) opening in ischemia-damaged mitochondria. *PLoS One* 10:e0118834. doi: 10.1371/journal.pone.0118834

Chen, J. (2014). Heme oxygenase in neuroprotection: from mechanisms to therapeutic implications. *Rev. Neurosci.* 25, 269–280. doi: 10.1515/revneuro-2013-0046

Christophe, M., and Nicolas, S. (2006). Mitochondria: a target for neuroprotective interventions in cerebral ischemia-reperfusion. *Curr. Pharm. Des.* 12, 739–757. doi: 10.2174/138161206775474242

Donnan, G. A., Fisher, M., Macleod, M., and Davis, S. M. (2008). Stroke. *Lancet* 371, 1612–1623. doi: 10.1016/S0140-6736(08)60694-7

Du, Y., Bales, K. R., Dodel, R. C., Hamilton-Byrd, E., Horn, J. W., Czilli, D. L., et al. (1997). Activation of a caspase 3-related cysteine protease is required for glutamate-mediated apoptosis of cultured cerebellar granule neurons. *Proc. Natl. Acad. Sci. U.S.A.* 94, 11657–11662. doi: 10.1073/pnas.94.21.11657

Feissner, R. F., Skalska, J., and Gaum, W. E. (2009). Crosstalk signaling between mitochondrial Ca2+ and ROS. *Front. Biosci.* 14:1197–1218. doi: 10.2741/3303

Floyd, R. A., Castro, Faria Neto HC, Zimmerman, G. A., Hensley, K., and Towner, R. A. (2013). Nitrone-based therapeutics for neurodegenerative diseases: their use alone or in combination with lanthionines. *Free Radic. Biol. Med.* 62, 145–156. doi: 10.1016/j.freeradbiomed.2013.01.033

Ghosh, N., Ghosh, R., Bhat, Z. A., Mandal, V., Bachar, S. C., Nima, N. D., et al. (2014). Advances in herbal medicine for treatment of ischemic brain injury. *Nat. prod. commun.* 9, 1045–1055.

Grupke, S., Hall, J., Dobbs, M., Bix, G. J., and Fraser, J. F. (2014). Understanding history, and not repeating it. Neuroprotection for acute ischemic stroke: from review to preview. *Clin. Neurol. Neurosurg.* 129, 1–9. doi: 10.1016/j.clineuro.2014.11.013

Jing, Y., Liu, L. Z., Jiang, Y., Zhu, Y., Guo, N. L., Barnett, J., et al. (2012). Cadmium increases HIF-1 and VEGF expression through ROS, ERK, and AKT signaling pathways and induces malignant transformation of human bronchial epithelial cells. *Toxicol. Sci.* 125, 10–19. doi: 10.1093/toxsci/kfr256

Jo, H., Mondal, S., Tan, D., Nagata, E., Takizawa, S., Sharma, A. K., et al. (2012). Small molecule-induced cytosolic activation of protein kinase Akt rescues ischemia-elicited neuronal death. *Proc. Natl. Acad. Sci. U.S.A.* 109, 10581–10586. doi: 10.1073/pnas.1202810109

Kim, H. K., Song, I. S., Lee, S. Y., Jeong, S. H., Lee, S. R., Heo, H. J., et al. (2014). B7-H4 downregulation induces mitochondrial dysfunction and enhances doxorubicin sensitivity via the cAMP/CREB/PGC1-α signaling pathway in HeLa cells. *Pflugers Arch.* 466, 2323–2338. doi: 10.1007/s00424-014-1493-3

Lai, T. W., Zhang, S., and Wang, Y. T. (2014). Excitotoxicity and stroke: identifying novel targets for neuroprotection. *Prog. Neurobiol.* 115, 157–188. doi: 10.1016/j.pneurobio.2013.11.006

Lau, A., and Tymianski, M. (2010). Glutamate receptors, neurotoxicity and neurodegeneration. *Pflugers Arch.* 460, 525–542. doi: 10.1007/s00424-010-0809-1

Lee, D. S., Cha, B. Y., Woo, J. T., Kim, Y. C., and Jang, J. H. (2015). Acerogenin a from acer nikoense maxim prevents oxidative stress-induced neuronal cell death through Nrf2-mediated heme oxygenase-1 expression in mouse hippocampal HT22 cell line. *Molecules* 20, 12545–12557. doi: 10.3390/molecules200712545

Lim, J. L., Wilhelmus, M. M., de, Vries HE, Drukarch, B., Hoozemans, J. J., and van, Horssen J (2014). Antioxidative defense mechanisms controlled by Nrf2: state-of-the-art and clinical perspectives in neurodegenerative diseases. *Arch. Toxicol.* 88, 1773–1786. doi: 10.1007/s00204-014-1338-z

Liu, X., Zhang, R., Xu, W., Li, C., Zhao, Q., and Wang, X. (2003). Synthesis of the novel liqustrazine derivatives and their protective effect on injured vascular endothelial cell damaged by hydrogen peroxide. *Bioorg. Med. Chem. Lett.* 13, 2123–2126. doi: 10.1016/S0960-894X(03)00359-7

Maurer, U., Preiss, F., Brauns-Schubert, P., Schlicher, L., and Charvet, C. (2014). GSK-3 - at the crossroads of cell death and survival. *J. Cell Sci.* 127, 1369–1378. doi: 10.1242/jcs.138057

Nguyen, T., Nioi, P., and Pickett, C. B. (2009). The Nrf2-antioxidant response element signaling pathway and its activation by oxidative stress. *J. Biol. Chem.* 284, 13291–13295. doi: 10.1074/jbc.R900010200

Pang, T., Wang, Y. J., Gao, Y. X., Xu, Y., Li, Q., Zhou, Y. B., et al. (2016). A novel GSK-3β inhibitor YQ138 prevents neuronal injury induced by glutamate and brain ischemia through activation of the Nrf2 signaling pathway. *Acta Pharmacol. Sin.* 37, 741–752. doi: 10.1038/aps.2016.3

Paoletti, P. (2011). Molecular basis of NMDA receptor functional diversity. *Eur. J. Neurosci.* 33, 1351–1365. doi: 10.1111/j.1460-9568.2011.07628.x

Pita-Almenar, J. D., Collado, M. S., Colbert, C. M., and Eskin, A. (2006). Different mechanisms exist for the plasticity of glutamate reuptake during early long-term potentiation (LTP) and late LTP. *J. Neurosci.* 26, 10461–10471. doi: 10.1523/JNEUROSCI.2579-06.2006

Robinson, A., Grösgen, S., and Mett, J. (2014). Upregulation of PGC-1α expression by Alzheimer's disease-associated pathway: presenilin 1/amyloid precursor protein (APP)/intracellular domain of APP. *Aging Cell* 13, 263–272. doi: 10.1111/acel.12183

Sano, M., and Fukuda, K. (2008). Activation of mitochondrial biogenesis by hormesis. *Circ. Res.* 103, 1191–1193. doi: 10.1161/CIRCRESAHA.108.189092

Shah, S. A., Lee, H. Y., Bressan, R. A., Yun, D. J., and Kim, M. O. (2014). Novel osmotin attenuates glutamate-induced synaptic dysfunction and neurodegeneration via the JNK/PI3K/Akt pathway in postnatal rat brain. *Cell Death Dis.* 5, e1026. doi: 10.1038/cddis.2013.538

Shin, J. H., Ko, H. S., Kang, H., Lee, Y., Lee, Y. I., Pletinkova, O., et al. (2011). PARIS (ZNF746) repression of PGC-1α contributes to neurodegeneration in Parkinson's disease. *Cell* 144, 689–702. doi: 10.1016/j.cell.2011.02.010S0092-8674(11)00124-3

Touaibia, M., Jean-Francois, J., and Doiron, J. (2011). Caffeic Acid, a versatile pharmacophore: an overview. *Mini Rev. Med. Chem.* 11, 695–713. doi: 10.2174/138955711796268750

Wahl, F., Obrenovitch, T. P., Hardy, A. M., Plotkine, M., Boulu, R., and Symon, L. (1994). Extracellular glutamate during focal cerebral ischaemia in rats: time course and calcium dependency. *J. Neurochem.* 63, 1003–1011. doi: 10.1046/j.1471-4159.1994.63031003.x

Wallgren, M., Lidman, M., Pedersen, A., Brännström, K., Karlsson, B. G., and Gröbner, G. (2013). Reconstitution of the anti-apoptotic Bcl-2 protein into lipid membranes and biophysical evidence for its detergent-driven association with the pro-apoptotic bax protein. *PLoS One* 8:e61452. doi: 10.1371/journal.pone.0061452

Wang, L., Chen, Y., Sternberg, P., and Cai, J. (2008). Essential roles of the PI3 kinase/Akt pathway in regulating Nrf2-dependent antioxidant functions in the RPE. *Invest. Ophthalmol. Vis. Sci.* 49, 1671–1678. doi: 10.1167/iovs.07-1099

Wang, Y., and Qin, Z. H. (2010). Molecular and cellular mechanisms of excitotoxic neuronal death. *Apoptosis* 15, 1382–1402. doi: 10.1007/s10495-010-0481-0

Wareski, P., Vaarmann, A., Choubey, V., Safiulina, D., Liiv, J., Kuum, M., et al. (2009). PGC-1α and PGC-1β regulate mitochondrial density in neurons. *J. Biol. Chem.* 284, 21379–21385. doi: 10.1074/jbc.M109.018911

Xu, D., Chen, H., Mak, S., Hu, S., Tsim, K. W. K., Hu, Y., et al. (2016). Neuroprotection against glutamate-induced excitotoxicity and induction of neurite outgrowth by T-006, a novel multifunctional derivative of tetramethylpyrazine in neuronal cell models. *Neurochem. Int.* 99, 194–205. doi: 10.1016/j.neuint.2016.07.006

Xue, Y., Tie, C. R., Li, J., Tian, T., and Li, Q. X. (2011). Ligustrazine inhibits lipopolysaccharide-induced proliferation by affecting P27, Bcl-2 expression in rat mesangial cells. *Eur. J. Pharmacol.* 665, 8–12. doi: 10.1016/j.ejphar.2011.05.004

Yin, X., Wang, X., Fan, Z., Peng, C., Ren, Z., Huang, L., et al. (2015). Hyperbaric oxygen preconditioning attenuates myocardium ischemia-reperfusion injury through upregulation of heme oxygenase 1 expression: PI3K/Akt/Nrf2 pathway involved. *J. Cardiovasc. Pharmacol. Ther.* 20, 428–438. doi: 10.1177/1074248414568196

Zhang, J., Li, Y., Chen, X., Pan, Y., Zhang, S., and Wang, Y. (2014). Systems pharmacology dissection of multi-scale mechanisms of action for herbal medicines in stroke treatment and prevention. *PLoS One* 9:e102506. doi: 10.1371/journal.pone.0102506

Zhang, R., Chae, S., Lee, J. H., and Hyun, J. W. (2012). The cytoprotective effect of butin against oxidative stress is mediated by the up-regulation of manganese superoxide dismutase expression through a PI3K/Akt/Nrf2-dependent pathway. *J. Cell. Biochem.* 113, 1987–1997. doi: 10.1002/jcb.24068

7

Inhibition of Connexin 43 Hemichannels Alleviates Cerebral Ischemia/Reperfusion Injury via the TLR4 Signaling Pathway

Yingzhu Chen[1,2†], *Liangzhu Wang*[2,3†], *Lingling Zhang*[1,2], *Beilei Chen*[1,2], *Liu Yang*[2,3], *Xiaobo Li*[1,2,4], *Yuping Li*[1,2] *and Hailong Yu*[1,2,4,5*]

[1]*Clinical Medical College of Yangzhou University, Yangzhou, China,* [2]*Department of Neurology, Northern Jiangsu People's Hospital, Yangzhou, China,* [3]*Dalian Medical University, Dalian, China,* [4]*Institute of Neuroscience, Northern Jiangsu People's Hospital, Yangzhou, China,* [5]*Drum Tower Hospital, Medical School of Nanjing University, Nanjing, China*

Correspondence:
Hailong Yu
hailongyu1982tg@163.com

[†]*These authors have contributed equally to this work*

Connexin 43 (Cx43) widely exists in all components of the neurovascular unit (NVU) and is a constituent of gap junctions and hemichannels. In physiological states, gap junctions are open for regular intercellular communication, and the hemichannels present low open probability in astrocytes. After cerebral ischemia, a large number of hemichannels are unusually opened, leading to cell swelling and even death. Most known hemichannel blockers also inhibit gap junctions and sequentially obstruct normal electrical cell-cell communication. In this study, we tested the hypothesis that Gap19, a selective Cx43-hemichannel inhibitor, exhibited neuroprotective effects on cerebral ischemia/reperfusion (I/R). An obvious improvement in neurological scores and infarct volume reduction were observed in Gap19-treated mice after brain ischemia induced by middle cerebral artery occlusion (MCAO). Gap19 treatment attenuated white matter damage. Moreover, Gap19 treatment suppressed the expression of Cx43 and Toll-like receptor 4 (TLR4) pathway-relevant proteins and prevented the overexpression of tumour necrosis factor-α (TNF-α) and interleukin-1β (IL-1β). To further explore downstream signaling, we established an *in vitro* model–oxygen glucose deprivation (OGD) to simulate ischemic conditions. Immunofluorescence staining showed that Cx43 co-existed with TLR4 in astrocytes. The hemichannel activity was increased after OGD and Gap19 could inhibit this effect on astrocytes. Gap19 substantially improved relative cell vitality and decreased the expression of Cx43, TLR4 and inflammatory cytokines *in vitro*. In addition, in the lipopolysaccharide (LPS) stimulation OGD model, Gap19 also exhibited a protective effect via inhibiting TLR4 pathway activation. In summary, our results showed that Gap19 exerted a neuroprotective effect after stroke via inhibition of the TLR4-mediated signaling pathway.

Keywords: cerebral ischemia/reperfusion, hemichannel, inflammation, toll-like receptor 4, neurovascular unit, neuroprotection

INTRODUCTION

Stroke is the most common neurological disease, and it causes high disability and high mortality (Lo, 2010). An epidemiological study revealed that 70%–80% of all strokes are ischemic (Mozaffarian et al., 2015). Currently, intravenous tissue plasminogen activator (t-PA) is recognized as the most effective therapy for acute ischemic stroke (Powers et al., 2018). However, its clinical use is largely limited because of the narrow time window and strict inclusion criteria (Saver et al., 2013). Recent research has been devoted to the development of alternative neuroprotective agents, but almost no agents have been successful in clinical trials (Sahota and Savitz, 2011). The primary reason is that previous studies focus on single target neurons or white matter and ignore the communication between the components of the neurovascular unit (NVU; Girouard and Iadecola, 2006). NVU is a complex of neurons, astrocytes, and cerebrovascular endothelial cells, considered as the structural and functional unit of the brain (Zhang et al., 2012; Xue et al., 2013). NVU components are involved in the transport of substances via intercellular signal transduction and neurovascular coupling and regulate the steady state microenvironment of neurons (Guo et al., 2008). Abnormal NVU function may cause neurological disorders, such as stroke (Moskowitz et al., 2010).

Cell communication in the NVU primarily occurs via gap junctions (Islam and Mohamed, 2015). Gap junctional intercellular communication (GJIC) allows direct cell-to-cell communication, energy metabolites and diffusion of molecules to maintain homeostatic balance in the brain, such as K^+ or glutamate (Naus and Giaume, 2016). Gap junction is consisted by the aggregation of two connexons (or hemichannels), to form a direct pathway linking the cytoplasm of the neighboring cells (Bodendiek and Raman, 2010). Each hemichannel consists of six connexin proteins, and 11 subtypes are expressed in brain (Chew et al., 2010). The connexin 43 (Cx43) subtype is one of the most abundant connexin proteins in brain, widely exists in the component of NVU, predominately in astrocytes (Giaume et al., 2010). Connexins are four-time transmembrane proteins and exist on the plasma membranes. They own two extracellular loops (ELs) and one intracellular cytoplasmic loop (CL; Schulz et al., 2015). In the physiological state, gap junctions in astrocytes remain open, while the hemichannels still present low open probability (Kim et al., 2016). Hemichannels are primarily activated after cerebral ischemia, allowing the entry of Na^+ and Ca^{2+} and the release of adenosine triphosphate (ATP) and other small metabolites. These fluctuations cause Ca^{2+} overload, osmotic imbalance, energy exhaustion and even cell death (Sáez and Leybaert, 2014). Moreover, ATP released from hemichannels could mediate the microglia activation and induce inflammatory cytokines secretion from activated microglia, further upregulate the Cx43 hemichannels and form a vicious cycle (Shaikh et al., 2012; Sáez et al., 2013).

Hemichannels modulation was considered as a potential neuro-therapeutic target in cerebral ischemia/reperfusion (I/R) injury (De Bock et al., 2011). Connexin43 mimetic peptides could prevent the opening of hemichannels and further reduce the spread of harmful substance after ischemic injury (Evans and Leybaert, 2007; O'Carroll et al., 2008). Our previous study found that the Gap26 and Gap27 could significantly reduce infarct size and promote neurological function recovery after hypoxia/ischemia injury in neonatal rats (Li et al., 2015). However, when applied for several hours, these agents also prevented the joining of hemichannels and affected gap junction communication due to their poor specificity (Decrock et al., 2009). Another mimetic peptide, Gap19, consists of nine amino acids KQIEIKKFK (Schulz et al., 2015), and it inhibits the opening of hemichannels without interference the gap junction communication in astrocytes (Abudara et al., 2014). Selective inhibition of Cx43 hemichannels using Gap19 protects against myocardial I/R injury *in vitro* and *in vivo* (Wang N. et al., 2013). Given the higher specificity, we can hypothesis that Gap19 may alleviate cerebral I/R injury. Restoration of blood supply and reoxygenation are usually associated with deterioration of tissue injury and a profound inflammation called reperfusion injury (Kim et al., 2014). Subsequent reperfusion further activates of innate and adaptive immune responses and cell death programmes (Eltzschig and Eckle, 2011). Recently study shows that Cx43 hemichannel opening could be triggered by treatment with pro-inflammatory cytokines in astrocytes (Retamal et al., 2007). Nevertheless, whether Gap19 influences cerebral I/R injury via disruption of inflammatory responses is not clear.

In the present study, we established middle cerebral artery occlusion (MCAO) and oxygen glucose deprivation (OGD) models to assess the role and relevant mechanisms of Gap19 in cerebral ischemia. We found that Gap19 exerted a protective role in cerebral I/R injury via inhibition of Toll-like receptor 4 (TLR4) signaling *in vitro* and *in vivo*. Therefore, Gap19 is a promising new drug candidate for the treatment of ischemic stroke.

MATERIALS AND METHODS

Animals and Experimental Groups

Adult male ICR mice (8–10 weeks, 25–35 g) were purchased from the Comparative Medical Centre of Yangzhou University. Animals were housed in an appropriate environment at $22 \pm 2°C$ and 60% humidity with a 12-h light/dark cycle. All experiment protocols were approved by the Animal Ethics Committee of the Yangzhou University (license number: YIACUC-15-0013). Animals were randomly separated into five groups ($n = 6–15$ each): (I) sham; (II) Gap19 group; (III) I/R group; (IV) I/R + Gap19 group; and (V) I/R + Gap26 group. In the I/R group, the animals were assigned to several subgroups with different reperfusion time points (4 h, 12 h, 24 h, 72 h and 7 days).

The Middle Cerebral Artery Occlusion (MCAO) Model

The MCAO was established as described previously (Wang et al., 2014). Briefly, after anesthetize mice with 5.0% isoflurane, made a small incision on the neck skin, and carefully exposed the left common carotid artery (CCA), external carotid artery (ECA), and internal carotid artery (ICA). The ECA was ligated to block blood flow, and aneurysm clips were used to clamp the left CCA and ICA. A small incision was created at 2 mm proximal end of the CCA bifurcation. Through the incision, the filament was inserted into the ICA, and about 9–11 mm was inserted to block the MCA. The filament was gently removed (onset of reperfusion) after 45 min of focal cerebral ischemia. Tight the ICA with suture line and close the neck incision. Sham group only accepted neck incision and ligation of the

ECA without occluding MCA. The mice went back to the cages with closely monitored and keep the body temperature at 36.5–37.5°C by the electric blanket until they recovered from anesthesia.

Drug Preparation and Treatment Schedule

Gap19 was purchased from TOCRIS (catalog No. 5353) and dissolved in sterilized double distilled water (ddH_2O). Gap19 was injected into the right lateral cerebral ventricle (coordinates: 0.5 mm posterior to Bregma, 1.0 mm right of the midline, and depth is 2.5 mm) 1 h after MCAO as described previously (Meller et al., 2005). The optimal dose was selected based on previous studies (Li et al., 2015) and 10 μg Gap19/Gap26 in 10 μl ddH_2O was slowly injected over 10 min.

Evaluation of Neurological Deficit

A researcher who was unclear of animal grouping assessed neurological deficits at 24 h after reperfusion. A 5-point method of neurological deficit scores was applied to assess neurological behavior, as described previously (Yu H. et al., 2012): 0, no deficit; 1, failure to fully extend right paw; 2, circling to right; 3, falling to right; 4, no spontaneous walking with depressed consciousness. Score of 0–2 manifested mild neurological impairment, and 3–4 manifested severe neurological impairment. Remove the animals with no deficit after MCAO.

Measurement of Infarct Volume

Infarct volume was measured with 0.2% (w/v) 2,3,5-triphenyltetrazolium chloride (TTC, Sigma-Aldrich) as described previously (Tsubokawa et al., 2007; Yu H. et al., 2012). Briefly, mice were decapitated after neurological evaluation, and quickly removed and frozen the brain. After cut the brains into 2 mm coronal sections, slices were stained with 0.2% TTC for 30 min at 37°C, then fixed with 4% paraformaldehyde overnight. The infarct tissue area was not stained (white), and normal tissue was stained red. Then all brain slices were photographed in one picture and the infarct volume in each slice was determined by a computerized image analysis system (AlphaEase Image Analysis Software V 3.1.2). The percent hemispheric infarct volume was calculated as described previously (Xiong et al., 2011; Li et al., 2015), calculated the ratio (%) of the infarction area to the contralateral area of the same brain.

Luxol Fast Blue Myelin Staining

Luxol fast blue staining (Sigma) and Cresyl violet was used as a counterstain to assess the myelin damage at 7 days after reperfusion. Washed the slices in ddH_2O for 2 min, and incubated in 95% ethanol for 1 min. Sections were then incubated in a preheated solution of 1% LFB (60°C) for 2 h. After washed, differentiate sections with a 0.05% lithium carbonate solution and 70% ethyl alcohol each for 10 s. Repeated this step twice and stained with a 0.1% cresyl violet for 1 min. Tissues were gradually dehydrated in an ethanol gradient (70%, 95% and 100%) and fixed with xylene. Quantitative analyses of Luxol fast blue-stained sections were performed as described previously (Jing et al., 2014). White matter damage was calculated as the percentage of blue area in the ipsilateral striatum.

Isolation and Purification of Three Kinds of Mice Cerebral Cells

Brain microvascular endothelial cells (BMECs) were collected from 2-week-old mice, as previously described (Gauthier et al., 2012; Ruck et al., 2014). Briefly, gray matter was minced into small pieces in ice-cold 20 mM HEPES in Dulbecco's Modified Eagle Medium (DMEM). Tissue was digested at 37°C for 30 min in 0.05% collagenase/dispase. Isolated BMECs with 17% dextran and ultracentrifuged at 4°C 10,000× *g* for 30 min. Autoclaved glass beads were used to collect the cells. Precipitates were resuspended in DMEM supplemented with 10% FBS, 100 U/ml penicillin, 100 mg/ml streptomycin, 2 mM L-glutamine, 50 mg/ml DNase I and 0.1 mM nonessential amino-acids. Seed the cells on 6-well culture plates pre-coated with 1% gelatin and incubate at 37°C in 5% CO_2. The purified endothelial cells were used for following experiments.

Astrocytes were prepared from mice brain cortices within 24 h of birth, as previously described (Nakagawa et al., 2009). Gray cortices were minced, digested 0.25% trypsin and centrifuged. Sediments were resuspended in DMEM supplemented with 10% FBS and 100 U/ml penicillin, and 100 mg/ml streptomycin. Cells were seeded at a density of 4.5×10^6 cells/flask onto 75-cm^2 flasks pre-coated with 20 μg/ml poly-D-lysine. Change the culture medium every 2 days. After 12–14 days of culture, shake the flasks to discard microglia and collect the purified astrocytes. Astrocytes could be digested with 0.25% trypsin and seeded on different culture plates for further experiments.

Neurons were obtained from mice embryos at 15–16 days of gestation, as previously described, using a modified protocol (Zhu et al., 2014). Briefly, remove the embryos and separate the cerebral cortex quickly, strip meninges in the sterile filter papers. Put the acquired tissues into a Ca^{2+}/Mg^{2+}-free Hank's balanced saline solution (HBSS) solution. Then digest in 2-mg/ml papain for 30 min and centrifuged. Cells were seeded at 5×10^5 cells/cm^2 into 6-well culture plates pre-coated with 100 μg/ml poly-D-lysine and cultured with Neurobasal medium including 4.5 g/L glucose, Glutamax and 2% B27. Replace half of the medium with new medium after 2 days and maintain in culture 3 days prior to each experiment.

Establishment of *in vitro* NVU Model

NVU model was constructed by using the transwell system (Corning Incorporated) according to previous report (Xue et al., 2013; Tian et al., 2016). Briefly, the neurons were first seeded into the 6-well culture plate to 0.5×10^5 cells/cm^2 for 5 days. Then seed the purified astrocytes on the external of the transwell insert membrane with a density of 5×10^5 cells/cm^2. After astrocytes were adhered for 4 h, and the insert was transferred into the well to co-culture with neurons. After 1 day, BMECs were plated to the internal of the transwell insert membrane with 1.0×10^5 cells/cm^2 and co-cultured for 2–3 days. After co-culture, medium was replaced with DMEM-F12 supplemented with 10% FBS, L-glutamine, penicillin (100 U/ml) and streptomycin (100 mg/ml). The NVU model was prepared for next experiments. Lipopolysaccharide (LPS; 1 μg/ml, Sigma) and Gap19 were added to the medium below the transwell at the beginning of OGD to construct the model.

Oxygen-Glucose Deprivation

To simulate ischemia *in vitro*, OGD treatment was established as described previously (Rowe et al., 2014) with small modification. First, removed the original culture medium and replaced with glucose/serum-free DMEM. Then, transfer the plates into an anaerobic chamber for 4 h at 37°C, which already balanced with 5% CO_2 and 95% N_2. Cells were returned to completely normal conditions for 24 h. Groups as follows: (1) control; (2) Gap19 group; (3) OGD group; (4) OGD + Gap19 group; (5) OGD + LPS group; and (6) OGD + LPS + Gap19 group. Control cells were incubated in the normoxic incubator. Gap19 (100 μM) were treated into system at the beginning of OGD.

Cytotoxicity Assay

The 3-(4,5-dimethyl-thiazol-2-yl)-2,5-diphenyltetrazolium bromide (MTT) assay was used to assess the cell viability (Jiang et al., 2014). Briefly, purified astrocytes were seeded in 96-well plates with DMEM without serum. Cells were disposed with different concentrations (10 μM, 50 μM, 100 μM, 150 μM and 200 μM) of Gap19 at the beginning of OGD. Then the medium was removed, and the MTT assay was conducted according to the manufacturer's protocols. The formation of formazan crystals was detected at 490 nm by a microplate reader. Cell viability was showed as a percentage of the control that had not undergone Gap19 treatment.

Immunofluorescence Staining

Immunofluorescence was performed as described in a previous study (Tian et al., 2016). Briefly, different cell types were seeded on coverslips. Cells were gently washed after reaching 70% confluency and fixed with 4% paraformaldehyde for 20 min. Then block with 3% bovine serum for 1 h and incubate with primary antibody at 4°C overnight. BMECs were incubated with CD31 (anti-rabbit, 1:20, Abcam), and neurons were incubated with tubulin β-III isoform (anti-mouse, 1:200, Millipore). Astrocytes were incubated with GFAP (anti-mouse, 1:100, Millipore; anti-rabbit, 1:500, Cell Signaling), Cx43 (anti-rabbit, 1:1,000, Cell Signaling; anti-mouse, 1:100, Abcam) and TLR4 (anti-mouse, 1:500, Proteintech). Cells were washed and incubated with anti-rabbit IgG labeled with Alexa-594 (Invitrogen) or anti-mouse IgG labeled with Alexa-488 (Invitrogen). Finally, stain the nuclei with 4',6-diamidino-2- phenylindole (DAPI, C1006; Beyotime, Shanghai, China). The coverslips were viewed by the fluorescence microscope (LSM780, Zeiss, Jena, Germany).

Ethidium Bromide Uptake

To evaluate the hemichannels activity after OGD and the effect of Gap19, astrocytes, neurons and BMECs were respectively cultured on 24-well plates. After OGD, the cultured cells were washed with HBSS twice and incubated with 5 μM ethidium bromide (EtBr; Giaume et al., 2012) in 37°C for10 min. Then washed the cells again, fixed with 4% paraformaldehyde and visualized by the fluorescence microscope. Pictures were analyzed through counting the number of EtBr-positive cells per field by ImageJ software.

Enzyme-Linked Immunosorbent Assay (ELISA) Analysis

Carefully collect the cell culture supernatants after OGD and centrifuge at 12,000× *g* 4°C for 15 min. Tumor necrosis factor-α (TNF-α) and interleukin-1β (IL-1β) concentrations were evaluated by Enzyme-Linked Immunosorbent Assay (ELISA) assay kits. All procedures were performed following the directions provided in the kit. The absorbance of each sample was detected by a microplate reader at 490 nm. The concentration of cell cytokines is described as picograms per milliliter.

Western Blot Analysis

At different reperfusion times, protein was extracted from the infarcted hemispheres and cultured cells by a protein extraction kit (Beyotime Biotech) as described in our previous report (Li et al., 2015). Protein samples were next electrophoresed and transferred to polyvinylidene difluoride filter (PVDF) membranes. Then block the membrane with 5% fat-free milk at room temperature for 2 h, and incubate with primary antibodies as follows: anti-Tubulin (Cell Signaling), anti-Cx43 (Cell Signaling), anti-TLR4 (Proteintech), anti-MyD88 (Cell Signaling), anti-NF-κB p65 (Proteintech), anti-IL-1β (Bioss), and anti-TNF-α (Bioss) at 4°C overnight. Next day, incubate with secondary horse anti-mouse or goat anti-rabbit antibodies conjugated with horseradish peroxidase (Cell Signaling) for 2 h and visualize by an enhanced chemiluminescence system (ECL). Relative protein levels were quantified after normalization to Tubulin.

Statistical Analysis

All data were described as the mean ± SEM. Pictures were analyzed by ImageJ software. Data from all experiments were quantified and analyzed by GraphPad Prism 7.0 software. $P < 0.05$ was regarded as statistically significant.

RESULTS

Gap19 Decreased Infarct Volume and Prevented the Deterioration of Neurological Deficit

Animals were euthanized after 24 h reperfusion, and the brain infarction volume was analyzed using TTC staining to determine whether Gap19 was protective after cerebral I/R injury. Results demonstrated I/R group has a large infarct volume (56.06 ± 1.77%). Gap26 and Gap19 treatment groups exhibited a significantly smaller infarct volume than I/R group ($P < 0.05$, **Figures 1A,B**). Furthermore, the infarct volume of the I/R + Gap19 group (27.9 ± 0.93%) was significantly smaller than that of the I/R + Gap26 group (40.12 ± 0.95%; $P < 0.05$, **Figures 1A,B**). This result demonstrated that Gap19 had a better neuroprotective effect. As shown in **Figure 1C**, no obvious neurological deficits were generated in the sham

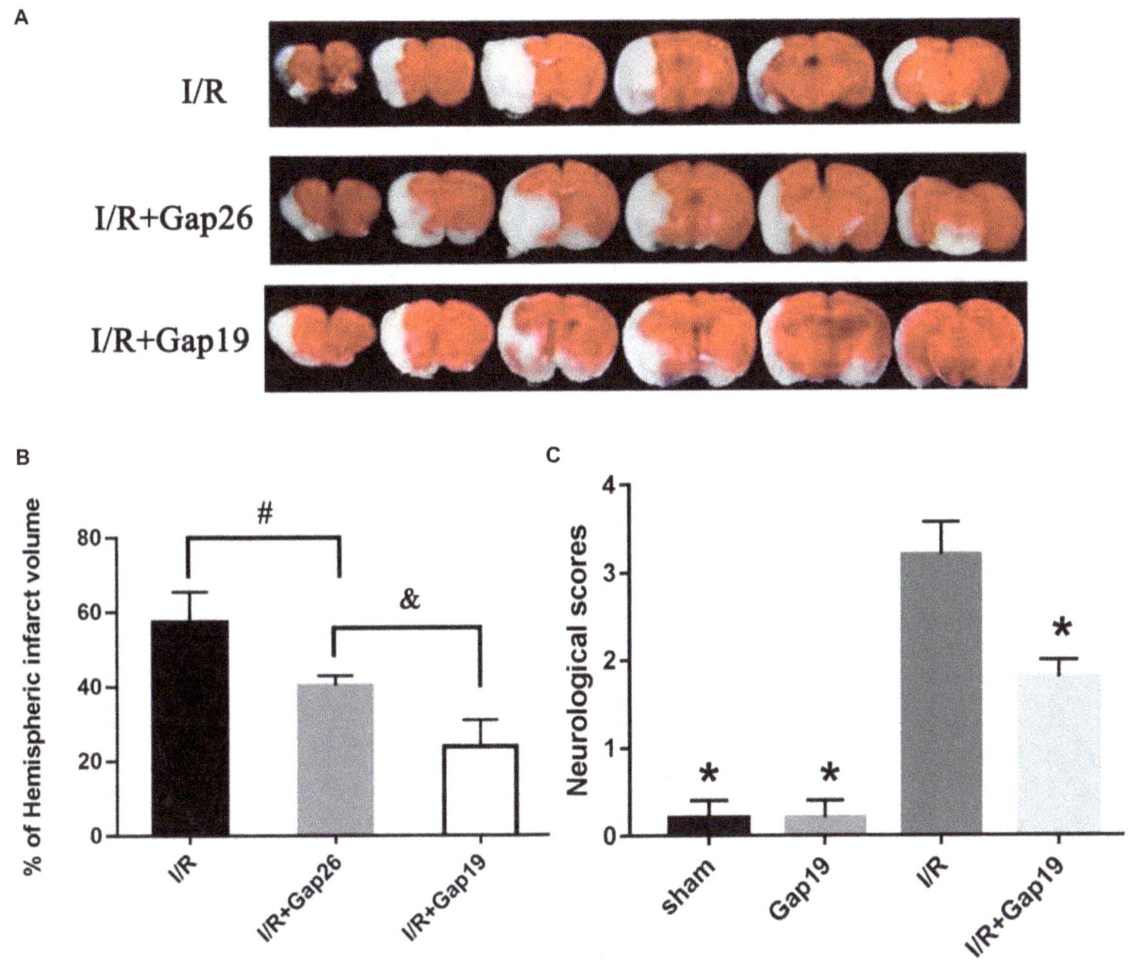

FIGURE 1 | Gap19 decreased infarct volume and prevented the deterioration neurological deficit after ischemia/reperfusion (I/R) injury. Mice were administered Gap26 or Gap19 1 h after middle cerebral artery occlusion (MCAO). 2,3,5-triphenyltetrazolium chloride chloride (TTC) staining and neurological scores were examined at 24 h after reperfusion. **(A)** Representative TTC-stained slices of different treatment groups after MCAO. The infarct tissue area was not stained (white), and normal tissue was stained (red). **(B,C)** Statistical analyses of infarct volume of different treatment groups were shown. **(C)** Neurological scores were assessed with a 5-point scale system. Gap19 treatment observably decreased neurological deficits. Data represent mean ± SEM of five brains. $^{*}P < 0.05$ vs. I/R group, $^{\#,\&}P < 0.05$.

or Gap19 groups, whereas severe deficits could be observed in I/R group. Consistent with this result, we also found that Gap19 treatment remarkably reduced neurological scores and prevented the deterioration of the neurological function ($P < 0.05$, **Figure 1C**).

Gap19 Ameliorated White Matter Injury After Cerebral I/R Injury

We euthanized mice at 7 days after reperfusion, and the brains were prepared for frozen sectioning, stained with LFB to examine the influence of Gap19 on white matter after I/R injury. We chose the white matter-enriched area of the striatum for LFB stain and analyzed the blue area in the striatum. Striatum staining was shallow in the I/R group, and the cells were swollen and disorganized (**Figures 2A,B**). The blue area in I/R + Gap19 group was obviously larger than the area in I/R group ($P < 0.05$, **Figure 2C**). This result demonstrated that Gap19 alleviated the white matter injury in the MCAO model.

The Relative Amount of Cx43 and TLR4 Increased After Cerebral I/R Injury

Western blots analyzed the expression levels of Cx43 and TLR4 at different reperfusion time points. The infarcted hemispheres were extracted from the sham group and groups with different reperfusion times (4 h, 12 h, 24 h, 72 h and 7 days). Upon I/R 4 h, it was observed an increase in the abundance of Cx43. Expression increased 4 h after reperfusion, peaked 24 h after reperfusion, and declined but remained higher than normal until 7 days ($P < 0.05$, **Figures 3A,C**). TLR4 level increased obviously in the infarcted region at 24 h after reperfusion and reached a maximum at 72 h post-reperfusion ($P < 0.05$, **Figures 3A,B**). This trend correlated with Cx43 expression. At 24 h after cerebral I/R injury, the level of Cx43 protein in I/R + Gap19 group was lower than that in the

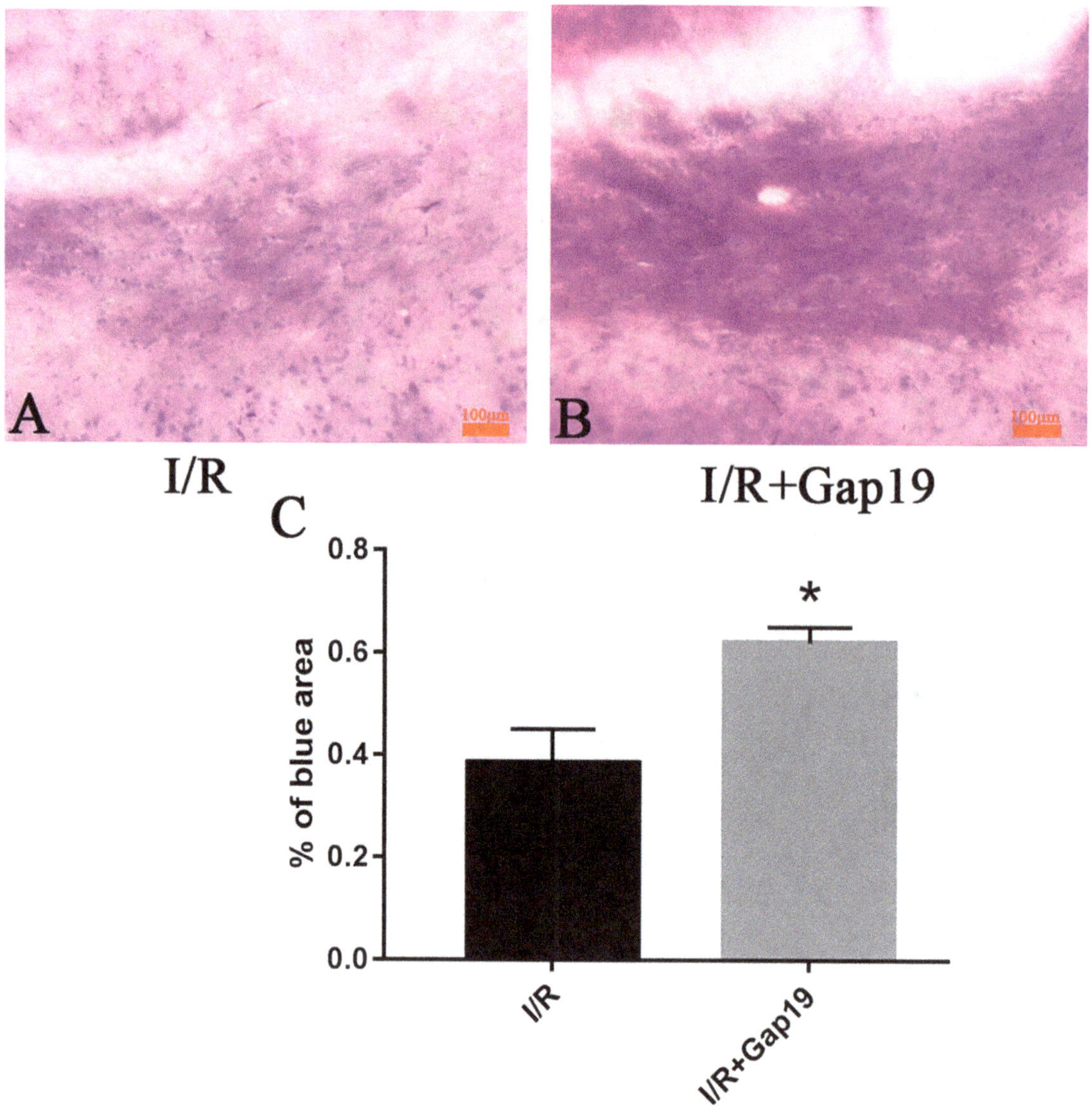

FIGURE 2 | Gap19 ameliorated white matter injury. **(A,B)** Representative pictures of LFB stain at 7 days after cerebral ischemia. **(C)** The percentage of blue area in I/R + Gap19 group was increased compared to I/R group. *$P < 0.05$ vs. I/R group. Data represent the mean ± SEM (n = 3 mice/group). Scar bar = 100 μm.

I/R group, which indicated that Gap19 effectively prevented the increase in the abundance of Cx43 ($P < 0.05$, **Figures 3D,E**).

Gap19 Inhibited Activation of the TLR4 Pathway and Reduced Inflammatory Cytokines *in vivo*

The secondary inflammatory response is the main reason for secondary injury after cerebral I/R, and TLR4-mediated innate immunity plays an important role (Wang Y. et al., 2013). We found that the expression of TLR4 was remarkably increased after MCAO than sham group or Gap19 group ($P < 0.05$, **Figures 4A,B**). TLR4 level was significantly lower in I/R + Gap19 group than I/R group. Gap19 also inhibited the expression of the TLR4 downstream protein MyD88 and NF-κB ($P < 0.05$, **Figures 4A,C,E**). Furthermore, proinflammatory cytokines as TNF-α and IL-1β released from ischemic tissue are associated with neurotoxic effects by inducing apoptosis of neuronal cells (Boutin et al., 2001; Shichita et al., 2012). Previous studies showed that these cytokines could also affect Cx43 abundance in both astrocytes (Même et al., 2006; Retamal et al., 2007) and microglia (Eugenín et al., 2001). Our study demonstrated that Gap19 treatment remarkably decreased the expression of IL-1β and TNF-α ($P < 0.05$, **Figures 4D,F,G**), which could further decreasing the Cx43 expression. These results revealed that Gap19 could effectively inhibited TLR4 pathway and decreased inflammation in a mouse cerebral I/R model.

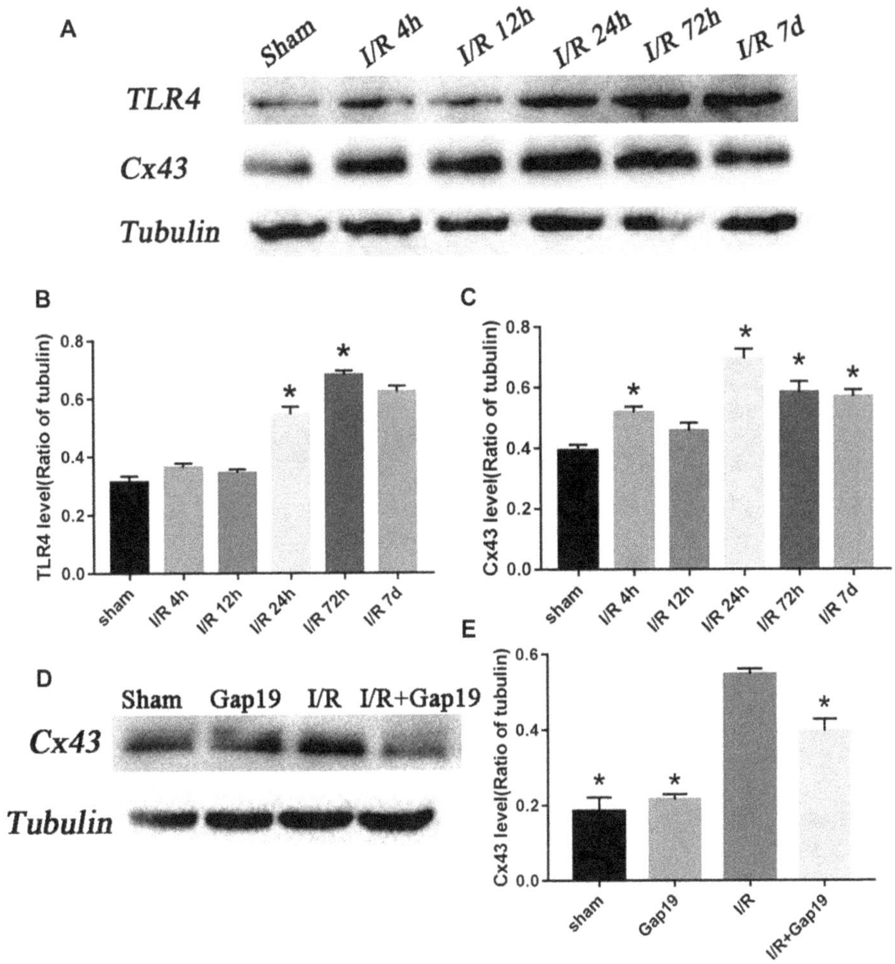

FIGURE 3 | The relative amount of connexin 43 (Cx43) and Toll-like receptor 4 (TLR4) increased after cerebral I/R injury. **(A)** Photomicrographs showed Cx43 and TLR4 tubulin levels in the sham group and 4 h, 12 h, 24 h, 72 h and 7 days after cerebral I/R injury. **(B,C)** Quantitative analyses revealed the variation tendency of Cx43 and TLR4 after cerebral I/R injury. **(D)** Photomicrographs showed Cx43 levels at 24 h after cerebral I/R injury. **(E)** Quantitative analysis of Cx43. Data represent the mean ± SEM ($n = 3$ mice/group). $^*P < 0.05$ vs. I/R group.

Cx43 Co-existed With TLR4 in Astrocytes

We performed immunofluorescence staining for Cx43 and TLR4 in primary astrocytes to further determine the relationship between the protective effect of Gap19 and the TLR4 signaling pathway in cerebral ischemic injury. We could saw both TLR4 and Cx43 existed on astrocytes in the OGD model. Cx43 was primarily expressed in the cytoplasm (yellow arrow), and TLR4 was expressed in the cell membrane (red arrow; **Figure 5**).

Gap19 Increased Cell Viability After OGD and Inhibited Cx43 Expression

We performed MTT assay in primary astrocytes to determine the optimal concentration of Gap19 in the cell OGD model. Different concentrations of Gap19 were selected to intervention in the onset of OGD, and cell viability was determined. The results demonstrated that Gap19 effectively improved the relative vitality of co-cultured cells at 50 μM, 100 μM, 150 μM and 200 μM ($P < 0.05$, **Figure 6A**), and we chose optimal concentration—100 μM ($P < 0.01$) for subsequent experiments. The expression level of Cx43 was increased in the cell OGD model, and the expression was reduced after Gap19 intervention, which was consistent with the *in vitro* results ($P < 0.05$, **Figures 6B,C**).

Gap19 Decreased the Hemichannels Activity After OGD on Astrocytes

Previous study showed that Gap19 can inhibit Cx43 hemichannel activity in astrocytes after treatment with pro-inflammatory cytokines (Abudara et al., 2014). In this study, we targeted the Cx43 hemichannels after brain ischemia, so we conducted the EtBr uptake assay to evaluate the hemichannels activity in different cells after OGD. First, we identified the three cell types with specific cellular markers. Neuron was verified by anti-β-III tubulin antibody (**Figure 7A**), BMECs were characterized by anti-CD31 antibody (**Figure 7B**) and astrocytes

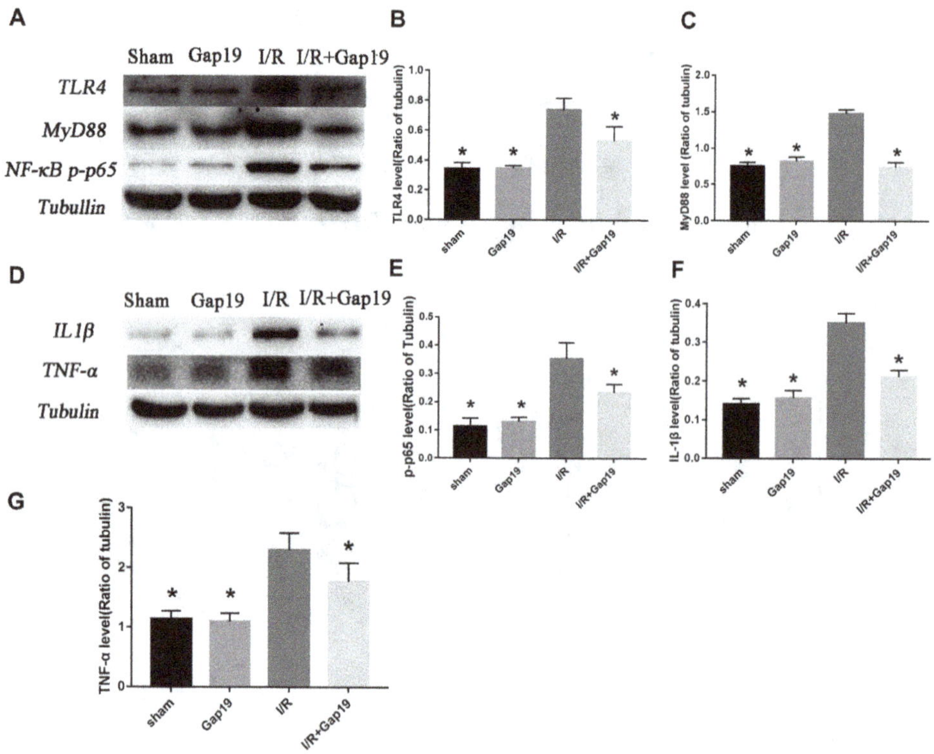

FIGURE 4 | Gap19 suppressed the TLR4 signaling pathway and inflammatory cytokines expression *in vivo*. **(A)** Brain tissues were collected after 24 h reperfusion, and TLR4, MyD88 and NF-κB p-p65 levels were determined by Western blot. Gap19 treatment inhibited the increment of TLR4 **(B)**, MyD88 **(C)** and NF-κB p-p65 **(E)** expression. **(D)** Interleukin-1β (IL-1β) and tumor necrosis factor-α (TNF-α) protein expression was also lower in Gap19-treated mice than I/R mice 24 h post-reperfusion **(F,G)**. Data represent the mean ± SEM (n = 3 mice/group). *P < 0.05 vs. I/R group.

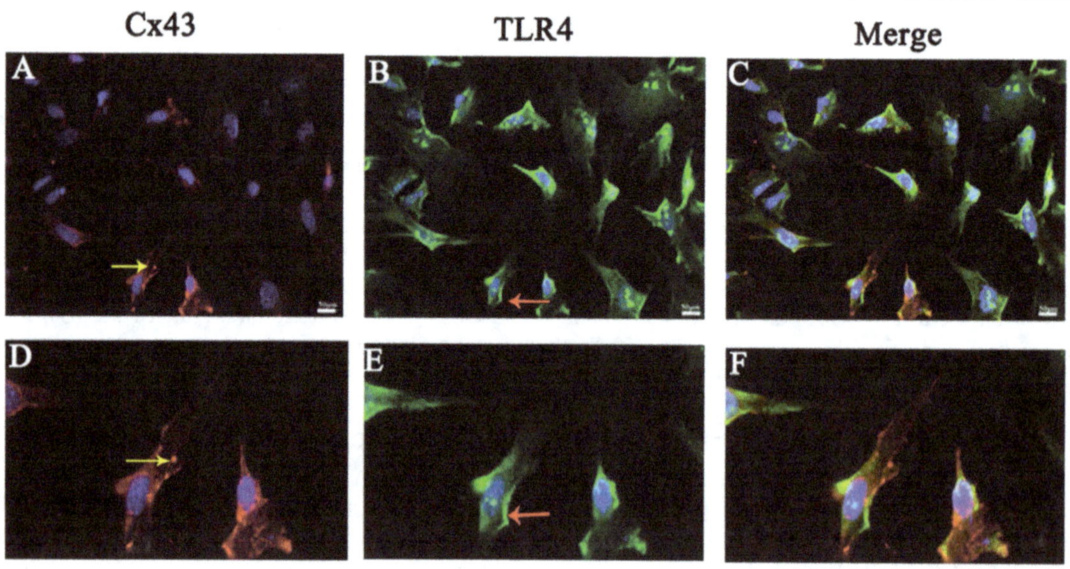

FIGURE 5 | Cx43 co-existed with TLR4 in astrocytes. **(A–C)** Double immunofluorescence staining showed the Cx43 (yellow arrow) and TLR4 (red arrow) in cultured astrocytes after oxygen glucose deprivation (OGD). **(D–F)** The pictures were the amplification of the cell with the arrow above. Scar bar = 50 μm.

were identified by anti-GFAP antibody (**Figure 7C**). Then, we observed that EtBr uptake was increased in three type cells after OGD (**Figures 7G–I**) than the control group (**Figures 7D–F**). There was slightly reduction of hemichannels

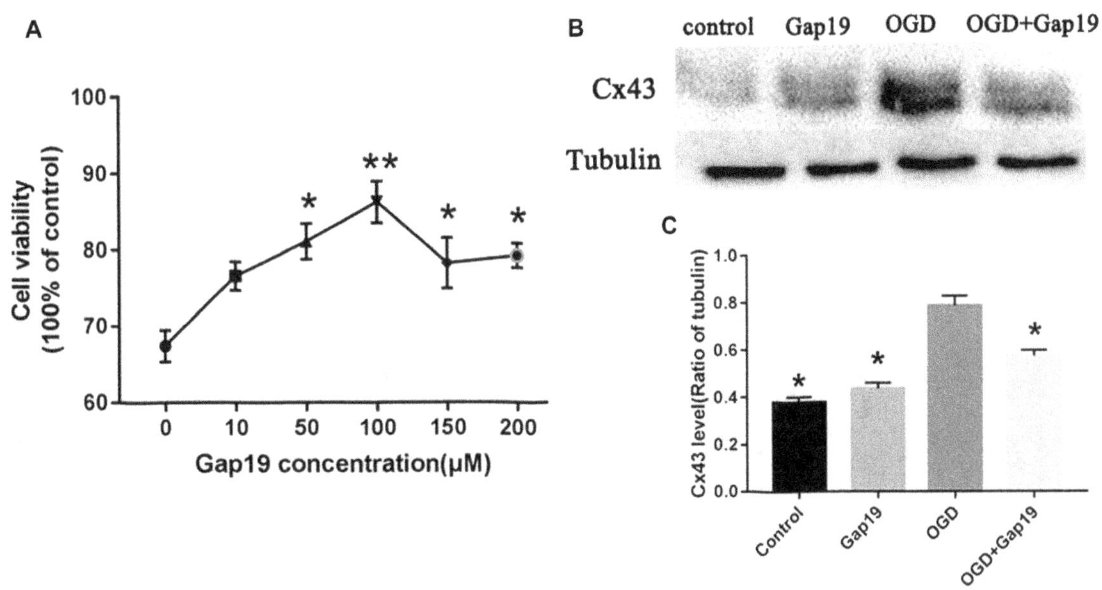

FIGURE 6 | Gap19 increased cell viability after OGD and inhibited Cx43 expression. **(A)** Cell viability following different concentrations of Gap19 after OGD. **(B)** Astrocytes were deprived oxygen-glucose for 4 h following 24 h reoxygenation, and the level of Cx43 was detected using Western blot. **(C)** Quantitative analysis confirmed that Gap19 treatment at the beginning of OGD significantly decreased Cx43 expression. Data represent the mean ± SEM (n = 3). *$P < 0.05$, **$P < 0.01$ vs. OGD group.

activity in neurons and BMECs after treatment with Gap19, but without statistical difference (**Figures 7J,K,M,N**). Meanwhile, Gap19 could obviously inhibit the hemichannels opening after OGD in astrocytes (**Figures 7L,O**). This result was consistent with a recently study. Walrave et al. (2018) found that Gap19 inhibited the hemichannels open induced by Pilocarpine and exerted anticonvulsant effects. Based on these result, we think astrocytes are the most critical cell type in this triple co-culture system.

Gap19 Also Prevented the Activation of TLR4 Pathway and Reduced Inflammatory Cytokines *in vitro*

We constructed a triple cell co-culture system to verify the role of Gap19 *in vitro* cerebral I/R model. Gap19 reduced the activation of TLR4 ($P < 0.05$, **Figures 8A,B**) compared to the levels in the triple cell co-culture OGD group. MyD88 and NF-κB level were also lower in the OGD + Gap19 group ($P < 0.05$, **Figures 8A,C,D**). We conducted ELISA to analyze the levels of inflammatory factors in the culture supernatant. The secretion of TNF-α and IL-1β in the Gap19 treatment group was decreased ($P < 0.05$, **Figures 8E,F**). These results were similar to those in the *in vitro* study. To further identify the anti-inflammation role of Gap19, we use the neutralizing antibodies of TNF-α to treat the astrocytes after OGD and detect the cell viability. We qualitatively found both TNF-α and p-P65 expression was inhibited through Western blot (**Figure 8G**). The MTT assay revealed that neutralization of TNF-α can also increase the astrocytes viability after OGD, just like Gap19 ($P < 0.05$, **Figure 8H**). This is a very interesting result, which further confirmed that Gap19 could alleviate the inflammatory response by inhibiting the opening of Cx43 hemichannels.

Gap19 Attenuated LPS-Induced TLR4 Activation and Inflammation *in vitro*

Based on the above results, we hypothesized that Gap19 protected against cerebral I/R injury via downregulation of TLR4 signaling. LPS is one of the pathogen-associated molecular pattern that can specifically activate TLR4 signaling (Shao et al., 2013), and increase Cx43 hemichannels activity in astrocytes (Retamal et al., 2007). We conducted the LPS-induced experiment to further verify this hypothesis. The expression of TLR4 after LPS treatment was increased compared to the OGD group in the triple cell co-culture system ($P < 0.05$, **Figures 9A,B**). Gap19 treatment significantly attenuated TLR4 expression after LPS stimulation in OGD model. We further detected proinflammatory cytokine levels in the cell supernatant using ELISA. Gap19 treatment decreased the release of TNF-α and IL-1β in the culture medium after LPS stimulation ($P < 0.05$, **Figures 9C,D**). These results further corroborate that the protective effect of Gap19 occurred via downregulation of the TLR4 pathway.

DISCUSSION

The concept of the NVU was first proposed in 2003 by Lo and colleagues (Lo et al., 2003). Cerebrovascular disease research has gradually shifted focus from merely neurons or astrocytes to the NVU integral components, and it is considered a precondition for the screening of novel drugs and therapeutic

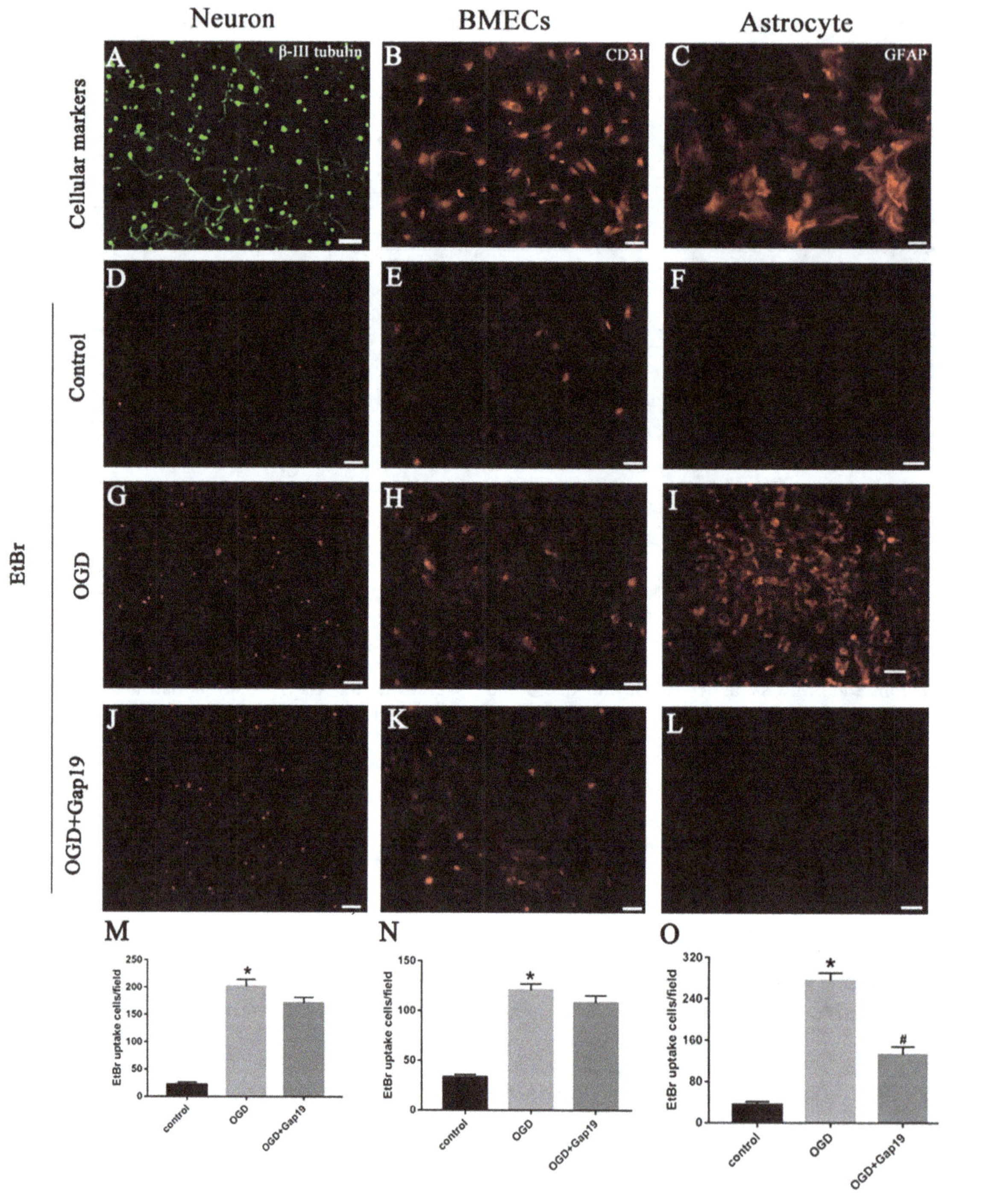

FIGURE 7 | Gap19 decreased the hemichannels activity after OGD on astrocytes. **(A–C)** Immunophenotyping of three cells were identified by β-III tubulin, CD31 and GFAP. **(D–L)** Representative pictures showed ethidium bromide (EtBr) uptake via hemichannels in the three groups of different cells. **(M–O)** EtBr uptake was increased after OGD injury, and Gap19 could remarkably inhibited hemichannels activity. *$P < 0.05$ vs. control group. #$P < 0.05$ vs. OGD group. Scar bar = 100 μm.

target for stroke (Hu et al., 2017). Glial cells (astrocytes and oligodendrocytes) and BMECs are damaged via similar injury pathways, including glutamate toxicity, during ischemic injury (George and Steinberg, 2015). Ischemic damage also activates endogenous immune cells such as microglia (Kim et al., 2014). This study successfully established the cerebral I/R model *in vivo/vitro* and examined the role of Gap19 in cerebral I/R injury. Our results suggested that Gap19 reduced the infarct size and prevented the deterioration of the neurological function after cerebral ischemia and alleviated brain white matter damage.

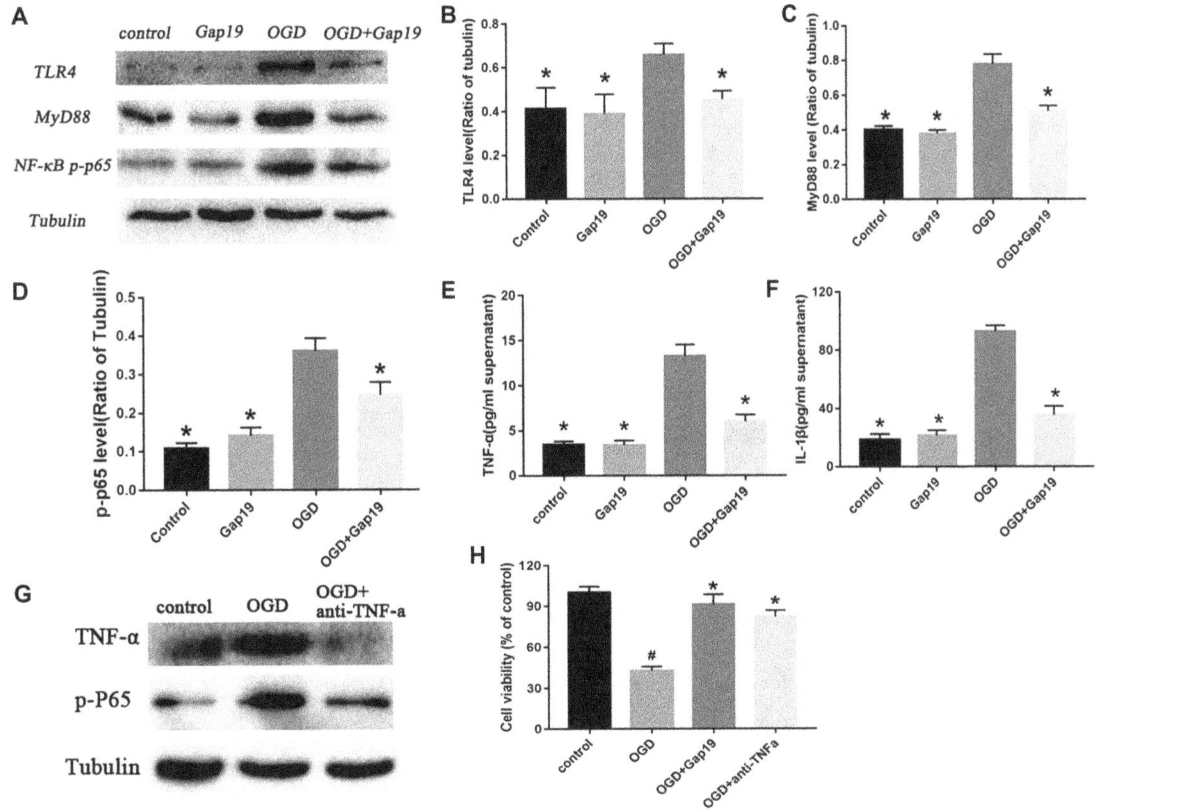

FIGURE 8 | Gap19 prevented the activation of TLR4 pathway and reduced inflammatory cytokines *in vitro*. **(A–D)** Western blot and quantitative analysis showed the expression of TLR4, MyD88 and NF-κB p-p65 were decreased by Gap19 after OGD. **(E,F)** Enzyme-linked immunosorbent assay (ELISA) revealed that Gap19-treated cells exhibited altered release of IL-1β and TNF-α 24 h after reoxygenation. **(G,H)** The neutralizing antibodies of TNF-α decrease the p-P65 expression and increased the astrocytes viability after OGD. Values (mean ± SEM) are representative of at least three independent experiments. $^{*}P < 0.05$ vs. the OGD group. $^{\#}P < 0.05$ vs. the control group.

We further investigated the protection mechanism of Gap19. Result showed that Gap19 reduced the expression levels of Cx43, TLR4, MyD88 and NF-κB after ischemic injury and reduced the inflammatory response secondary to reperfusion.

We also investigated the mechanism about how Gap19 alleviating inflammation following stroke. We cultured primary neurons, astrocytes and cerebrovascular endothelial cells and constructed an NVU model for OGD treatment to simulate the *in vivo* process of cerebral I/R injury. Our result showed that when the concentration of Gap19 over 150 μM, the cell viability decreased compared with 100 μM. We think that high concentration strongly inhibits the Cx43 expression and decrease the gap junction formation, further interfering cell-to-cell communication. We detected the change of hemichannels activity on different treatment by EtBr uptake assay. Results showed that the opening of hemichannels increased after OGD and Gap19 could inhibit this effect on astrocytes. We also observed that Gap19 inhibited activation of the TLR4 pathway after OGD and inhibited the expression of pathway-related proteins, reduced the release of TNF-α and IL-1β, which was similar with the role of neutralization of TNF-α. Gap19 also decreased the expression of TLR4 in the LPS administration OGD model. Our results are the first to demonstrate that specific blocker of Cx43 hemichannels-Gap19 plays a vital role in protecting cerebral ischemia via inhibition of activation of the TLR4 pathways.

NVU consists of neurons, astrocytes and cerebrovascular endothelial cells, pericytes, basal membranes, and extracellular matrix (Stanimirovic and Friedman, 2012). Nerve cells are primarily connected with each other via gap junctions to communicate electrical signals, transmit chemical signals and metabolites to support the normal function of NVU cells (Giaume et al., 2010). Our study considered the NVU as the main research object and gap junctions as the main target. Cx43 is the main connexin protein that forms the gap junctions and hemichannels, and these proteins are expressed abundantly in brain, especially in astrocytes (D'hondt et al., 2014). Large amounts of hemichannels are opened after ischemia, causing ion disorders, loss of important metabolic substances, cell swelling and even death. Previous studies have shown that the use of gap junction inhibitors, such as glycyrrhetinic acid and its derivative carbenoxolone, improve blood-brain barrier permeability in mice, but the specificity is poor, and glycyrrhetinic acid interferes with other types of junctions

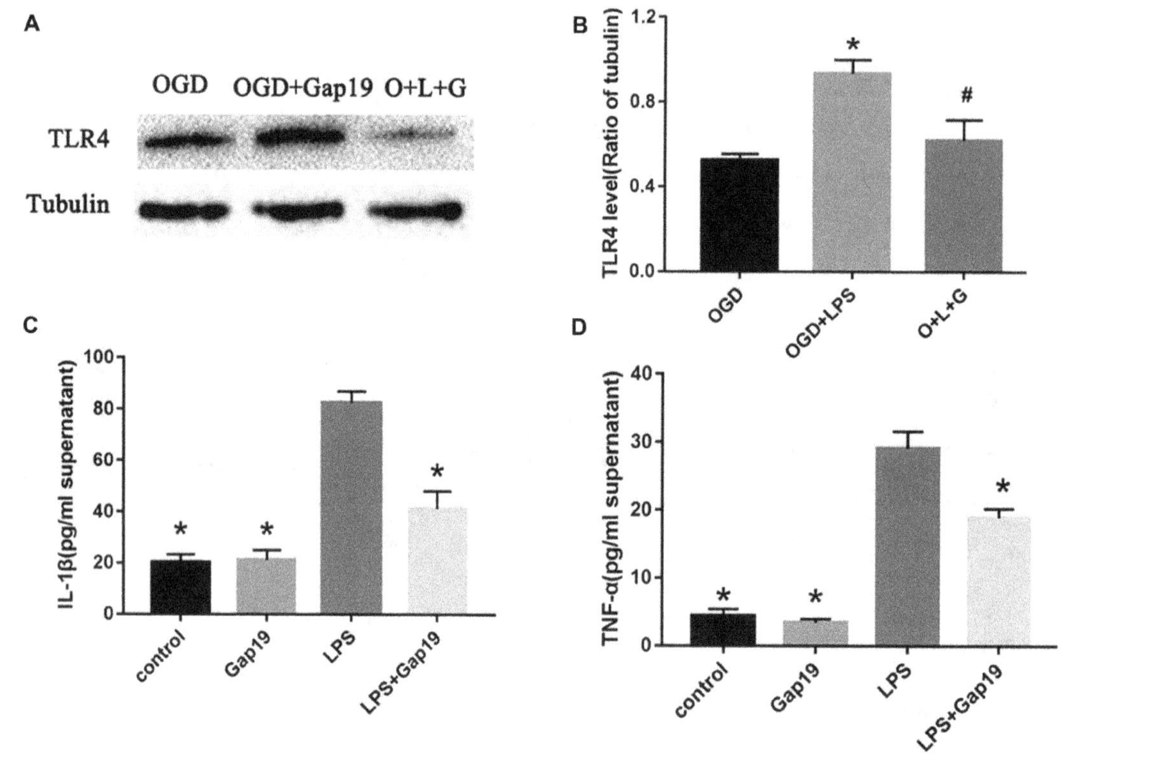

FIGURE 9 | Gap19 attenuated LPS-induced TLR4 activation and inflammation *in vitro*. **(A)** Photomicrographs show TLR4 levels after LPS treatment using Western blot. The group O + L + G means OGD + LPS + Gap19 group. **(B)** Quantitative analysis confirmed that Gap19 treatment decreased TLR4 expression after LPS stimulation. **(C,D)** ELISA showed that Gap19 inhibited the release of IL-1β and TNF-α after LPS administration. Data represent the mean ± SEM (n = 3). $^*P < 0.05$ vs. OGD group, $^{\#}P < 0.05$ vs. OGD + LPS group.

(Takeuchi et al., 2011). Our previous studies demonstrated that the Cx43 mimetic peptides Gap26/Gap27 exhibited protective effects on the hypoxia/ischemia model in neonatal rats (Li et al., 2015). Hawat et al. (2010) found that Gap26 reduced infarct volume in myocardial ischemia reperfusion injury in rats. However, Gap26/27 also affected the formation of gap junctions when hemichannels are blocked.

Gap19 is a mimetic peptide that corresponds to a sequence in the CL of Cx43, which may disturb the interaction of C-terminal tail and CL of Cx43 (Abudara et al., 2014). The peptide may keep the gap junction open and hemichannel closed after ischemia with high specificity (Delmar et al., 2004). Wang N. et al. (2013) verified that Gap19 decreased the infarct volume after myocardial I/R in mice and alleviated cell oedema. Vicario et al. (2017) found that Gap19 specifically inhibited damage to human neuroblastoma cells after hypoxia/reoxygenation injury. Walrave et al. (2016) reported that TAT-Gap19 impaired hippocampal short-term spatial memory via inhibition of Cx43 hemichannels. Treatment with Gap19 decreased Cx43 expression in our study, which could further decrease the formation of Cx43 hemichannels. Our previous study found that Gap26 could decrease both total and dephosphorylated Cx43, and promote the internalization of Cx43 and the degradation of Cx43 in cytoplasm through the ubiquitin proteasome pathway (Li et al., 2015). In this study, Gap19 reduced infarction volume more than Gap26, exhibited better specificity and played a neuroprotective role in brain ischemia, and our results identified that Gap19 could significantly decrease the hemichannels activity on astrocytes but not on neurons and BMECs. Previous studies showed that Cx43 mainly expressed in astrocytes, rarely on neurons (Liu et al., 2012; Schulz et al., 2015), and could increase in BMECs after inflammation (Danesh-Meyer et al., 2012). In this NVU model, astrocytes were the critical one as bridge to connect the different components.

I/R is a pathological process that interrupts the blood flow of an organ, subsequent with reperfusion and reoxidation. Blood recirculation further aggravates tissue damage, which leads to a more severe inflammatory response, known as reperfusion injury (Eltzschig and Eckle, 2011). This injury occurs in a sterile environment and involves signaling events through pattern-recognition receptors (PRRs), such as TLRs, and the infiltration of blood immune cells of the innate and adaptive immune systems (Shichita et al., 2012). As we all know, microglia is the primary immune effector and can be activated by ischemia, releasing inflammatory cytokines (Morioka et al., 1993). And in brain, TLRs are constitutively expressed in microglia, but also in astrocyte and can be activated by endogenous damage-associated molecular patterns (DAMPs), such as ATP (Zhang et al., 2010), high mobility group box 1 protein (Yang et al., 2011), heat shock proteins, extracellular matrix proteins and so on. They are released from damaged brain cells after ischemia (Kim et al., 2014; Molteni et al., 2016). Increasing evidence suggests that TLR4 plays an important role in secondary brain injury following ischemia (Brea et al., 2011). A recent study demonstrated that $TLR4^{-/-}$ mice decreased neuronal damage and apoptosis after global cerebral I/R (Hua et al., 2007). Hua et al. (2015) found that TLR4 blocker TAK-242 alleviated the inflammation after brain ischemia and played a neuroprotective role. Although TLR4 was primarily expressed in microglia in the central nervous system, these receptors are also expressed in astrocytes (Carpentier et al., 2008), neurons (Tang et al., 2007), and cerebrovascular endothelial cells (Grace et al., 2014) in some pathological environments. Our study demonstrated that Gap19 inhibited activation of the TLR4 signaling by MyD88-dependent pathway. Previous studies showed that treatment with TNF-α or IL-1β could increase membrane permeability through Cx43 hemichannels in astrocytes (Retamal et al., 2007) and upregulate the expression of Cx43 in microglia (Shaikh et al., 2012; Sáez et al., 2013). Our results revealed that Gap19 attenuated the expression of TNF-α and IL-1β after cerebral I/R injury which further suggests that the protective effect may occur via inhibition of the inflammatory response after reperfusion. Previous researches showed that after inflammation stimulation, microglia can also express Cx43 and communicate with each other through the gap junction (Eugenín et al., 2001; Shaikh et al., 2012; Sáez et al., 2013). In the future study, it will be valuable to add the microglia in this system for further study.

A recent study demonstrated that the Cx43 hemichannel may be a novel mediator of sterile inflammatory diseases (Li et al., 2018), which is consistent with the results of our study. This research further indicates that Cx43 is associated with inflammation. LPS is the main component of the cytoderm of Gram-negative bacteria and specifically activated the TLR4 pathway to induce an inflammatory response (Kawai and Akira, 2010). The *in vitro* model found that Gap19 reduced TLR4 and inflammatory cytokines expression after LPS stimulation. Previous studies reported that IL-1β and TNF-α released by activated microglia can inhibit the gap junction communication and increase the hemichannels activity on astrocyte (Même et al., 2006; Retamal et al., 2007). In other words, Gap19 may also decrease the opening of Cx43 hemichannels. All these data demonstrated that the inhibitory effect of Gap19 on the inflammation secondary to I/R injury may be associated with the inhibition of TLR4 signaling pathway. However, how the interaction of Gap19 and Cx43 causes inhibition of the TLR4 pathway remains unknown. We think that the mechanism may be similar to the treatment with Gap26. Previous study showed that the decrease of Cx43 expression after DNA hyper-methylation further activates the transcriptional activation of apoptosis suppressor genes (Yu S. C. et al., 2012). Li et al. (2016) found that hypoxia during pregnancy may lead to continuous whole-brain hypo-methylation in the fetal brain. Hence, does it affect the methylation of Cx43 DNA promoter region? This still requires further study.

CONCLUSION

Our results indicate that Gap19 can decrease the brain infarct volume, prevent the deterioration of neurological deficit and alleviate white matter damage, and that Gap19 can also remarkably reduce the inflammatory response via inhibition of the TLR4 signaling pathway following *in vivo* MCAO and *in vitro* OGD. Therefore, Gap19 may be a potential therapeutic drug for cerebral ischemic injury which associated with NVU disruption.

However, whether Gap19 affects TRIF-mediated inflammatory responses, which is the other pathway of TLR4, is not known. Future experiments should address this relationship. We did not verify the inhibition of Gap19 on the TLR4 pathway at the gene expression level, and more studies are required to further validate these results.

AUTHOR CONTRIBUTIONS

YC, LW and HY: conceived and designed the experiments; contributed to the writing of the manuscript. LW, LZ and LY: performed the experiments. HY, YL and LW: analyzed the data. LW, XL and BC: contributed reagents, materials and analysis tools. All authors approved the final manuscript.

FUNDING

This study was supported by National Natural Science Foundation of China (Grant nos. 81400963 and 81371377), 333 project of Jiangsu Province (the grant number: BRA2015187 and BRA2017168) and Jiangsu Provincial Medical Youth Talent (Grant #QNRC2016327 and QNRC2016328, QNRC2016326) and Six big talent peak fund in Jiangsu Province (grant #2016-WSN-274).

ACKNOWLEDGMENTS

All authors have contributed significantly, and all authors are in agreement with the content of the manuscript. We gratefully thank YC, XL, BC, YL and HY for their generous assistance.

REFERENCES

Abudara, V., Bechberger, J., Freitas-Andrade, M., De Bock, M., Wang, N., Bultynck, G., et al. (2014). The connexin43 mimetic peptide Gap19 inhibits hemichannels without altering gap junctional communication in astrocytes. *Front. Cell. Neurosci.* 8:306. doi: 10.3389/fncel.2014.00306

Bodendiek, S. B., and Raman, G. (2010). Connexin modulators and their potential targets under the magnifying glass. *Curr. Med. Chem.* 17, 4191–4230. doi: 10.2174/092986710793348563

Boutin, H., LeFeuvre, R. A., Horai, R., Asano, M., Iwakura, Y., and Rothwell, N. J. (2001). Role of IL-1α and IL-1β in ischemic brain damage. *J. Neurosci.* 21, 5528–5534. doi: 10.1523/JNEUROSCI.21-15-05528.2001

Brea, D., Blanco, M., Ramos-Cabrer, P., Moldes, O., Arias, S., Perez-Mato, M., et al. (2011). Toll-like receptors 2 and 4 in ischemic stroke: outcome and therapeutic values. *J. Cereb. Blood Flow Metab.* 31, 1424–1431. doi: 10.1038/jcbfm.2010.231

Carpentier, P. A., Duncan D', A. S., and Miller, S. D. (2008). Glial toll-like receptor signaling in central nervous system infection and autoimmunity. *Brain Behav. Immun.* 22, 140–147. doi: 10.1016/j.bbi.2007.08.011

Chew, S. S., Johnson, C. S., Green, C. R., and Danesh-Meyer, H. V. (2010). Role of connexin43 in central nervous system injury. *Exp. Neurol.* 225, 250–261. doi: 10.1016/j.expneurol.2010.07.014

Danesh-Meyer, H. V., Kerr, N. M., Zhang, J., Eady, E. K., O'Carroll, S. J., Nicholson, L. F., et al. (2012). Connexin43 mimetic peptide reduces vascular leak and retinal ganglion cell death following retinal ischaemia. *Brain* 135, 506–520. doi: 10.1093/brain/awr338

De Bock, M., Culot, M., Wang, N., Bol, M., Decrock, E., De Vuyst, E., et al. (2011). Connexin channels provide a target to manipulate brain endothelial calcium dynamics and blood-brain barrier permeability. *J. Cereb. Blood Flow Metab.* 31, 1942–1957. doi: 10.1038/jcbfm.2011.86

Decrock, E., De Vuyst, E., Vinken, M., Van Moorhem, M., Vranckx, K., Wang, N., et al. (2009). Connexin 43 hemichannels contribute to the propagation of apoptotic cell death in a rat C6 glioma cell model. *Cell Death Differ.* 16, 151–163. doi: 10.1038/cdd.2008.138

Delmar, M., Coombs, W., Sorgen, P., Duffy, H. S., and Taffet, S. M. (2004). Structural bases for the chemical regulation of connexin43 channels. *Cardiovasc. Res.* 62, 268–275. doi: 10.1016/j.cardiores.2003.12.030

D'hondt, C., Iyyathurai, J., Himpens, B., Leybaert, L., and Bultynck, G. (2014). Cx43-hemichannel function and regulation in physiology and pathophysiology: insights from the bovine corneal endothelial cell system and beyond. *Front. Physiol.* 5:348. doi: 10.3389/fphys.2014.00348

Eltzschig, H. K., and Eckle, T. (2011). Ischemia and reperfusion—from mechanism to translation. *Nat. Med.* 17, 1391–1401. doi: 10.1038/nm.2507

Eugenín, E. A., Eckardt, D., Theis, M., Willecke, K., Bennett, M. V., and Saez, J. C. (2001). Microglia at brain stab wounds express connexin 43 and *in vitro* form functional gap junctions after treatment with interferon-γ and tumor necrosis factor-α. *Proc. Natl. Acad. Sci. U S A* 98, 4190–4195. doi: 10.1073/pnas.051634298

Evans, W. H., and Leybaert, L. (2007). Mimetic peptides as blockers of connexin channel-facilitated intercellular communication. *Cell Commun. Adhes.* 14, 265–273. doi: 10.1080/15419060801891034

Gauthier, S. A., Sahoo, S., Jung, S. S., and Levy, E. (2012). Murine cerebrovascular cells as a cell culture model for cerebral amyloid angiopathy: isolation of smooth muscle and endothelial cells from mouse brain. *Methods Mol. Biol.* 849, 261–274. doi: 10.1007/978-1-61779-551-0_18

George, P. M., and Steinberg, G. K. (2015). Novel stroke therapeutics: unraveling stroke pathophysiology and its impact on clinical treatments. *Neuron* 87, 297–309. doi: 10.1016/j.neuron.2015.05.041

Giaume, C., Koulakoff, A., Roux, L., Holcman, D., and Rouach, N. (2010). Astroglial networks: a step further in neuroglial and gliovascular interactions. *Nat. Rev. Neurosci.* 11, 87–99. doi: 10.1038/nrn2757

Giaume, C., Orellana, J. A., Abudara, V., and Saez, J. C. (2012). Connexin-based channels in astrocytes: how to study their properties. *Methods Mol. Biol.* 814, 283–303. doi: 10.1007/978-1-61779-452-0_19

Girouard, H., and Iadecola, C. (2006). Neurovascular coupling in the normal brain and in hypertension, stroke and Alzheimer disease. *J. Appl. Physiol.* 100, 328–335. doi: 10.1152/japplphysiol.00966.2005

Grace, P. M., Ramos, K. M., Rodgers, K. M., Wang, X., Hutchinson, M. R., Lewis, M. T., et al. (2014). Activation of adult rat CNS endothelial cells by opioid-induced toll-like receptor 4 (TLR4) signaling induces proinflammatory, biochemical, morphological and behavioral sequelae. *Neuroscience* 280, 299–317. doi: 10.1016/j.neuroscience.2014.09.020

Guo, S., Kim, W. J., Lok, J., Lee, S. R., Besancon, E., Luo, B. H., et al. (2008). Neuroprotection via matrix-trophic coupling between cerebral endothelial cells and neurons. *Proc. Natl. Acad. Sci. U S A* 105, 7582–7587. doi: 10.1073/pnas.0801105105

Hawat, G., Benderdour, M., Rousseau, G., and Baroudi, G. (2010). Connexin 43 mimetic peptide Gap26 confers protection to intact heart against myocardial ischemia injury. *Pflugers Arch.* 460, 583–592. doi: 10.1007/s00424-010-0849-6

Hu, X., De Silva, T. M., Chen, J., and Faraci, F. M. (2017). Cerebral vascular disease and neurovascular injury in ischemic stroke. *Circ. Res.* 120, 449–471. doi: 10.1161/circresaha.116.308427

Hua, F., Ma, J., Ha, T., Xia, Y., Kelley, J., Williams, D. L., et al. (2007). Activation of toll-like receptor 4 signaling contributes to hippocampal neuronal death following global cerebral ischemia/reperfusion. *J. Neuroimmunol.* 190, 101–111. doi: 10.1016/j.jneuroim.2007.08.014

Hua, F., Tang, H., Wang, J., Prunty, M. C., Hua, X., Sayeed, I., et al. (2015). TAK-242, an antagonist for toll-like receptor 4, protects against acute cerebral ischemia/reperfusion injury in mice. *J. Cereb. Blood Flow Metab.* 35, 536–542. doi: 10.1038/jcbfm.2014.240

Islam, M. M., and Mohamed, Z. (2015). Computational and pharmacological target of neurovascular unit for drug design and delivery. *Biomed Res. Int.* 2015:731292. doi: 10.1155/2015/731292

Jiang, M., Li, J., Peng, Q., Liu, Y., Liu, W., Luo, C., et al. (2014). Neuroprotective effects of bilobalide on cerebral ischemia and reperfusion injury are associated with inhibition of pro-inflammatory mediator production and down-regulation of JNK1/2 and p38 MAPK activation. *J. Neuroinflammation* 11:167. doi: 10.1186/s12974-014-0167-6

Jing, Z., Xing, J., Chen, X., Stetler, R. A., Weng, Z., Gan, Y., et al. (2014). Neuronal NAMPT is released after cerebral ischemia and protects against white matter injury. *J. Cereb. Blood Flow Metab.* 34, 1613–1621. doi: 10.1038/jcbfm.2014.119

Kawai, T., and Akira, S. (2010). The role of pattern-recognition receptors in innate immunity: update on toll-like receptors. *Nat. Immunol.* 11, 373–384. doi: 10.1038/ni.1863

Kim, Y., Davidson, J. O., Gunn, K. C., Phillips, A. R., Green, C. R., and Gunn, A. J. (2016). Role of hemichannels in CNS inflammation and the inflammasome pathway. *Adv. Protein Chem. Struct. Biol.* 104, 1–37. doi: 10.1016/bs.apcsb.2015.12.001

Kim, J. Y., Kawabori, M., and Yenari, M. A. (2014). Innate inflammatory responses in stroke: mechanisms and potential therapeutic targets. *Curr. Med. Chem.* 21, 2076–2097. doi: 10.2174/0929867321666131228205146

Li, W., Bao, G., Chen, W., Qiang, X., Zhu, S., Wang, S., et al. (2018). Connexin 43 hemichannel as a novel mediator of sterile and infectious inflammatory diseases. *Sci. Rep.* 8:166. doi: 10.1038/s41598-017-18452-1

Li, Y., Ma, Q., Halavi, S., Concepcion, K., Hartman, R. E., Obenaus, A., et al. (2016). Fetal stress-mediated hypomethylation increases the brain susceptibility to hypoxic-ischemic injury in neonatal rats. *Exp. Neurol.* 275, 1–10. doi: 10.1016/j.expneurol.2015.10.007

Li, X., Zhao, H., Tan, X., Kostrzewa, R. M., Du, G., Chen, Y., et al. (2015). Inhibition of connexin43 improves functional recovery after ischemic brain injury in neonatal rats. *Glia* 63, 1553–1567. doi: 10.1002/glia.22826

Liu, X., Sun, L., Torii, M., and Rakic, P. (2012). Connexin 43 controls the multipolar phase of neuronal migration to the cerebral cortex. *Proc. Natl. Acad. Sci. U S A* 109, 8280–8285. doi: 10.1073/pnas.1205880109

Lo, E. H. (2010). Degeneration and repair in central nervous system disease. *Nat. Med.* 16, 1205–1209. doi: 10.1038/nm.2226

Lo, E. H., Dalkara, T., and Moskowitz, M. A. (2003). Mechanisms, challenges and opportunities in stroke. *Nat. Rev. Neurosci.* 4, 399–415. doi: 10.1038/nrn1106

Meller, R., Stevens, S. L., Minami, M., Cameron, J. A., King, S., Rosenzweig, H., et al. (2005). Neuroprotection by osteopontin in stroke. *J. Cereb. Blood Flow Metab.* 25, 217–225. doi: 10.1038/sj.jcbfm.9600022

Même, W., Calvo, C. F., Froger, N., Ezan, P., Amigou, E., Koulakoff, A., et al. (2006). Proinflammatory cytokines released from microglia inhibit gap junctions in astrocytes: potentiation by β-amyloid. *FASEB J.* 20, 494–496. doi: 10.1096/fj.05-4297fje

Molteni, M., Gemma, S., and Rossetti, C. (2016). The role of toll-like receptor 4 in infectious and noninfectious inflammation. *Mediators Inflamm.* 2016:6978936. doi: 10.1155/2016/6978936

Morioka, T., Kalehua, A. N., and Streit, W. J. (1993). Characterization of microglial reaction after middle cerebral artery occlusion in rat brain. *J. Comp. Neurol.* 327, 123–132. doi: 10.1002/cne.903270110

Moskowitz, M. A., Lo, E. H., and Iadecola, C. (2010). The science of stroke: mechanisms in search of treatments. *Neuron* 67, 181–198. doi: 10.1016/j.neuron.2010.07.002

Mozaffarian, D., Benjamin, E. J., Go, A. S., Arnett, D. K., Blaha, M. J., Cushman, M., et al. (2015). Heart disease and stroke statistics—2015 update: a report from the American Heart Association. *Circulation* 131, e29–e322. doi: 10.1161/CIR.0000000000000152

Nakagawa, S., Deli, M. A., Kawaguchi, H., Shimizudani, T., Shimono, T., Kittel, A., et al. (2009). A new blood-brain barrier model using primary rat brain endothelial cells, pericytes and astrocytes. *Neurochem. Int.* 54, 253–263. doi: 10.1016/j.neuint.2008.12.002

Naus, C. C., and Giaume, C. (2016). Bridging the gap to therapeutic strategies based on connexin/pannexin biology. *J. Transl. Med.* 14:330. doi: 10.1186/s12967-016-1089-0

O'Carroll, S. J., Alkadhi, M., Nicholson, L. F., and Green, C. R. (2008). Connexin 43 mimetic peptides reduce swelling, astrogliosis and neuronal cell death after spinal cord injury. *Cell Commun. Adhes.* 15, 27–42. doi: 10.1080/15419060802014164

Powers, W. J., Rabinstein, A. A., Ackerson, T., Adeoye, O. M., Bambakidis, N. C., Becker, K., et al. (2018). 2018 Guidelines for the early management of patients with acute ischemic stroke: a guideline for healthcare professionals from the American Heart Association/American Stroke Association. *Stroke* 49, e46–e110. doi: 10.1161/STR.0000000000000158

Retamal, M. A., Froger, N., Palacios-Prado, N., Ezan, P., Saez, P. J., Saez, J. C., et al. (2007). Cx43 hemichannels and gap junction channels in astrocytes are regulated oppositely by proinflammatory cytokines released from activated microglia. *J. Neurosci.* 27, 13781–13792. doi: 10.1523/jneurosci.2042-07.2007

Rowe, D. D., Collier, L. A., Seifert, H. A., Chapman, C. B., Leonardo, C. C., Willing, A. E., et al. (2014). Leukemia inhibitor factor promotes functional recovery and oligodendrocyte survival in rat models of focal ischemia. *Eur. J. Neurosci.* 40, 3111–3119. doi: 10.1111/ejn.12675

Ruck, T., Bittner, S., Epping, L., Herrmann, A. M., and Meuth, S. G. (2014). Isolation of primary murine brain microvascular endothelial cells. *J. Vis. Exp.* 93:e52204. doi: 10.3791/52204

Sáez, J. C., and Leybaert, L. (2014). Hunting for connexin hemichannels. *FEBS Lett.* 588, 1205–1211. doi: 10.1016/j.febslet.2014.03.004

Sáez, P. J., Shoji, K. F., Retamal, M. A., Harcha, P. A., Ramirez, G., Jiang, J. X., et al. (2013). ATP is required and advances cytokine-induced gap junction formation in microglia *in vitro*. *Mediators Inflamm.* 2013:216402. doi: 10.1155/2013/216402

Sahota, P., and Savitz, S. I. (2011). Investigational therapies for ischemic stroke neuroprotection and neurorecovery. *Neurotherapeutics* 8, 434–451. doi: 10.1007/s13311-011-0040-6

Saver, J. L., Fonarow, G. C., Smith, E. E., Reeves, M. J., Grau-Sepulveda, M. V., Pan, W., et al. (2013). Time to treatment with intravenous tissue plasminogen activator and outcome from acute ischemic stroke. *JAMA* 309, 2480–2488. doi: 10.1001/jama.2013.6959

Schulz, R., Görge, P. M., Görbe, A., Ferdinandy, P., Lampe, P. D., and Leybaert, L. (2015). Connexin 43 is an emerging therapeutic target in ischemia/reperfusion injury, cardioprotection and neuroprotection. *Pharmacol. Ther.* 153, 90–106. doi: 10.1016/j.pharmthera.2015.06.005

Shaikh, S. B., Uy, B., Perera, A., and Nicholson, L. F. (2012). AGEs-RAGE mediated up-regulation of connexin43 in activated human microglial CHME-5 cells. *Neurochem. Int.* 60, 640–651. doi: 10.1016/j.neuint.2012.02.023

Shao, J., Liu, T., Xie, Q. R., Zhang, T., Yu, H., Wang, B., et al. (2013). Adjudin attenuates lipopolysaccharide (LPS)- and ischemia-induced microglial activation. *J. Neuroimmunol.* 254, 83–90. doi: 10.1016/j.jneuroim.2012.09.012

Shichita, T., Sakaguchi, R., Suzuki, M., and Yoshimura, A. (2012). Post-ischemic inflammation in the brain. *Front. Immunol.* 3:132. doi: 10.3389/fimmu.2012.00132

Stanimirovic, D. B., and Friedman, A. (2012). Pathophysiology of the neurovascular unit: disease cause or consequence? *J. Cereb. Blood Flow Metab.* 32, 1207–1221. doi: 10.1038/jcbfm.2012.25

Takeuchi, H., Mizoguchi, H., Doi, Y., Jin, S., Noda, M., Liang, J., et al. (2011). Blockade of gap junction hemichannel suppresses disease progression in mouse models of amyotrophic lateral sclerosis and Alzheimer's disease. *PLoS One* 6:e21108. doi: 10.1371/journal.pone.0021108

Tang, S. C., Arumugam, T. V., Xu, X., Cheng, A., Mughal, M. R., Jo, D. G., et al. (2007). Pivotal role for neuronal toll-like receptors in ischemic brain injury and functional deficits. *Proc. Natl. Acad. Sci. U S A* 104, 13798–13803. doi: 10.1073/pnas.0702553104

Tian, X., Peng, J., Zhong, J., Yang, M., Pang, J., Lou, J., et al. (2016). β-Caryophyllene protects *in vitro* neurovascular unit against oxygen-glucose deprivation and re-oxygenation-induced injury. *J. Neurochem.* 139, 757–768. doi: 10.1111/jnc.13833

Tsubokawa, T., Jadhav, V., Solaroglu, I., Shiokawa, Y., Konishi, Y., and Zhang, J. H. (2007). Lecithinized superoxide dismutase improves outcomes and attenuates focal cerebral ischemic injury via antiapoptotic mechanisms in rats. *Stroke* 38, 1057–1062. doi: 10.1161/01.str.0000257978.70312.1d

Vicario, N., Calabrese, G., Zappala, A., Parenti, C., Forte, S., Graziano, A. C. E., et al. (2017). Inhibition of Cx43 mediates protective effects on hypoxic/reoxygenated human neuroblastoma cells. *J. Cell. Mol. Med.* 21, 2563–2572. doi: 10.1111/jcmm.13177

Walrave, L., Pierre, A., Albertini, G., Aourz, N., De Bundel, D., Van Eeckhaut, A., et al. (2018). Inhibition of astroglial connexin43 hemichannels with TAT-Gap19 exerts anticonvulsant effects in rodents. *Glia* doi: 10.1002/glia.23341 [Epub ahead of print].

Walrave, L., Vinken, M., Albertini, G., De Bundel, D., Leybaert, L., and Smolders, I. J. (2016). Inhibition of connexin43 hemichannels impairs spatial short-term memory without affecting spatial working memory. *Front. Cell. Neurosci.* 10:288. doi: 10.3389/fncel.2016.00288

Wang, N., De Vuyst, E., Ponsaerts, R., Boengler, K., Palacios-Prado, N., Wauman, J., et al. (2013). Selective inhibition of Cx43 hemichannels by Gap19 and its impact on myocardial ischemia/reperfusion injury. *Basic Res. Cardiol.* 108:309. doi: 10.1007/s00395-012-0309-x

Wang, P. F., Fang, H., Chen, J., Lin, S., Liu, Y., Xiong, X. Y., et al. (2014). Polyinosinic-polycytidylic acid has therapeutic effects against cerebral ischemia/reperfusion injury through the downregulation of TLR4 signaling via TLR3. *J. Immunol.* 192, 4783–4794. doi: 10.4049/jimmunol.1303108

Wang, Y., Ge, P., and Zhu, Y. (2013). TLR2 and TLR4 in the brain injury caused by cerebral ischemia and reperfusion. *Mediators Inflamm.* 2013:124614. doi: 10.1155/2013/124614

Xiong, X., Barreto, G. E., Xu, L., Ouyang, Y. B., Xie, X., and Giffard, R. G. (2011). Increased brain injury and worsened neurological outcome in interleukin-4 knockout mice after transient focal cerebral ischemia. *Stroke* 42, 2026–2032. doi: 10.1161/STROKEAHA.110.593772

Xue, Q., Liu, Y., Qi, H., Ma, Q., Xu, L., Chen, W., et al. (2013). A novel brain neurovascular unit model with neurons, astrocytes and microvascular endothelial cells of rat. *Int. J. Biol. Sci.* 9, 174–189. doi: 10.7150/ijbs.5115

Yang, Q. W., Lu, F. L., Zhou, Y., Wang, L., Zhong, Q., Lin, S., et al. (2011). HMBG1 mediates ischemia-reperfusion injury by TRIF-adaptor independent toll-like receptor 4 signaling. *J. Cereb. Blood Flow Metab.* 31, 593–605. doi: 10.1038/jcbfm.2010.129

Yu, S. C., Xiao, H. L., Jiang, X. F., Wang, Q. L., Li, Y., Yang, X. J., et al. (2012). Connexin 43 reverses malignant phenotypes of glioma stem cells by modulating E-cadherin. *Stem Cells* 30, 108–120. doi: 10.1002/stem.1685

Yu, H., Zhang, Z. L., Chen, J., Pei, A., Hua, F., Qian, X., et al. (2012). Carvacrol, a food-additive, provides neuroprotection on focal cerebral ischemia/reperfusion injury in mice. *PLoS One* 7:e33584. doi: 10.1371/journal.pone.0033584

Zhang, J. H., Badaut, J., Tang, J., Obenaus, A., Hartman, R., and Pearce, W. J. (2012). The vascular neural network—a new paradigm in stroke pathophysiology. *Nat. Rev. Neurol.* 8, 711–716. doi: 10.1038/nrneurol.2012.210

Zhang, Q., Raoof, M., Chen, Y., Sumi, Y., Sursal, T., Junger, W., et al. (2010). Circulating mitochondrial DAMPs cause inflammatory responses to injury. *Nature* 464, 104–107. doi: 10.1038/nature08780

Zhu, H. T., Bian, C., Yuan, J. C., Chu, W. H., Xiang, X., Chen, F., et al. (2014). Curcumin attenuates acute inflammatory injury by inhibiting the TLR4/MyD88/NF-κB signaling pathway in experimental traumatic brain injury. *J. Neuroinflammation* 11:59. doi: 10.1186/1742-2094-11-59

8

Targeting MAPK Pathways by Naringenin Modulates Microglia M1/M2 Polarization in Lipopolysaccharide-Stimulated Cultures

Bei Zhang, Yi-Zheng Wei, Guo-Qing Wang, Dai-Di Li, Jing-Shan Shi and Feng Zhang*

Key Laboratory of Basic Pharmacology of Ministry of Education, Joint International Research Laboratory of Ethnomedicine of Ministry of Education, Zunyi Medical University, Zunyi, China

***Correspondence:**
Feng Zhang
zhangfengzmc@163.com

Neuroinflammation is considered to be an important and inevitable pathological process associated with all types of damages to, and disorders of, the central nervous system. The hallmark of neuroinflammation is the microglia activation. In response to different micro-environmental disturbances, microglia could polarize into either an M1 pro-inflammatory phenotype, exacerbating neurotoxicity, or an M2 anti-inflammatory phenotype, exerting neuroprotection. Therefore, shifting the polarization of microglia toward the M2 phenotype could possess a more viable strategy for the neuroinflammatory disorders treatment. Naringenin (NAR) is naturally a grapefruit flavonoid and possesses various kinds of pharmacological activities, such as anti-inflammatory and neuroprotective activities. In the present study, we aimed to investigate the potential effects of NAR on microglial M1/M2 polarization and further reveal the underlying mechanisms of actions. First, NAR inhibited lipopolysaccharide (LPS)-induced microglial activation. Then, NAR shifted the M1 pro-inflammatory microglia phenotype to the M2 anti-inflammatory M2 microglia state as demonstrated by the decreased expression of M1 markers (i.e., inducible TNF-α and IL-1β) and the elevated expression of M2 markers (i.e., arginase 1, IL-4, and IL-10). In addition, the effects of NAR on microglial polarization were dependent on MAPK signaling, particularly JNK inactivation, as evidenced by the fact that the selective activator of JNK abolished NAR-promoted M2 polarization and further NAR-inhibited microglial activation. Together, this study demonstrated that NAR promoted microglia M1/M2 polarization, thus conferring anti-neuroinflammatory effects via the inhibition of MAPK signaling activation. These findings might provide new alternative avenues for neuroinflammation-related disorders treatment.

Keywords: neuroinflammation, microglia polarization, lipopolysaccharide, naringenin, MAPK signaling

INTRODUCTION

Accumulating evidence has confirmed that central nervous system (CNS) is an immunologically privileged site due to the limited inflammatory capacity with the presence of blood-brain barrier and the lack of lymphatic infiltration (Hanisch and Kettenmann, 2007). Recently, neuroinflammation is considered to be an important and inevitable pathological process associated with all types of damages to, and disorders of, the CNS (Gemma, 2010). As the major cellular elements of neuroinflammation, microglia execute specific immune functions to maintain physiological homoeostasis (Dhama et al., 2015). In response to the pathogenic insult to the CNS, microglia become activated and undergo morphological changes with hypertrophy as well as functional transformations (Ji et al., 2013; Huo et al., 2018). Several lines of studies have indicated that microglia activation plays a pivotal role in the pathogenesis of neurological disorders, including trauma, brain infections coma stroke, ischemia, and neurodegenerative diseases (Nimmo and Vink, 2009). Furthermore, the activated microglia consist of two cell populations which have distinct and even opposing functions. These two microglial polarization extremes are termed as the classically activated M1 (pro-inflammatory) and alternatively activated M2 (anti-inflammatory) phenotypes (Hu et al., 2015). In addition, the two microglial distinct functional polarization states were discerned in the neurodegenerative diseases, such as Parkinson's disease (Bok et al., 2018). Generally, the activated M1 phenotype microglia are characterized by the increased production of pro-inflammatory factors, including tumor necrosis factor-α (TNF-α), interleukin-1β (IL-1β) and the upregulation of inducible nitric oxide synthase (iNOS), CD16, and CD68 (David and Kroner, 2011). Conversely, the activated M2 state microglia are demonstrated to upregulate anti-inflammatory mediators, such as arginase-1 (Arg-1), CD206, and transforming growth factor-β (TGF-β) (Saijo and Glass, 2011). Functionally, the microglia M1 phenotype exacerbates neuronal damage and impedes cellular repair during CNS trauma and disorders. On the contrary, the M2 microglia exert neuroprotection and promote neuronal recovery and remodeling (Mantovani et al., 2013). Therefore, shifting the polarization of microglia toward the M2 phenotype could possess a more viable strategy for the neuroinflammatory disorders treatment.

Naringenin (NAR) is naturally a grapefruit flavonoid and possesses various kinds of pharmacological activities, such as anti-oxidant, anti-inflammatory, cardioprotective and anti-tumor activities (Al-Dosari et al., 2017). The anti-inflammatory effects of NAR are well verified in several different models. NAR protected against airway remodeling after mycoplasma pneumoniae infection via the inhibition of autophagy-mediated lung inflammation and fibrosis (Lin et al., 2018). Also, NAR suppressed the development of precancerous lesions through controlling hyperproliferation and inflammation in the colon of rats (Rehman et al., 2018). Recently, in addition to these beneficial actions, growing interests have been focused on its neuroprotective actions (Kara et al., 2014). First, NAR conferred neuroprotection in Parkinson's disease animal models and attenuated neuroinflammatory reactions (Magalingam et al., 2015). Moreover, NAR produced analgesic effects via inhibiting oxidative stress and oxidation cytokine production (Manchope et al., 2016). However, whether NAR could promote microglial polarization to M2 phenotype and the mechanisms underlying NAR-mediated anti-neuroinflammatory effects remain unilluminated.

In the present study, we aimed to investigate the potential effects of NAR on microglial M1/M2 polarization and further reveal the underlying mechanisms of actions. Specifically, these findings might provide new alternative avenues for neuroinflammation-related disorders treatment.

MATERIALS AND METHODS

Reagents

Naringenin, lipopolysaccharide (LPS) and Anisomycin (ANI) were purchased from Sigma-Aldrich (St. Louis, MO, United States). Enzyme-linked Immunosorbent Assay (ELISA) kits were obtained from R&D Systems (Minneapolis, MN, United States). The fluorescence probe dichlorodihydrofluorescein diacetate (DCFH-DA) were bought from Sangon Biotech (San Diego, CA, United States). SYBR green polymerase chain reaction (PCR) master mix was purchased from Bio-Rad (CA, United States). Anti-mitogen-activated protein kinase (MAPK) signaling pathway antibodies were purchased from Cell signaling Technology (Beverly, MA, United States). Anti-ionize calcium binding adapter molecule 1 (Iba-1), anti-TNF-α, anti-Arg-1, and anti-β-actin antibodies were obtained from Proteintech Group (Chicago, IL, United States).

Cell Culture and Treatment

BV-2 cells, an immortalized murine microglial cell line, were obtained from Wuhan University Cell Library (Wuhan, China). Cells were cultured in DMEM/F12 medium with 10% FBS and 1% penicillin/streptomycin at 37°C in a humidified atmosphere containing 95% air and 5% CO_2. Cells were seeded into 24-well plates at 5×10^5/well or 96-well plates at 1×10^5/well. Cultures were pretreated with NAR (50 μM) for 1 h, and then incubated with or without ANI (5 nM) for another 1 h. Finally, LPS (100 ng/ml) were added to cultures for 24 h. The corresponding indexes were tested.

MTT Assay

Cells were seeded into 96-well plates at 1×10^5/well. MTT (5 mg/ml) solution was added to each well and continued incubation for 4 h at 37°C. After removing the upper medium, dimethyl sulfoxide (DMSO) was added to each well at 37°C to solubilize formazon. Absorbance values were measured at 490 nm.

ELISA

Cells were seeded into 24-well plates at 5×10^5/well. The TNF-α and IL-10 levels in the supernatant were detected using ELISA kit according to the manufacturer's instructions.

Real-Time RT-PCR Assay

Total RNA was extracted with Trizol agent and purified with RNeasy kit. Iba-1, TNF-α, IL-1β, Arg-1, IL-10, and β-actin genes were amplified using the forward and reverse primers. Real-time PCR was performed using a SYBR Green Supermix according to the instruction and then determined on a CFX96 real-time PCR detection system (Bio-Rad, CA, United States). The target gene expression levels were normalized with that of β-actin using the data analysis software provided with the system.

Western Blotting

Cells were lysed in RIPA buffer and the lysates were incubated on ice for 15 min and then centrifuged at 12,000 × g for 15 min at 4°C. The protein concentrations were quantified by BCA assay. A total of 10 μg protein were resolved on 10% Bis-Tris Nu-PAGE gels and transferred to the polyvinylidene difluoride (PVDF) membranes and blocked in 5% fat-free milk at room temperature for 2 h. Membranes were incubated with following primary antibodies: anti-phosphorylated c-Jun Nterminal kinase (p-JNK,1:1000), anti-JNK (1:1000), anti-phosphorylated extracellular signal-regulated kinasel/2 (p-ERK1/2,1:2000), anti-ERK1/2 (1:1000), anti-phosphorylated p38 (p-p38,1:1000), anti-p38 (1:1000), anti-Iba-1 (1:1000), and anti-β-actin (1:2000). The membranes were then incubated with horseradish peroxidase (HRP)-conjugated secondary antibodies at 1:2000 for 1 h. The proteins were detected with ECL substrate.

Immunocytochemical Staining

BV-2 cells were fixed with 4% paraformaldehyde for 30 min at room temperature followed by permeabilization using 0.3% Triton X-100 for 15 min. Cells were then blocked with goat serum at 37°C for 40 min. Cells were concentrated with anti-Iba-1 (1:300), anti-TNF-α (1:300) and anti-Arg-1 (1:300) at 4°C overnight, respectively. The next day, cells were incubated with anti-rabbit-IgG (1: 1500) or anti-mouse-IgG (1: 1500) at 37°C for 1 h. Subsequently, cells were incubated with DAPI for 2 min at room temperature.

Statistical Analysis

Data were presented as mean ± standard error of the mean (SEM). Statistical significance was analyzed by one-way ANOVA through the GraphPad Prism software (GraphPad Software Inc., San Diego, CA, United States). After ANOVA demonstrated the significant differences, pairwise comparisons between means were accessed by Bonferroni's *post hoc* tests with correction. $p < 0.05$ was considered as statistically significant.

RESULTS

NAR Attenuated LPS-Induced Microglial Activation

As shown in **Figures 1A,B**, MTT assay indicated that NAR (100 μM) decreased BV2 cell viability and had cytotoxicity up to the concentration of 200 μM.BV-2 cells were exposed to NAR (50 μM) and LPS (100 ng/ml) for 24 h, cell morphology and cell viability were first determined. In addition, both NAR (50 μM) and LPS (100 ng/ml) had no significant toxic effects on the cell viability. Meanwhile, LPS and NAR had no effect on BV2 cells proliferation (**Supplementary Figure S1**). To discern the effects of NAR on LPS-induced microglial activation, the morphological changes were evaluated via immunostaining using an anti-Iba-1 (a specific microglial marker) antibody. As indicated in **Figure 1C**, in LPS-treated cultures, activated microglia illustrated irregular shapes and amoeboid status. However, NAR attenuated LPS-induced morphological changes of microglia with exhibiting resting round and small cells. In addition, western blot analysis provided quantitative estimation of microglial activation. As shown in **Figures 1D,E**, NAR inhibited LPS-induced increase of Iba-1 mRNA level and protein expression.

NAR Switched Microglial M1 to M2 Polarization

It is well known that TNF-α and IL-1β were used as the marker of M1 polarization, whereas Arg-1 and IL-10 was applied as the marker of M2 polarization. The above observations prompted us to explore whether NAR directly switches microglial M1 to M2 phenotype. As shown in **Figure 2A**, less TNF-α and Arg-1 immunoreactivity was detected in control cultures. Notably, strong TNF-α immunoreactivity and less Arg-1 immunoreactivity were indicated in LPS-treated cultures. After NAR treatment, TNF-α immunoreactivity was decreased, and Arg-1 immunoreactivity was increased. As expected, the increased mRNA and extracellular protein expressions of TNF-α and IL-1β were observed in LPS-treated cultures. NAR-treated microglia expressed higher levels of mRNA and extracellular protein of anti-inflammatory cytokine Arg-1 and IL-10 than those exposed to LPS shown in **Figures 2B,C**. In addition, NAR alone had no significant effect on M1/M2 polarization (**Supplementary Figure S2**).

NAR Inhibited MAPK Signaling Pathway Activation

To determine whether NAR could modulate the MAPK signaling pathway activation, the protein expressions of JNK, p-JNK, ERK1/2, p-ERK1/2, p38 and p-p38 were measured. As shown in **Figure 3**, NAR counteracted the LPS-induced phosphorylation of JNK and ERK1/2. Interestingly, NAR had the most obvious inhibitory effects on JNK activation. However, NAR didn't show the recovery effects on LPS-induced activation of p38. Besides, NAR alone had no significant effect on MAPK signaling pathway (**Supplementary Figure S2**).

NAR Promoted Microglial M1/M2 Polarization Through JNK Inactivation

Naringenin promoted microglia from M1 to M2 polarization and inhibited JNK and ERK1/2 phosphorylation, especially JNK phosphorylation. However, the specific target mediating this action was still unclear. Anisomycin (ANI), a selective agonist of JNK, was thus used to verify the role of JNK activation in NAR-mediated microglial M1/M2 polarization. First, as shown in **Figure 4A**, MTT assay indicated that ANI (5 nM) didn't affect cell viability. In addition, ANI specifically counteracted NAR-elicited downregulation of phosphorylated-JNK but not phosphorylated-ERK1/2 and phosphorylated-p38 as shown in **Figure 4B**.

Next, we assessed and compared the functional recovery between NAR-treated cultures and NAR-ANI co-treated cultures to further determine the role of JNK on NAR-suppressed microglial activation. As shown in **Figure 5A**, NAR and ANI co-treated cultures exhibited irregular shapes and amoeboid status, parallel to the morphological changes in LPS-treated

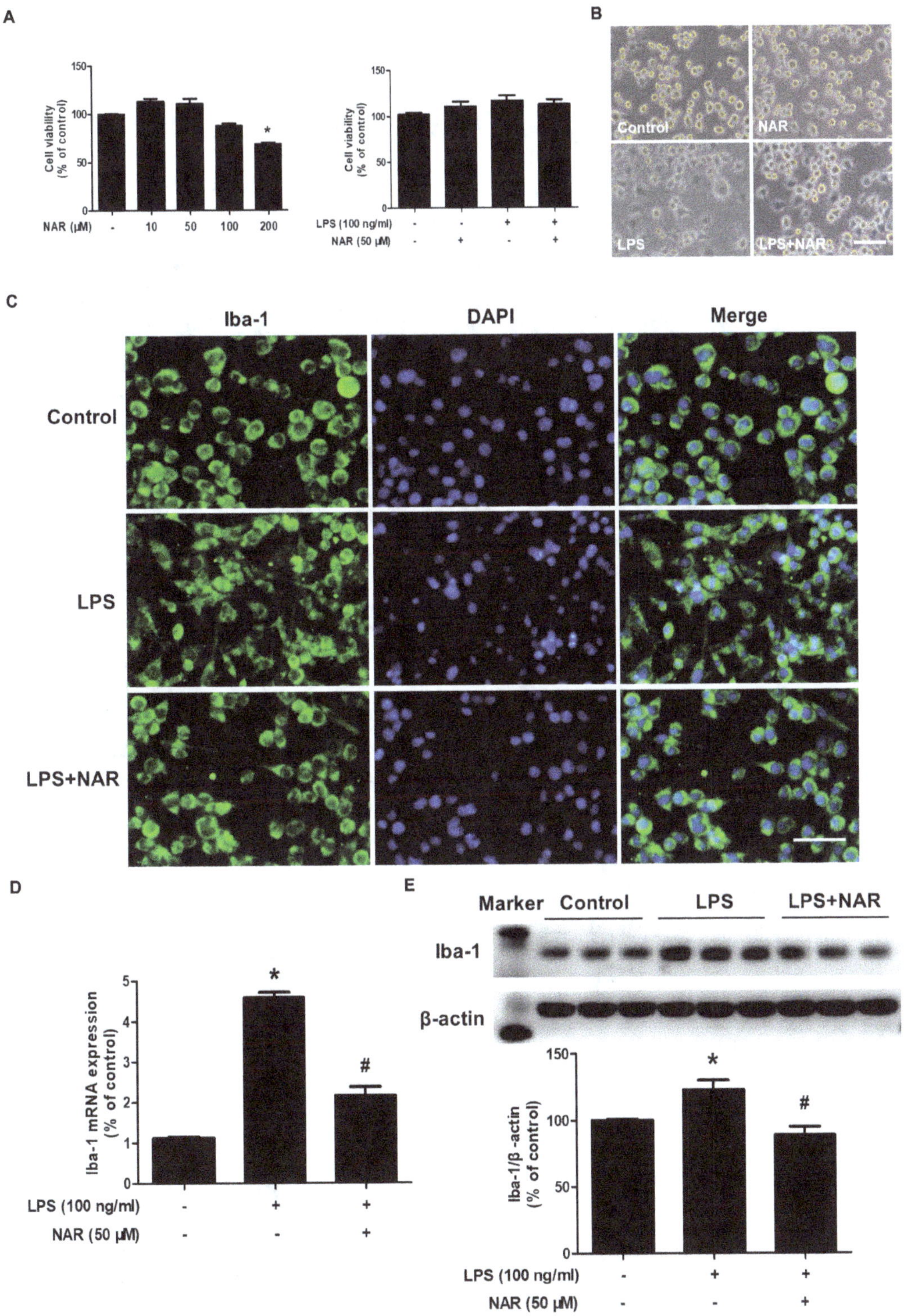

FIGURE 1 | NAR attenuated LPS-induced microglial activation. BV-2 cells were treated with different concentrations of NAR for 24 h, cell viability was measured by MTT assay **(A)**. In addition, BV-2 cells were pretreated with NAR (50 μM) for 1 h and then incubated with LPS (100 ng/ml) for 24 h, cell viability were determined by MTT assay **(A)** and cell morphology was observed via an optical microscopeand **(B)**. Microglial activation was visualized by immunostaining with an anti-Iba-1 antibody **(C)**. Activation of microglia was quantitated by RT-PCR **(D)** and western blot analysis **(E)**. The ratio of densitometry values of Iba1 with β-actin was analyzed and normalized to each respective control cultures. Results were the mean ± SEM from three independent experiments performed in triplicate. $^{*}p < 0.05$ compared to the control cultures. $^{\#}p < 0.05$ compared to LPS-treated cultures. Scale bar = 50 μm.

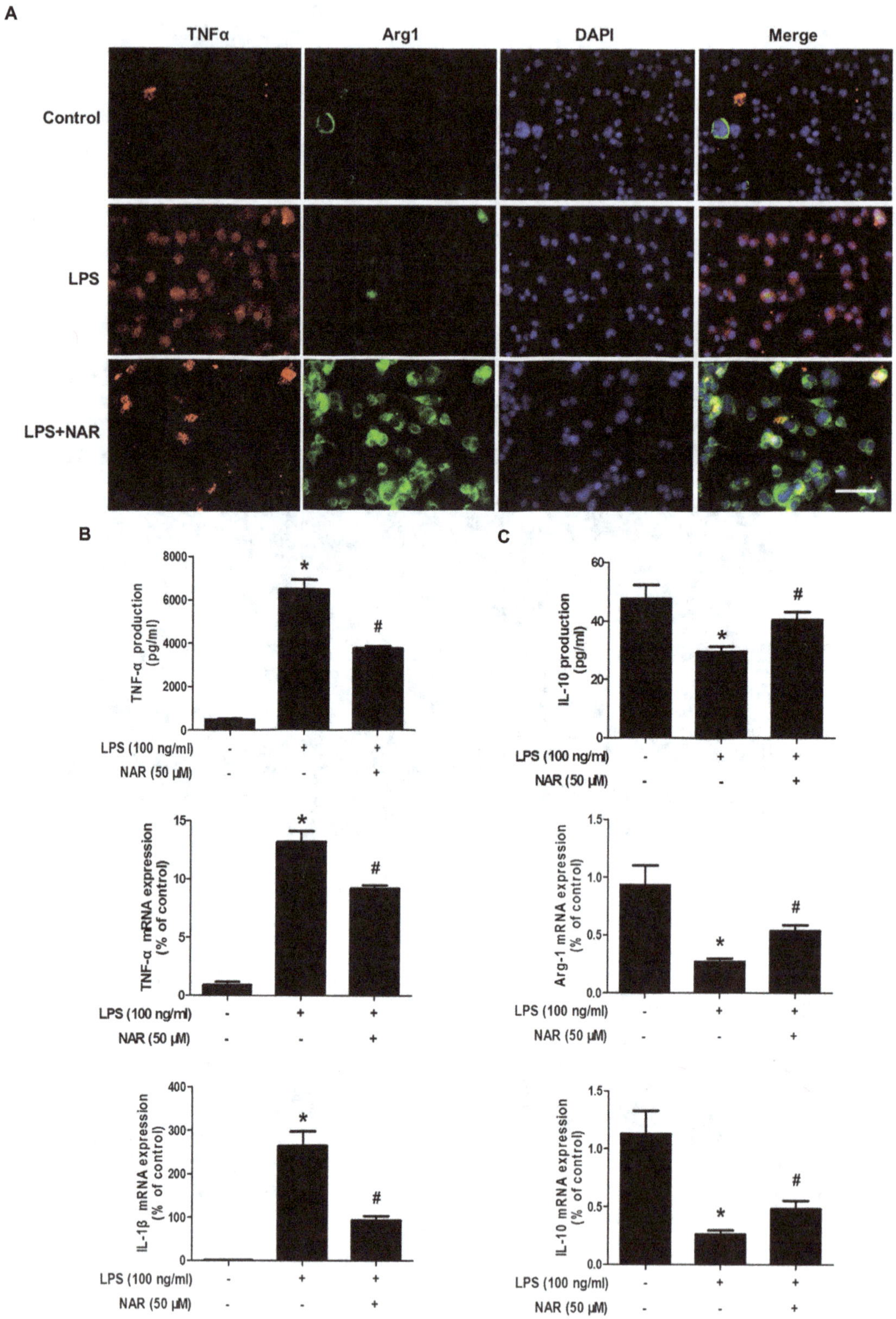

FIGURE 2 | NAR switched microglial M1 to M2 polarization. BV-2 cells were pretreated with NAR (50 μM) for 1 h followed by LPS (100 ng/ml) adminstration for 24 h. Cultures were visualized by immunostaining with anti-TNF-α and Arg-1 antibodies **(A)**. The levels of TNF-α and IL-10 in supernatant were detected by ELISA and the whole cells were collected to detect the gene expressions of TNF-α, IL-1β, Arg-1, and IL-10 by real time RT-PCR **(B,C)**. Results were the mean ± SEM from three independent experiments performed in triplicate. *$p < 0.05$ compared to the control cultures. #$p < 0.05$ compared to LPS-treated cultures. Scale bar = 50 μm.

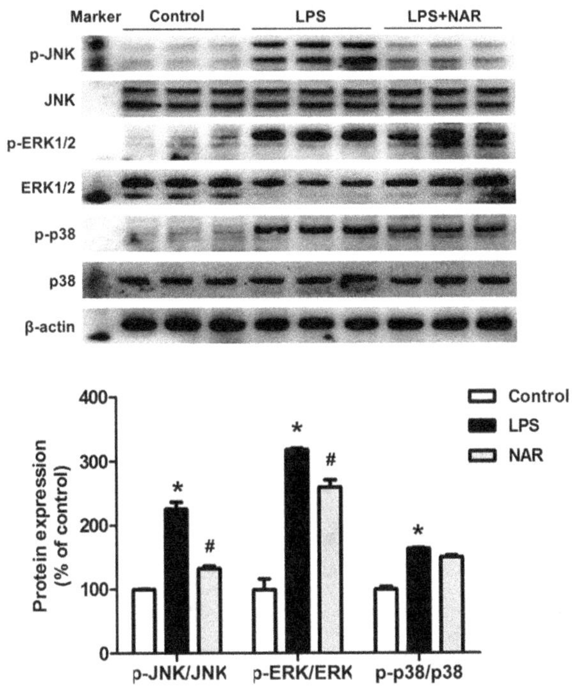

FIGURE 3 | NAR inhibited MAPK signaling pathway activation. BV-2 cells were treated with NAR (50 μM) for 1 h prior to LPS (100 ng/ml) treatment. After LPS (100 ng/ml) stimulation for 24 h, cultures were harvested to detect the protein expressions of JNK, p-JNK, ERK1/2, p-ERK1/2, p38, p-p38 by western blot assay. The ratio of densitometry values of p-ERK1/2, p-JNK and p-p38 with total ERK1/2, JNK and p38 was assessed and normalized to each respective control group. Results were the mean ± SEM from three independent experiments performed in triplicate. $^{*}p < 0.05$ compared to the control cultures. $^{\#}p < 0.05$ compared to LPS-treated cultures.

cultures. Western blot analysis further indicated that NAR-inhibited microglia activation was abrogated by ANI treatment shown in **Figure 5B**. These results pointed out a critical role of the activation of JNK in NAR-inhibited microglial activation.

Further studies were then conducted to evaluate the role of JNK on microglia M1/M2 polarization. As shown in **Figure 6A**, NAR and ANI co-treated cultures exhibited strong TNF-α (M1) immunoreactivity and less Arg-1(M2) immunoreactivity compared with NAR-treated culture. Furtherly, NAR-mediated reversal of LPS-induced downregulation of the M2 marker (Arg-1 and IL-10) and upregulation of the M1 marker (TNF-α and IL-1β) was abrogated by ANI administration as shown in **Figures 6B,C**. Thus, NAR switched microglial M1 to M2 polarization via a JNK-dependent pathway.

DISCUSSION

The current study indicated that NAR shifted the M1 pro-inflammatory microglia phenotype to the M2 anti-inflammatory M2 microglia state, thus inhibiting microglia-mediated neuroinflammation. In addition, the effects of NAR on microglial polarization was dependent on MAPK signaling, particularly JNK inactivation, as evidenced by the fact that the selective activator of JNK abolished NAR-promoted M2 polarization and further NAR-inhibited microglial activation. Together, this study demonstrated that NAR promoted microglia M1/M2 polarization, thus conferring anti-neuroinflammatory effects via MAPK-dependent inactivation.

To date, oxidative stress, mitochondrial dysfunction and environmental exposure have been characterized to be closely associated with the pathogenesis of neurological disorders. However, the underlying mechanisms remain unelucidated. Growing evidence has confirmed that neuroinflammation is involved in the pathogenesis of neurological disorders. The hallmark of neuroinflammation is the glial activation, especially microglial activation (Tentillier et al., 2016). Once activated by brain injury or inflammogen, microglia could release various types of pro-inflammatory and cytotoxic factors. The accumulation of these neurotoxic factors contributed to the surrounding neuronal damage. However, the continuous dying of neurons, in turn induced the secondary activation of microglia and the activated microglia further elicited neuronal damage (Block et al., 2007). Taken together, a vicious cycle leading to the prolonged neuroinflammation and the progressive neuronal loss was created (Gao and Hong, 2008). Thus, inhibition of microglial activation-mediated neuroinflammation might be promising therapeutic strategy for neuroprotection. The present study indicated that NAR inhibited microglia activation-mediated neuroinflammation. These results were consistent with the previous studies that NAR alleviated neuropathic pain through inhibiting microglia-induced neuroinflammation (Hu and Zhao, 2014).

In addition, a great number of studies set out to consider that microglia were highly plastic cells that could assume two diverse phenotypes and participate in different functional programs in response to the pathology of CNS. Recently, similar to the classical M1 phenotype versus the alternative M2 phenotype paradigm defined for macrophages, microglial M1/M2 polarization has been coined and recognized in various neurological disorders, such as traumatic brain injury, stroke, and neurodegenerative diseases (Wang et al., 2013; Wu et al., 2016; Cheon et al., 2017). Typically, the activated M1 phenotype microglia produce various destructive pro- inflammatory factors that result in neuronal damage. As one of the most interesting M1 microglial polarization markers, TNF-α has been confirmed to be implicated in the pathology of neurological disorders (Makuch et al., 2013). IL-1β could be released by activated M1 microglia and the intrathecal administration of IL-1β was discerned to exert algesic actions (Kawasaki et al., 2008). In contrast, the alternatively activated M2 phenotype microglia generate numerous protective and neurotrophic factors and then underly the neuroprotective properties (Prinz and Priller, 2014). Therefore, the pro- and anti-inflammatory responses of microglia phenotype need to be balanced to prevent the potential detrimental activities of an uncontrolled and prolonged inflammation. So far, several lines of evidence presented for the role of neuroinflammation on neurodegenerative diseases pointed to a prolonged and uncontrolled activated microglia M1 state which led to additional continuous neuronal damage (Mantovani et al., 2013). Nevertheless, based on previous

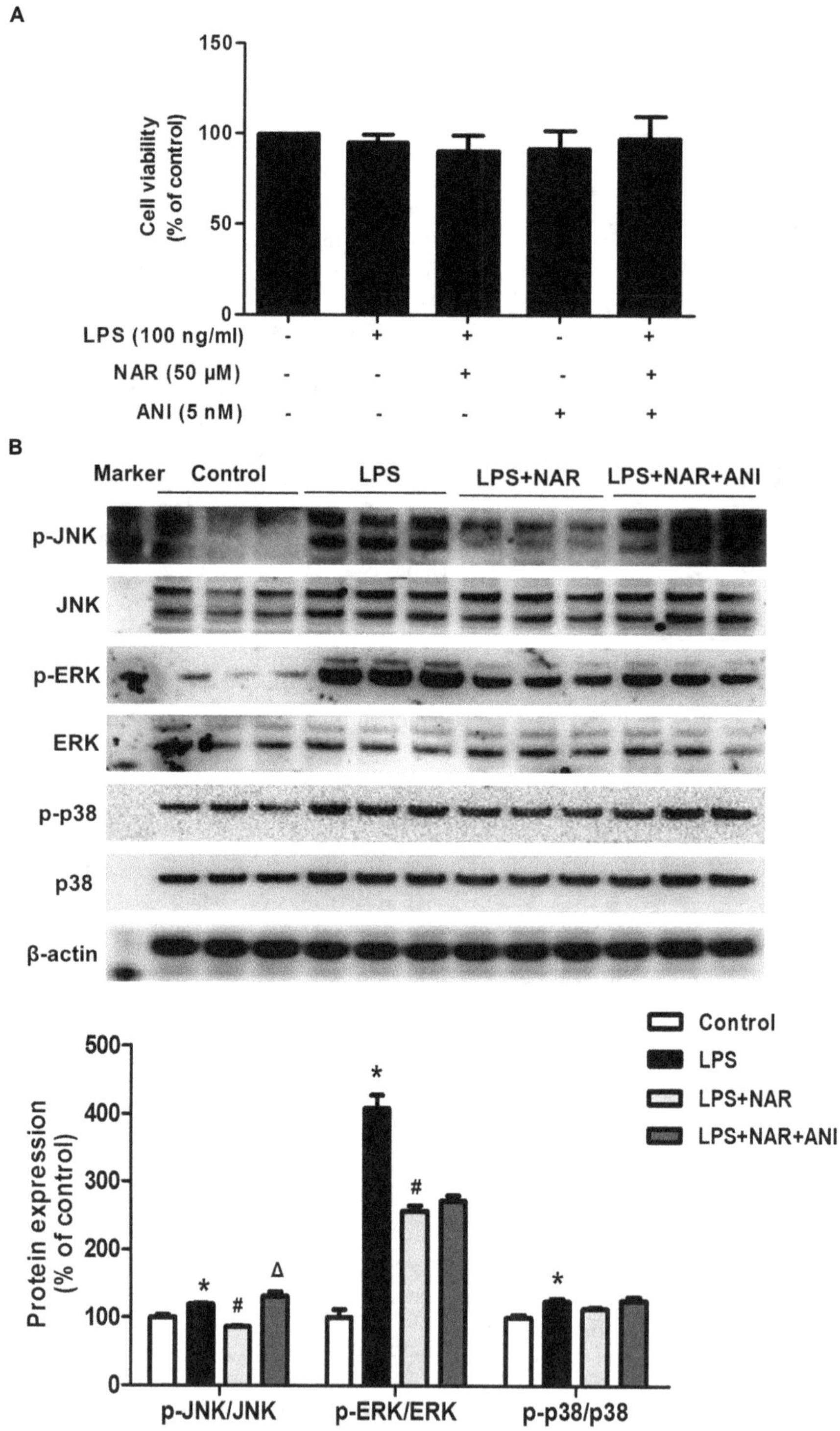

FIGURE 4 | JNK activator attenuated NAR-suppressed JNK activation. BV-2 cells were treated with NAR (50 μM) for 1 h and then ANI (5 nM) for 1 h followed by LPS (100 ng/ml) application for 24 h. Cell viability was determined by MTT assay **(A)**. The protein expressions of JNK, p-JNK, ERK1/2, p-ERK1/2, p38 and p-p38 were detected by western blot assay **(B)**. The ratio of densitometry values of p-ERK1/2, p-JNK and p-p38 with total ERK1/2, JNK and p38 was normalized to each respective control group. Results were the mean ± SEM from three independent experiments performed in triplicate. $^{*}p < 0.05$ compared to the control cultures. $^{\#}p < 0.05$ compared to LPS-treated cultures. $^{\Delta}p < 0.05$ compared to LPS and NAR co-treated cultures.

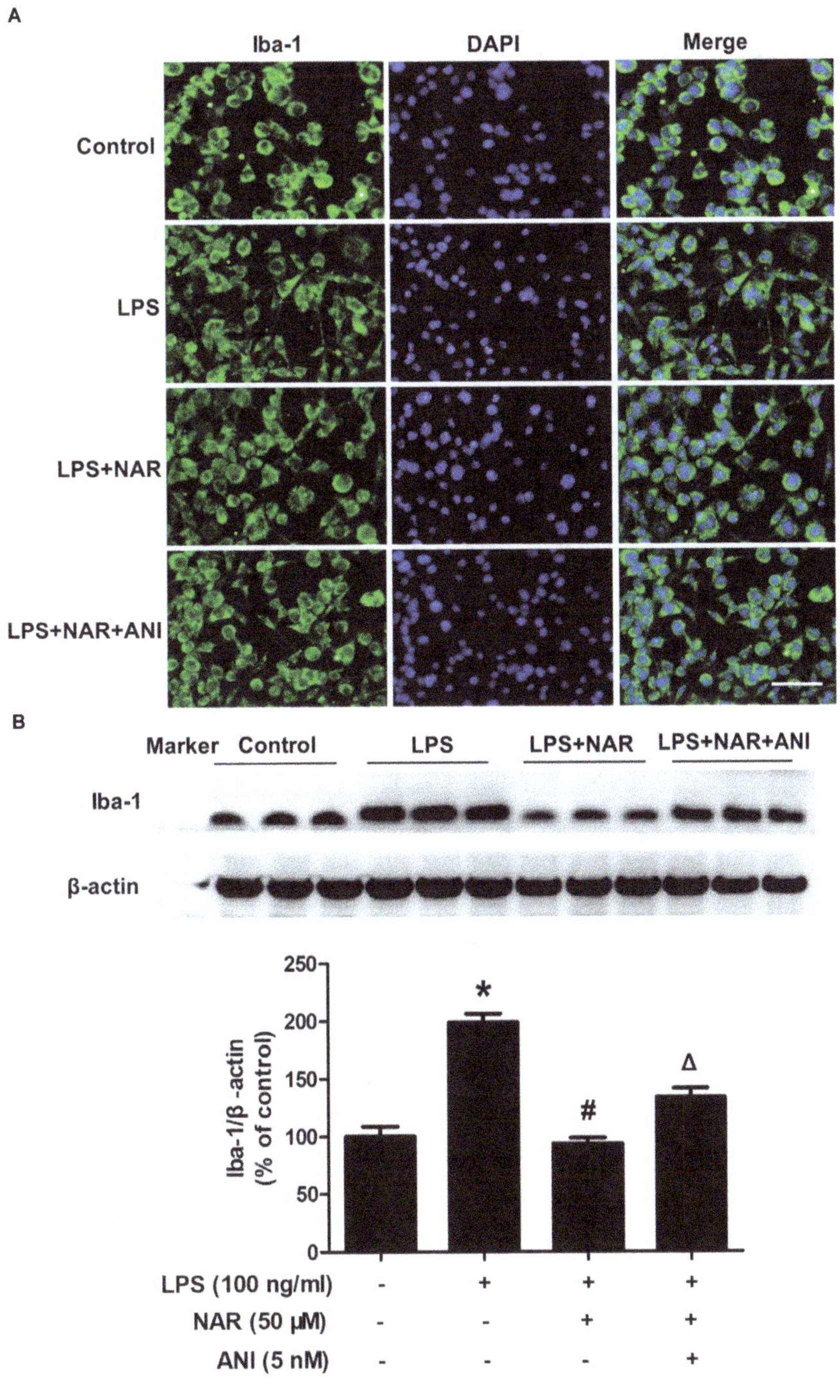

FIGURE 5 | NAR inhibited microglia activation through JNK inactivation. BV-2 cells were treated with ANI (5 nM) for 1h after NAR pretreatment for 1 h. Then, LPS (100 ng/ml) were added into cultures. After LPS stimulation for 24 h, microglial activation was visualized by immunostaining **(A)** and quantitated by western blot analysis **(B)** using an anti-Iba-1 antibody. The ratio of densitometry values of Iba1 with β-actin was analyzed and normalized to each respective control cultures. $^{*}p < 0.05$ compared to the control cultures. $^{\#}p < 0.05$ compared to LPS-treated cultures. $^{\Delta}$ $p < 0.05$ compared to LPS and NAR co-treated cultures. Scale bar = 50 μm.

non-steroidal anti-inflammatory drug and Alzheimer's disease anti-inflammatory prevention trial studies, simply suppressing inflammation via inhibiting M1 activation would likely not exert overall benefits (Becker et al., 2011). On the contrary, promoting the shift of microglial M1 to M2 phenotype while inhibiting microglia M1 state has been emerged as a more promising strategy for neuroinflammation-related disorders treatment (Li et al., 2018). Currently, most of the compounds

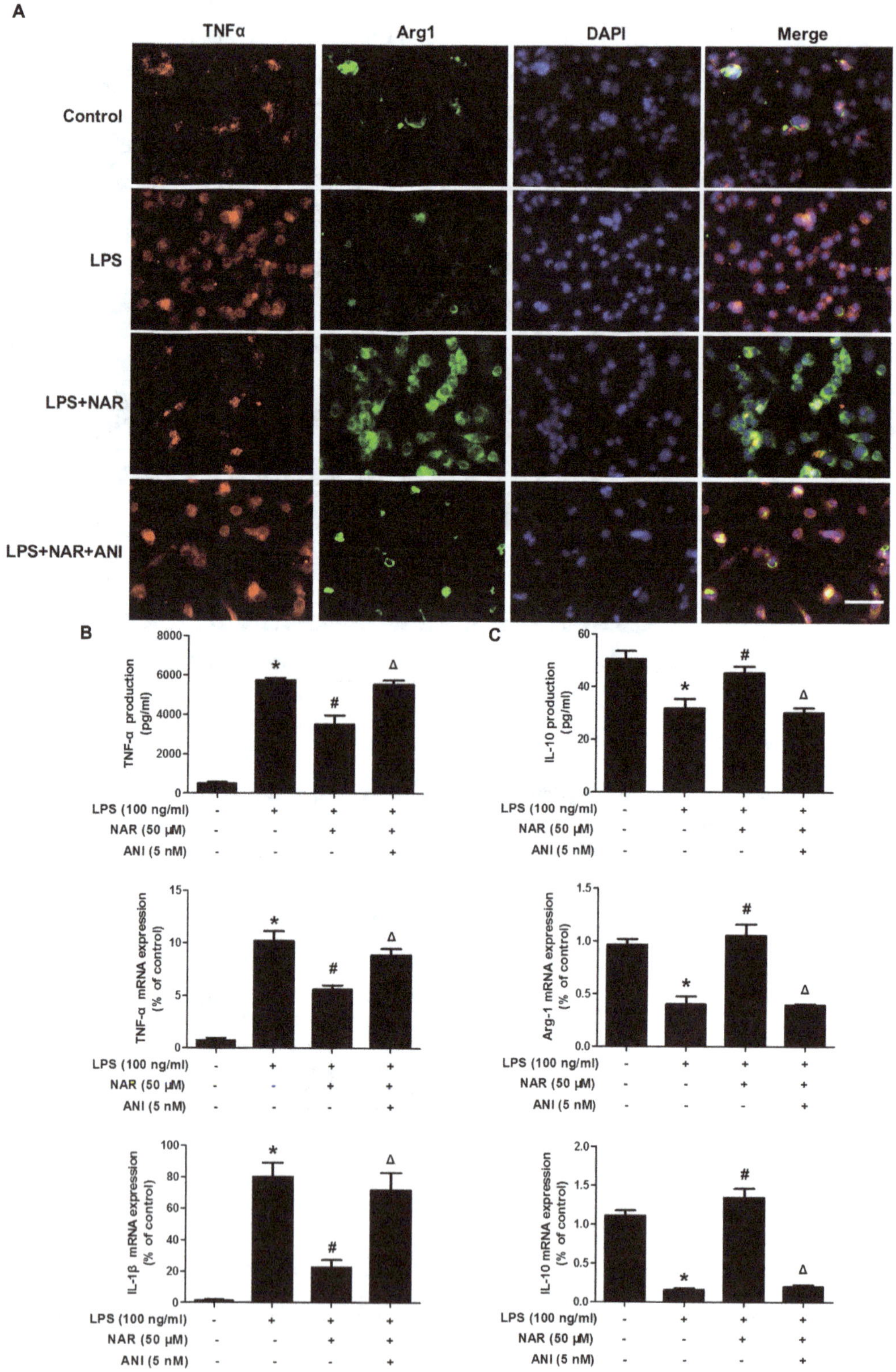

FIGURE 6 | NAR promoted microglial M1/M2 polarization via the inhibition of JNK activation. BV-2 cells were treated with NAR (50 μM) for 1 h and ANI (5 nM) for another 1 h and then stimulated by LPS (100 ng/ml) for 24 h. Cultures were immunostained with anti-TNF-α and anti-Arg-1 antibodies **(A)**. Culture medium was collected to detect the contents of TNF-α and IL-10 by ELISA and the whole cells were collected to measure the gene expressions of TNF-α, IL-1β, Arg-1, and IL-10 by real time RT-PCR **(B,C)**. Results were the mean ± SEM from three independent experiments performed in triplicate. $^*p < 0.05$ compared to the control cultures. $^\#p < 0.05$ compared to LPS-treated cultures. $^\Delta\ p < 0.05$ compared to LPS and NAR co-treated cultures. Scale bar = 50 μm.

suppressed neuroinflammation via simply inhibiting microglial M1 phenotype. However, few compounds were verified to promote microglial polarization to the M2 phenotype (Huang et al., 2017). Since NAR attenuated neuroinflammatory response, it is of significance to investigate the role of NAR on the modulation of microglial polarization. This study indicated that NAR robustly inhibited microglial M1 phenotype markers expressions and promoted microglia polarization toward the M2 anti-inflammatory phenotype, which might contribute to NAR-mediated neuroprotective actions against neuroinflammation.

Further analysis of cascade signaling events underlying NAR-mediated microglial polarization demonstrates the involvement of mitogen-activated protein kinases (MAPK) signaling pathway. MAPK pathway is a highly conserved family of serine/threonine kinases, including ERK1/2, p38 and JNK isoforms. MAPK signaling not only participates in the regulation of inflammatory responses, but also promotes macrophage/microglia polarization into the M2 stage (Quero et al., 2017). For instance, activation of ERK1/2 and p38 was implicated in the regulation of pro-inflammatory factors production in activated microglia (Zhang et al., 2010a). Moreover, p38 played a crucial role in allowing Ecto-5′-nucleotidase to modulate microglial M1/M2 polarization (Xu et al., 2018). In addition, a common involvement of JNK has also been studied in the regulation of both microglial iNOS and IL-1β expressions (Zhang et al., 2010b). Also, JNK was involved in exosomes-triggered macrophage polarization (Xiao et al., 2018). Thus, MAPK signaling is considered as an attractive target for inflammatory diseases treatment. Recently, some synthetic and natural compounds that could activate MAPK to exert anti-inflammatory effects and promote microglial M2 polarization (Bhatia et al., 2016; Xiang et al., 2018). Therefore, it was of interest to investigate the relationship between NAR-mediated anti-neuroinflammatory actions and MAPK activation. In the present study, we first found that NAR suppressed the phosphorylation of JNK and ERK1/2 in BV-2 cells, while p38 was not altered by NAR after LPS stimulation. Next, we tested whether NAR-mediated microglia polarization toward M2 state was dependent on JNK inactivation. Of note, the specific JNK activator abolished NAR-promoted microglia polarization further inhibiting microglial activation. The current data suggested that NAR-mediated microglial M1/M2 polarization was dependent on the inactivation of MAPK signaling.

In summary, this study demonstrated that NAR administration inhibited the microglial M1 phenotype and shifted the microglial polarization toward M2 state via the inhibition of MAPK signaling activation, which was accompanied by the reduced neuroinflammatory response. The current results supported the potential pharmaceutical application of NAR in neuroinflammation-related neurological disorders therapies.

CONCLUSION

This study illustrates that NAR promoted microglial polarization toward the M2 phenotype through MAPK-dependent inactivation. These findings provide a new evidence that NAR might have considerable value as a potent agent for neuroinflammatory diseases treatment.

AUTHOR CONTRIBUTIONS

FZ conceived and designed the experiments. BZ, G-QW, and Y-ZW participated in the experiments performance. G-QW, D-DL, J-SS, and FZ finished the data analysis. FZ and G-QW wrote, revised, and checked the article. All authors have reviewed the contents of the manuscript, validated the accuracy of the data, and approved the submitted manuscript.

FUNDING

This study was supported by the National Natural Science Foundation of China (Nos. 81460556 and 81760658), the foundation for High-Level Innovative Talents of Guizhou Province (No. 20164027), the Innovation Research Group Project of Education Department of Guizhou Province (No. 2016038), and the Foundation for Excellent Young Talents of Zunyi Medical University (No. 201603).

SUPPLEMENTARY MATERIAL

FIGURE S1 | The effects of NAR on cell proliferation. BV-2 cells were treated with NAR (50 μM) for 1 h prior to LPS (100 ng/ml) treatment. After LPS (100 ng/ml) stimulation for 24 h, cultures were harvested to detect the protein expressions of PCNA by western blot assay.

FIGURE S2 | The effects of NAR alone on M1/M2 polarization and MAPK signaling pathway. BV-2 cells were treated with NAR (50 μM) for 24 h. The gene expressions of TNF-α, IL-1β, Arg-1, and IL-10 were detected by real time RT-PCR. The protein expressions of JNK, p-JNK, ERK1/2, p-ERK1/2, p38, p-p38 were measured by western blot assay.

REFERENCES

Al-Dosari, D. I., Ahmed, M. M., Al-Rejaie, S. S., Alhomida, A. S., and Ola, M. S. (2017). Flavonoid naringenin attenuates oxidative stress, apoptosis and improves neurotrophic effects in the diabetic rat retina. *Nutrients* 9:E1161. doi: 10.3390/nu9101161

Becker, C., Jick, S. S., and Meier, C. R. (2011). NSAID use and risk of Parkinson disease: a population-based case-control study. *Eur. J. Neurol.* 18, 1336–1342. doi: 10.1111/j.1468-1331.2011.03399.x

Bhatia, H. S., Baron, J., Hagl, S., Eckert, G. P., and Fiebich, B. L. (2016). Rice bran derivatives alleviate microglia activation: possible involvement of MAPK pathway. *J. Neuroinflammation* 13:148. doi: 10.1186/s12974-016-0615-6

Block, M. L., Zecca, L., and Hong, J. S. (2007). Microglia-mediated neurotoxicity: uncovering the molecular mechanisms. *Nat. Rev. Neurosci.* 8, 57–69. doi: 10.1038/nrn2038

Bok, E., Chung, Y. C., Kim, K. S., Baik, H. H., Shin, W. H., and Jin, B. K. (2018). Modulation of M1/M2 polarization by capsaicin contributes to the survival of dopaminergic neurons in the lipopolysaccharide-lesioned substantia nigra in vivo. *Exp. Mol. Med.* 50:76. doi: 10.1038/s12276-018-0111-4

Cheon, S. Y., Kim, E. J., Kim, J. M., Kam, E. H., Ko, B. W., and Koo, B. N. (2017). Regulation of microglia and macrophage polarization via apoptosis signal-regulating kinase 1 silencing after ischemic/hypoxic injury. *Front. Mol. Neurosci.* 10:261. doi: 10.3389/fnmol.2017.00261

David, S., and Kroner, A. (2011). Repertoire of microglial and macrophage responses after spinal cord injury. *Nat. Rev. Neurosci.* 12, 388–399. doi: 10.1038/nrn3053

Dhama, K., Kesavan, M., Karthik, K., Amarpal, Tiwari, R., Sunkara, L. T., et al. (2015). Neuroimmunomodulation countering various diseases, disorders, infections, stress and aging. *Int. J. Pharmacol.* 11, 76–94. doi: 10.3923/ijp.2015.76.94

Gao, H. M., and Hong, J. S. (2008). Why neurodegenerative diseases are progressive: uncontrolled inflammation drives disease progression. *Trends. Immunol.* 29, 357–365. doi: 10.1016/j.it.2008.05.002

Gemma, C. (2010). Neuroimmunomodulation and aging. *Aging Dis.* 1, 169-172.

Hanisch, U. K., and Kettenmann, H. (2007). Microglia: active sensor and versatile effector cells in the normal and pathologic brain. *Nat. Neurosci.* 10, 1387–1394. doi: 10.1038/nn1997

Hu, C. Y., and Zhao, Y. T. (2014). Analgesic effects of naringenin in rats with spinal nerve ligation-induced neuropathic pain. *Biomed. Rep.* 2, 569–573. doi: 10.3892/br.2014.267

Hu, X., Leak, R. K., Shi, Y., Suenaga, J., Gao, Y., Zheng, P., et al. (2015). Microglial and macrophage polarization-new prospects for brain repair. *Nat. Rev. Neurol.* 11, 56–64. doi: 10.1038/nrneurol.2014.207

Huang, X. P., Peng, J. H., Pang, J. W., Tian, X. C., Li, X. S., Wu, Y., et al. (2017). Peli1 contributions in microglial activation, neuroinflammatory responses and neurological deficits following experimental subarachnoid hemorrhage. *Front. Mol. Neurosci.* 10:398. doi: 10.3389/fnmol.2017.00398

Huo, W., Zhang, Y., Liu, Y., Lei, Y., Sun, R., Zhang, W., et al. (2018). Dehydrocorydaline attenuates bone cancer pain by shifting microglial M1/M2 polarization toward the M2 phenotype. *Mol. Pain* 14:1744806918781733. doi: 10.1177/1744806918781733

Ji, R. R., Berta, T., and Nedergaard, M. (2013). Glia and pain: is chronic pain a gliopathy? *Pain* 154, S10–S28. doi: 10.1016/j.pain.2013.06.022

Kara, S., Gencer, B., Karaca, T., Tufan, H. A., Arikan, S., Ersan, I., et al. (2014). Protective effect of hesperetin and naringenin against apoptosis in ischemia/reperfusion-induced retinal injury in rats. *The Sci. World J.* 2014:797824. doi: 10.1155/2014/797824

Kawasaki, Y., Zhang, L., Cheng, J. K., and Ji, R. R. (2008). Cytokine mechanisms of central sensitization: distinct and overlapping role of interleukin-1beta, interleukin-6, and tumor necrosis factor-alpha in regulating synaptic and neuronal activity in the superficial spinal cord. *J. Neurosci.* 28, 5189–5194. doi: 10.1523/JNEUROSCI.3338-07.2008

Li, C., Zhang, C., Zhou, H., Feng, Y., Tang, F., Hoi, M. P. M., et al. (2018). Inhibitory effects of betulinic acid on LPS-induced neuroinflammation involve M2 microglial polarization via CaMKKβ-dependent AMPK activation. *Front. Mol. Neurosci.* 11:98. doi: 10.3389/fnmol.2018.00098

Lin, Y., Tan, D., Kan, Q., Xiao, Z., and Jiang, Z. (2018). The protective effect of naringenin on airway remodeling after mycoplasma pneumoniae infection by inhibiting autophagy-mediated lung inflammation and fibrosis. *Mediators Inflamm.* 2018, 1–10. doi: 10.1155/2018/8753894

Magalingam, K. B., Radhakrishnan, A. K., and Haleagrahara, N. (2015). Protective mechanisms of flavonoids in Parkinson's Disease. *Oxid. Med. Cell. Longev.* 2015:314560. doi: 10.1155/2015/314560

Makuch, W., Mika, J., Rojewska, E., Zychowska, M., and Przewlocka, B. (2013). Effects of selective and non-selective inhibitors of nitric oxide synthase on morphine-and endomorphin-1-induced analgesia in acute and neuropathic pain in rats. *Neuropharmacology* 75, 445–457. doi: 10.1016/j.neuropharm.2013.08.031

Manchope, M. F., Calixto-Campos, C., Coelho-Silva, L., Zarpelon, A. C., Pinho-Ribeiro, F. A., Georgetti, S. R., et al. (2016). Naringenin inhibits superoxide anion-induced inflammatory pain: role of oxidative stress, cytokines, Nrf-2 and the NO-cGMP-PKG-KATP channel signaling pathway. *PloS One.* 11:e0153015. doi: 10.1371/journal.pone.0153015

Mantovani, A., Biswas, S. K., Galdiero, M. R., Sica, A., and Locati, M. (2013). Macrophage plasticity and polarization in tissue repair and remodeling. *J. Pathol.* 229, 176–185. doi: 10.1002/path.4133

Nimmo, A. J., and Vink, R. (2009). Recent patents in CNS drug discovery: the management of inflammation in the central nervous system. *Recent Pat. CNS Drug Discov.* 4, 86–95. doi: 10.2174/157488909788452997

Prinz, M., and Priller, J. (2014). Microglia and brain macrophages in the molecular age: from origin to neuropsychiatric disease. *Nat. Rev. Neurosci.* 15, 300–312. doi: 10.1038/nrn3722

Quero, L., Hanser, E., Manigold, T., Tiaden, A. N., and Kyburz, D. (2017). TLR2 stimulation impairs anti-inflammatory activity of M2-like macrophages, generating a chimeric M1/M2 phenotype. *Arthritis Res. Ther.* 19:245. doi: 10.1186/s13075-017-1447-1

Rehman, M. U., Rahman Mir, M. U., Farooq, A., Rashid, S. M., Ahmad, B., Bilal Ahmad, S., et al. (2018). Naringenin (4,5,7-trihydroxyflavanone) suppresses the development of precancerous lesions via controlling hyperproliferation and inflammation in the colon of wistar rats. *Environ. Toxicol.* 33, 422–435. doi: 10.1002/tox.22528

Saijo, K., and Glass, C. K. (2011). Microglial cell origin and phenotypes in health and disease. *Nat. Rev. Immunol.* 11, 775–787. doi: 10.1038/nri3086

Tentillier, N., Etzerodt, A., Olesen, M. N., Rizalar, F. S., Jacobsen, J., Bender, D., et al. (2016). Anti-inflammatory modulation of microglia via CD163-targeted glucocorticoids protects dopaminergic neurons in the 6-OHDA Parkinson's disease model. *J. Neurosci.* 36, 9375–9390. doi: 10.1523/JNEUROSCI.1636-16.2016

Wang, G., Zhang, J., Hu, X., Zhang, L., Mao, L., Jiang, X., et al. (2013). Microglia/macrophage polarization dynamics in white matter after traumatic brain injury. *J. Cereb. Blood Flow Metab.* 33, 1864–1874. doi: 10.1523/JNEUROSCI.1636-16.2016

Wu, L. H., Lin, C., Lin, H. Y., Liu, Y. S., Wu, C. Y., Tsai, C. F., et al. (2016). Naringenin suppresses neuroinflammatory responses through inducing suppressor of cytokine signaling 3 expression. *Mol. Neurobiol.* 53, 1080–1091. doi: 10.1007/s12035-014-9042-49

Xiang, B., Xiao, C., Shen, T., and Li, X. (2018). Anti-inflammatory effects of anisalcohol on lipopolysaccharide-stimulated BV2 microglia via selective modulation of microglia polarization and down-regulation of NF-κB p65 and JNK activation. *Mol. Immunol.* 95, 39–46. doi: 10.1016/j.molimm.2018.01.011

Xiao, M., Zhang, J., Chen, W., and Chen, W. (2018). M1-like tumor-associated macrophages activated by exosome-transferred THBS1 promote malignant migration in oral squamous cell carcinoma. *J. Exp. Clin. Cancer Res.* 3:143. doi: 10.1186/s13046-018-0815-2

Xu, S., Zhu, W., Shao, M., Zhang, F., Guo, J., Xu, H., et al. (2018). Ecto-5'-nucleotidase (CD73) attenuates inflammation after spinal cord injury by promoting macrophages/microglia M2 polarization in mice. *Front. J. Neuroinflammation* 15:3155. doi: 10.1186/s12974-018-1183-8

Zhang, F., Qian, L., Flood, P. M., Shi, J. S., Hong, J. S., and Gao, H. M. (2010a). Inhibition of ikappaB kinase-beta protects dopamine neurons against lipopolysaccharide-induced neurotoxicity. *J. Pharmacol. Exp. Ther.* 333, 822–833. doi: 10.1124/jpet.110.165829

Zhang, F., Shi, J. S., Zhou, H., Wilson, B., Hong, J. S., and Gao, H. M. (2010b). Resveratrol protects dopamine neurons against LPS-induced neurotoxicity through its anti-inflammatory actions. *Mol. Pharmacol.* 78, 466–477. doi: 10.1124/mol.110.064535

9

Adeno-Associated Viral Vector Serotype DJ-Mediated Overexpression of N171-82Q-Mutant Huntingtin in the Striatum of Juvenile Mice is a New Model for Huntington's Disease

*Minhee Jang [1], Seung Eun Lee [2] and Ik-Hyun Cho [1,3]**

[1]Department of Convergence Medical Science, College of Korean Medicine, Kyung Hee University, Seoul, South Korea,
[2]Virus Facility, Research Animal Resource Center, Korea Institute of Science and Technology (KIST), Seoul, South Korea,
[3]Brain Korea 21 Plus Program and Institute of Korean Medicine, College of Korean Medicine, Kyung Hee University, Seoul, South Korea

***Correspondence:**
Ik-Hyun Cho
ihcho@khu.ac.kr

Huntington's disease (HD) is an autosomal-dominant inherited neurodegenerative disorder characterized by motor, psychiatric and cognitive symptoms. HD is caused by an expansion of CAG repeats in the huntingtin (*HTT*) gene in various areas of the brain including striatum. There are few suitable animal models to study the pathogenesis of HD and validate therapeutic strategies. Recombinant adeno-associated viral (AAV) vectors successfully transfer foreign genes to the brain of adult mammalians. In this article, we report a novel mouse model of HD generated by bilateral intrastriatal injection of AAV vector serotype DJ (AAV-DJ) containing N171-82Q mutant *HTT* (82Q) and N171-18Q wild type *HTT* (18Q; sham). The AAV-DJ-82Q model displayed motor dysfunctions in pole and rotarod tests beginning 4 weeks after viral infection in juvenile mice (8 weeks after birth). They showed behaviors reflecting neurodegeneration. They also showed increased apoptosis, robust glial activation and upregulated representative inflammatory cytokines (tumor necrosis factor-alpha (TNF-α) and interleukin (IL)-6), mediators (cyclooxygenase-2 and inducible nitric oxide synthase) and signaling pathways (nuclear factor kappa B and signal transducer and activator of transcription 3 (STAT3)) in the striatum at 10 weeks after viral infection (14 weeks after birth) via successful transfection of mutant *HTT* into neurons, microglia, and astrocytes in the striatum. However, little evidence of any of these events was found in mice infected with the AAV-DJ-18Q expressing construct. Intrastriatal injection of AAV-DJ-82Q might be useful as a novel *in vivo* model to investigate the biology of truncated N-terminal fragment (N171) in the striatum and to explore the efficacy of therapeutic strategies for HD.

Keywords: Huntington's disease, adeno-associated viral vector serotype DJ, mutant huntingtin, N171-82Q, polyglutamine expansion

INTRODUCTION

Huntington's disease (HD) is an inherited progressive neurodegenerative disorder characterized by involuntary abnormal movements (chorea), cognitive decline and emotional as well as psychiatric disturbances (Damiano et al., 2010; Jacobsen et al., 2011; Gil-Mohapel et al., 2014). HD typically becomes apparent at 35–45 years of age and progresses toward death within 15–20 years after the appearance of the first clinical symptoms (Ceccarelli et al., 2016). HD is caused by an abnormal expansion of a CAG codon ≥36 repeats located in exon one of the huntingtin gene (*HTT*) on chromosome 4 that confers a toxic function to the protein (Damiano et al., 2010; Jacobsen et al., 2011; Gil-Mohapel et al., 2014). The expansion encodes a prolonged polyglutamine sequence that results in conformational change of the *HTT* protein and induces the formation of intranuclear inclusions of mutant *HTT* in various areas of the brain. This mutation leads to neuronal loss and neuronal degeneration, most prominently in the striatum (Damiano et al., 2010; Jacobsen et al., 2011; Gil-Mohapel et al., 2014). On postmortem analysis, ubiquitinated intranuclear inclusions are observed, suggesting abnormal processing/folding of the polyglutamine domain in affected cells. However, the pathogenic mechanisms leading to neurodegeneration are unclear.

There is no established treatment to prevent or to delay the onset or forestall the progression of HD (Wyant et al., 2017). A critical aspect for drug discovery is the creation of *in vivo* models that recapitulating the genetic and molecular mechanisms underlying the neurodegenerative processes and that present symptoms of the HD patient. With the convergence of the genetic theory of the disease and gene transfer technology, various *in vivo* models of HD have been manufactured (Pouladi et al., 2013). Invertebrate models (*Drosophila and Caenorhabditis elegans*) have been used to effectively and rapidly screen potential therapeutic interventions and to investigate genetic/molecular pathogenesis of HD (Faber et al., 1999; Parker et al., 2001). Toxin models, which were the first animal models of HD, clarified the role of mitochondrial dysfunction and excitotoxicity, two events that have been characterized in the brains of individuals with HD (Beal et al., 1993; Pouladi et al., 2013). However, whether these models recapitulate HD biology is still uncertain (Pouladi et al., 2013). Transgenic (Tg) mouse models including R6/2, BACHD and YAC128 have been generated by introducing truncated N-terminal fragment or full-length of a juvenile HD patient's *HTT* gene into the mouse genome (Pouladi et al., 2013; Menalled and Brunner, 2014). The Tg models revealed behavioral deficits, such as motor symptoms, electrophysiological alterations, striatal neurodegenerations, presence of intranuclear *HTT* inclusions, or alteration of transcriptional factors. However, some Tg models have various phenotypes. They do not reproduce some major features of HD pathology, such as serious neuronal degeneration in the striatum (Crook and Housman, 2011; Pouladi et al., 2013; Menalled and Brunner, 2014). R6/2 mice are well known to have limited lifespan (Perry et al., 2010). Nonetheless, these models have been widely used to study HD pathogenesis and for therapeutic trials (Crook and Housman, 2011; Pouladi et al., 2013; Menalled and Brunner, 2014). Drug discovery trials using these models are a labor-, time-, and cost-intensive efforts. Recent advances in viral-vector technology have provided promising alternatives based on direct transfer of genes to selected sub-regions of the brain (Ruiz and Déglon, 2012; Blessing and Déglon, 2016; Saraiva et al., 2016).

Recombinant adeno-associated viral (AAV) vectors have been successfully used to locally or systemically enhance or silence gene expression in a variety of tissues, including brain tissues, in adult animals or human clinical trials (de Backer et al., 2010; Ruiz and Déglon, 2012; Blessing and Déglon, 2016; Saraiva et al., 2016). The AAV vectors are reportedly more effective than lentiviral vectors at regulating the expression of specific genes at specific brain regions (de Backer et al., 2010; Ruiz and Déglon, 2012; Blessing and Déglon, 2016; Saraiva et al., 2016). Thus far, 11 serotypes of AAV have been identified. These serotypes differ in their tropism or the type of cells they infect (Kwon and Schaffer, 2008). Hybrid capsids derived from multiple different serotypes can also alter viral tropism. AAV serotype DJ (AAV-DJ), one common hybrid example, contains a hybrid capsid derived from eight serotypes. AAV-DJ displays a higher transduction efficiency *in vitro* than any wild type serotype. *In vivo*, it displays very high infectivity across a broad range of cell types (Grimm et al., 2008).

An AAV-induced animal model was first manufactured to express expanded polyglutamine tracts (97Q) fused to green fluorescence protein (GFP) in the adult rat brain. The model revealed the rapid formation of fibrillar, cytoplasmic and ubiquitinated nuclear polyglutamine aggregates in neurons (Senut et al., 2000). Recently, a rat HD model obtained by AAV serotype 2/9 containing Exon 1-Q138 mutant *HTT* (Q138) was reported as a short-term model for *in vivo* studies in drug discovery (Ceccarelli et al., 2016). Although these models are useful in HD studies, more models would provide more options to researchers. In the present study, we used AAV-DJ expressing N-terminal truncated fragment (N171) carrying 82 or 18 CAG repeats (mutant *HTT* and wild type, respectively) to establish and optimize a mouse model of HD. AAV-DJ-N171-82Q (AAV-DJ-82Q) and AAV-DJ-N171–18Q (AAV-DJ-18Q) as control were stereotaxically injected in the bilateral striata of juvenile mice. As a result, we demonstrate that this AAV-DJ-82Q model could be valuable as a new tool for drug efficacy trials through confirming reduced motor activity, striatal cell death and increased *HTT* aggregation.

MATERIALS AND METHODS

AAV Vector Production

To generate AAV-*HTT*-N171-82Q, we used HD-N171-82Q cDNA construct in pBluescript to generate N171-82Q mouse model of HD (Schilling et al., 1999, 2004). The construct with first three exons (171 amino acids) of human *HTT* and 82 CAG gene repeats (*HTT*-N171-82Q) was obtained from Dr. David R. Borchelt (Santa Fe Health Care Alzheimer's Disease Research Center, University of Florida). The *HTT*-N171-82Q construct was double digested with EcoRI/XhoI and inserted into multi-cloning sites of an AAV-MCS expression vector (Cell Biolabs Inc., cat# VPK-410). This vector was created by expression under cytomegalovirus (CMV) immediate early enhancer and promoter. As a control vector, *HTT* cDNA containing 18Q CAG repeats was used. All plasmid constructs were verified by nucleotide sequencing. These viral vectors used in this study were pseudo-typed where the transgene was flanked by inverted terminal repeats of AAV2 packaged in an AAV-DJ capsid. AAV-DJ was engineered using a DNA family shuffling technology to create a hybrid capsid from eight AAV serotypes. Additionally, AAV-DJ-*HTT*-N171-82Q and AAV-DJ-*HTT*-N171–18Q vectors were purified by iodixanol gradient ultracentrifugation by Korea Institute of Science and Technology (KIST) Virus Facility[1]. The production titer was 1.3×10^{13} genome copies/ml (GC/ml) for AAV-DJ-*HTT*-N171-82Q and 1.6×10^{13} GC/ml for AAV-DJ-*HTT*-N171–18Q.

Animals and Ethical Statement

Male C57BL/6 mice (Narabiotec Co., Ltd., Seoul, South Korea; Seed mice were originated from Taconic Biosciences Inc., Cambridge, IN, USA) were kept at a constant temperature of 23 ± 2°C with a 12-h light-dark cycle (light on 08:00–20:00) and fed food and water *ad libitum*. The animals were allowed to habituate to the housing facilities for 1 week before the experiments. This study was carried out in accordance with the recommendations of a NIH Workshop on preclinical models of neurological diseases (Landis et al., 2012). The protocol was approved by the Institutional Animal Care and Use Committee at Kyung Hee University. In this process, proper randomization of laboratory animals and handling of data were performed in a blinded manner.

Experimental Groups

To confirm the effect of AAV-DJ-82Q-infection, 4-week-old male juvenile mice were selected from a 5-day preliminary behavioral test. The selected mice were randomly divided into sham ($n = 5$), AAV-DJ-18Q (7.9×10^{12} GC/ml, $n = 7$), AAV-DJ-82Q (0.62×10^{12} GC/ml, $n = 7$), and AAV-DJ-82Q (1.23×10^{12} GC/ml, $n = 7$) groups.

Stereotactic Brain Surgery

Mice (4 weeks; body weight, 14–15 g) were deeply anesthetized (2%–3% isoflurane, 60% O_2, 40% N_2O), placed on a stereotaxic apparatus (myNeuroLab, St. Louis, MO, USA), and gently fixed with ear bars and head holder. Two microliters of AAV-DJ-18Q (7.9×10^{12} GC/ml) and AAV-DJ-82Q (0.62×10^{12} GC/ml and 1.23×10^{12} GC/ml) were injected at a speed of 0.5 μl/min into the mid-coronal level of the bilateral striatum (stereotaxic coordinates in mm with reference to the bregma were anteroposterior, +0.8; mediolateral, ±2.0; dorsoventral, −2.5; Paxinos and Watson, 1998) using a Hamilton syringe (Sigma-Aldrich, St. Louis, MO, USA) equipped with a 30 gauge sharp-tipped needle. After 5 min, the needle was removed in three intermediate steps for 3 min to minimize the backflow. After surgical suturing, the mice were kept on a warm pad until being awakened.

Behavioral Assessment

To investigate whether AAV-DJ-82Q injection induces neurological impairment (reduced motor coordination and imbalance), we measured body weight and accomplished pole and rota-rod performance tests (Choi et al., 2018) a weekly during 10 weeks from 1 day before AAV-DJ-82Q injection. Briefly, for the pole test, each mouse was placed on the top of a pole with a rough surface (1 cm in diameter and 50 cm in height) with its head facing upwards. The time in which the mouse completely turned downwards on the top of the pole and climbed down to the floor was recorded. At 1 h after pole test, each mouse was placed on the rotating rod (diameter = 4 cm) and tested at 16 rpm/s for 5 min. The latency to fall off the rota-rod apparatus within this time was recorded by magnetic trip plates. The assessment was accomplished by an experimenter who was unaware of the experimental condition under constant conditions of temperature (23 ± 2°C) and humidity (55 ± 5%) in a quiet room. Mice were acclimated to the pole and rota-rod apparatuses for 5 days before the first test. Mice that turned downwards on the top of the pole and climbed down to the floor within 2 min and that stayed on the rod without falling during training (for 5 min) were selected and randomly divided into the experimental groups.

Western Blot Analysis

Western blot analysis was performed as previously described (Jang et al., 2013, 2014; Jang and Cho, 2016; Lee et al., 2016a,b). Briefly, 10 weeks (14 weeks after birth) after the AAV-DJ-82Q-injection, mice ($n = 7$ per group) were anesthetized and the striatum was immediately removed with lysis buffer. The protein (30 μg) from each striatum was transferred to polyvinylidene fluoride membranes and blocked. These membranes were probed with mouse anti-*HTT* (1:500; catalog LS-C24591-100, a.a. 181–810, clone 2Q75; LifeSpan BioSciences, Seattle, WA, USA), mouse anti-*HTT* protein (1:200; catalog MAB5374, clone EM48; Millipore, Darmstadt, Germany), rabbit anti-NeuN (1:2000; Abcam, Cambridge, MA, USA), mouse anti-dopamine- and cAMP-regulated neuronal phosphoprotein (DARPP-32) (1:2000; BD Biosciences, San Jose, CA, USA), rabbit anti-cleaved caspase-3 (1:1000; Cell Signaling Technology, Beverly, MA, USA), rabbit anti-ionized calcium-binding adapter molecule 1 (Iba-1) (1:1000; WAKO, Chuo-Ku, Japan), rabbit anti-glial fibrillary acidic protein (GFAP) (1:2000; DACO, Carpinteria, CA, USA), rabbit anti-oligodendrocyte transcription factor 2 (Olig2) (1:500; Abcam), rabbit anti-tumor necrosis factor-alpha (TNF-α) (1:500; Cell Signaling Technology), rabbit anti-interleukin (IL)-6 (1:500; Cell Signaling Technology), mouse anti-inducible nitric oxide synthases (iNOS) (1:500; Santa Cruz Biotechnology, Santa Cruz, CA, USA), mouse anti-cyclooxygenase-2 (COX-2) (1:500, BD Biosciences), rabbit anti-phospho (p)-IkappaB-alpha (IκBα) (1:500; Cell Signaling Technology), rabbit anti-p-nuclear factor kappa B (NF-κB) (1:500; Cell Signaling Technology), rabbit anti-p-signal transducer and activator of transcription 3 (STAT3) (1:500; Cell Signaling Technology), and mouse anti-GFAP (1:2000; Millipore) followed by incubation with an horseradish peroxidase-conjugated secondary antibody prior to enhanced chemiluminescence (Amersham Pharmacia Biotech, Piscataway, NJ, USA). To normalize the level of protein expression, the membranes were stripped and reprobed with mouse anti-gyceraldehyde 3-phosphate dehydrogenase (GAPDH) (1:10,000; Cell Signaling Technology). After Western blots were performed three times, the density of each band was converted

[1] http://virus.kist.re.kr

into numerical values using the Photoshop CS2 program (Adobe, San Jose, CA, USA), subtracting background values from an area of film immediately adjacent to the stained band. Data are expressed as the ratio of protein to total GAPDH for each sample.

Tissue Preparation and Immunofluorescence Procedure

To examine the histopathological changes in the striatum, 10 weeks (14 weeks after birth) after AAV-DJ-82Q injection, the mice ($n = 7$ per group) were deeply anesthetized with diethyl ether and then intracardially perfused with saline and cold 4% paraformaldehyde in 0.1 M phosphate buffer (PB, pH 7.4). Brains were removed and post-fixed for 24 h and cryoprotected in 10, 20 and 30% sucrose in PBS serially at 4°C. Serial coronal slices (30-μm thickness) of striatum were acquired on a model CM3050S freezing microtome (Leica, Wetzlar, Germany) and collected in sequence as free-floating sections on PBS. The sections from the mid-coronal level of the striatum (Franklin and Paxinos, 2008) were processed for immunofluorescence stain as previously described (Lee et al., 2016a). Briefly, the brain sections from each group ($n = 3$ per brain) were incubated with mouse anti-*HTT* protein (1:400; catalog MAB5374, clone EM48; Millipore), rabbit anti-NeuN (1:5,000; Abcam), rabbit anti-cleaved caspase-3 (1:500; Cell Signaling Technology), rabbit anti-Iba-1 (1:2,000; WAKO), mouse anti-GFAP (1:5,000; Millipore) and rabbit anti-Olig2 (1:500; Abcam) overnight with gentle agitation at room temperature. The sections were followed with a mixture of secondary antibodies and examined with confocal imaging system (LSM five PASCAL; Carl Zeiss, Germany).

Statistical Analysis

Statistical analysis was performed by using the SPSS 21.0 package (SPSS Inc., Chicago, IL, USA) for Windows. Multiple comparisons were made using one-way ANOVA with Tukey *post hoc* test. All data are presented as means ± SEM and statistical difference was accepted at the 5% level unless otherwise indicated.

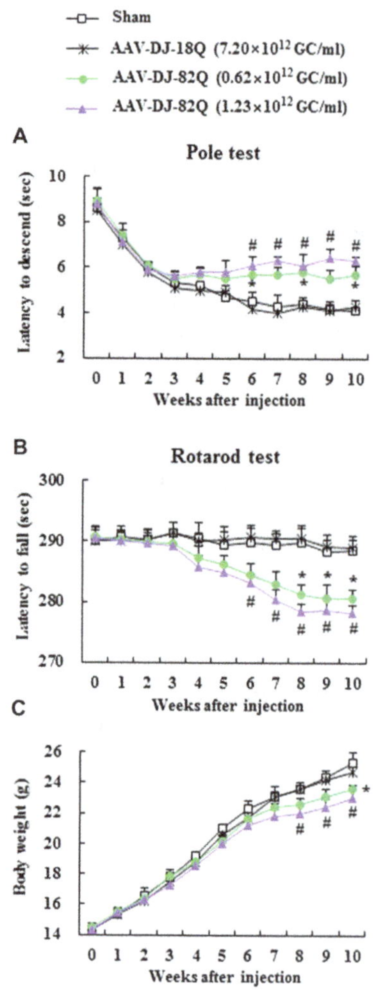

FIGURE 1 | Adeno-associated viral (AAV)-DJ-82Q-injection induces neurological impairment. Two microliters of AAV-DJ-82Q (0.62 × 10^{12} GC/ml and 1.23 × 10^{12} GC/ml) and AAV-DJ-18Q (7.9 × 10^{12} GC/ml) were stereotaxically injected into the mid-striatum of male juvenile mice (4 weeks old). Sham group received the same dose of vehicle. Pole **(A)** and rota-rod performance tests **(B)** and alteration of body weight **(C)** were measured weekly. ANOVA test; $^{*}p < 0.05$ and $^{\#}p < 0.05$ vs. sham group and AAV-DJ-18Q groups.

RESULTS

AAV-DJ-82Q-Injection Induces Neurological Impairment

First, to confirm whether AAV-DJ-82Q injection induced neurological symptoms and to select a more effective dose of the viral vector, motor coordination and balance activities were measured weekly after AAV-DJ-82Q-injetion using pole and rotarod performance tests. In the pole test, beginning at week 4 after AAV-DJ-82Q injection (8 weeks after birth), the average descent time to the bottom of the pole was increased (5.7 ± 0.3 and 6.3 ± 0.2 s in the 0.62 × 10^{12} GC/ml and 1.23 × 10^{12} GC/ml groups, respectively) 8 weeks after injection (12 weeks after birth) compared to the sham group (4.3 ± 0.5 s at 8 weeks after injection) and AAV-DJ-18Q (4.0 ± 0.3 s at 8 weeks after injection) groups (**Figure 1A**). In the rotarod test, the average latency to fall was reduced since week 4 after the AAV-DJ-82Q injection (282.9 ± 2.3 and 280.3 ± 1.7 s in the 0.62 × 10^{12} GC/ml and 1.23 × 10^{12} GC/ml groups, respectively, 8 weeks after injection) compared with the sham group (289.5 ± 1.9 s, 8 weeks after injection) and AAV-DJ-18Q (290.5 ± 1.3 s, 8 weeks after injection; **Figure 1B**). Body weight was significantly decreased since week 8 after AAV-DJ-82Q injection (1.23 × 10^{12} GC/ml), partially corresponding to both behavioral symptoms (**Figure 1C**). There were no significant differences in behavioral tests or change in body weight between low and high doses of vector groups (**Figures 1A–C**). At the end of experiment, all mice were alive. These results suggest that AAV-DJ-82Q-injection can successfully induce neurological impairment.

AAV-DJ-82Q Injection Enhances Mutant *HTT* Expression and Induces Neurodegeneration in Striatum

Since 1.23 × 10^{12} GC/ml of AAV-DJ-82Q more effectively induced neurological impairment than 0.62 × 10^{12} GC/ml of AAV, we further investigated whether the neurological impairments were associated with the level of AAV-DJ-82Q-infection into the striatum at the same dose. The level of AAV-DJ-82Q infection was measured by Western blot and immunohistochemical analysis against *HTT* and *HTT* aggregates with LS-C24591-100 and EM48 antibodies, respectively. Protein expression by anti-*HTT* antibody showed two bands. The *HTT* expression (~75 KDa) was increased clearly in the striatum of sham and AAV-DJ-18Q groups while mutant *HTT* expression was increased clearly in the striatum of AAV-DJ-82Q group (**Figures 2A,D**). Expression level of mutant *HTT* aggregates by using EM48 antibody was not detected in the striatum from the sham or the AAV-DJ-18Q group. However, its expression was markedly increased in the striatum of the AAV-DJ-82Q group (**Figures 2B,D**). In agreement with these results, many EM48-immunnoreactive cells were detected in the striatum from the AAV-DJ-82Q group, while they were not detected in the striatum from the sham and AAV-DJ-18Q groups (**Figures 2E–G**). Subsequently, we confirmed whether the AAV-DJ-82Q-infection induced neurodegeneration in striatum. The protein expressions of NeuN (a neuron marker) AND DARPP-32 (a marker for medium spiny neurons) were significantly reduced and cleaved caspase-3 (apoptotic cell marker) were significantly enhanced in the striatum from the AAV-DJ-82Q group compared to the sham and AAV-DJ-18Q groups (**Figures 2C,D**) consistent with the expression pattern of NeuN and cleaved caspase-3-immunoreactive cells (**Figures 2E–M**). These results suggested that AAV-DJ-82Q-injection can over-express mutant *HTT* in the striatum, resulting in neurodegeneration associated with apoptosis.

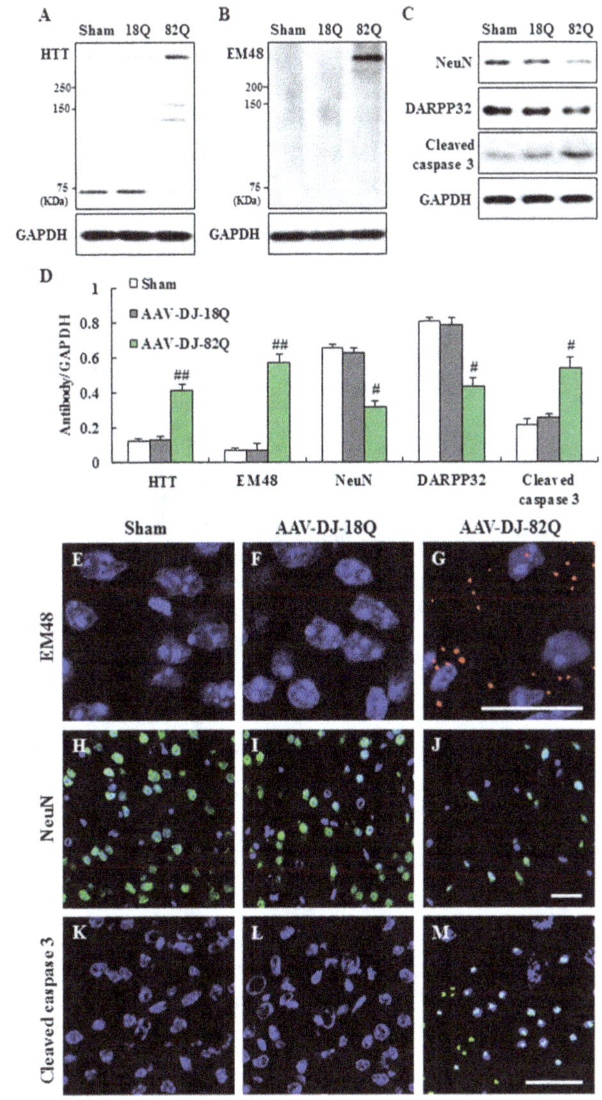

FIGURE 2 | AAV-DJ-82Q injection enhances mutant *huntingtin (HTT)* expression and induces neurodegeneration in the striatum. **(A–E)** Eight weeks after AAV-DJ-82Q-injection, the striata from sham, AAV-DJ-18Q, and AAV-DJ-82Q groups (n = 7 per group) were analyzed by Western blot to investigate change in protein expression of *HTT* (clone, 2Q75 and EM48), NeuN, DARPP32 and cleaved caspase-3 **(A–C)** and then quantified concerning the ratio of protein to total GAPDH for each sample **(D)**. **(A–C)** show a representative Western blot. ANOVA test; $^{\#}p < 0.05$ and $^{\#\#}p < 0.01$ vs. sham and AAV-DJ-18Q groups. **(E–M)** Striatal sections (n = 2 per brain) from each group (n = 7 per group) were accomplished by immunofluorescence stain using anti-*HTT* (clone, EM48, red) **(E–G)**, NenN (green) **(H–J)**, and cleaved caspase-3 (green) **(K–M)** antibodies. Scale bar denotes 100 μm.

AAV-DJ-82Q-Infection Induces Microglial and Astroglial Activation and Inflammation in Striatum

We examined whether AAV-DJ-82Q infection in the striatum affects the features of neuroglia (**Figure 3**). The protein expressions of Iba-1 (microglia marker) and GFAP (astrocyte marker) by Western blot analysis were significantly enhanced in striatal lesions from the AAV-DJ-82Q group compared to the sham and AAV-DJ-18Q groups (**Figures 3A,B**). In agreement with these results, the intensity of Iba-1-immunoreactive microglia was increased within or around striatal lesions from AAV-DJ-82Q group and the immunoreactive cells displayed activated forms with an enlarged cell body and short and thick processes, as compared to the sham and AAV-DJ-82Q groups, which generally displayed the typical morphology of resting cells with small cell bodies and thin processes (**Figures 3C–E**), as previous described (Cho et al., 2008; Jang et al., 2013, 2014; Jang and Cho, 2016; Lee et al., 2016a). The intensity of GFAP-immunoreactive astrocytes was also increased within or around striatal lesions from the AAV-DJ-82Q group, as compared with those of the sham and AAV-DJ-18Q groups (**Figures 3F–H**). However, AAV-DJ-82Q-injection did not significantly affect the protein expression of Olig2 (a marker of oligodendrocytes) (**Figures 3A,B**). Since activated microglia and astrocytes are involved in the inflammatory response (Lobsiger and Cleveland, 2007), we measured the level of expression of representative inflammatory mediators in the

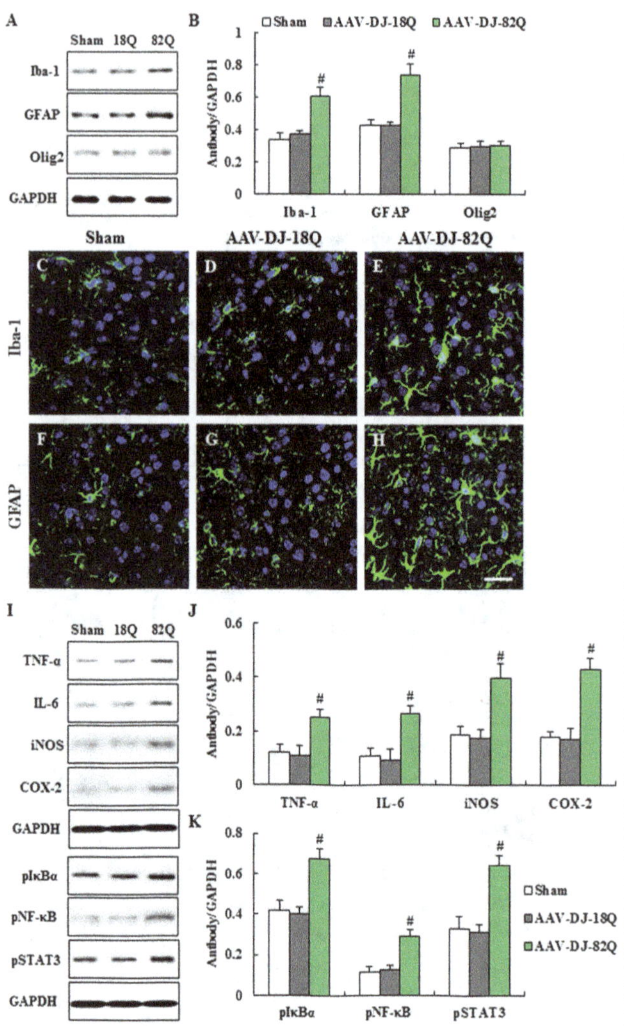

FIGURE 3 | AAV-DJ-82Q-infection induces microglial and astroglial activation and 263–270 inflammation in the striatum. **(A–F)** Eight weeks after the AAV-DJ-82Q-injection, the striata from sham, AAV-DJ-18Q, and AAV-DJ-/82Q groups (n = 7 per group) were analyzed by Western blot to investigate change in protein expression of Iba-1, glial fibrillary acidic protein (GFAP), and Olig2 **(A)** and then quantified as the ratio of protein to total GAPDH for each sample **(B)** ANOVA test; $^{\#}p < 0.05$ vs. sham and AAV-DJ-18Q groups. **(C–H)** Striatal sections (n = 2 per brain) from each group (n = 7 per group) were accomplished by immunofluorescence stain using anti-Iba-1 **(C–E)**, and GFAP **(F–H)** antibodies. Scale bar denotes 100 μm. **(I–K)** Eight weeks after AAV-DJ-82Q-injection, the striata from sham, AAV-DJ-18Q, and AAV-DJ-82Q groups (n = 7 per group) were analyzed by Western blot to investigate change in protein expression of TNF-α, IL-6, iNOS, COX-2, p-IκBα, p-NF-κB, p-signal transducer and activator of transcription (STAT3) and GAPDH **(I)** and then quantified concerning the ratio of protein to total GAPDH for each sample **(J,K)**. **(I)** show a representative Western blot. ANOVA test; $^{\#}p < 0.05$ vs. sham and AAV-DJ-18Q groups.

striatum 8 weeks after AAV-DJ-82Q injection by Western blot analysis (**Figures 3I–K**). Little or no expression of TNF-α, IL-6, iNOS and COX-2 proteins were detected in the striatum of sham and AAV-DJ-18Q groups, whereas their expressions were significantly enhanced in the striatum from the AAV-DJ-82Q group (**Figures 3I,J**). Additionally, we measured levels of activation of NF-κB and STAT3 pathways as representative inflammatory pathways. As expected, expression levels of p-IκBα, p-NF-κB, and p-STAT3 were significantly increased in the striatum of the AAV-DJ-82Q group (**Figures 3I–K**). These findings suggest that the AAV-DJ-82Q-infection may produce striatal cell death and neurological dysfunction by inducing the activation of microglia, astrocytes and the inflammatory response.

AAV-DJ-82Q Vector Infects Neurons, Microglia and Astrocytes, but Not Oligodendrocytes

The EM48-immunoreactive mutant *HTT* aggregates were densely spread in the striatal area from the AAV-DJ-82Q group (**Figure 2G**). However, it is unclear whether the aggregates are expressed in specific cell types. To investigate this, immunofluorescence staining was done using NeuN, Iba-1, GFAP, and Olig2 antibodies, as a marker of neurons, microglia, astrocytes, and oligodendrocytes, respectively. EM48-positive aggregates were predominantly expressed in the nucleus and cytoplasm of neurons, microglia, and astrocytes (**Figures 4A–C**). These aggregates were co-stained with NeuN (23.1 ± 1.5%; 45.4 ± 5.2 co-stained cells of 193.0 ± 8.7 NeuN-positive cells), Iba-1 (19.5 ± 1.3%; 14.0 ± 1.5 co-stained cells of 71.0 ± 3.6 Iba-1-positive cells), and GFAP (11.8 ± 1.1%; 8.1 ± 1.2 co-stained cells of 67.3 ± 3.9 GFAP-positive cells) antibodies (**Figures 4A–C**). However, these aggregates were not co-stained with Olig2 antibody (**Figure 4D**). These results indicate that AAV-DJ-82Q can infect specific cell types in striatum and induce HD-like pathology.

DISCUSSION

In the development of new therapeutic strategies for neurodegenerative disorders such as HD, animal models recapitulating the etiology, pathology and molecular mechanisms described in patients are positively necessary. However, currently a lot of animal models do not reproduce the critical therapeutic mechanisms/targets of the diseases (Crook and Housman, 2011; Pouladi et al., 2013; Menalled and Brunner, 2014). To help these challenges, various viral vectors for gene delivery and gene therapy within the nervous system have been developed over the past several decades. The studies have revealed the seemingly unlimited possibilities for viral vector systems in deciphering the nature of neurodegenerative disorders, such as HD, and so for the development of eradication regimens (Ruiz and Déglon, 2012). Despite several published reports using lentiviral and AAV vectors to model HD by over-expression of mutant *HTT*, neuroscientists in the field of HD have a much smaller selection of vectors to choose from. In the present study, we developed a novel animal model that was based on over-expression of human mutant *HTT* via a bilateral intrastriatal injection by AAV-DJ-82Q into juvenile mice. The mice over-express the transgene in the striatum beginning as juveniles and extending into adulthood. Our findings demonstrated that, after intrastriatal injection of mutant *HTT* into juvenile mice,

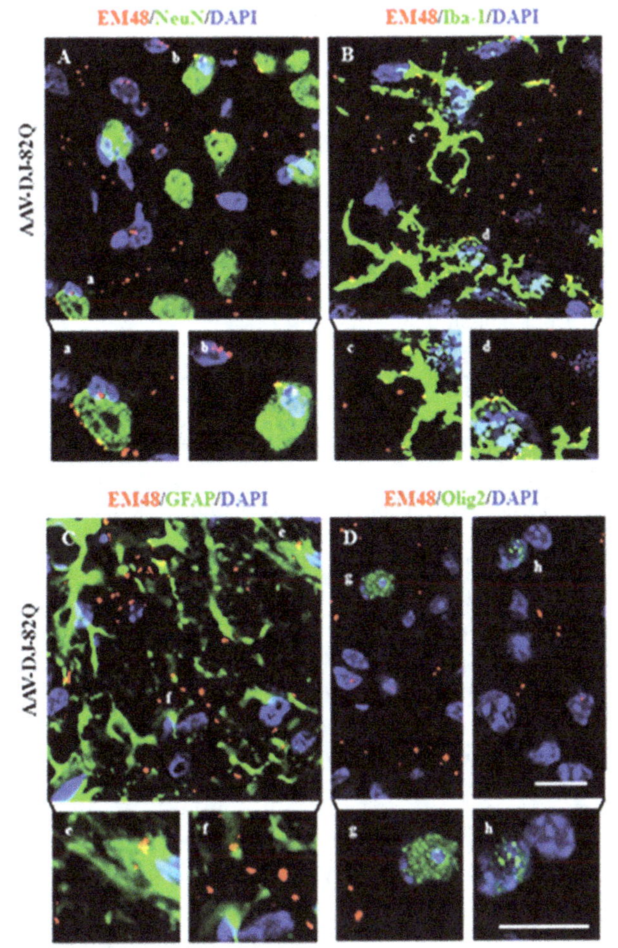

FIGURE 4 | AAV-DJ-82Q vector successfully infects neurons, microglia and astrocytes. Eight weeks after the AAV-DJ-82Q-injection, the striatal sections (*n* = 2 per brain) from sham, AAV-DJ-18Q and AAV-DJ-82Q groups (*n* = 7 per group) were analyzed by double immunofluorescence stain using anti-EM48, NeuN, Iba-1, GFAP and Olig2 antibodies **(A–D)**. Lower panels in **(A–D)** display high magnification micrographs of the areas marked with **(a–h)** in upper panels. Scale bar denotes 50 μm.

adult mice over-expressed mutant *HTT*, displayed neuronal loss, and showed striatal neuroinflammation, resulting in motor dysfunction. In particular, mutant *HTT* predominantly infected neurons, microglia, and astrocytes. Our findings suggest that the AAV-DJ-82Q-injected mouse model may be a helpful tool to study the pathophysiology of mutant *HTT*-associated disease and to develop efficacious therapeutic strategies in translational research.

Several types of N-terminal Tg (R6/1, R6/2, N171-82Q), full-length (YAC128, BACHD) and knock-in (Hdh^{Q111}) models have been generated to investigate the pathogenicity of HD and to discover therapeutic approaches (Pouladi et al., 2013; Menalled and Brunner, 2014). The *in vivo* models have revealed behavioral disorders including movement deficits, striatal neurodegeneration, electrophysiological dysfunctions, intracellular aggregates, and alteration of transcriptional factors (Pouladi et al., 2013; Menalled and Brunner, 2014). However, each model has different characteristics and so their results are not absolutely reproducible concerning some critical characteristics of HD pathology, such as clear neurodegeneration in the striatum or reduced life span (Crook and Housman, 2011). In addition, the research can experience difficulty in maintaining the animal strains. Problems include breeding failure and the high cost of maintaining the animals in the long-term. Our AAV-DJ-82Q model displayed clear motor deficits by pole and rota-rod tests, which were evident in the short term (at least 4–5 weeks following injection) by the onset of behavioral dysfunction as well as striatal degeneration and cellular aggregates. These results suggest that AAV-DJ-82Q model may be more helpful than others.

In the last two decades, there have been several attempts to develop the ideal vector (vehicle) for gene transfer to the central nervous system (CNS). Presently, recombinant AAVs are one of the preferred vectors, because their stable transduction of dividing and non-dividing cells, strong neural tropism, low risk of insertional mutagenesis, and reduced immune responses (Blessing and Déglon, 2016; Grieger et al., 2016; Saraiva et al., 2016). According to many studies that measured the ability of AAV serotypes to target the CNS, when administrated into the brain parenchyma of rodents, most of the serotypes (1, 2, 4, 5, 8 and 9) transduced neurons and glia in the CNS areas including striatum, hippocampus and neocortex (Ruiz and Déglon, 2012; Watakabe et al., 2015; Ceccarelli et al., 2016; Saraiva et al., 2016). Other serotypes, such as AAV-DJ, are potentially useful but have been less well examined (Cearley and Wolfe, 2006; Klein et al., 2008; Aschauer et al., 2013; Holehonnur et al., 2014). AAV-DJ is a synthetic serotype with a chimeric capsid of AAV-2, 8 and 9. AAV-DJ contains a heparin-binding domain in its capsid, which may efficiently transduce a broad range of cell types and escape from immune neutralization (Grimm et al., 2008). However, AAV-DJ has been available only recently and so relatively little is known about its optimal preparation/purification and application. In present study, we injected the striatum bilaterally with 0.62×10^{12} GC and 1.23×10^{12} GC in 2.0 ul of AAV-DJ-82Q per side, as is done with other vectors. The higher dose of viral injections produced more serious movement disorder in the pole and rota-rod performance tests (**Figures 1A,B**). The movement disorder progressively increased beginning 4–5 weeks following injection and lasted at least by 8 weeks after the injection. However, features of movement disorder were different to that of N171-82Q Tg mice (expressing a mutant N-terminal fragment of *HTT*), which displayed loss of coordination, hunched posture, tremors, abnormal gait, and clasping of hindlimbs (Schilling et al., 1999). In the present study, *HTT* aggregates were observed only in the striatum, similar to the *in vivo* rat HD model obtained by stereotaxic injection of AAV serotype nine containing Exon1-Q138 mutant *HTT* (AAV-9-Q138) (Ceccarelli et al., 2016). However, the expression pattern was different to that of N171-82Q Tg mice (Schilling et al., 1999). In the latter, nuclear inclusions were observed in various areas of the brain including the cerebral cortex, striatum, hippocampus, and amygdala. Furthermore, neuritic aggregates were seen in several areas of the brain including the medial amygdala and subthalamic nucleus (Schilling et al., 1999). In the present study, *HTT* aggregates were observed in the nucleus and cytoplasm of neurons, microglia and astrocytes, but not in oligodendrocytes of striatum (**Figure 4**). However, in three HD mouse models that express either full-length *HTT* (Hdh^{Q150}, zQ175) or an N-terminal exon1 fragment (R6/2) of mutant HTT, the nuclear inclusions were observed in neurons, microglia, astrocytes, and oligodendrocytes (Jansen et al., 2017). In the present study, mutant *HTT* aggregates were observed in 23.1 ± 1.5% of the NeuN-positive neurons, 19.5 ± 1.3% of the Iba-1-positive microglia, and 11.8 ± 1.1% of the GFAP-positive astrocytes 8 weeks after AAV-DJ-82Q injection. However, in the three HD mouse models, at late stages of the disease, nuclear inclusions were found in 30%–50% of the neurons, 30% of the S100B-positive glial cells, 4%–10% of the GFAP-positive astrocytes, 3%–10% of the oligodendrocytes, and 0%–2% of the microglia (Jansen et al., 2017). Nuclear inclusions were also present in neurons and all studied glial cell types in human patient material (Jansen et al., 2017). Like this, in our AAV-DJ-82Q model, the expression pattern of mutant *HTT* aggregates was nearly the same with the Tg mouse models previous reported. The small differences may be explained by fundamental difference between Tg model (congenital) and AAV model (acquired) or among the AAV vector serotypes. Taken together, our results demonstrate that the AAV-DJ-82Q vector can possibly infect most functional classes of CNS, although our current data do not discriminate endothelial cell and immature/undifferentiated neural cells.

In the neurodegenerative diseases, microglia, resident immunocompetent and phagocytic cells, are activated and recruited/infiltrated around or into the lesions and serves as scavenger cell (Lobsiger and Cleveland, 2007; Kabba et al., 2018). Circulating peripheral immune cells (macrophages) may surpass a compromised blood–brain barrier and encounter neurons and microglia (Kadiu et al., 2005; Main and Minter, 2017). Although this response is initiated to protect the CNS from the harmful agents, the effect may be detrimental via releasing toxic mediators in neurodegenerative lesions (Lobsiger and Cleveland, 2007). Astrocytes can be activated by products from dead cells or infiltrated/activated immune cells within or around the lesion (Lobsiger and Cleveland, 2007). Interestingly, AAV-DJ-82Q injection clearly induced microglial and astroglial activation and protein expression of representative proinflammatory cytokines (TNF-α, IL-6) and inflammatory mediators (COX-2 and iNOS) in striatum at 14 weeks after injection, corresponding to enhanced expression of p-IκBα, p-NF-κB and p-STAT3 as representative inflammatory pathways. Whether glial activation protects against mutant *HTT* aggregates (toxicity) after the injection of AAV-DJ-82Q into normal mice is unclear. Nonetheless, our results provide the first demonstration that the AAV-DJ-82Q may induce neuroinflammatory response related to neurodegeneration in striatum.

CONCLUSION

An *in vivo* model recapitulating some cardinal pathogenesis of HD needs to be generated. Here, intrastriatal injection of AAV-DJ-82Q to juvenile mice successfully induced mutant *HTT* aggregation, neurodegeneration, and neuroinflammatory response in adult striatum, resulting in HD-like symptoms. Our findings suggest that AAV-DJ-82Q vector might be a helpful tool to better understand neuropathological mechanisms in the striatum of HD patients and develop new therapeutic strategies for HD-like symptoms.

AUTHOR CONTRIBUTIONS

MJ performed the stereotaxic injection, behavioral experiment, immunohistochemistry and Western blots and prepared the figures. SEL developed viral vector and produced AAV virus. I-HC conceived all experiments, analyzed the results and wrote the manuscript. All authors have read and approved the final manuscript.

FUNDING

This research was supported by Basic Science Research Program and Brain Research Program through the National Research Foundation of Korea (NRF) funded by the Ministry of Science and ICT (NRF-2017R1A2A2A05069493 and NRF-2016M3C7A1905074).

REFERENCES

Aschauer, D. F., Kreuz, S., and Rumpel, S. (2013). Analysis of transduction efficiency, tropism and axonal transport of AAV serotypes 1, 2, 5, 6, 8 and 9 in the mouse brain. *PLoS One* 8:e76310. doi: 10.1371/journal.pone.0076310

Beal, M. F., Brouillet, E., Jenkins, B. G., Ferrante, R. J., Kowall, N. W., Miller, J. M., et al. (1993). Neurochemical and histologic characterization of striatal excitotoxic lesions produced by the mitochondrial toxin 3-nitropropionic acid. *J. Neurosci* 13, 4181–4192. doi: 10.1523/jneurosci.13-10-04181.1993

Blessing, D., and Déglon, N. (2016). Adeno-associated virus and lentivirus vectors: a refined toolkit for the central nervous system. *Curr. Opin. Virol.* 21, 61–66. doi: 10.1016/j.coviro.2016.08.004

Cearley, C. N., and Wolfe, J. H. (2006). Transduction characteristics of adeno-associated virus vectors expressing cap serotypes 7, 8, 9, and Rh10 in the mouse brain. *Brain Mol. Ther.* 13, 528–537. doi: 10.1016/j.ymthe.2005.11.015

Ceccarelli, I., Fiengo, P., Remelli, R., Miragliotta, V., Rossini, L., Biotti, I., et al. (2016). Recombinant Adeno Associated Viral (AAV) vector type 9 delivery of Ex1-Q138-mutant huntingtin in the rat striatum as a short-time model for *in vivo* studies in drug discovery. *Neurobiol. Dis.* 86, 41–51. doi: 10.1016/j.nbd.2015.11.019

Cho, I. H., Hong, J., Suh, E. C., Kim, J. H., Lee, H., Lee, J. E., et al. (2008). Role of microglial IKKβ in kainic acid-induced hippocampal neuronal cell death. *Brain* 131, 3019–3033. doi: 10.1093/brain/awn230

Choi, J. H., Jang, M., Nah, S. Y., Oh, S., and Cho, I. H. (2018). Multitarget effects of Korean red ginseng in animal model of Parkinson's disease: antiapoptosis, antioxidant, antiinflammation and maintenance of blood-brain barrier integrity. *J. Ginseng Res.* In Press. doi: 10.1016/j.jgr.2018.01.002

Crook, Z. R., and Housman, D. (2011). Huntington's disease: can mice lead the way to treatment? *Neuron* 69, 423–435. doi: 10.1016/j.neuron.2010.12.035

Damiano, M., Galvan, L., Déglon, N., and Brouillet, E. (2010). Mitochondria in Huntington's disease. *Biochim. Biophys. Acta* 1802, 52–61. doi: 10.1016/j.bbadis.2009.07.012

de Backer, M. W., Fitzsimons, C. P., Brans, M. A., Luijendijk, M. C., Garner, K. M., Vreugdenhil, E., et al. (2010). An adeno-associated viral vector transduces the rat hypothalamus and amygdala more efficient than a lentiviral vector. *BMC Neurosci.* 11:81. doi: 10.1186/1471-2202-11-81

Faber, P. W., Alter, J. R., MacDonald, M. E., and Hart, A. C. (1999). Polyglutamine-mediated dysfunction and apoptotic death of a *Caenorhabditis elegans* sensory neuron. *Proc. Natl. Acad. Sci. U S A* 96, 179–184. doi: 10.1073/pnas.96.1.179

Franklin, K. B. J., and Paxinos, G. (2008). *The Mouse Brain in Stereotaxic Coordinates*. San Diego, CA: Elsevier Academic Press.

Gil-Mohapel, J., Brocardo, P. S., and Christie, B. R. (2014). The role of oxidative stress in Huntington's disease: are antioxidants good therapeutic candidates? *Curr. Drug Targets* 15, 454–468. doi: 10.2174/13894501156661401151l3734

Grieger, J. C., Soltys, S. M., and Samulski, R. J. (2016). Production of recombinant adeno-associated virus vectors using suspension HEK293 cells and continuous harvest of vector from the culture media for gmp fix and flt1 clinical vector. *Mol. Ther.* 24, 287–297. doi: 10.1038/mt.2015.187

Grimm, D., Lee, J. S., Wang, L., Desai, T., Akache, B., Storm, T. A., et al. (2008). *In vitro* and *in vivo* gene therapy vector evolution via multispecies interbreeding and retargeting of adeno-associated viruses. *J. Virol.* 82, 5887–5911. doi: 10.1128/JVI.00254-08

Holehonnur, R., Luong, J. A., Chaturvedi, D., Ho, A., Lella, S. K., Hosek, M. P., et al. (2014). Adeno-associated viral serotypes produce differing titers and differentially transduce neurons within the rat basal and lateral amygdala. *BMC Neurosci.* 15:28. doi: 10.1186/1471-2202-15-28

Jacobsen, J. C., Gregory, G. C., Woda, J. M., Thompson, M. N., Coser, K. R., Murthy, V., et al. (2011). HD CAG-correlated gene expression changes support a simple dominant gain of function. *Hum. Mol. Genet.* 20, 2846–2860. doi: 10.1093/hmg/ddr195

Jang, M., and Cho, I. H. (2016). Sulforaphane Ameliorates 3-Nitropropionic Acid-Induced Striatal Toxicity by Activating the Keap1-Nrf2-ARE pathway and inhibiting the MAPKs and NF-κB pathways. *Mol. Neurobiol.* 53, 2619–2635. doi: 10.1007/s12035-015-9230-2

Jang, M., Lee, M. J., and Cho, I. H. (2014). Ethyl pyruvate ameliorates 3-nitropropionic acid-induced striatal toxicity through anti-neuronal cell death and anti-inflammatory mechanisms. *Brain Behav. Immun.* 38, 151–165. doi: 10.1016/j.bbi.2014.01.015

Jang, M., Lee, M. J., Kim, C. S., and Cho, I. H. (2013). Korean Red Ginseng Extract Attenuates 3-Nitropropionic Acid-Induced Huntington's-Like Symptoms. *Evid. Based Complement Alternat. Med.* 2013:237207. doi: 10.1155/2013/237207

Jansen, A. H., van Hal, M., Op den Kelder, I. C., Meier, R. T., de Ruiter, A. A., Schut, M. H., et al. (2017). Frequency of nuclear mutant huntingtin inclusion formation in neurons and glia is cell-type-specific. *Glia* 65, 50–61. doi: 10.1002/glia.23050

Kabba, J. A., Xu, Y., Christian, H., Ruan, W., Chenai, K., Xiang, Y., et al. (2018). Microglia: housekeeper of the central nervous system. *Cell Mol. Neurobiol.* 38, 53–71. doi: 10.1007/s10571-017-0504-2

Kadiu, I., Glanzer, J. G., Kipnis, J., Gendelman, H. E., and Thomas, M. P. (2005). Mononuclear phagocytes in the pathogenesis of neurodegenerative diseases. *Neurotox Res.* 8, 25–50. doi: 10.1007/bf03033818

Klein, R. L., Dayton, R. D., Tatom, J. B., Henderson, K. M., and Henning, P. P. (2008). AAV8, 9, Rh10, Rh43 vector gene transfer in the rat brain: effects of serotype, promoter and purification method. *Mol. Ther.* 16, 89–96. doi: 10.1186/1471-2202-15-28

Kwon, I., and Schaffer, D. V. (2008). Designer gene delivery vectors: molecular engineering and evolution of adeno-associated viral vectors for enhanced gene transfer. *Pharm. Res.* 25, 489–499. doi: 10.1007/s11095-007-9431-0

Landis, S. C., Amara, S. G., Asadullah, K., Austin, C. P., Blumenstein, R., Bradley, E. W., et al. (2012). A call for transparent reporting to optimize the predictive value of preclinical research. *Nature* 490, 187–191. doi: 10.1038/nature11556

Lee, M. J., Bing, S. J., Choi, J., Jang, M., Lee, G., Lee, H., et al. (2016a). IKKβ-mediated inflammatory myeloid cell activation exacerbates experimental autoimmune encephalomyelitis by potentiating Th1/Th17 cell activation and compromising blood brain barrier. *Mol. Neurodegener.* 11:54. doi: 10.1186/s13024-016-0116-1

Lee, M. J., Jang, M., Choi, J., Lee, G., Min, H. J., Chung, W. S., et al. (2016b). Bee venom acupuncture alleviates experimental autoimmune encephalomyelitis by upregulating regulatory T cells and suppressing Th1 and Th17 responses. *Mol. Neurobiol.* 53, 1419–1445. doi: 10.1007/s12035-014-9012-2

Lobsiger, C. S., and Cleveland, D. W. (2007). Glial cells as intrinsic components of non-cell-autonomous neurodegenerative disease. *Nat. Neurosci.* 10, 1355–1360. doi: 10.1038/nn1988

Main, B. S., and Minter, M. R. (2017). Microbial immuno-communication in neurodegenerative diseases. *Front. Neurosci.* 11:151. doi: 10.3389/fnins.2017.00151

Menalled, L., and Brunner, D. (2014). Animal models of Huntington's disease for translation to the clinic: best practices. *Mov. Disord.* 29, 1375–1390. doi: 10.1002/mds.26006

Parker, J. A., Connolly, J. B., Wellington, C., Hayden, M., Dausset, J., and Neri, C. (2001). Expanded polyglutamines in *Caenorhabditis elegans* cause axonal abnormalities and severe dysfunction of PLM mechanosensory neurons without cell death. *Proc. Natl. Acad. Sci. USA* 98, 13318–13323. doi: 10.1073/pnas.231476398

Perry, G. M., Tallaksen-Greene, S., Kumar, A., Heng, M. Y., Kneynsberg, A., van Groen, T., et al. (2010). Mitochondrial calcium uptake capacity as a therapeutic target in the R6/2 mouse model of Huntington's disease. *Hum. Mol. Genet.* 19, 3354–3371. doi: 10.1093/hmg/ddq247

Pouladi, M. A., Morton, A. J., and Hayden, M. R. (2013). Choosing an animal model for the study of Huntington's disease. *Nat. Rev. Neurosci.* 14, 708–721. doi: 10.1038/nrn3570

Ruiz, M., and Déglon, N. (2012). Viral-mediated overexpression of mutant huntingtin to model HD in various species. *Neurobiol. Dis.* 48, 202–211. doi: 10.1016/j.nbd.2011.08.023

Saraiva, J., Nobre, R. J., and Pereira de Almeida, L. (2016). Gene therapy for the CNS using AAVs: The impact of systemic delivery by AAV9. *J. Control Release* 241, 94–109. doi: 10.1016/j.jconrel.2016.09.011

Schilling, G., Becher, M. W., Sharp, A. H., Jinnah, H. A., Duan, K., Kotzuk, J. A., et al. (1999). Intranuclear inclusions and neuritic aggregates in transgenic mice expressing a mutant N-terminal fragment of huntingtin. *Hum. Mol. Genet.* 8, 397–407. doi: 10.1093/hmg/8.3.397

Schilling, G., Savonenko, A. V., Klevytska, A., Morton, J. L., Tucker, S. M., Poirier, M., et al. (2004). Nuclear-targeting of mutant huntingtin fragments produces Huntington's disease-like phenotypes in transgenic mice. *Hum. Mol. Genet.* 13, 1599–1610. doi: 10.1093/hmg/ddh175

Senut, M. C., Suhr, S. T., Kaspar, B., and Gage, F. H. (2000). Intraneuronal aggregate formation and cell death after viral expression of expanded polyglutamine tracts in the adult rat brain. *J. Neurosci.* 20, 219–229. doi: 10.1523/jneurosci.20-01-00219.2000

Watakabe, A., Ohtsuka, M., Kinoshita, M., Takaji, M., Isa, K., Mizukami, H., et al. (2015). Comparative analyses of adeno-associated viral vector serotypes 1, 2, 5, 8 and 9 in marmoset, mouse and macaque cerebral cortex. *Neurosci. Res.* 93, 144–157. doi: 10.1016/j.neures.2014.09.002

Wyant, K. J., Ridder, A. J., and Dayalu, P. (2017). Huntington's disease-update on treatments. *Curr. Neurol. Neurosci. Rep.* 17:33. doi: 10.1007/s11910-017-0739-9

10

Antiphospholipid Antibodies Overlapping in Isolated Neurological Syndrome and Multiple Sclerosis: Neurobiological Insights and Diagnostic Challenges

Chiara D'Angelo [1,2,3], *Oriol Franch* [4], *Lidia Fernández-Paredes* [1,2], *Celia Oreja-Guevara* [5], *María Núñez-Beltrán* [1], *Alejandra Comins-Boo* [1,2], *Marcella Reale* [3] *and Silvia Sánchez-Ramón* [1,2]*

[1] Department of Clinical Immunology and IdISSC, Hospital Clínico San Carlos, Madrid, Spain, [2] Department of Immunology, Ophthalmology and ENT, Complutense University School of Medicine, Madrid, Spain, [3] Department of Medical, Oral and Biotechnological Sciences, University "G. d'Annunzio" Chieti-Pescara, Chieti, Italy , [4] Department of Neurology, Hospital Ruber Internacional, Madrid, Spain, [5] Department of Neurology, Hospital Clínico San Carlos, Madrid, Spain

***Correspondence:**
Silvia Sánchez-Ramón
ssramon@salud.madrid.org

Antiphospholipid syndrome (APS) is characterized by arterial and venous thrombosis, pregnancy morbidity and fetal loss caused by pathogenic autoantibodies directed against phospholipids (PL) and PL-cofactors. Isolated neurological APS may represent a significant diagnostic challenge, as epidemiological, clinical and neuroimaging features may overlap with those of multiple sclerosis (MS). In an open view, MS could be considered as an organ-specific anti-lipid (phospholipid and glycosphingolipid associated proteins) disease, in which autoreactive B cells and CD8+ T cells play a dominant role in its pathophysiology. In MS, diverse autoantibodies against the lipid-protein cofactors of the myelin sheath have been described, whose pathophysiologic role has not been fully elucidated. We carried out a review to select clinical studies addressing the prevalence of antiphospholipid (aPL) autoantibodies in the so-called MS-like syndrome. The reported prevalence ranged between 2% and 88%, particularly aCL and aβ2GPI, with predominant IgM isotype and suggesting worse MS prognosis. Secondarily, an updated summary of current knowledge on the pathophysiological mechanisms and events responsible for these conditions is presented. We draw attention to the clinical relevance of diagnosing isolated neurological APS. Prompt and accurate diagnosis and antiaggregant and anticoagulant treatment of APS could be vital to prevent or at least reduce APS-related morbidity and mortality.

Keywords: antiphospholipid syndrome, pathogenesis, MS-like syndrome, thrombosis, vasculopathy

CURRENT CHALLENGES IN THE DIAGNOSIS AND MANAGEMENT OF THE ANTIPHOSPHOLIPID SYNDROME

The antiphospholipid syndrome (APS) is a systemic autoimmune disorder characterized by the presence of peripheral procoagulant autoantibodies together with the occurrence of recurrent thrombosis (venous, arterial or both) and/or pregnancy morbidity and fetal loss (Miyakis et al., 2006). The sole presence of autoantibodies does not always lead to thrombosis. APS can indeed be caused by a diverse array of antiphospholipid (aPL) antibodies that recognize cell surface proteins linked to phospholipids as "non self" within a pro-inflammatory context that has been described as a "second hit" (after infection or tissue damage). This combined effect would in turn activate the clotting cascade in a wide variety of mechanisms that lead to the development of thrombosis (Giannakopoulos and Krilis, 2013; Meroni et al., 2018).

The routine diagnostic aPL antibodies, used according to the 2006 Sydney revised APS classification criteria, are anticardiolipin (aCL), antiβ2-glycoprotein-I (aβ2GPI) and lupus anticoagulant (LA). The non-classic aPL antibodies include anti-phosphatidylserine (aPS), anti-phosphatidylserine-β2GPI (aPS-β2), anti-phosphatidylethanolamine (aPE), anti-prothrombin-prothrombin complex (aPT-PT), anti-phosphatidylserine-prothrombin complex (aPS-PT) and anti-annexin V (aAnV; Shoenfeld et al., 2008).

According to Sydney revision, classification of APS requires at least one clinical manifestation of vascular thrombosis or obstetrical events and the presence of at least two positive laboratory criteria (aCL IgG or IgM and/or aβ2GPI IgG or IgM at moderate titers and/or LA positivity) on two separate occasions at least 12 weeks apart (Miyakis et al., 2006). Persistence of positive aPL was introduced in order to differentiate the aPL antibodies appearing in the setting of infections or other unspecific conditions, in which aPL are transient and non-thrombogenic. Indeed, it is also well known that aPL antibodies fluctuate in blood, which hampers their interpretation (Donohoe et al., 2002; Fonseca and D'Cruz, 2008). To make the picture more complicated, besides the well-recognized obstetric and thrombotic hallmarks, APS can encompass an exceedingly variable clinical spectrum of multiorgan non-thrombotic manifestations, in the so called "extra-criteria" or "non-criteria" manifestations. Among these are the neurological manifestations, such as epilepsy, myelitis, chorea and migraine; hematological manifestations, such as thrombocytopenia and hemolytic anemia; livedo reticularis; pulmonary and osteoarticular manifestations; valvular heart disease; and nephropathy, to mention a few examples that cannot be exclusively explained by prothrombotic phenomena (Gómez-Puerta and Cervera, 2014; Negrini et al., 2017; Garcia and Erkan, 2018). In addition, the extra-criteria manifestations, as well as the classical ones, can occur in the setting of APS without fulfilling the serological criteria, as for instance with low titers' aCL or aβ2GPI antibodies (Cobo-Soriano et al., 1999; Micheloud et al., 2005) or even in the absence of detectable aPL in the so-called "seronegative APS."

APS may be diagnosed as an isolated disease (primary APS) or associated to other autoimmune disorders, mainly systemic lupus erythematous (SLE), rheumatoid arthritis, Sjögren syndrome, autoimmune thyroid disease, systemic sclerosis, systemic vasculitis, dermatopolymyositis, primary biliary cirrhosis and autoimmune hepatitis. It has been estimated that approximately 50% of patients who suffer from APS will develop SLE (Salmon et al., 2007). Nowadays, because of potentially recurrent thrombosis and the hypercoagulability scenario, there is consensus in treating APS patients with long-term oral anticoagulants and, in order to prevent obstetric manifestations, with a combination of low dose aspirin and low molecular weight heparin (LMWH; Empson et al., 2005).

There is a heated debate on the clinically significant titers of aPL antibodies. Investigators are strongly advised to classify patients as affected by APS, when more than one laboratory criterion is present alone or in combination. Specifically, LA presence in plasma; medium or high titer of IgG and/or IgM aCL antibody in serum or plasma (i.e., >40 GPL or MPL, or >the 99th percentile); IgG and/or IgM aβ2GPI antibody in serum or plasma (in titer >the 99th percentile; Miyakis et al., 2006). Growing evidences claim to consider the clinical impact of low level positive aPL antibodies and the necessity to set new cut-off levels, basically—though not exclusively—in obstetric APS (Devreese et al., 2010; Mekinian et al., 2012). The proposal to modify the APS classification criteria, mostly referring to laboratory requirements, is reinforced also by consideration that no differences were observed on obstetric complications, gestational period, arterial and/or venous thrombosis, when comparing pregnant women with aPL-related obstetric complications not fulfilling the Sydney criteria, with those fulfilling them (Arachchillage et al., 2015; Alijotas-Reig et al., 2018). Considering that also atypical (low or non-persistent), aPL antibodies presence may be associated with neurological disorders, such as transient ischemic attacks and migraine, but also epilepsy, transverse myelitis, multiple sclerosis (MS)-like syndrome, visual symptoms, dementia and chorea as well (Islam et al., 2016). The "rigid" adhesion to such criteria in clinical practice might exclude patients with "non-criteria" manifestations of APS in face of diagnostic uncertainty (Abreu et al., 2015; Aggarwal et al., 2015; Joseph and Habboush, 2018; Limper et al., 2018).

Whether anti-aggregant prophylaxis is needed in subjects with persistent positive aPL but without thrombosis history is still unclear. For the identification of the actual thrombotic risk, additional factors should be taken into consideration, such as hypertension, smoking, hypercholesterolemia, overweight or treatment with estrogens. Coexisting SLE and positivity to two or more aPL antibodies should be assessed too (Khamashta et al., 2016).

Isolated Involvement of the Central Nervous System in the Antiphospholipid Syndrome

Neurological features, already predicted in the first description of APS in 1983 (Hughes, 1983), have not been included yet in the APS classification criteria. According to the 2006 APS classification criteria (Miyakis et al., 2006), only transient ischemic attack and stroke have been included as neurological manifestations. Nevertheless, a wide variety of neurological symptoms including cognitive dysfunction, psychosis, chorea and epilepsy cannot be solely explained by thrombotic events or hypercoagulability. These manifestations represent thus an important challenge in diagnostic practice, with a growing demand to recognize these "non-criteria" neurological manifestations in the classification of the disease (Abreu et al., 2015; Islam et al., 2016; Joseph and Habboush, 2018; Zhang and Pereira, 2018). A special case is the isolated central nervous system (CNS) involvement of APS, given the overlapping clinical and radiological features with MS (Achiron et al., 2004). In fact, isolated CNS APS usually occurs ranging from optical neuritis, chronic headache, migraine, cerebral ischemia, chorea, epilepsy, transverse myelopathy, to dementia and cognitive impairment (Hughes, 2003; Rodrigues et al., 2010). Most of these symptoms are usually referred as MS-like syndrome.

CNS APS and MS may be difficult to distinguish also from an immunological perspective, as the aPL antibody isotypes may involve IgG, IgM or IgA and therefore not always detected as the characteristic mirror pattern (positivity in serum and cerebrospinal fluid, CSF) or even of oligoclonal bands (OCB; predominant intrathecal antibody production; Cuadrado et al., 2000; Vilisaar et al., 2005). The two diseases resemble each other also for the epidemiological features of affected population, the relapsing-remitting course and for their appearance in neuroimaging (**Figure 1**). For both diseases, multifocal white matter lesions in magnetic resonance imaging (MRI) are the most common manifestation within the CNS (Chapman, 2004; Ferreira et al., 2005). In APS subjects, small strokes can occur in the white matter of brain and spinal cord, resulting in lesions that resemble the MS demyelinating plaques. The preferential localization is the subcortical area, and in a recent study, multiple subcortical and cortical infarcts with demyelination, involving both lobes of the brain, have been classified as characteristic MRI features for APS patients. White matter lesions were found in the periventricular area of the brain in almost the totality of the studied cases (Zhu et al., 2014).

Significant correlation between cognitive dysfunction and MRI lesions in primary APS patients has been reported, also in patients without CNS involvement (Tektonidou et al., 2006). In addition, vasculitis and inflammatory changes were also prevalent (Renaud et al., 2014).

Nowadays, the management and the treatment of APS patients with CNS involvement is still a matter of debate. There is good evidence of the benefit of anticoagulation in the typical thrombotic complications of APS, but there is still no consensus on the management with immunosuppression vs. anticoagulant therapy for non-thrombotic complications observed in MS-like syndrome. One might naturally wonder why, in the absence of any evident thrombotic injury on brain imaging, anticoagulant therapy should be used. In a case report by Zhang and Pereira (2018) an elderly woman with 6 months history of headache and intermittent choreiform movements of the face and arm, dramatically improved with warfarin therapy. Her blood tests showed positive LA, weakly positive aCL and negative aβ2GPI, with neither history of pregnancy loss or thrombosis. She received a trial of warfarin in the setting of probable APS, even if further investigation excluded potential secondary APS. After 2 weeks, her aberrant movements resolved as did her headaches, and since then she was symptom free for 18 months (Zhang and Pereira, 2018).

The evidence on how to manage movement disorders associated with APS are insufficient and no superiority of one drug to another has been demonstrated. In the reported case, a clear improvement of the patient's life quality was achieved with anticoagulation, although the pathophysiology of movement disorders in APS, including chorea, as well as of other non-criteria neurological symptoms, remains poorly understood (Joseph and Habboush, 2018).

No standard treatment exists for non-thrombotic neurological manifestations of APS and available evidence mostly derives from retrospective non-randomized trials or

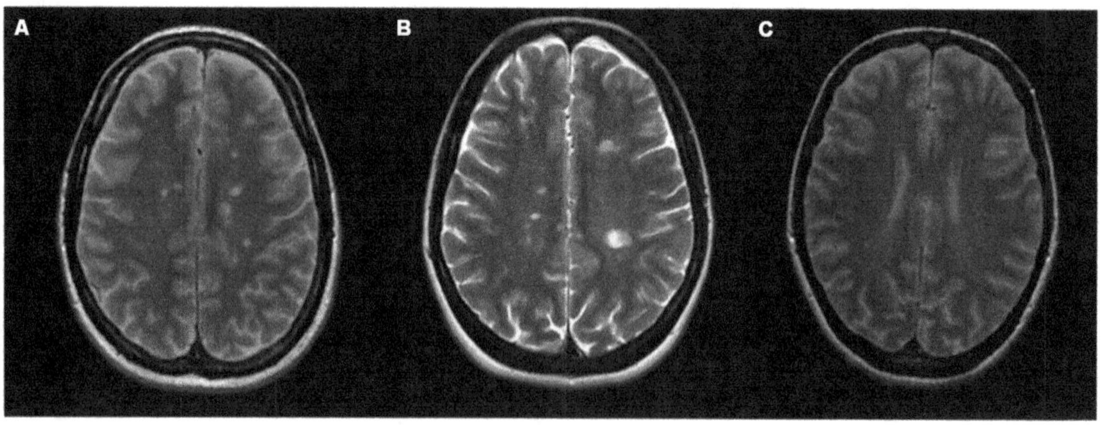

FIGURE 1 | Conventional magnetic resonance imaging (MRI) showing similar demyelinating lesions in: **(A)** multiple sclerosis (MS) and **(B)** antiphospholipid syndrome (APS). **(A)** Gadolinium-enhanced T2-weighted sequence of a patient with MS showing multiple demyelinating lesions in the *supra* and infratentorial white matter, predominantly periventricular, without evidence of postcontrast enhancement. **(B)** T2-weighted sequence of a patient with APS that shows multiple focal demyelinating lesions in periventricular, juxtacortical posterior left parietal (by confluence of several lesions) white matter. that are hyperintense relative to the normal appearing brain tissue, indicating increased permeability of the blood–brain barrier. **(C)** Normal T2 MRI.

case reports. In these studies anticoagulants have proven to be effective for the treatment of conditions that are not primarily thrombotic, such as migraine, transverse myelitis, and neuropsychiatric disturbances (Asherson et al., 2007; Roie et al., 2013).

According to the present state of knowledge, one might consider, under specific conditions, immunosuppressive treatment with corticosteroids, azathioprine and cyclophosphamide in addition to antithrombotic therapy, and combination with symptomatic management with neuroleptics (Cervera et al., 2014; Espinosa and Cervera, 2015; Yelnik et al., 2016). Rituximab, a monoclonal anti-CD20 antibody that depletes B cells, is currently used to treat various autoimmune diseases and hematological malignancies. Several case reports describe the use of rituximab in patients with APS, suggesting a beneficial role in the treatment and monitoring of refractory thrombocytopenia (Gamoudi et al., 2017) and recurrent thrombotic events in APS secondary to SLE (Emmi et al., 2017; Diószegi et al., 2018). The pilot therapeutic trial RITAPS that was designed to evaluate the efficacy and safety of rituximab in non-criteria APS manifestations (cognitive dysfunction, thrombocytopenia, cardiac valve disease, skin ulcers, nephropathy) did not show significant improvement of aPL profiles but a beneficial effect for a few of that conditions, given the small sample size. RITAPS was the first attempt to investigate immunosuppressive treatment in the management of cognitive dysfunction in aPL-positive patients without other systemic autoimmune diseases. The obtained findings indicated improvement in attention, visuomotor speed and flexibility (Erkan et al., 2013).

On the other hand, the rationale for the use of immunosuppressive and/or anticoagulant therapy could be given by the potential aPL-mediated damage considering each specific clinical case and clinical manifestations (Espinosa and Cervera, 2015).

ANTIPHOSPHOLIPID SYNDROME PATHOPHYSIOLOGY

aβ2GPI antibodies are central in many pathogenic APS mechanisms and, although the full pathogenesis of APS is not clear yet, the binding of these aPL antibodies to the antigens on the cell surface of platelets, monocytes, endothelial cells and trophoblasts, triggers intracellular signaling with subsequent activation and alteration of diverse cell functions. Monocytes and endothelial cells' activation determine a pro-aggregation status due to up-regulated expression of adhesion molecules, such as E-selectin, and release of tissue factor (TF) and proinflammatory cytokines (**Figure 2**). Platelets' activation and the subsequent release of thromboxane favor their aggregation. Cellular activation starts after the binding of the complex aβ2GPI antibody/β2GPI to the toll-like or annexin II receptors. Thrombosis at the fine vasculature of the target organ, such as retina or in the CNS, is thought to be more dependent from antibodies against the anticoagulant AnV. The resulting pathological and clinical events include inflammation and vasculitis, thrombus formation and arterial and/or venous vessel-occlusive disease (Pierangeli et al., 2006; Muscal and Brey, 2007; Merashli et al., 2015).

Although APS is considered an autoimmune condition mediated by specific production of autoantibodies and autoreactive T cells, innate immunity defects have been described as essential trigger factors within a multifactorial etiopathogenic scenario. As in most autoimmune diseases, genetically predisposed subjects, exposed to certain environmental agents could develop a specific immune response against self-proteins-binding phospholipids with a subsequent autoantibody production, together with the contribution of innate immunity mediators. Intrinsic alterations of the CNS myelin lipids or their cofactors (target tissue) could play a role in etiopathogenesis as well (Reale and Sanchez-Ramon, 2017). Coming up next, we summarize the events taking place in both innate and adaptive responses concerning APS.

Innate Immune System in Antiphospholipid Syndrome Pathophysiology

APS is characterized by the presence of autoantibodies, but as previously mentioned, aPL antibodies is a necessary but not sufficient condition for the onset of the disease. Additional factors or a "second hit," mediated by innate immunity, would be necessary to trigger the pathogenesis of the disease in the presence of autoantibodies, according to the current accepted theory (Pengo et al., 2011). In this context, certain environmental, proinflammatory or non-immunological procoagulant factors could induce the development of the disease, in genetically susceptible subjects (for instance, HLA-DR4 and HLA-Drw53 are risk factors; Matthey et al., 1989).

It must be also considered that, similarly to MS, several pathogens have been long described as potential triggers of the autoimmune response in APS. Molecular mimicry, with a modified-β2GPI from bacterial or viral structures may contribute to the development of the autoimmune response and the selection of autoantibodies (Cruz-Tapias et al., 2012).

aPL antibodies could be responsible of the specific activation of other innate immune cells and even non-immune cells. Presence of aβ2GPI antibodies induces up-regulation of TLR7 and TLR8 in plasmacytoid dendritic cells (pDCs; Prinz et al., 2011) and activates specific cells through the binding to relevant targets, such as TLR2, 4 and annexin A2 on monocytes and endothelial cells (Lambrianides et al., 2010; Satta et al., 2011; Allen et al., 2012); or ApoE receptor and glycoprotein Iba on platelets (Urbanus et al., 2008), promoting the development of a prothrombotic phenotype. It has indeed been demonstrated that knockout mice for these innate receptors, show a reduced thrombotic response following aPL antibodies administration (Pierangeli et al., 2007; Ramesh et al., 2011).

In addition, aPL antibodies directly promote up-regulation of the TF synthesis in monocytes (Sorice et al., 2007), neutrophils (Ritis et al., 2006) and endothelial cells (Kornberg et al., 2000). This procoagulant condition, not present under normal circumstances, plays an important role in contributing to the

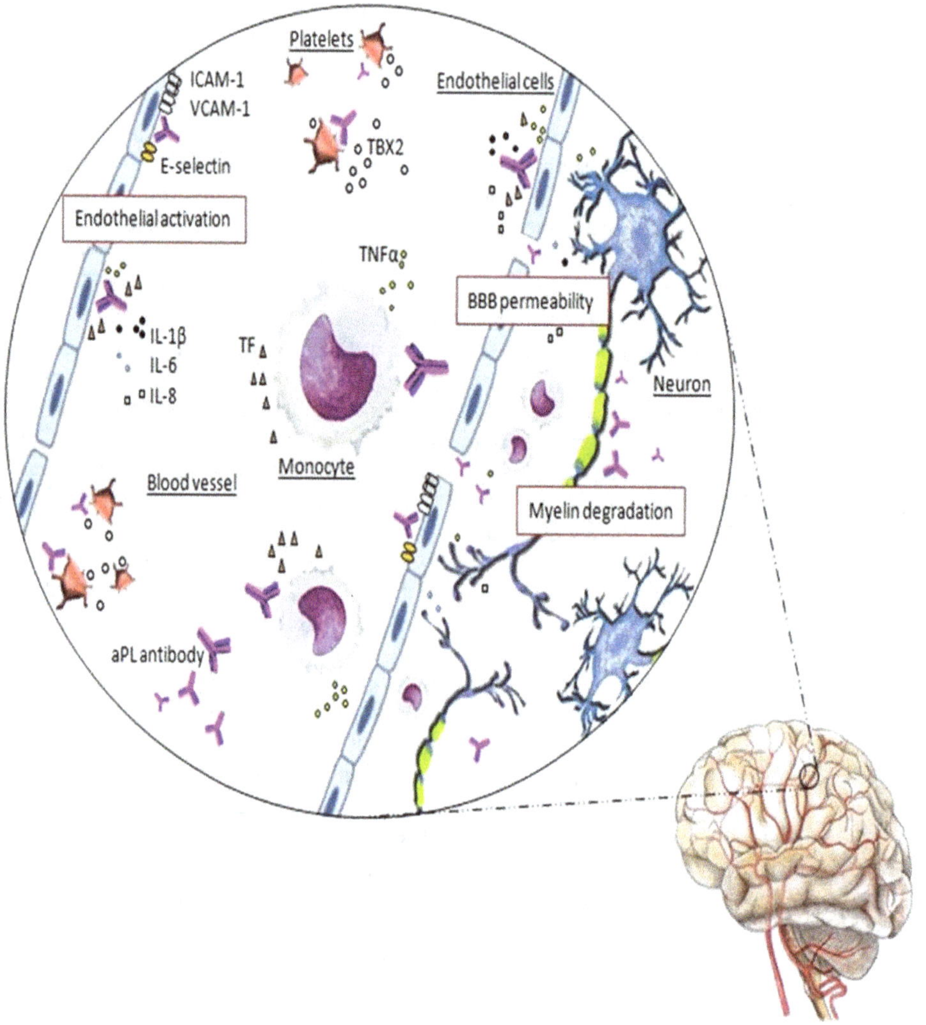

FIGURE 2 | Schematic representation of the autoreactive response in APS in which the thrombus formation is mediated by the interaction of antiphospholipid (aPL) antibodies with the anticoagulant annexinV (AnV) on the surface of the endothelial cells, which are destroyed, accelerating coagulation cascade. Moreover, the binding of aPL antibodies promotes the endothelial cells activation determining an increased expression of adhesion molecules (ICAM-1, VCAM-1, E-selectin) and the release of tissue factor (TF), TNFα, IL-1β, IL-6 and IL-8 proinflammatory cytokines. aPL antibodies promote also platelets and monocytes activation. On the platelets membrane, anti-β2GP1 antibodies lead to platelets activation and thromboxane B2 (TBX2) release. In monocytes, aPL antibodies induce TF expression and TNFα production.The inflammatory condition determined by these events causes a vascular endothelium dysfunction with increased permeability of the blood-brain barrier (BBB). The neurons and myelin become now accessible to the aPL antibodies and their binding may trigger the myelin destruction and the neurodegeneration found in APS with MS-like syndrome.

onset of thrombotic events in cancer, inflammation, angiogenesis and embryogenesis (Mackman, 2009).

aPL antibodies also interfere with the protein C function, especially through the competition for the phospholipid binding site, and therefore predispose to the development of venous thromboembolism (de-Groot et al., 1996).

Activation of the complement pathway is closely linked with thrombosis. Indeed, inhibition of the alternative complement pathway improves clinical outcomes reducing thrombosis risk (Chapin et al., 2016). aPL antibodies have shown to induce complement activation and to promote the upregulation of TF expression on neutrophils mediated by C5a (Ritis et al., 2006).

On the other hand, recent experimental studies on mice models suggest that natural killer T (NKT) cells play an important role in the regulation of aCL antibody production. NKT cells are characterized by their ability to recognize lipid antigens presented by CD1d molecules. Among a wide variety of self- and non-self lipids linked to CD1d in NKT cells, cardiolipin has been identified (Cox et al., 2009). NKT cells expansion was suggested to have a beneficial role in several autoimmune disorders through the release of immunomodulatory cytokines after antigen recognition (Godfrey and Kronenberg, 2004). This recognition of lipids, in the absence of exogenous antigens, is a hallmark of NKT cells and could account for activation and increased numbers of peripheral NKT cells described in several oncological and autoimmune diseases (Brigl et al., 2003; Darmoise et al., 2010). Although the exact mechanism is not well understood, it has been demonstrated that NKT cells can regulate the activation of autoreactive B cells in a CD1d-dependent manner (Wermeling et al., 2010; Yang et al., 2011). In contrast, absence or reduction of NKT cells or of CD1d-expression on B cells have been related with an increased autoreactive B cells activation and higher aPL release, which raised the hypothesis that aPL antibodies could result from imbalanced NKT population. These data point to NKT cells as an intriguing therapeutic strategy to establish tolerance, a key element for ameliorating autoimmune diseases (Wermeling et al., 2010).

Adaptive Immune System in APS Pathophysiology

Undoubtedly, aPL auto-antibodies production by autoreactive B cells is the key feature of APS, although little is known about their emergence, their overactivation, regulation and about all their pathological effects. In line with the second hit theory, molecular mimicry has been proposed as a potential underlying mechanism for aPL antibodies production (Blank et al., 2002; Gharavi et al., 2002, 2003; Shoenfeld et al., 2006; Martin et al., 2011). In humans, many viral or bacterial infections have been associated with the production of IgM and IgG aPL, which can be persistent in time. As β2GPI has a similar aminoacidic sequence to that of several bacterial and viral components, it has been postulated that subjects with a certain genetic background may produce cross-reactive antibodies (Abdel-Wahab et al., 2016). For many years, aPL antibodies have been considered natural antibodies because of their polyspecific repertoire and other similar characteristics to those produced by B1 cells (Youinou and Renaudineau, 2004; Merrill, 2006). Conversely, aPL antibodies have been shown to be mainly of IgG and IgA isotype (Fanopoulos et al., 1998), hence probably their secretion needs to be T-cell dependent. In fact, a specific T cell-response against β2GPI in APS patients has been reported by several investigators (Kuwana, 2003; Yamaguchi et al., 2007). An increase in IL-17/IL-23 indicating a Th17 response has been described in APS as well (Meroni et al., 2011; Popovic-Kuzmanovic et al., 2013; Jakiela et al., 2016). Although there is no definitive evidence to prove these concepts, it has been demonstrated that antigen driven maturation increases the pathogenic potential of aPL antibodies, although it is not an indispensable prerequisite for pathogenicity (Lieby et al., 2004). In fact, aPL antibodies production induced by infection has not shown to be pathogenic, even if significantly higher number of infected patients with aPL antibodies titer develop thrombotic events. Further, serum collected from healthy individuals can present these autoantibodies too (Uthman et al., 1999; Justo et al., 2011; Nakayama et al., 2014; Abdel-Wahab et al., 2016). To date, it is universally accepted that aPL antibodies cause the typical clinical manifestations of APS, but the causal relationship with the thrombotic events remains speculative.

Besides the diverse effects previously described on innate immune cells, aPL antibodies appear to interfere with the natural antithrombotic processes, by recognition and binding to β2GPI, expressed on the surface membranes of several cell types involved in the coagulation cascade, as well as decidual stromal cells, throphoblast cells, glial cells and neurons (Borghi et al., 2007; Lavazza et al., 2007). The former have been reported to induce defective *in vitro* trophoblast proliferation and differentiation as well as increased apoptosis (Di Simone et al., 2007).

aPL antibodies' prothrombotic effects have also been observed in the CNS. Intrathecal synthesis of aPL antibodies or the disruption of the blood-brain barrier (BBB) could allow aPL autoantibodies to enter the CNS (Martínez-Cordero et al., 1997). Prothrombotic events could be triggered by direct interaction between aPL antibodies and CNS-resident cells. aPL antibodies have been related to astrocyte proliferation and nonspecific permeabilization and depolarization of synaptoneurosomes *in vitro* (Chapman et al., 1999).

The most characteristic features of APS affecting CNS, have been reported to be the connective dysfunction disorder and demyelinization (Espinosa and Cervera, 2008), but the specific role of aPL antibodies in non-thrombotic CNS manifestations of APS or transverse myelitis, remains to be established. Even though studies on small cohorts of patients have shown specific non-thrombogenic effects of aPL antibodies on CNS, with both vascular and non-vascular damage involved in the neurological manifestations of the disease. Data suggest a direct binding of aPL antibodies within the CNS, inducing activation of astrocytes, neurons and brain endotheliocytes (**Figure 2**). However, the binding of aPL antibodies to the membrane phospholipids within the brain has not been extensively studied. Caronti et al. (1998a,b) demonstrated that the neuronal damage might occur by a direct interaction of aPL antibodies with neurons or by functional impairment after their interaction with astrocytes, endothelial cell activation and adherence to CNS cells. These authors showed by indirect immunofluorescence that aβ2GPI antibodies purified from the serum of a patient with SLE/APS specifically bound CNS cells, in particular astrocytes and neurons in culture and in histological sections of human and monkey brain, and to cerebral vascular endothelium.

aCL antibodies' binding was demonstrated also in a cell line of rat astrocytes. In these cells, aCL antibodies exerted an inhibitory effect by decreasing the cells' viability and by depolarizing the cell membrane, impairing the signal transduction (Sun et al., 1992).

Chapman et al. (1999) in 1999 speculated about the potential target site of aPL antibodies at the neuronal synapses. They examined aPL antibodies effects on the plasma membrane function of rat synaptoneurosomes with IgG aPL purified from APS patients' sera. The study was a proof-of-concept describing the functional interaction of IgG purified aPL antibodies from APS subjects with neuronal cell membranes, showing increased depolarization and permeabilization of synaptoneurosomes.

Moreover, it should be considered that by targeting antigens at the BBB and compromising its integrity, aPL antibodies in APS patients gain access to the CNS (**Figure 2**). Further, supporting the hypothesis of a direct role of these autoantibodies in the pathogenesis of neurological manifestations, *in vivo* mice behavioral tests were performed by Shoenfeld et al. (2003).

After direct injection of IgG aPL purified from APS patients into mice brain, worst performances were demonstrated in the animals.

Despite these studies were conducted long-time ago, whether neurological hyperexcitatory manifestations, such as epilepsy and chorea could result from aPL-induced synaptic depolarization or whether the neuronal depolarization might explain the dementia and cognitive dysfunction found in APS, remains unknown.

The CNS involvement in APS might be additionally mediated by a direct neurotoxic effect of aPL antibodies that leads to impaired basal ganglion cell function with the development of neuroinflammation. Possibly, the aPL antibody bond to the cerebral endothelium could also cause endothelial dysfunction and lead to microthrombosis and inflammation of the blood vessels as well. This hypothesis might provide an explanation of why anticoagulation or immunosuppression therapy can represent at present an effective treatment in these aPL positive patients with neurological features. The above-mentioned mechanisms may be relevant not only in APS but in aPL positive MS patients, given the parallel mechanisms that cross between the two conditions.

In addition, a hypothesis proposes that the already described MS-like manifestations in APS patients could depend on the direct reactivity of aPL antibodies and myelin antigens by "molecular mimicry" and cross-reacting with myelin, myelin-related proteins and the cerebral phospholipids cephalin and sphingomyelin (**Figure 2**; Rombos et al., 1990; Karussis et al., 1998; Cikes et al., 2008). MRI studies of APS patients frequently show multiple T2-hyperintense brain lesions. Thus, typical demyelinating lesions of MS, transverse myelitis and optic neuritis, may also be present in the pathological spectrum of APS (Cikes et al., 2008). Moreover, preliminary data showed that the molecular mimicry of aPL-target antigens with myelin, myelin-related proteins and brain phospholipids may lead to cross-reactivity and predispose to a prothrombotic state (Koudriavtseva et al., 2014; Uthman et al., 2015).

PREVALENCE OF NON ORGAN-SPECIFIC ANTIPHOSPHOLIPID ANTIBODIES IN MULTIPLE SCLEROSIS

MS is an autoimmune mediated inflammatory and neurodegenerative disease characterized by multifocal areas of inflammation, due to autoreactive T and B lymphocytes and macrophage infiltrations, which cause demyelination, axonal damage with neuronal loss and gliosis, within both the white and gray matter of the CNS (Machado-Santos et al., 2018). These events lead to the formation of lesions, called plaques, which interfere with nerve impulses' transmission. The nervous transmission alteration accounts for the clinical MS features, such as autonomic and sensory defects, loss or reduction of motor functions and paralysis, fatigue, speech disorders, ataxia, difficulties in concentrating/thinking, learning and memory impairment and psychological problems (Compston and Coles, 2008).

The well-known heterogeneity of MS reflects a myriad of pathogenic mechanisms contributing to the disease. MS pathogenesis is mainly considered to be mediated by Th1 and Th17 autoreactive T cells infiltrating the CNS, which initiate an inflammatory cascade causing destruction of myelin sheath, oligodendrocyte and microglia damage, and finally axonal and neuronal destruction. Lipid-reactive NKT cells have been suggested to primarily drive Th1 and Th17 responses, after activation between certain myelin glycosphingolipids (particularly the derivatives of galactosylceramides) and CD1d glycoprotein (De Libero et al., 2007; Blewett, 2008; Hogan et al., 2013). Phospholipids and glycosphingolipids are the major components of CNS myelin sheath that, under certain circumstances, could become immunogenic and trigger autoimmune responses (Reale and Sanchez-Ramon, 2017). Moreover, invariant NKT (iNKT) cells seem to have a dual proinflammatory vs. counter-regulatory role in MS responses (Podbielska et al., 2018).

To date, B cells and humoral response in MS pathogenesis have reached more importance based on clonally expanded memory B cells and anti-myelin-specific lipids autoantibodies detected in MS patients, as indicated by the diagnostic use of OCB. The presence of the characteristic OCBs in the CSF is one of the main hallmarks of MS although not specific, together with antibody deposition, complement activation and demyelination.

The first and the most common detected autoantibodies in MS recognize the complexes of membrane proteins assembled to myelin lipids, like the transmembrane proteolipid protein (PLP), the extrinsic myelin basic protein (MBP), the myelin oligodendrocyte glycoprotein (MOG) and the myelin associated glycoprotein (MAG; Kanter et al., 2006; Podbielska and Hogan, 2009). Antibodies directed against glycolipids like ganglioside have been reported too (Stevens et al., 1992). Specific autoreactive T-cells and autoantibodies' reactivity directed against lipids such as sulfatide, phosphatidylcholine and sphingomyelin, and also against lipids that are altered by oxidative processes within the brain tissue of MS patients, including cholesterol, phosphatidylcholine, phosphatidyl ethanolamine and lysophosphatidyl ethanolamine have been described (Kanter et al., 2006; Fraussen et al., 2014). These antigenic stimuli from oxidized lipids, may overlap with those involved in the pathophysiology of APS. In MS, it has been evoked the role of capillary and venous hemorrhages that result in extracellular release of hemoglobin and reactive molecules that could induce local oxidative stress, inflammation and tissue damage. In fact, oxidized extracellular hemoglobin cause direct oxidative damage to myelin components, specifically to MBP (Bamm et al., 2017). In this context, vascular pathology could exert a primary event in the induction of a subsequent immunogenic response in MS. In an open view, MS could be considered as an organ-specific aPL disease, in which autoreactive B cells and $CD8^+$ T-cells play a major role in its pathophysiology (Machado-Santos et al., 2018).

The use of MRI and the paramagnetic element gadolinium (Gd) in MS is useful to detect CNS plaques with active inflammation and lesion burden. Gd can only cross the damaged BBB at sites of tissue destruction or inflammation. However, the correlation between Gd-enhancing lesions and cognitive deficit is weak or absent in MS (Rocca et al., 2015).

Different MS clinical forms have been described, including relapsing remitting (RRMS), the most common subtype (approximately affects 87% of patients), primary progressive (PPMS), secondary progressive (SPMS) and progressive relapsing (PRMS). RRMS is characterized by acute inflammatory attacks, known as exacerbations or relapses, followed by periods of remission between relapses. During every attack, destruction of myelin and nerve fibers occur and accumulate in the long-term. Nearly 65% of patients with RRMS will subsequently develop SPMS, which is considered the second phase of the disease (Ghasemi et al., 2017).

MS different clinical forms are considered to translate into variable pathophysiological pathways, determining different patients' prognosis and treatment decisions. To-date, there is no cure for primary progressive MS, while there are diverse disease-modifying treatments (DMTs) for RRMS and SPMS in current use. The most common strategy of MS management is the "escalation therapy" beginning with interferon-β, glatiramer acetate, and corticosteroids for acute relapses. In patients with demonstrated moderate-to-high-disease activity, early initiation of "high-efficacy" DMTs, such as fingolimod, monoclonal antibodies such as natalizumab and alemtuzumab and new generation monoclonal anti-CD20 antibodies such as ocrelizumab may help to better control the disease (Merkel et al., 2017). These immunomodulatory and anti-inflammatory treatments can partially diminish disease progression and alleviate MS symptoms, by exerting inhibition of immune cell activation and migration through the BBB, lymphocyte proliferation and macrophage-mediated myelin degradation and blocking secretion of proinflammatory cytokines, among other effects (Torkildsen et al., 2016; Ghasemi et al., 2017; Nandoskar et al., 2017).

The hypothesis that aPL antibodies may be involved in the pathogenesis of MS, and the potential association between their presence and specific MS clinical subtypes or clinical phase is not recent (Marchiori et al., 1990; Sugiyama and Yamamoto, 1996; Karussis et al., 1998; Roussel et al., 2000; Horstman et al., 2009). Interestingly, PL/PL-linked cofactor antigens are clinically relevant in MS. We carried out a review in several steps: (1) articles were identified and revised by a computer assisted search of published reports (PubMed, US National Library of Medicine, National Institutes of Health) to locate all cases of MS in which aPL antibodies were analyzed and their positivity was reported. Bibliographies of each article were also scanned for references not identified in the initial search. Only cases with well documented clinical summaries and relevant information were included in the review. Data from these articles were summarized using a standardized data form, including population size, diagnosis and MS clinical phase, sample type, and the percentage of positivity for the specific antibody. According to our review, non organ-specific aPL autoantibodies, particularly aCL and aβ2GPI, that could account for APS patients with MS-like syndrome, occur within a range between 2% and 88% according to the different studies, with predominant IgM over IgG isotype, both in serum and CSF (**Table 1**). Due to the conflicting published levels, the exact prevalence, pathogenic role

TABLE 1 | Summary of relevant studies on the prevalence of aPL in MS patients.

Study	Population	aPL antibodies positivity
Filippidou et al. (2016)	127 MS (Serum); 88 RR, 11 PP, 28 SP	RR: aCL: 10.2% IgM, 18.2% IgG PP: aCL: 36.4% IgM, 18.2% IgG SP: aCL: 35.7% IgM, 32.1% IgG
Mandoj et al. (2015)	100 MS (Serum); 58 REM, 26 REL, 16 SP	REM: aCL: 1.7% IgM, 1.7% IgG, aβ2GPI: 1.7% IgM, aPT: 3.4% IgM, 5.2% IgG, aAnV: 1.7% IgM, 6.9% IgG REL: aCL: 7.7% IgM, 11.5% IgG, aβ2GPI: 26.9% IgM, aPT: 15.4% IgM, 19.2%IgG, aAnV: 3.8% IgM,15.4% IgG SP: aCL: 6.3% IgM, 6.3% IgG, aβ2GPI: 6.3% IgM, aPT: 6.3% IgM, aAnV: 6.3% IgM, 18.8% IgG
Shor et al. (2015)	98 MS (Serum)	aPS-β2: 14.6% IgM, 22.4% IgG, aPT: 46.9% IgM, aPT-PT: 71.4% IgG
Koudriavtseva et al. (2014)	100 MS (Serum)	aCL: 4% IgM, 5% IgG, aβ2GPI: 9% IgM, aPT: 7% IgM, 8% IgG, aAnV: 3% IgM, 11% IgG
Szmyrka-Kaczmarek et al. (2012)	85 MS (Serum)	aβ2GPI: 20% IgM, aCL: 4.7% IgM, 1% IgG
Stosic et al. (2010)	49 MS (Serum)	aCL: 18.4%, aβ2GPI: 10.2%, aPS: 18.4%, aPE: 32.6%
Garg et al. (2007)	111 MS, 27 CIS (Serum)	MS: aCL: 6%, aβ2GPI: 2%, CIS: aβ2GPI: 4%
Bidot et al. (2007)	24 RRMS (Serum); 7 REM, 17 REL	REM: aβ2GPI: 28% IgM, aCL: 28% IgM, aPS: 14% IgM, aPE: 28% IgM, aPC: 14% IgM REL: aβ2GPI: 82% IgM, aCL: 82% IgM, aFVIIa: 59% IgM, aPS: 71% IgM, aPE: 82% IgM, aPC: 76% IgM
Roussel et al. (2000)	89 MS (Serum)	aCL: 4.5% IgM, 16.9% IgG aβ2GPI: 13.5% IgM, 2.2% IgG
Karussis et al. (1998)	170 MS (Serum); 100 atypical, 70 classical	aCL: 27% atypical MS aCL: 5.7% classical MS
Sugiyama and Yamamoto (1996)	32 MS (Serum)	aCL: 44% IgM, 9% IgG
Marchiori et al. (1990)	33 MS (Serum, CSF)	aCL: 46.2% IgG (CSF)

MS, multiple sclerosis; RR, relapsing remitting; PP, primary progressive; SP, secondary progressive; REM, remission; REL, relaps; CIS, clinically isolated syndrome; CSF, cerebrospinal fluid; Acl, anti-cardiolipin; aβ2GPI, anti-β2glycoprotein I; aAnV, anti-annexin V; aPS-β2, anti-phosphatidylserine-β2GPI complex; aPT, anti-prothrombin; aPT-PT, anti-prothrombin complex; aPE, anti-phosphatidylethanolamine; aPS, anti-phosphatidylserine; aPC, anti-phosphatidylcholine; aFVIIa, anti-factor VII activated.

and clinical significance of aPL antibodies in MS remain still unclear and highly debated.

In 2007, two studies found higher aPL antibodies titer in later MS phases, aCL and PE were more common in SPMS when compared to RRMS (Bidot et al., 2007; Garg et al., 2007). By studying MS during the exacerbation phase, Bidot et al. (2007) found a higher titer of IgM aβ2GPI and aCL in 82% of patients with respect to those in remission phase (28%).

Koudriavtseva et al. (2014) found significantly higher frequency of aPL antibodies in MS subjects (32%) compared to healthy controls (7%), with a higher titer in RRMS patients (53.8%). Increased prevalence of IgM β2GPI in MS patients (20%) vs. controls (3.3%), was detected also by Szmyrka-Kaczmarek et al. (2012) of whom 33% were in SPMS patients and 21% in RRMS patients.

More recent studies have focused as well on aPL autoantibodies incidence in MS patients in different clinical phases of the disease, showing at least one IgM aPL or IgG isotype elevated in MS subjects, in RRMS or SPMS phases (Mandoj et al., 2015; Shor et al., 2015; Filippidou et al., 2016).

Positive aPL in the setting of local inflammatory status may induce any of the diverse pathogenetic mechanisms previously mentioned. aPL antibodies may account for antibody-mediated complement deposition in a portion of MS demyelinating lesions and might underline a proportion of approximately 30% of MS patients in which hypoxia-like pathological findings are found (Lucchinetti et al., 2000). Presence of aPL antibodies in SPMS or at later stages of MS might be indicative of a more chronic and worst course of CNS injury. Therefore, positive aPL antibodies in MS might associate to MRI lesions, as their detection could reveal more severe lesions in MS patients with aPL antibodies positivity with respect to those with lower or absent aPL titers (Stosic et al., 2010). However, these correlations still remain to be further investigated.

OVERLAP BETWEEN ANTIPHOSPHOLIPID SYNDROME AND MULTIPLE SCLEROSIS: CLINICAL AND PROGNOSTIC IMPLICATIONS

Nowadays, there are no definite diagnostic tools for distinguishing atypical MS and neurological APS cases, and the occurrence of positive aPL autoantibodies in patients with MS, in the absence of systemic manifestations of autoimmune disease or APS, is of particular concern. Therefore, it seems probable that a small percentage of patients diagnosed with MS, do in fact have a primary neurological APS, a condition with an entirely different pharmacological treatment and that would condition prognosis too. APS misdiagnosis as MS makes a crucial point for the therapeutic approach, given the increased prothrombotic risk (Fernández-Fernández et al., 2006; Donnan and McDonald, 2009; Ahbeddou et al., 2012). Finally, the coexistence of both autoimmune diseases, like APS secondary to MS, could also be possible.

An acute clinical isolated neurological syndrome (CIS) poses the biggest diagnostic challenge, since it is the most common onset of MS, but can also be the only feature or the first manifestation in APS before the occurrence of other features, such as thrombosis or miscarriages (Ferreira et al., 2005). An article published in The Times newspaper reported the results of a survey of the London Lupus Centre suggesting that at least 5% of MS patients were misdiagnosed and suffer from APS instead of MS (Rose, 2006).

APS patients have a generally good clinical outcome under anticoagulant treatment; manifestations such as headache and memory loss often improve drastically, with no further neurological events, when they are properly anticoagulated (Cuadrado et al., 2000).

For the above reasons, APS is recognized as a severe but potentially treatable condition, considering also the neurological complications. However, no standard treatment is available yet for the aPL-associated neurologic manifestations not included in the APS classification criteria, and the effects of immunosuppressive and anti-inflammatory agents, usually used in MS, is unknown in these patients (Espinosa and Cervera, 2015). A careful and correct diagnosis could be vital to avoid or at least reduce APS-related morbidity and mortality.

Despite MS is an incurable neuroinflammatory and neurodegenerative disease, a prompt and adequate treatment, focused on control of MS relapses, partially ameliorates accumulation of physical and neurological disability in the long-term. In fact, relapses timing is unpredictable but during every attack, destruction of myelin occurs and destroyed axonal fibers accumulate in CNS with worsening of patient's clinical condition. The early initiation of DMTs leads to improved stability control of MS disease, when compared to delayed therapy onset (Kavaliunas et al., 2017; Merkel et al., 2017). The presence of aPL antibodies in MS may herald a misdiagnosis of APS or the coexistence with APS, implying the establishment of anticoagulant therapy and the improvement of the prognosis for the individual patient.

CONCLUSION

APS and MS may be both considered as anti-lipid autoimmune diseases with specific pathophysiological mechanisms and events, given the direct role of antiphospholipid in the coagulation cascade, which can cross in the individual patient. Since the time they have been defined, clinical findings cannot clearly distinguish between atypical MS and neurological APS; basic and clinical research is still needed to reduce the misdiagnosis in these difficult cases. In these patients, to date, an accurate diagnosis may only emerge after long-term follow-up. Primary or secondary APS has to be considered an essential differential diagnosis from MS because prompt and correct treatment can improve quality of life and may also reduce morbidity and mortality in the affected patients. Understanding the possible associations between aPL antibodies and non-stroke neurological disabilities warrants further research. The knowledge of new pathogenic mechanisms of aPL might identify novel therapeutic targets and therefore improve the clinical management of atypical APS and aPL-positive MS patients.

AUTHOR CONTRIBUTIONS

CDA and SS-R designed the work and wrote the first draft of the article. LF-P and MR substantially contributed to writing. All authors have revised and approved the manuscript.

ACKNOWLEDGMENTS

We would like to thank the reviewers for their thoughtful comments and efforts towards improving our manuscript.

REFERENCES

Abdel-Wahab, N., Lopez-Olivo, M. A., Pinto-Patarroyo, G. P., and Suarez-Almazor, M. E. (2016). Systematic review of case reports of antiphospholipid syndrome following infection. *Lupus* 25, 1520–1531. doi: 10.1177/0961203316640912

Abreu, M. M., Danowski, A., Wahl, D. G., Amigo, M. C., Tektonidou, M., Pacheco, M. S., et al. (2015). The relevance of "non-criteria" clinical manifestations of antiphospholipid syndrome: 14th international congress on antiphospholipid antibodies technical task force report on antiphospholipid syndrome clinical features. *Autoimmun. Rev.* 14, 401–414. doi: 10.1016/j.autrev.2015.01.002

Achiron, A., Mandel, M., and Shoenfeld, Y. (2004). Multiple sclerosis and anti-phospholipid syndrome—one or two diseases? *Harefuah* 143, 724–766, 766, 765.

Aggarwal, R., Ringold, S., Khanna, D., Neogi, T., Johnson, S. R., Miller, A., et al. (2015). Distinctions between diagnostic and classification criteria? *Arthritis Care Res.* 67, 891–897. doi: 10.1002/acr.22583

Ahbeddou, N., Ait Ben Haddou, E., Hammib, S., Slimani, C., Regragui, W., Benomar, A., et al. (2012). Multiple sclerosis associated with antiphospholipid syndrome: diagnostic and therapeutic difficulties. *Rev. Neurol.* 168, 65–69. doi: 10.1016/j.neurol.2011.01.021

Alijotas-Reig, J., Esteve-Valverde, E., Ferrer-Oliveras, R., LLurba, E., Ruffatti, A., Tincani, A., et al. (2018). Comparative study between obstetric antiphospholipid syndrome and obstetric morbidity related with antiphospholipid antibodies. *Med. Clin.* 151, 215–222. doi: 10.1016/j.medcli.2017.11.017

Allen, K. L., Fonseca, F. V., Betapudi, V., Willard, B., Zhang, J., and McCrae, K. R. (2012). A novel pathway for human endothelial cell activation by antiphospholipid/anti-β2 glycoprotein I antibodies. *Blood* 119, 884–893. doi: 10.1182/blood-2011-03-344671

Arachchillage, D. R., Machin, S. J., Mackie, I. J., and Cohen, H. (2015). Diagnosis and management of non-criteria obstetric antiphospholipid syndrome. *Thromb. Haemost.* 113, 13–19. doi: 10.1160/th14-05-0416

Asherson, R. A., Giampaulo, D., Singh, S., and Sulman, L. (2007). Dramatic response of severe headaches to anticoagulation in a patient with antiphospholipid syndrome. *J. Clin. Rheumatol.* 13, 173–174. doi: 10.1097/rhu.0b013e3180690af6

Bamm, V. V., Henein, M. E. L., Sproul, S. L. J., Lanthier, D. K., and Harauz, G. (2017). Potential role of ferric hemoglobin in MS pathogenesis: effects of oxidative stress and extracellular methemoglobin or its degradation products on myelin components. *Free Radic. Biol. Med.* 112, 494–503. doi: 10.1016/j.freeradbiomed.2017.08.022

Bidot, C. J., Horstman, L. L., Jy, W., Jimenez, J. J., Bidot, C. Jr., Ahn, Y. S., et al. (2007). Clinical and neuroimaging correlates of antiphospholipid antibodies in multiple sclerosis: a preliminary study. *BMC Neurol.* 7:36. doi: 10.1186/1471-2377-7-36

Blank, M., Krause, I., Fridkin, M., Keller, N., Kopolovic, J., Goldberg, I., et al. (2002). Bacterial induction of autoantibodies to β2-glycoprotein-I accounts for the infectious etiology of antiphospholipid syndrome. *J. Clin. Invest.* 109, 797–804. doi: 10.1172/jci200212337

Blewett, M. M. (2008). Hypothesized role of galactocerebroside and NKT cells in the etiology of multiple sclerosis. *Med Hypotheses* 70, 826–830. doi: 10.1016/j.mehy.2007.07.037

Borghi, M. O., Raschi, E., Scurati, S., Grossi, C., Chen, P. P., Pierangeli, S. S., et al. (2007). Effects of Toll-like receptor antagonist and anti-annexin A2 antibodies on binding and activation of decidual cells by anti-b2-glycoprotein I antibodies. Proceedings of the 12th international congress on antiphospholipid antibodies; 2007 Apr 18–21; Florence, Italy. *Clin. Exp. Rheumatol.* 25:157.

Brigl, M., Bry, L., Kent, S. C., Gumperz, J. E., and Brenner, M. B. (2003). Mechanism of CD1d- restricted natural killer T cell activation during microbial infection. *Nat. Immunol.* 4, 1230–1237. doi: 10.1038/ni1002

Caronti, B., Calderaro, C., Alessandri, C., Conti, F., Tinghino, R., Pini, C., et al. (1998a). Serum anti- β2-glycoprotein I antibodies from patients with antiphospholipid antibody syndrome bind central nervous system cells. *J. Autoimmun.* 11, 425–429. doi: 10.1006/jaut.1998.0214

Caronti, B., Pittoni, V., Palladini, G., and Valesini, G. (1998b). Anti-β2-glycoprotein I antibodies bind to central nervous system. *J. Neurol. Sci.* 156, 211–219. doi: 10.1016/s0022-510x(98)00027-6

Cervera, R., Rodríguez-Pintó, I., Colafrancesco, S., Conti, F., Valesini, G., Rosário, C., et al. (2014). 14th international congress on antiphospholipid antibodies task force report on catastrophic antiphospholipid syndrome. *Autoimmun. Rev.* 13, 699–707. doi: 10.1016/j.autrev.2014.03.002

Chapin, J., Terry, H. S., Kleinert, D., and Laurence, J. (2016). The role of complement activation in thrombosis and hemolytic anemias. *Transfus. Apher. Sci.* 54, 191–198. doi: 10.1016/j.transci.2016.04.008

Chapman, J. (2004). The interface of multiple sclerosis and antiphospholipid antibodies. *Thromb. Res.* 114, 477–481. doi: 10.1016/j.thromres.2004.06.016

Chapman, J., Cohen-Armon, M., Shoenfeld, Y., and Korczyn, A. D. (1999). Antiphospholipid antibodies permeabilize and depolarize brain synaptoneurosomes. *Lupus* 8, 127–133. doi: 10.1191/096120399678847524

Cikes, N., Bosnic, D., and Sentic, M. (2008). Non-MS autoimmune demyelination. *Clin. Neurol. Neurosurg.* 110, 905–912. doi: 10.1016/j.clineuro.2008.06.011

Cobo-Soriano, R., Sánchez-Ramón, S., Aparicio, M. J., Teijeiro, M. A., Vidal, P., Suárez-Leoz, M., et al. (1999). Antiphospholipid antibodies and retinal thrombosis in patients without risk factors: a prospective case-control study. *Am. J. Ophthalmol.* 128, 725–732. doi: 10.1016/s0002-9394(99)00311-6

Compston, A., and Coles, A. (2008). Multiple sclerosis. *Lancet* 372, 1502–1517. doi: 10.1016/S0140-6736(08)61620-7

Cox, D., Fox, L., Tian, R., Bardet, W., Skaley, M., Mojsilovic, D., et al. (2009). Determination of cellular lipids bound to human CD1d molecules. *PLoS One* 4:e5325. doi: 10.1371/journal.pone.0005325

Cruz-Tapias, P., Blank, M., Anaya, J. M., and Shoenfeld, Y. (2012). Infections and vaccines in the etiology of antiphospholipid syndrome. *Curr. Opin. Rheumatol.* 24, 389–393. doi: 10.1097/bor.0b013e32835448b8

Cuadrado, M. J., Khamashta, M. A., Ballesteros, A., Godfrey, T., Simon, M. J., and Hughes, G. R. (2000). Can Hughes (antiphospholipid) syndrome be distinguished from multiple sclerosis? Analysis of 27 patients and review of the literature. *Medicine* 79, 57–68. doi: 10.1097/00005792-200001000-00006

Darmoise, A., Teneberg, S., Bouzonville, L., Brady, R. O., Beck, M., Kaufmann, S. H. E., et al. (2010). Lysosomal α-galactosidase controls the generation of self lipid antigens for natural killer T cells. *Immunity* 33, 216–228. doi: 10.1016/j.immuni.2010.08.003

De Libero, G., Macdonald, H. R., and Dellabona, P. (2007). T cell recognition of lipids: quo vadis? *Nat. Immunol.* 8, 223–227. doi: 10.1038/ni0307-223

de-Groot, P. G., Horbach, D. A., and Derksen, R. H. (1996). Protein C and other cofactors involved in the binding of antiphospholipid antibodies: relation to the pathogenesis of thrombosis. *Lupus* 5, 488–493. doi: 10.1177/096120339600500532

Devreese, K., Peerlinck, K., and Hoylaerts, M. F. (2010). Thrombotic risk assessment in the antiphospholipid syndrome requires more than the quantification of lupus anticoagulants. *Blood* 115, 870–878. doi: 10.1182/blood-2009-09-244426

Di Simone, N., Meroni, P. L., D'Asta, M., Di Nicuolo, F., D'Alessio, M. C., and Caruso, A. (2007). Pathogenic role of anti-β2-glycoprotein I antibodies on human placenta: functional effects related to implantation and roles of heparin. *Hum. Reprod. Update* 13, 189–196. doi: 10.1093/humupd/dml051

Diószegi, Á., Tarr, T., Nagy-Vincze, M., Nánásy-Vass, M., Veisz, R., Bidiga, L., et al. (2018). Microthrombotic renal involvement in an SLE patient with concomitant catastrophic antiphospholipid syndrome: the beneficial effect of rituximab treatment. *Lupus* 27, 1552–1558. doi: 10.1177/0961203318768890

Donnan, P. T., and McDonald, M. J. (2009). Patients' experiences of a diagnosis of Hughes' syndrome. *Clin. Rheumatol.* 28, 1091–1100. doi: 10.1007/s10067-009-1196-x

Donohoe, S., Quenby, S., Mackie, I., Panal, G., Farquharson, R., Malia, R., et al. (2002). Fluctuations in levels of antiphospholipid antibodies and increased coagulation activation markers in normal and heparin-treated antiphospholipid syndrome pregnancies. *Lupus* 11, 11–20. doi: 10.1191/0961203302lu132oa

Emmi, G., Urban, M. L., Scalera, A., Becatti, M., Fiorillo, C., Silvestri, E., et al. (2017). Repeated low-dose courses of rituximab in SLE-associated antiphospholipid syndrome: data from a tertiary dedicated centre. *Semin. Arthritis Rheum.* 46, e21–e23. doi: 10.1016/j.semarthrit.2016.08.002

Empson, M., Lassere, M., Craig, J., and Scott, J. (2005). Prevention of recurrent miscarriage for women with antiphospholipid antibody or lupus anticoagulant. *Cochrane Database Syst. Rev.* 2:CD002859. doi: 10.1002/14651858.cd002859.pub2

Erkan, D., Vega, J., Ramón, G., Kozora, E., and Lockshin, M. D. (2013). A pilot open-label phase II trial of rituximab for non-criteria manifestations of antiphospholipid syndrome. *Arthritis Rheum.* 65, 464–471. doi: 10.1002/art.37759

Espinosa, G., and Cervera, R. (2008). Antiphospholipid syndrome. *Arthritis Res. Ther.* 10:230. doi: 10.1186/ar2536

Espinosa, G., and Cervera, R. (2015). Current treatment of antiphospholipid syndrome: lights and shadows. *Nat. Rev. Rheumatol.* 11, 586–596. doi: 10.1038/nrrheum.2015.88

Fanopoulos, D., Teodorescu, M. R., Varga, J., and Teodorescu, M. (1998). High frequency of abnormal levels of IgA anti-β2-glycoprotein I antibodies in patients with systemic lupus erythematosus: relationship with antiphospholipid syndrome. *J. Rheumatol.* 25, 675–680.

Fernández-Fernández, F. J., Rivera-Gallego, A., de la Fuente-Aguado, J., Pérez-Fernández, S., and Muñoz-Fernández, D. (2006). Antiphospholipid syndrome mimicking multiple sclerosis in two patients. *Eur. J. Intern. Med.* 17, 500–502. doi: 10.1016/j.ejim.2006.02.018

Ferreira, S., D'Cruz, D. P., and Hughes, G. R. (2005). Multiple sclerosis, neuropsychiatric lupus and antiphospholipid syndrome: where do we stand? *Rheumatology* 44, 434–442. doi: 10.1093/rheumatology/keh532

Filippidou, N., Krashias, G., Pericleous, C., Rahman, A., Ioannou, Y., Giles, I., et al. (2016). The association between IgG and IgM antibodies against cardiolipin, 2-glycoprotein I and Domain I of 2-glycoprotein I with disease profile in patients with multiple sclerosis. *Mol. Immunol.* 75, 161–167. doi: 10.1016/j.molimm.2016.05.022

Fonseca, A. G., and D'Cruz, D. P. (2008). Controversies in the antiphospholipid syndrome: can we ever stop warfarin? *J. Autoimmune Dis.* 5:6. doi: 10.1186/1740-2557-5-6

Fraussen, J., Claes, N., de Bock, L., and Somers, V. (2014). Targets of the humoral autoimmune response in multiple sclerosis. *Autoimmun. Rev.* 13, 1126–1137. doi: 10.1016/j.autrev.2014.07.002

Gómez-Puerta, J. A., and Cervera, R. (2014). Diagnosis and classification of the antiphospholipid syndrome. *J. Autoimmun.* 48–49, 20–25. doi: 10.1016/j.jaut.2014.01.006

Gamoudi, D., Cutajar, M., Gamoudi, N., Camilleri, D. J., and Gatt, A. (2017). Achieving a satisfactory clinical and biochemical response in antiphospholipid syndrome and severe thrombocytopenia with rituximab: two case reports. *Clin. Case Rep.* 5, 845–848. doi: 10.1002/ccr3.946

Garcia, D., and Erkan, D. (2018). Diagnosis and management of the antiphospholipid syndrome. *N. Engl. J. Med.* 378, 2010–2021. doi: 10.1056/NEJMra1705454

Garg, N., Zivadinov, R., Ramanathan, M., Vasiliu, I., Locke, J., Watts, K., et al. (2007). Clinical and MRI correlates of autoreactive antibodies in multiple sclerosis patients. *J. Neuroimmunol.* 187, 159–165. doi: 10.1016/j.jneuroim.2007.04.008

Gharavi, A. E., Pierangeli, S. S., Espinola, R. G., Liu, X., Colden-Stanfield, M., and Harris, E. N. (2002). Antiphospholipid antibodies induced in mice by immunization with a cytomegalovirus-derived peptide cause thrombosis and activation of endothelial cells *in vivo*. *Arthritis Rheum.* 46, 545–552. doi: 10.1002/art.10130

Gharavi, A. E., Pierangeli, S. S., and Harris, E. N. (2003). Viral origin of antiphospholipid antibodies: endothelial cell activa-tion and thrombus enhancement by CMV peptide-induced APL antibodies. *Immunobiology* 207, 37–42. doi: 10.1078/0171-2985-00216

Ghasemi, N., Razavi, S. H., and Nikzad, E. (2017). Multiple sclerosis: pathogenesis, symptoms, diagnoses, and cell-based therapy. *Cell J.* 19, 1–10. doi: 10.22074/cellj.2016.4867

Giannakopoulos, B., and Krilis, S. A. (2013). The pathogenesis of the antiphospholipid syndrome. *N. Engl. J. Med.* 368, 1033–1044. doi: 10.1056/NEJMra1112830

Godfrey, D. I., and Kronenberg, M. (2004). Going both ways: immune regulation via CD1d-dependent NKT cells. *J. Clin. Invest.* 114, 1379–1388. doi: 10.1172/jci23594

Hogan, E. L., Podbielska, M., and O'Keeffe, J. (2013). Implications of lymphocyte anergy to glycolipids in multiple sclerosis (MS): iNKT cells may mediate the MS infectious trigger. *J. Clin. Cell. Immunol.* 4:144. doi: 10.4172/2155-9899.1000144

Horstman, L. L., Yj, W., Bidot, C. J., Ahn, Y. S., Kelley, R. E., Zivadinov, R., et al. (2009). Antiphospholipid antibodies: paradigm in transition. *J. Neuroinflammation* 6:3. doi: 10.1186/1742-2094-6-3

Hughes, G. R. V. (1983). Thrombosis, abortion, cerebral disease, and the lupus anticoagulant. *Br. Med. J.* 287, 1088–1089. doi: 10.1136/bmj.287.6399.1088

Hughes, G. R. V. (2003). Migraine, memory loss, and "multiple sclerosis". Neurological features of the antiphospholipid (Hughes') syndrome. *Postgrad. Med. J.* 79, 81–83. doi: 10.1136/pmj.79.928.81

Islam, M. A., Alam, F., Kamal, M. A., Wong, K. K., Sasongko, T. H., and Gan, S. H. (2016). 'Non-criteria' neurologic manifestations of antiphospholipid syndrome: a hidden kingdom to be discovered. *CNS Neurol. Disord. Drug Targets* 15, 1253–1265. doi: 10.2174/1871527315666160920122750

Jakiela, B., Iwaniec, T., Plutecka, H., Celinska-Lowenhoff, M., Dziedzina, S., and Musial, J. (2016). Signs of impaired immunoregulation and enhanced effector T-cell responses in the primary antiphospholipid syndrome. *Lupus* 25, 389–398. doi: 10.1177/0961203315618267

Joseph, F. G., and Habboush, H. W. (2018). The antiphospholipid syndrome and its 'non-criteria' manifestations. *Pract. Neurol.* 18, 82–83. doi: 10.1136/practneurol-2017-001846

Justo, D., Finn, T., Atzmony, L., Guy, N., and Steinvil, A. (2011). Thrombosis associated with acute cytomegalo-virus infection: a meta-analysis. *Eur. J. Intern. Med.* 22, 195–199. doi: 10.1016/j.ejim.2010.11.006

Kanter, J. L., Narayana, S., Ho, P. P., Catz, I., Warren, K. G., Sobel, R. A., et al. (2006). Lipid microarrays identify key mediators of autoimmune brain inflammation. *Nat. Med.* 12, 138–143. doi: 10.1038/nm1344

Karussis, D., Leker, R. R., Ashkenazi, A., and Abramsky, O. (1998). A subgroup of multiple sclerosis patients with anticardiolipin antibodies and unusual clinical manifestations: do they represent a new nosological entity? *Ann. Neurol.* 44, 629–634. doi: 10.1002/ana.410440408

Kavaliunas, A., Manouchehrinia, A., Stawiarz, L., Ramanujam, R., Agholme, J., Hedstrom, A. K., et al. (2017). Importance of early treatment initiation in the clinical course of multiple sclerosis. *Mult. Scler.* 23, 1233–1240. doi: 10.1177/1352458516675039

Khamashta, M., Taraborelli, M., Sciascia, S., and Tincani, A. (2016). Antiphospholipid syndrome. *Best Pract. Res. Clin. Rheumatol.* 30, 133–148. doi: 10.1016/j.berh.2016.04.002

Kornberg, A., Renaudineau, Y., Blank, M., Youinou, P., and Shoenfeld, Y. (2000). Anti-β 2-glycoprotein I antibodies and anti-endothelial cell antibodies induce tissue factor in endothelial cells. *Isr. Med. Assoc. J.* 2, 27–31.

Koudriavtseva, T., D'Agosto, G., Mandoj, C., Sperduti, I., and Cordiali-Fei, P. (2014). High frequency of antiphospholipid antibodies in relapse of multiple sclerosis: a possible indicator of inflammatory-thrombotic processes. *Neurol. Sci.* 35, 1737–1741. doi: 10.1007/s10072-014-1823-4

Kuwana, M. (2003). Autoreactive $CD4^{+}$ T cells to β_2-glycoprotein I in patients with antiphospholipid syndrome. *Autoimmun. Rev.* 2, 192–198. doi: 10.1016/s1568-9972(03)00007-7

Lambrianides, A., Carroll, C. J., Pierangeli, S. S., Pericleous, C., Branch, W., Rice, J., et al. (2010). Effects of polyclonal IgG derived from patients with different clinical types of the antiphospholipid syndrome on monocyte signaling pathways. *J. Immunol.* 184, 6622–6628. doi: 10.4049/jimmunol.0902765

Lavazza, T., Dipinto, A., Borghi, M. O., Usuelli, V., Bergamaschi, A., Zimarino, V., et al. (2007). Antiphospholipid antibodies and central nervous system involvement: direct autoantibody binding to neuronal cells. Proceedings of the 12th international congress on antiphospholipid antibodies; 2007 Apr 18–21; Florence, Italy. *Clin. Exp. Rheumatol.* 25:147.

Lieby, P., Poindron, V., Roussi, S., Klein, C., Knapp, A. M., Garaud, J. C., et al. (2004). Patho-genic antiphospholipid antibody: an antigen-selected needle in a haystack. *Blood* 104, 1711–1715. doi: 10.1182/blood-2004-02-0462

Limper, M., Scirè, C. A., Talarico, R., Amoura, Z., Avcin, T., Basile, M., et al. (2018). Antiphospholipid syndrome: state of the art on clinical practice guidelines. *RMD Open* 4:e000785. doi: 10.1136/rmdopen-2018-000785

Lucchinetti, C., Brück, W., Parisi, J., Scheithauer, B., Rodriguez, M., and Lassmann, H. (2000). Heterogeneity of multiple sclerosis lesions: implications for the pathogenesis of demyelination. *Ann. Neurol.* 47, 707–717. doi: 10.1002/1531-8249(200006)47:6<707::aid-ana3>3.0.co;2-q

Machado-Santos, J., Saji, E., Tröscher, A. R., Paunovic, M., Liblau, R., Gabriely, G., et al. (2018). The compartmentalized inflammatory response in the multiple sclerosis brain is composed of tissue-resident CD8+ T lymphocytes and B cells. *Brain* 41, 2066–2082. doi: 10.1093/brain/awy151

Mackman, N. (2009). The many faces of tissue factor. *J. Thromb. Haemost.* 7, 136–139. doi: 10.1111/j.1538-7836.2009.03368.x

Mandoj, C., Renna, R., Plantone, D., Sperduti, I., Cigliana, G., Conti, L., et al. (2015). Anti-annexin antibodies, cholesterol levels and disability in multiple sclerosis. *Neurosci. Lett.* 606, 156–160. doi: 10.1016/j.neulet.2015.08.054

Marchiori, P. E., Dos Reis, M., Quevedo, M. E., Callegaro, D., Hirata, M. T., Scaff, M., et al. (1990). Cerebrospinal fluid and serum antiphospholipid antibodies in multiple sclerosis, Guillain-Barre syndrome and systemic lupus erythematosus. *Arq. Neuropsiquiatr.* 48, 465–468. doi: 10.1590/s0004-282x1990000400010

Martin, E., Winn, R., and Nugent, K. (2011). Catastrophic antiphospholipid syndrome in a community-acquired methicillin-resistant Staphylococcus aureus infection: a review of pathogenesis with a case for molecular mimicry. *Autoimmun. Rev.* 10, 181–188. doi: 10.1016/j.autrev.2010.09.023

Martínez-Cordero, E., Rivera García, B. E., and Aguilar León, D. E. (1997). Anticardiolipin antibodies in serum and cerebrospinal fluid from patients with systemic lupus erythematosus. *J. Investig. Allergol. Clin. Immunol.* 7, 596–601.

Matthey, F., Walshe, K., Mackie, I. J., and Machin, S. J. (1989). Familial occurrence of the antiphospholipid syndrome. *J. Clin. Pathol.* 42, 495–497. doi: 10.1136/jcp.42.5.495

Mekinian, A., Loire-Berson, P., Nicaise-Roland, P., Lachassinne, E., Stirnemann, J., Boffa, M. C., et al. (2012). Outcomes and treatment of obstetrical antiphospholipid syndrome in women with low antiphospholipid antibody levels. *J. Reprod. Immunol.* 94, 222–226. doi: 10.1016/j.jri.2012.02.004

Merashli, M., Noureldine, M. H., Uthman, I., and Khamashta, M. (2015). Antiphospholipid syndrome: an update. *Eur. J. Clin. Invest.* 45, 653–662. doi: 10.1111/eci.12449

Merkel, B., Butzkueven, H., Traboulsee, A. L., Havrdova, E., and Kalincik, T. (2017). Timing of high-efficacy therapy in relapsingremitting multiple sclerosis: a systematic review. *Autoimmun. Rev.* 16, 658–665. doi: 10.1016/j.autrev.2017.04.010

Meroni, P. L., Borghi, M. O., Grossi, C., Chighizola, C. B., Durigutto, P., and Tedesco, F. (2018). Obstetric and vascular antiphospholipid syndrome: same antibodies but different diseases? *Nat. Rev. Rheumatol.* 14, 433–440. doi: 10.1038/s41584-018-0032-6

Meroni, P. L., Borghi, M. O., Raschi, E., and Tedesco, F. (2011). Pathogenesis of antiphos- pholipid syndrome: understanding the antibodies. *Nat. Rev. Rheumatol.* 7, 330–339. doi: 10.1038/nrrheum.2011.52

Merrill, J. T. (2006). Do antiphospholipid antibodies develop for a purpose? *Curr. Rheumatol. Rep.* 8, 109–113. doi: 10.1007/s11926-006-0050-2

Micheloud, D., Sánchez-Ramón, S., Carbone, J., Rodríguez Molina, J. J., Fernández-Cruz, E., López-Longo, F. J., et al. (2005). Discordance between anti-β2-glycoprotein-I and anti-cardiolipin antibodies in patients with clinical criteria of antiphospholipid syndrome. *Clin. Exp. Rheumatol.* 23, 525–528.

Miyakis, S., Lockshin, M. D., Atsumi, T., Branch, D. W., Brey, R. L., Cervera, R., et al. (2006). International consensus statement on an update of the classification criteria for definite antiphospholipid syndrome (APS). *J. Thromb. Haemost.* 4, 295–306. doi: 10.1111/j.1538-7836.2006.01753.x

Muscal, E., and Brey, R. L. (2007). Neurological manifestations of the antiphospholipid syndrome: risk assessments and evidence-based medicine. *Int. J. Clin. Pract.* 61, 1561–1568. doi: 10.1111/j.1742-1241.2007.01478.x

Nakayama, T., Akahoshi, M., Irino, K., Kimoto, Y., Arinobu, Y., Niiro, H., et al. (2014). Transient antiphospholipid syndrome associated with primary cytomegalovirus infection: a case report and literature review. *Case Rep. Rheumatol.* 2014:271548. doi: 10.1155/2014/271548

Nandoskar, A., Raffel, J., Scalfari, A. S., Friede, T., and Nicholas, R. S. (2017). Pharmacological approaches to the management of secondary progressive multiple sclerosis. *Drugs* 77, 885–910. doi: 10.1007/s40265-017-0726-0

Negrini, S., Pappalardo, F., Murdaca, G., Indiveri, F., and Puppo, F. (2017). The antiphospholipid syndrome: from pathophysiology to treatment. *Clin. Exp. Med.* 17, 257–267. doi: 10.1007/s10238-016-0430-5

Pengo, V., Ruffatti, A., Legnani, C., Testa, S., Fierro, T., De Marongiu, F., et al. (2011). Incidence of a first thromboembolic event in asymptomatic carriers of high-risk antiphospholipid antibody profile: a multicenter prospective study. *Blood* 118, 4714–4718. doi: 10.1182/blood-2011-03-340232

Pierangeli, S. S., Chen, P. P., and González, E. B. (2006). Antiphospholipid antibodies and the antiphospholipid syndrome: an update on treatment and pathogenic mechanisms. *Curr. Opin. Hematol.* 13, 366–375. doi: 10.1097/01.moh.0000239710.47921.d2

Pierangeli, S. S., Vega-Ostertag, M. E., Raschi, E., Liu, X., Romay-Penabad, Z., De Micheli, V., et al. (2007). Toll-like receptor and antiphospholipid mediated thrombosis: *in vivo* studies. *Ann. Rheum. Dis.* 66, 1327–1333. doi: 10.1136/ard.2006.065037

Podbielska, M., and Hogan, E. L. (2009). Molecular and immunogenic features of myelin lipids: incitants or modulators of multiple sclerosis? *Pharmacol. Res.* 15, 1011–1029. doi: 10.1177/1352458509106708

Podbielska, M., O'Keeffe, J., and Hogan, E. L. (2018). Autoimmunity in multiple sclerosis: role of sphingolipids, invariant NKT cells and other immune elements in control of inflammation and neurodegeneration. *J. Neurol. Sci.* 385, 198–214. doi: 10.1016/j.jns.2017.12.022

Popovic-Kuzmanovic, D., Novakovic, I., Stojanovich, L., Aksentijevich, I., Zogovic, N., Tovilovic, G., et al. (2013). Increased activity of interleukin-23/interleukin-17 cytokine axis in primary antiphospholipid syndrome. *Immunobiology* 218, 186–191. doi: 10.1016/j.imbio.2012.03.002

Prinz, N., Clemens, N., Strand, D., Pütz, I., Lorenz, M., Daiber, A., et al. (2011). Antiphospholipid antibodies induce translocation of TLR7 and TLR8 to the endosome in human monocytes and plasmacytoid dendritic cells. *Blood* 118, 2322–2332. doi: 10.1182/blood-2011-01-330639

Ramesh, S., Morrell, C. N., Tarango, C., Thomas, G. D., Yuhanna, I. S., Girardi, G., et al. (2011). Antiphospholipid antibodies promote leukocyte-endothelial cell adhesion and thrombosis in mice by antagonizing eNOS via β2GPI and apoER2. *J. Clin. Invest.* 121, 120–131. doi: 10.1172/JCI39828

Reale, M., and Sanchez-Ramon, S. (2017). Lipids at the cross-road of autoimmunity in multiple sclerosis. *Curr. Med. Chem.* 24, 176–192. doi: 10.2174/0929867324666161123093606

Renaud, M., Aupy, J., Uring-Lambert, B., Chanson, J. B., Collongues, N., Blanc, F., et al. (2014). Isolated anti-β2-glycoprotein I antibodies in neurology: a frontier syndrome between multiple sclerosis and antiphospholipid syndrome? *Eur. J. Neurol.* 21, 901–906. doi: 10.1111/ene.12408

Ritis, K., Doumas, M., Mastellos, D., Micheli, A., Giaglis, S., Magotti, P., et al. (2006). A novel C5a receptor-tissue factor crosstalk in neutrophils links innate immunity to coagulation pathways. *J. Immunol.* 177, 4794–4802. doi: 10.4049/jimmunol.177.7.4794

Rocca, M. A., Amato, M. P., De Stefano, N., Enzinger, C., Geurts, J. J., Penner, I. K., et al. (2015). Clinical and imaging assessment of cognitive dysfunction in multiple sclerosis. *Lancet Neurol.* 14, 302–317. doi: 10.1016/S1474-4422(14)70250-9

Rodrigues, C. E., Carvalho, J. F., and Shoenfeld, Y. (2010). Neurological manifestations of antiphospholipid syndrome. *Eur. J. Clin. Invest.* 40, 350–359. doi: 10.1111/j.1365-2362.2010.02263.x

Roie, E. V., Labarque, V., Renard, M., Van Geet, C., and Gabriels, L. (2013). Obsessive-compulsive behavior as presenting symptom of primary antiphospholipid syndrome. *Psychosomat. Med.* 75, 326–330. doi: 10.1097/psy.0b013e31828acfbc

Rombos, A., Evangelopoulou-Katsiri, E., Leventakou, A., Voumvourakis, K., Triantafyllou, N., and Papageorgiou, C. (1990). Serum IgG and IgM anticardiolipin antibodies in neurological diseases. *Acta Neurol. Scand.* 81, 43–45. doi: 10.1111/j.1600-0404.1990.tb00975.x

Rose, D. (2006). *Hundreds Wrongly Told they are MS Sufferers.* The Times of London, August 22 2006. www.thesundaytimes.co.uk

Roussel, V., Yi, F., Jauberteau, M. O., Couderq, C., Lacombe, C., Michelet, V., et al. (2000). Prevalence and clinical significance of anti-phospholipid antibodies in multiple sclerosis: a study of 89 patients. *J. Autoimmun.* 14, 259–265. doi: 10.1006/jaut.2000.0367

Salmon, J. E., Girardi, G., and Lockshin, M. D. (2007). The antiphospholipid syndrome as a disorder initiated by inflammation: implications for the therapy of pregnant patients. *Nat. Clin. Pract. Rheumatol.* 3, 140–147. doi: 10.1038/ncprheum0432

Satta, N., Kruithof, E. K., Fickentscher, C., Dunoyer-Geindre, S., Boehlen, F., Reber, G., et al. (2011). Toll-like receptor 2 mediates the activation of human monocytes and endothelial cells by antiphospholipid antibodies. *Blood* 117, 5523–5531. doi: 10.1182/blood-2010-11-316158

Shoenfeld, Y., Blank, M., Cervera, R., Font, J., Raschi, E., and Meroni, P. L. (2006). Infectious origin of the antiphospholipid syndrome. *Ann. Rheum. Dis.* 65, 2–6. doi: 10.1136/ard.2005.045443

Shoenfeld, Y., Nahum, A., Korczyn, A. D., Dano, M., Rabinowitz, R., Beilin, O., et al. (2003). Neuronal-binding antibodies from patients with antiphospholipid syndrome induce cognitive deficits following intrathecal passive transfer. *Lupus* 12, 436–442. doi: 10.1191/0961203303lu409oa

Shoenfeld, Y., Twig, G., Katz, U., and Sherer, Y. (2008). Autoantibody explosion in antiphospholipid syndrome. *J. Autoimmun.* 30, 74–83. doi: 10.1016/j.jaut.2007.11.011

Shor, D. B.-A., Weiss, G. A., Barzilai, O., Ram, M., Anaya, L.-M., Shoenfeld, Y., et al. (2015). Prevalence of classic and non-classic antiphospholipid antibodies in multiple sclerosis. *Isr. Med. Assoc. J.* 17, 559–562.

Sorice, M., Longo, A., Capozzi, A., Garofalo, T., Misasi, R., Alessandri, C., et al. (2007). Anti-β2-glycoprotein I antibodies induce monocyte release of tumor necrosis factor α and tissue factor by signal transduction pathways involving lipid rafts. *Arthritis Rheum.* 56, 2687–2697. doi: 10.1002/art.22802

Stevens, A., Weller, M., and Wiethölter, H. (1992). CSF and serum ganglioside antibody patterns in MS. *Acta Neurol. Scand.* 86, 485–489. doi: 10.1111/j.1600-0404.1992.tb05129.x

Stosic, M., Ambrus, J., Garg, N., Weinstock-Guttman, B., Ramanathan, M., Kalman, B., et al. (2010). MRI characteristics of patients with antiphospholipid syndrome and multiple sclerosis. *J. Neurol.* 257, 63–71. doi: 10.1007/s00415-009-5264-6

Sugiyama, Y., and Yamamoto, T. (1996). Characterization of serum anti-phospholipid antibodies in patients with multiple sclerosis. *Tohoku J. Exp. Med.* 178, 203–215. doi: 10.1620/tjem.178.203

Sun, K. H., Liu, W. T., Tsai, C. Y., Liao, T. S., Lin, W. M., and Yu, C. L. (1992). Inhibition of astrocyte proliferation and binding to brain tissue of anticardiolipin antibodies purified from lupus serum. *Ann. Rheum. Dis.* 51, 707–712. doi: 10.1136/ard.51.6.707

Szmyrka-Kaczmarek, M., Pokryszko-Dragan, A., Pawlik, B., Gruszka, E., Korman, L., Podemski, R., et al. (2012). Antinuclear and antiphospholipid antibodies in patients with multiple sclerosis. *Lupus* 21, 412–420. doi: 10.1177/0961203311427550

Tektonidou, M. G., Varsou, N., Kotoulas, G., Antoniou, A., and Moutsopoulos, H. M. (2006). Cognitive deficits in patients with antiphospholipid syndrome: association with clinical, laboratory, and brain magnetic resonance imaging findings. *Arch. Intern. Med.* 166, 2278–2284. doi: 10.1001/archinte.166.20.2278

Torkildsen, Ø., Myhr, K. M., and Bø, L. (2016). Disease-modifying treatments for multiple sclerosis—a review of approved medications. *Eur. J. Neurol.* 23, 18–27. doi: 10.1111/ene.12883

Urbanus, R. T., Pennings, M. T., Derksen, R. H., and de Groot, P. G. (2008). Platelet activation by dimeric β2-glycoprotein I requires signalling via both glycoprotein Ibα and apolipoprotein E receptor 2'. *J. Thromb. Haemost.* 6, 1405–1412. doi: 10.1111/j.1538-7836.2008.03021.x

Uthman, I., Noureldine, M. H. A., Berjawi, A., Skaf, M., Haydar, A. A., Merashli, M., et al. (2015). Hughes syndrome and Multiple sclerosis. *Lupus* 24, 115–121. doi: 10.1177/0961203314555539

Uthman, I., Tabbarah, Z., and Gharavi, A. E. (1999). Hughes syndrome associated with cytomegalovirus infection. *Lupus* 8, 775–777. doi: 10.1191/096120399678841034

Vilisaar, J., Wilson, M., Niepel, G., Blumhardt, L. D., and Constantinescu, C. S. (2005). A comparative audit of anticardiolipin antibodies in oligoclonal band negative and positive multiple sclerosis. *Mult. Scler.* 11, 378–380. doi: 10.1191/1352458505ms1208oa

Wermeling, F., Lind, S. M., Jordö, E. D., Cardell, S. L., and Karlsson, M. C. I. (2010). Invariant NKT cells limit activation of autoreactive CD1d-positive B cells. *J. Exp. Med.* 207, 943–952. doi: 10.1084/jem.20091314

Yamaguchi, Y., Seta, N., Kaburaki, J., Kobayashi, K., Matsuura, E., and Kuwana, M. (2007). Excessive exposure to anionic surfaces maintains autoantibody response to b2-glycoprotein I in patients with antiphospholipid syndrome. *Blood* 110, 4312–4318. doi: 10.1182/blood-2007-07-100008

Yang, J.-Q., Wen, X., Kim, P. J., and Singh, R. R. (2011). Invariant NKT cells inhibit autoreactive B cells in a contact- and CD1d-dependent manner. *J. Immunol.* 186, 1512–1520. doi: 10.4049/jimmunol.1002373

Yelnik, C. M., Kozora, E., and Appenzeller, S. (2016). Non-stroke central neurologic manifestations in antiphospholipid syndrome. *Curr. Rheumatol. Rep.* 18:11. doi: 10.1007/s11926-016-0568-x

Youinou, P., and Renaudineau, Y. (2004). The antiphospholipid syndrome as a model for B cell-induced autoimmune diseases. *Thromb. Res.* 114, 363–369. doi: 10.1016/j.thromres.2004.06.019

Zhang, L., and Pereira, A. C. (2018). Oromandibular chorea in antiphospholipid syndrome. *Pract. Neurol.* 18, 132–133. doi: 10.1136/practneurol-2017-001824

Zhu, D.-S., Fu, J., Zhang, Y., Li, S. X., Zhang, G. X., Guan, Y. T., et al. (2014). Neurological antiphospholipid syndrome: clinical, neuroimaging, and pathological characteristics. *J. Neurol. Sci.* 346, 138–144. doi: 10.1016/j.jns.2014.08.010

Smilagenin Protects Dopaminergic Neurons in Chronic MPTP/Probenecid—Lesioned Parkinson's Disease Models

Xuan He[1†], *Shuangshuang Yang*[1†], *Rui Zhang*[1], *Lina Hou*[1], *Jianrong Xu*[1], *Yaer Hu*[1], *Rang Xu*[2*], *Hao Wang*[1*] *and Yongfang Zhang*[1*]

[1]*Department of Pharmacology, Institute of Medical Sciences, Shanghai JiaoTong University School of Medicine (SJTUSM), Shanghai, China,* [2]*Scientific Research Center, Xinhua Hospital, Shanghai JiaoTong University School of Medicine (SJTUSM), Shanghai, China*

Correspondence:
Yongfang Zhang
zhangyongfang1@yahoo.com
Hao Wang
angela_wanghao@hotmail.com
Rang Xu
rang_xu@hotmail.com

†These authors have contributed equally to this work

Current therapies for Parkinson's disease (PD) only offer limited symptomatic alleviation but fail to hamper the progress of the disease. Thus, it is imperative to establish new approaches aiming at protecting or reversing neurodegeneration in PD. Recent work elucidates whether smilagenin (abbreviated SMI), a steroidal sapogenin from traditional Chinese medicinal herbs, can take neuroprotective effect on dopaminergic neurons in a chronic model of 1-methyl-4-phenyl-1,2,3,6-tetrahydropyridine (MPTP) conjuncted with probenecid mice. We reported for the first time that SMI significantly improved the locomotor ability of chronic MPTP/probenecid–lesioned mice. SMI increased the tyrosine hydroxylase (TH) positive and Nissl positive neuron number in the substantia nigra pars compacta (SNpc), augmented striatal DA and its metabolites concentration and elevated striatal dopamine transporter density (DAT). In addition, dopamine receptor D2R not D1R was down-regulated by MPTP/probenecid and slightly raised by SMI prevention. What's more, we discovered that SMI markedly elevated striatal glial cell line-derived neurotrophic factor (GDNF) and brain-derived neurotrophic factor (BDNF) protein levels in SMI prevented mice. And we found that SMI increased GDNF and BDNF mRNA level by promoting CREB phosphorylation in 1-methyl-4-phenylpyridimium (MPP^+) treated SH-SY5Y cells. The results illustrated that SMI could prevent the impairment of dopaminergic neurons in chronic MPTP/probenecid-induced mouse model.

Keywords: brain-derived neurotrophic factor, Chinese herb, dopaminergic neurons, glial cell line-derived neurotrophic factor, Parkinson's disease

INTRODUCTION

Parkinson's disease (PD) is an age-related debilitating neurodegenerative disorder, characterized pathologically by selective loss of dopaminergic neurons in the substantia nigra pars compacta (SNpc) accompanied by a decrease in striatal dopamine level, and intracytoplasmic Lewy bodies aggregated by phosphorylated α-synuclein (αSyn). Additionally, the clinical symptoms such as resting tremor, rigidity, slowness of initial movement do not fully present until there is a loss of

Abbreviations: SMI, smilagenin; MPTP, 1-methyl-4-phenyl-1,2,3 6-tetrahydropyridine; DAT, dopamine transporter density; GDNF, glial cell line-derive neurotrophic factor; BDNF, brain-derived neurotrophic factor; SNpc, substantia nigra pars compacta; α-syn, α-synuclein; PD, Parkinson's disease; TH, tyrosine hydroxylase.

50%–60% SNpc neurons (Przedborski, 2017; Schapira et al., 2017). However current pharmacological therapies for PD, which dopamine replacement is a mainstay of therapeutic strategies, only alleviate symptoms but fail to hamper neurodegeneration process and restore dopaminergic dysfunction. What's worse, the existing therapies for PD after long-term treatment could cause severe adverse effects, such as motor response fluctuations and dyskinetic movements (Tarazi et al., 2014; Pires et al., 2017; Wong and Krainc, 2017). Thus, it is greatly imperative to establish neuroprotective therapy available for PD.

Administration of neurotrophic factors such as brain-derived neurotrophic factor (BDNF) and glial cell line-derived neurotrophic factor (GDNF) are generally recognized as powerful survival factors for the degenerated dopaminergic neurons and the nigro-triatal pathway in PD (Cass et al., 2006; Kramer and Liss, 2015; Sun et al., 2015). Although the potential neuroprotective effects of these neurotrophic factors are undisputed, unfortunately in a randomized controlled trial of intraputamenal infusion of recombinant human GDNF in patients with PD, there is no remarkable improvement in patients receiving GDNF (Lang et al., 2006; Ibáñez and Andressoo, 2017). Owing to its large polypeptide structure and consequent poor bioavailability, it is difficult for these neurotrophic factors to permeate the blood brain barrier (Tarazi et al., 2014; Fan et al., 2016).

Consequently, it is greatly urgent to implement some strategies to stimulate the endogenous expression of neurotrophic factors after oral administration to slow down or reverse the progression of neuronal degeneration. Traditional Chinese medicine have accumulated much knowledge in treatment of PD so that it might be feasible to develop drugs from Chinese medicinal herbs for curing PD (Zhang et al., 2015). Smilagenin (Cogane; 5β, 2α, 25R-spirostan-3β-ol, abbreviated as SMI), with a molecular weight of 416.63 daltons, is a lipid-soluble small-molecule steroidal sapogenin from *Rhizoma anemarrhenae* and *Radix asparagi* widely used in traditional Chinese medicine for treating chronic neurodegeneration diseases (Visanji et al., 2008; Sy et al., 2016). Our previous studies have confirmed that SMI could not only protect the cultures of rat embryonic mesencephalic neurons from 1-methyl-4-phenyl-1,2,3,6-tetrahydropyridine (MPTP) toxicity *in vitro* but also enhance GDNF release as well as motor function of aged rat *in vivo* (Zhang et al., 2008; Li et al., 2013). However, whether SMI could protect dopaminergic neurons *in vivo* in chronic MPTP/probenecid-lesioned mice are unknown. To clarify the protecting effect of SMI on dopaminergic neuron we adopted the chronic MPTP/probenecid mouse model to investigate locomotor ability and the effects of SMI on nigrostriatal dopaminergic system as well as GDNF and BDNF expression (Petroske et al., 2001; Schildknecht et al., 2017; Nonnekes et al., 2018).

MATERIALS AND METHODS

Materials

SMI with a purity of over 98 percent was supplied by Phytopharm plc. UK. One-methyl-4-phenyl-1,2,3,6-tetrahydropyridine hydrochloride (MPTP HCl), 1-methyl-4-phenylpyridimium (MPP^+) was from Sigma, Dulbecco's Modified Eagle Medium was from Gibco (Grand Island, NY, USA), probenecid, hydroxypropyl methyl cellulose (HPMC-Na), Ketanserin, SCH23390, fluoxetine and GBR-12909 and all reagents used in HPLC except acetonitrile were purchased from Sigma. Rabbit anti-mice tyrosine hydroxylase (TH) polyclonal antibody and 3,3′-diaminobenzidine (DAB) were from Chemicon. SABC kit was from Boster Bioengineering Co. Wuhan, China. [^{125}I]-FP-CIT was synthesized using Na[^{125}I] (from Chengdu Gaotong Isotope Co) and FP-CIT (from Jiangsu Institute of Nuclear Medicine) in our laboratory. [^{3}H] SCH23390 (specific activity 80.5 Ci/mmol) and [^{3}H] spiperone (specific activity 16.2 Ci/mmol) were purchased from Perkin Elmer Inc. Acetonitrile was from Merck. BDNF and GDNF ELISA kit were acquired from Promega company. Antibodies against the following proteins were used in the study: anti-BDNF (Abcam), anti-GDNF (Abcam), anti-DAT (Santa Cruz), anti-CREB (Santa Cruz), anti-pCREB (Santa Cruz), anti-D1 receptor (Millipore), anti-D2 receptor (Chemicon), anti-β-actin (Sigma). All primers used in qRT-PCR were designed using Primer Premier 5.0 software and synthesized by Shanghai Sangon Biotech Co. Ltd (Shanghai, China). The SYBR Green PCR Master Mix kit was from ABI (Warrington, UK).

Production of Animal Models and Drug Administration

Male C57BL/6 mice (10 weeks old, 23.80 ± 1.32 g, from Shanghai SIPPR-BK Laboratory Animal Company) were housed five per cage and maintained on a 12 h light-dark cycle in standard conditions. The room temperature and relative humidity were set at 22 ± 2°C and 55% ± 15% respectively, with food and water available *ad libitum*. This study was carried out in accordance with the recommendations of the NIH Guide, Shanghai JiaoTong University Animal Ethic Committee. The protocol was approved by the Shanghai JiaoTong University Animal Ethic Committee. One week period of acclimatization was allowed between delivery of mice and commencement of treatment.

The chronic PD model was produced according to the previous article with slight modifications (Petroske et al., 2001). In brief, 10 doses of MPTP HCL in saline plus probenecid in dimethyl sulfoxide were given in 5 weeks, with an interval of 3.5 days between consecutive injections. Each time, probenecid (250 mg/kg) was given by intraperitoneal injection 30 min prior to subcutaneous injection of MPTP (15 mg/kg; **Figure 1**). The normal control group was injected simultaneously with intraperitoneal injections of DMSO and 30 min later subcutaneous injections of saline. The mice were divided into four groups (seventeen in each group): normal control, MPTP/ probenecid (MPTP/P in figures) control, MPTP/ probenecid treated with SMI at dose of 10 and 26 mg/kg/day. From the third dose of MPTP injection, all mice were administered orally by intragastric administration either SMI or vehicle (HPMC) once daily for 60 days. For the last 3 days,

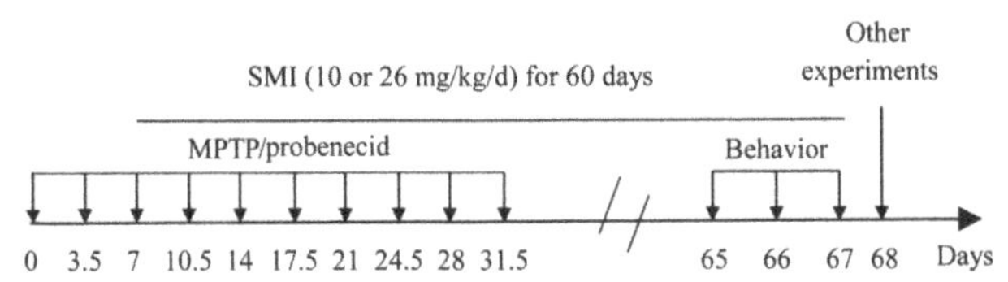

FIGURE 1 | Time schedule of experiments *in vivo*.

locomotor ability of mice is evaluated by the rotarod and open field test.

Rotarod and Open Field Test for Behavioral Assessment

We employed a modification of the procedure described by Rozas using a rotarod apparatus (IITC Life Science, Woodland Hills, CA, USA; Rozas et al., 1998). In general, all mice were trained to be accustomed to the rotarod apparatus at low speed rotation before formal experiment. Then each mouse was tested on rotating rods at a rate of six increments (8, 12, 16, 20, 24, 28 rpm) once per day for 3 days. Duration of each speed does not exceed 150 s. At least a 5 min resting period was required between each speed to alleviate mouse stress and fatigue. The overall rotarod performance for each mouse was obtained by plotting the average time on the rod at each speed vs. the rotating speed, and finally calculating the area under the curve (AUC) to evaluate the mice locomotor ability.

Next, we test spontaneous activity in a white open-field box. First the mice were put into the box to make it accustom to the environment for 5 min. Twenty-four hours later, the mice were placed into the same box and let them freely explore for 5 min. The locomotor activity was recorded by a video camera directly above the box and analyzed by a video track system (Noldus Ethovision).

Tyrosine Hydroxylase Immunohistochemistry and Nissl Staining in the SNpc and Stereological Counting

Coronal sections through the substantia nigra were processed for TH immunohistochemistry and Nissl staining as described previously with minor modifications (Xu et al., 2010). Briefly, mice were euthanized and fixed by 4% paraformaldehyde. Coronal frozen sections (50 μm) from mid brain SN were treated with 0.3% hydrogen peroxidase in methanol and subsequently in 0.3% Triton X-100 and 5% bovine serum albumin. For TH immunostaining, the sections were then incubated with rabbit anti-mouse TH polyclonal antibody (1:600) at 4°C overnight. The following day, sections were treated with biotinylated anti-mouse IgG and then processed with avidin–biotin peroxidase complex. The peroxidase reaction was visualized by 0.05% DAB with 0.03% H_2O_2. For Nissl staining, sections were immersed in Nissl staining solution for 10 min. Finally, TH-positive and Nissl staining areas in SNpc were photographed with a Nikon TE300 inverted microscope. Meanwhile the total number of TH-positive neurons of TH-immunostained sections was quantified by unbiased stereological counting. Briefly, neurons were quantified using an Olympus BX61 microscope with a monitored x-y-z stage linked to the stereo investigator software in every fourth section of each mouse for a total of 8–9 slides through the entire SNpc. As described previously, the software could calculate total numbers of TH-positive neurons automatically (Petroske et al., 2001; Xu et al., 2010).

HPLC Analysis of DA and Its Metabolites

The method adopted from Liang was made some modifications (Liang and Tang, 2006). In brief, striatum was rapidly dissected, weighed, homogenized and centrifuged. The final supernatant was stored at −70°C until HPLC assay. The concentrations of dopamine and its metabolites (DOPAC and HVA) were determined by a Waters 515 HPLC system (Milliford, MA, USA) with an electrochemical detector (HPLC-ECD) and a microbore ODS column (100 × 1 mm i.d.). The mobile phase consisted of 0.1 M NaH_2PO_4, 0.5 mM EDTA, 10 mM NaCl, 1 mM sodium octyl sulfate (pH 3.1) and 5% acetonitrile, and was pumped at 65 μl/min. The sample was diluted 1:4 with the mobile phase to neutralize the pH before chromatography. The calibration materials were assayed in parallel.

Autoradiography of Striatal Dopamine Transporter

Striatal dopamine transporter density (DAT) binding were estimated by $[^{125}I]$-FP-β-CIT binding autoradiography in coronal frozen sections (20 μm in thickness) prepared from right hemisphere including striatum region. Thawed sections were immersed in binding buffer (50 mM Tris, 120 mM NaCl, 5 mM KCl^-) for 2 × 15 min at room temperature, then incubated in the same buffer containing 50 pM $[^{125}I]$- FP-β-CIT and 100 nM fluoxetine (to inhibit serotonin binding to the $[^{125}I]$-FP-β-CIT) for 2 h at 25°C to determine the total binding. Non-specific binding (NSB) was assessed in parallel slices with the addition of 100 μM GBR 12909 (dopamine uptake inhibitor). All sections that were thoroughly washed and air-dried were exposed to X-ray film (Kodak, USA) for 2 d at 4°C. Then the film was developed and fixed. Finally, quantitative analysis of the autoradiographs was performed with a Gel Documentation System (Bio-Rad) by circumscribing the area of striatum on the digitized image and measuring the mean gray level. DAT density was expressed as the mean value of optical density unit.

Radioligand Binding Assay of Dopamine D1 and D2 Receptor Density in Striatum

Densities of Dl and D2 receptor were measured by the radioligand binding assay, using $[^3H]$ SCH23390 (SA: 80.5 Ci/mmol) for dopamine Dl receptor and $[^3H]$ spiperone (SA: 16.2 Ci/mmol) for dopamine D2 receptor binding, according to the method described previously with minor modifications (Popoli et al., 1998). In brief, the isolated striatum was homogenized in ice-cold buffer containing 50 mM Tris-HCl, 10 mM $MgCl_2$, 0.25 M sucrose, and subsequently centrifuged at 2,000 *g* for 15 min, then at 27,000 *g* for 15 min at 4°C. The precipitate was suspended with the above buffer without sucrose, and mixed as a membrane protein suspension. Micro-Lowry's method was utilized to quantify sample protein content. Dopamine receptor activity was measured in a parallel set of reaction tubes. A single dose of [^{3}H] SCH23390 at a saturation concentration of 5 nM was selected based on preliminary multipoint saturation analysis for all samples to detect D1 receptor. Parallel tubes with additional 5 μM unlabeled SCH23390 were used for measurement of NSB. D2 receptors were measured using 1.5 nM [^{3}H] spiperone combined with 50 nM ketanserin to block binding to serotonin receptors. NSB was determined in the presence of 80 nM haloperidol. The binding reaction system was incubated at 37°C for 50 min. The reaction was terminated by rinsing in ice-cold distilled water and harvested on a glass fiber filter which was then baked at 80°C, immersed in 0.6% b-PBD xylene scintillator and measured with a liquid scintillation counter (Beckman LS 6500). The density of receptors was determined using the following formula: Receptor density = (Total binding − NSB)/measure efficiency × 60 × specific × protein concentration).

Measurement of BDNF and GDNF Content by ELISA

BDNF and GDNF content were determined using BDNF or GDNF Emax Immunoassay System according to the manufacturer's guidelines. Briefly, the sample dissected from the striatum of unilateral hemisphere was sonicated in cold lysis buffer containing 137 mM NaCl, 20 mM Tris (pH 8.0), 0.5% TritonX-100, 10% glycerol and centrifuged at 10,000 *g* for 10 min at 4°C. Subsequently the supernatants were retained for assay. Then plates were coated with anti-BDNF or GDNF monoclonal antibody overnight. After nonspecific binding was blocked, each well added sample protein, BDNF or GDNF standards were incubated for 2 h (BDNF) or 6 h (GDNF) with shaking at room temperature. After washing, plates were incubated with polyclonal anti-human BDNF or anti-GDNF polyclonal antibody 2 h at room temperature or overnight at 4°C. Anti-IgY HRP-conjugated secondary antibody was added to the washed plates and incubated 1 h for BDNF and 2 h for GDNF at room temperature. Plates were then washed and incubated with TMB One Solution for 10 min or 15 min. Finally, plates were added 1 N hydrochloric acid to terminate the color change reaction and measured the absorbance at 450 nm using a plate reader. Data were expressed as picograms per milligram of protein.

Western Blot

Striatum tissues were homogenized by ultrasonication in 10 volumes of ice-cold RIPA lysis buffer respectively. The homogenates were then centrifuged at 12,000 *g* for 5 min at 4°C. The supernatants were collected and total protein concentration was determined according to the Micro bicinchoninic acid (BCA) procedure. Protein samples (40 μg) were separated by electrophoresis on a 10% PAGE and transferred to PVDF membranes. The membranes were blocked with 5% nonfat dried milk for 2 h at room temperature and then incubated with primary antibody overnight at 4°C. The membranes were rinsed three times with Tris-Buffered Saline with Tween-20 (TBST) and then followed by HRP-conjugated anti-rabbit/mouse IgG for 2 h at room temperature. After rinsing with TBST, the immunocomplexes were visualized by enhanced chemiluminescence using the ECL kit according to the manufacturer's instructions. Densitometric analyses were performed using ImageJ software.

Cell Culture and Treatment

The SH-SY5Y cell line was a kind gift from Dr. H. Zhang of the Shanghai Institute of Materia Medica who bought the cell line from ATCC (Manassas, VA, USA). The cells were seeded at 5×10^5 cells/ml in bottles containing DMEM cultured at 37°C with 5% CO_2. When the cells were 70–80% confluence, SMI was added at a final concentration of 10 μM. Twenty-four hours later, 1 mM MPP^+ was added.

Transfection of SH-SY5Y Cells With CREB siRNA

CREB siRNA and control siRNA were designed as previous described. CREB siRNA: 5′-UACAGCUGGCUAACAAUGG-3′; control siRNA: 5′-UUCUCCGAACGUGUCACGU-3′; Control siRNA showed no significant match and thus served as a non-functional control. Transfection was carried out using the Fugene 6 Transfection Reagent kit (Roche) following instructions in the kit protocol. In brief, when the cells were 70% confluent, 80 nM siRNA and 1 μl transfection reagent were added to 10^5 cells and were then incubated for 4 h to complete the transfection. GDNF and BDNF mRNA were examined 48 h later.

RT-PCR of GDNF and BDNF mRNA

In order to test the effects of MPP^+, SMI and CREB on the expression of GDNF and BDNF, qRT-PCR was carried out using the SYBR Green dye method as described previously (Zhang et al., 2008) with the following primers:

- GDNF; F-5′-CGGGACTCTAAGATGAAGTTATGGGAT GTCGTG-3′,
- R-5′-GGGTCAGATACATCCACACCGTTTAGCGG AATGC-3′,
- BDNF; F-5′-AGCTGAGCGTGTGTGACAGTATTAG-3′
- R-5′-ATTGCTTCAGTTGGCCTTTTGATAC-3′
- GAPDH; F-5′-GACCCCTTCATTGACCTCAACTACA-3′
- R-5′-TCTCGCTCCTGGAAGATGGTGATG-3′.

The amount of GDNF and BDNF mRNA in the SH-SY5Y cells were determined by real time qRT-PCR at 24 h after the addition of MPP^+. Data were finally normalized by respective GAPDH values from the same run and expressed as percent of the control sample.

Statistical Analysis

All data were represented as mean ± SEM. Statistical comparisons of data among the different groups were performed by an analyses of variance (ANOVA) followed by a *post hoc* Newman–Keuls using the SAS software package. $P < 0.05$ was judged to have statistical significance.

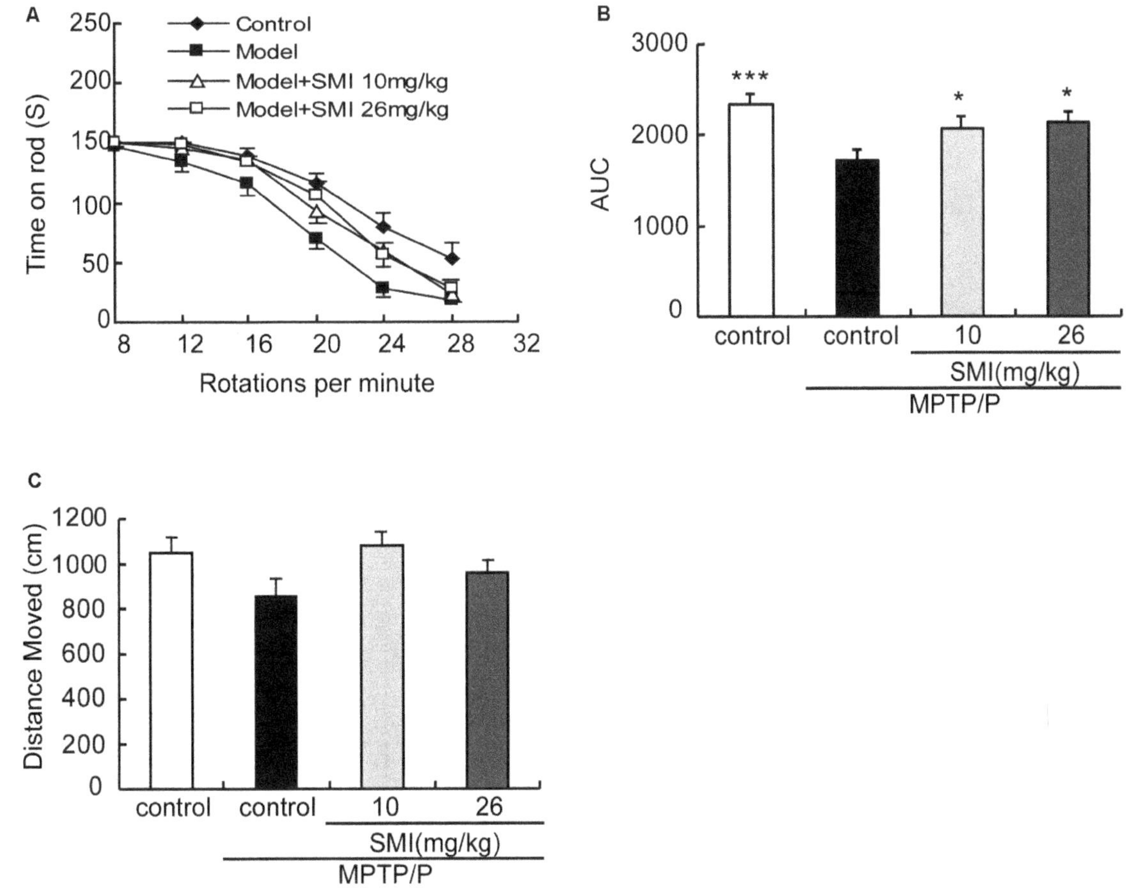

FIGURE 2 | Effects of smilagenin (SMI) on behavioral test of chronic 1-methyl-4-phenyl-1,2,3,6-tetrahydropyridine (MPTP)/probenecid-lesioned mice. **(A)** Time on the rod vs. rotation speed, each point was the mean ± SEM of 3 days consecutive tests. **(B)** Statistical comparisons of area under the curve (AUC) values between groups. **(C)** Total distance moved, measured as centimeters moved in 5 min, data are expressed as mean ± SEM, $n = 10$. *$P < 0.05$ and ***$P < 0.001$ respectively as compared with untreated model group, respectively.

RESULTS

Effect of SMI on Rotarod and Open Field Test for Behavioral Ability in Chronic MPTP/Probenecid-Lesioned Mice

In the present study, we adopted a commonly utilized rotarod test to measure motor coordination in animals and the AUC to reflect the mice on the rotarod movement. The time stayed on the rods for all mice declined with the increase of rotational speed from 8 to 28 rpm in the rotarod apparatus. Generally, the curve dropped most rapidly in the MPTP/probenecid models, followed by SMI treatment, and the normal control mice declined slowest (**Figure 2A**). As indicated in **Figure 2B**, the AUC was significantly declined in MPTP/probenecid-injured mice when compared with normal controls ($P < 0.001$). Meanwhile, SMI at dose of 10 or 26 mg/kg/day significantly ameliorated locomotor ability of MPTP/probenecid-lesioned mice ($P < 0.05$).

As shown in **Figure 2C**, in the open field test, the total distance of MPTP/probenecid injured mice was less than that of control group, but there was no statistically significant difference. There was also no significantly improved locomotor activity with SMI treatment ($P > 0.05$).

Effect of SMI on Tyrosine Hydroxylase Positive and Nissl Positive Neuron Number in Chronic MPTP/Probenecid-Lesioned Mice

According to **Figure 3A**, we can see that the TH-positive neuron number of SNpc was decreased in the model mice compared with normal controls and was increased both in treatment with SMI at 10 and 26 mg/kg/day compared with model mice. **Figure 3B** has indicated the statistical results of TH-positive neuron numbers. Compared with normal control mice, TH-positive neuron number in the SNpc was reduced by 74.4% in chronic MPTP/probenecid injured model mice ($P < 0.001$). Two months' treatment of 10 or 26 mg/kg/day SMI after three doses MPTP/probenecid injection increased TH (+) neurons by 104.1% and 228.8%, respectively when compared with MPTP/probenecid injection alone ($P < 0.01$, $P < 0.001$). On the other hand, Nissl staining showed that

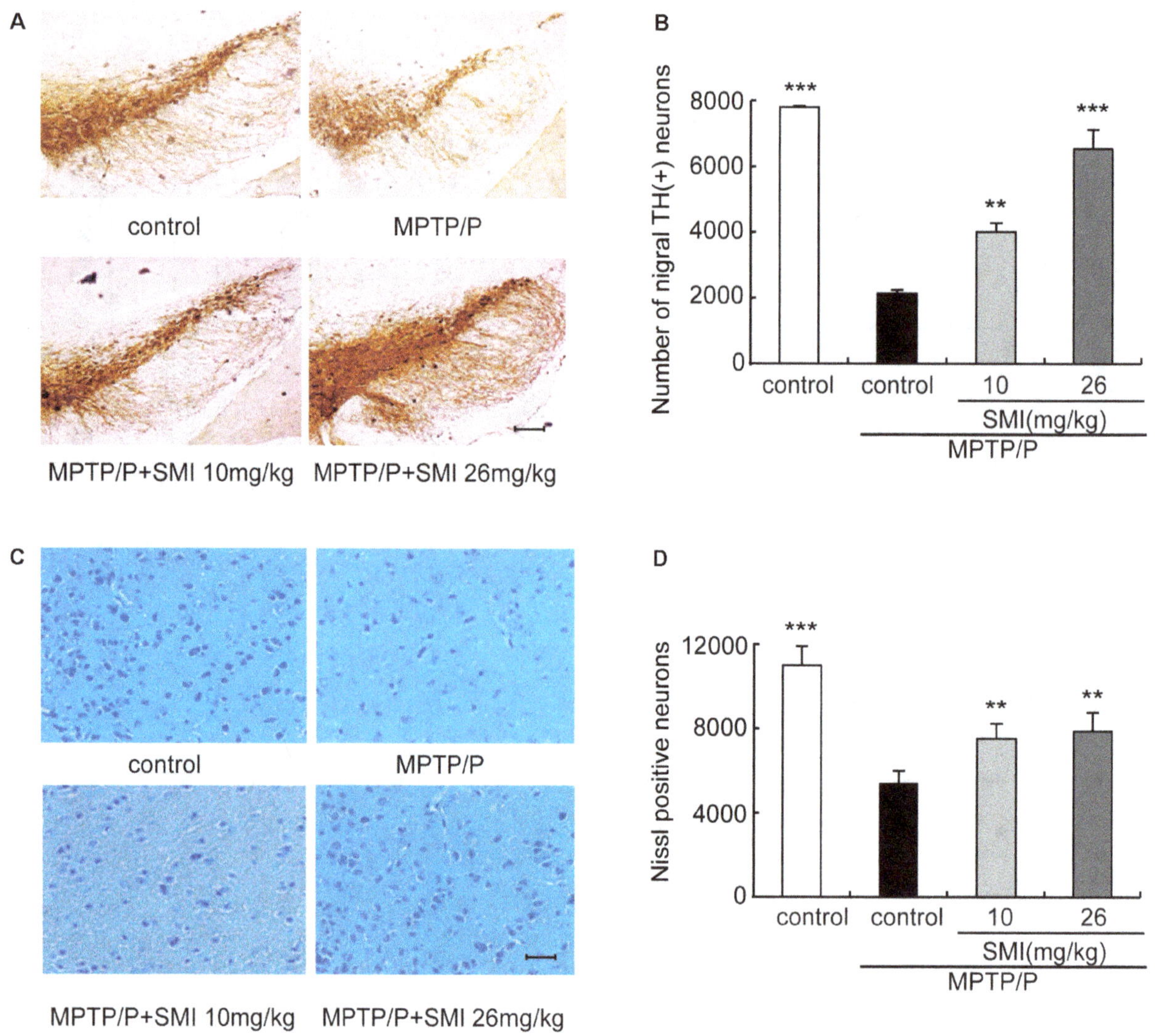

FIGURE 3 | Effect of SMI on tyrosine hydroxylase (TH)-positive and Nissl positive neuron number in chronic MPTP/probenecid-lesioned mice. Panel **(A)** shows the representative slices of the control mice, model mice treated with vehicle, 10 mg/kg/day, and 26 mg/kg/day SMI successively. (×100, scale bar = 100 μm). Panel **(B)** shows the statistical results. Panel **(C)** shows the representative images of Nissl-stained neurons in the substantia nigra pars compacta (SNpc) of the control mice, model mice treated with vehicle, 10 mg/kg/d, and 26 mg/kg/day SMI successively (×100, scale bar = 100 μm). Panel **(D)** shows quantification of Nissl-stained neurons. Number of nigral TH-positive neuron and Nissl-stained neurons in each mouse was quantified at ×100 magnification and then normalized to its corresponding control. Data are expressed as mean ± SEM, $n = 3$. $^{**}P < 0.01$ and $^{***}P < 0.001$, respectively as compared with untreated model group, respectively.

Nissl-stained neurons were reduced in the SNpc of chronic MPTP/probenecid injured model mice compared with controls and was increased after treatment with SMI in model mice (**Figures 3C,D**). These results suggest that administration of SMI may restore the loss of midbrain dopaminergic neurons caused by MPTP/probenecid.

Effect of SMI on Striatal DA and Its Metabolites Concentration in Chronic MPTP/Probenecid-Lesioned Mice

In the chronic PD model induced by MPTP/probenecid, the average concentrations of DA in striatum was only 35.7% of controls ($P < 0.05$). After treatment PD model with SMI for 2 months at dose of 10 or 26 mg/kg/day, DA concentration increased to 50.1% and 54.5% of normal ($P < 0.05$; **Figure 4A**). Besides, the concentrations of the metabolites DOPAC and HVA, which were decreased in the MPTP/probenecid model, were also elevated by SMI (**Figures 4B,C**). For DOPAC/DA, the ratios were 0.149 ± 0.004, 0.149 ± 0.009 and 0.153 ± 0.010, respectively for model and model treated with SMI at dose of 10 or 26 mg/kg/day (**Figure 4D**). For HVA/DOPAC, the ratios were 7.19 ± 0.34, 7.50 ± 0.41 and 7.91 ± 0.23, respectively ($P > 0.05$; **Figure 4E**). We can see SMI has no significant effect on the ratios of DOPAC/DA and HVA/DOPAC. This implicates that SMI did not change the catabolism of DA.

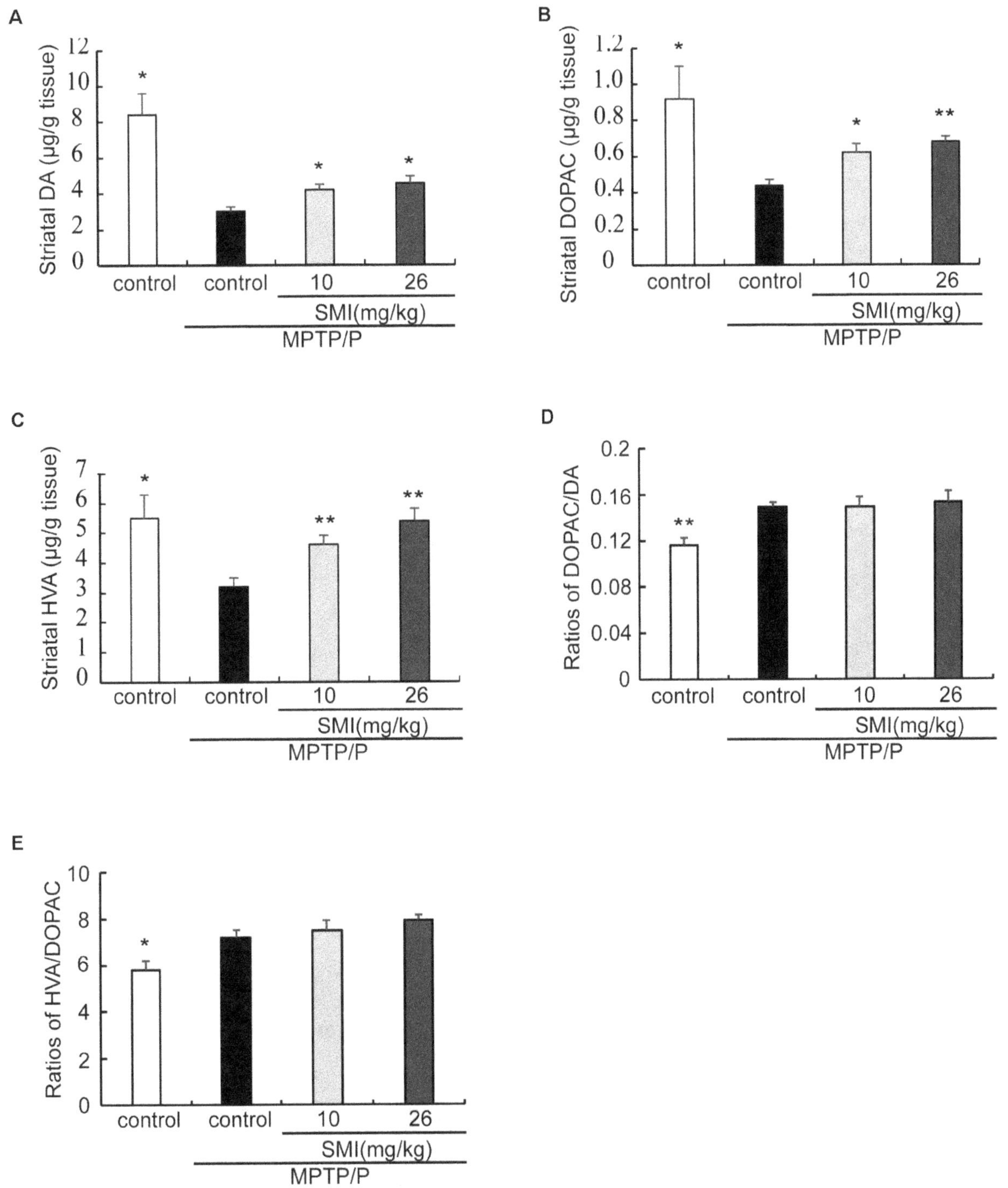

FIGURE 4 | Effect of SMI on striatal DA and its metabolites concentration in chronic MPTP/probenecid-lesioned mice. Panels **(A–C)** show amount of DA and its metabolites in striatum detected by HPLC-ECD. Panel **(D)** shows ratios of DAPOC/DA. Panel **(E)** shows ratios of HVA/DOPAC. Data are expressed as mean ± SEM, $n = 7$. $^{*}P < 0.05$ and $^{**}P < 0.01$, respectively as compared with untreated model group, respectively.

Effect of SMI on Striatal Dopamine Transporter Density and Protein Level in Chronic MPTP/Probenecid-Lesioned Mice

Autoradiography has been utilized to clarify striatal DAT. **Figure 5A** was the representative autoradiographic images. The statistical results revealed in **Figure 5B**, striatal DAT density in MPTP/probenecid-treated mice was significantly reduced by 30.03% ($P < 0.01$), as compared with normal control mice. Additionally, after administration of SMI whatever 10 or 26 mg/kg/day in MPTP/probenecid-injured mice, DAT density

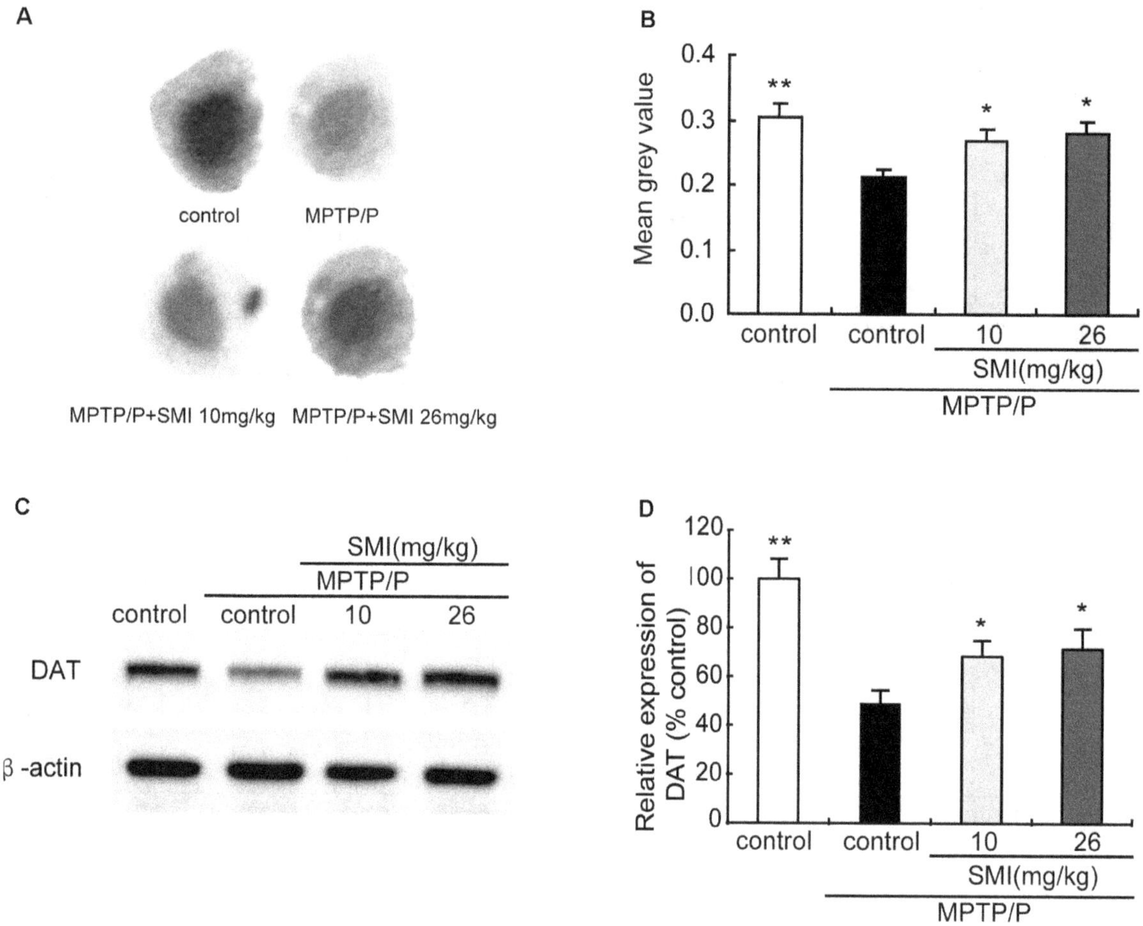

FIGURE 5 | Effect of SMI on striatal dopamine transporter (DAT) density and protein level in chronic MPTP/probenecid-lesioned mice. Panel **(A)** shows representative autoradiographic images of the control mice, model mice treated with vehicle, 10 mg/kg/d, and 26 mg/kg/d SMI successively. Panel **(B)** shows the statistical results (n = 7). Panel **(C)** shows representative western blot bands of DAT. Panel **(D)** shows relative protein expression levels were quantified by densitometry analysis using Image J software on DAT bands (n = 4). Data are expressed as mean ± SEM. *P < 0.05 and **P < 0.01, respectively as compared with untreated model group, respectively.

in striatum increased by 26.42% and 32.55%, respectively when compared with MPTP/probenecid mice model alone ($P < 0.05$, $P < 0.01$). As shown in **Figures 5C,D**, the same trend was also observed through the Western blot analysis. We found that protein level of DAT significantly downregulated in MPTP/probenecid-treated mice as compared to controls ($P < 0.01$), which was elevated after treatment of SMI ($P < 0.05$).

Effect of SMI on Striatal Dopamine D1 and D2 Receptor Density and Protein Level in Chronic MPTP/Probenecid-Lesioned Mice

Saturation radioligand binding on striatal membranes using ^{3}H-SCH23390 displayed increased D1 receptor density in the model mice compared with normal control and treatment with SMI at dose of 26 mg/kg/day ($P < 0.05$). SMI treatment produced D1 receptor downregulation from 196 to 164 fmol/mg protein in model mice (**Figure 6A**). Conversely, D2 receptor number in MPTP/probenecid-lesioned mice decreased compared with normal ($P < 0.05$); while after administration of SMI at dose of 26 mg/kg/day, there was a significantly increase ($P < 0.01$; **Figure 6B**). As shown in **Figures 6C,D**, we found that protein level of D1 receptor had no significant change through western blot and the reason might be antibody detection was not sensitive enough ($P > 0.05$). On the other hand, D2 receptor expression was downregulated in MPTP/probenecid-treated mice as compared to controls. Meanwhile, SMI at dose of 26 mg/kg/day, not 10 mg/kg/day, significantly restored D2 receptors protein level of MPTP/probenecid-lesioned mice ($P < 0.05$; **Figure 6E**).

Effect of SMI on Striatal GDNF and BDNF in Chronic MPTP/Probenecid-Lesioned Mice

Additionally, to further clarify the underlying mechanism of SMI's neuroprotective effect, we applied ELISA and Western blot to detect striatal GDNF and BDNF protein content. We found that there was a slight reduction but no significant difference in protein contents of GDNF and BDNF in the striatum between the MPTP/probenecid-treated mice and normal control

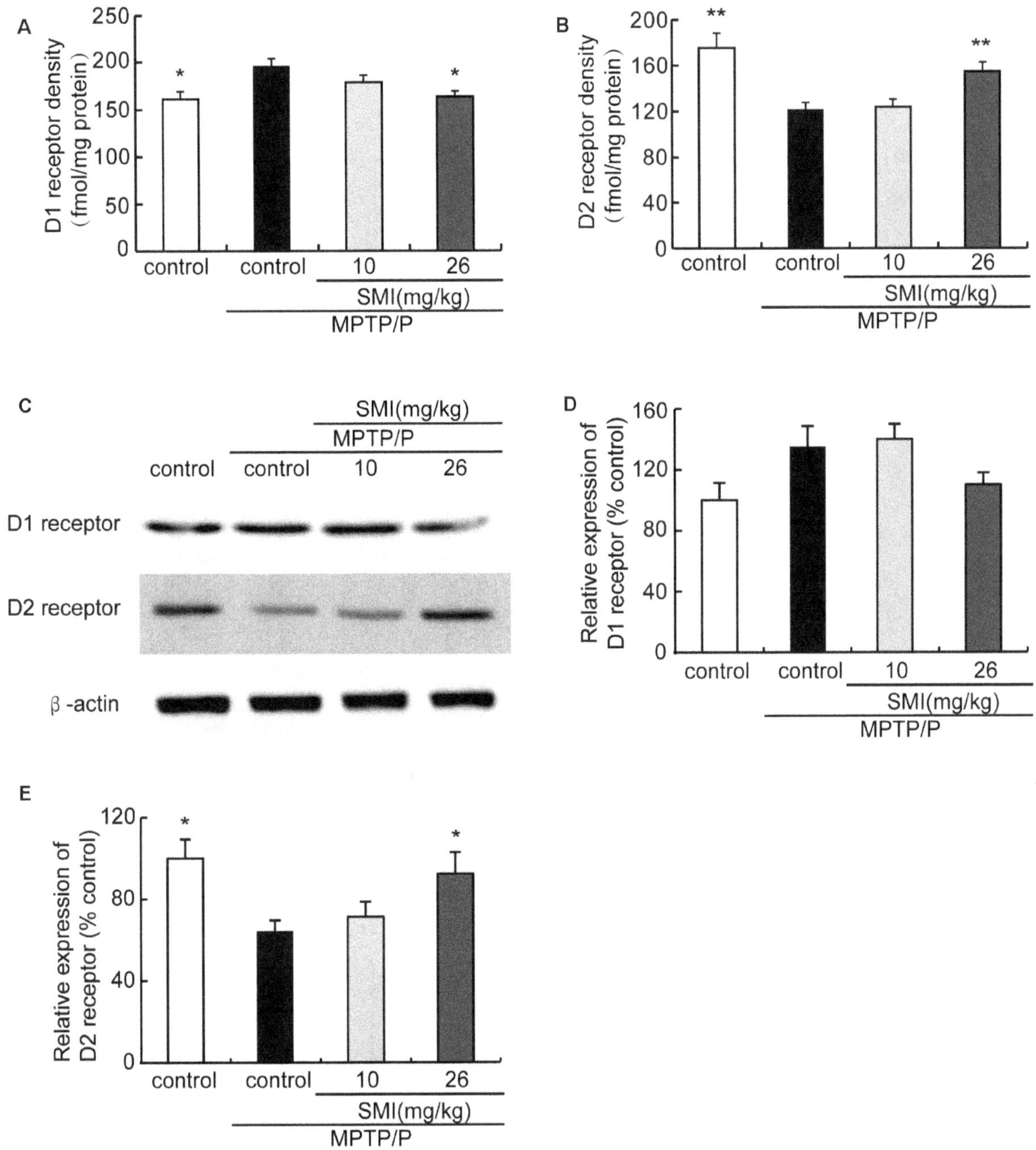

FIGURE 6 | Effect of SMI on striatal dopamine D1 and D2 receptor density and protein level in chronic MPTP/probenecid-lesioned mice. **(A)** D1 receptor density, assessed by ^{3}H-SCH23390 (n = 9). Panel **(B)** D2 receptor density, assessed by ^{3}H-spiperone (n = 9). Panel **(C)** shows representative western blot bands of D1 and D2 receptor. Panels **(D,E)** show relative protein expression levels were quantified by densitometry analysis using Image J software on D1 and D2 receptor bands (n = 4). Data are expressed as mean ± SEM. $^{*}P < 0.05$ and $^{**}P < 0.01$, respectively as compared with untreated model group, respectively.

mice ($P > 0.05$; **Figures 7A–F**). As shown in **Figures 7A,B**, SMI administration elevated the striatal GDNF and BDNF protein content of MPTP/probenecid-induced mice by ELISA analysis ($P < 0.01$). The same trend was also observed through the Western blot analysis. Meanwhile, we found SMI at dose of 26 mg/kg/day more significantly increased the protein level of GDNF compared with lower dose ($P < 0.001$; **Figure 7D**).

Effect of SMI on CREB Phosphorylation in Chronic MPTP/Probenecid-Lesioned Mice and CREB siRNA on mRNA Expression of GDNF and BDNF in MPP$^+$ Treated SH-SY5Y Cells

Cyclic AMP responsive element binding protein (CREB) is a transcription factor involved in regulation of genes associated

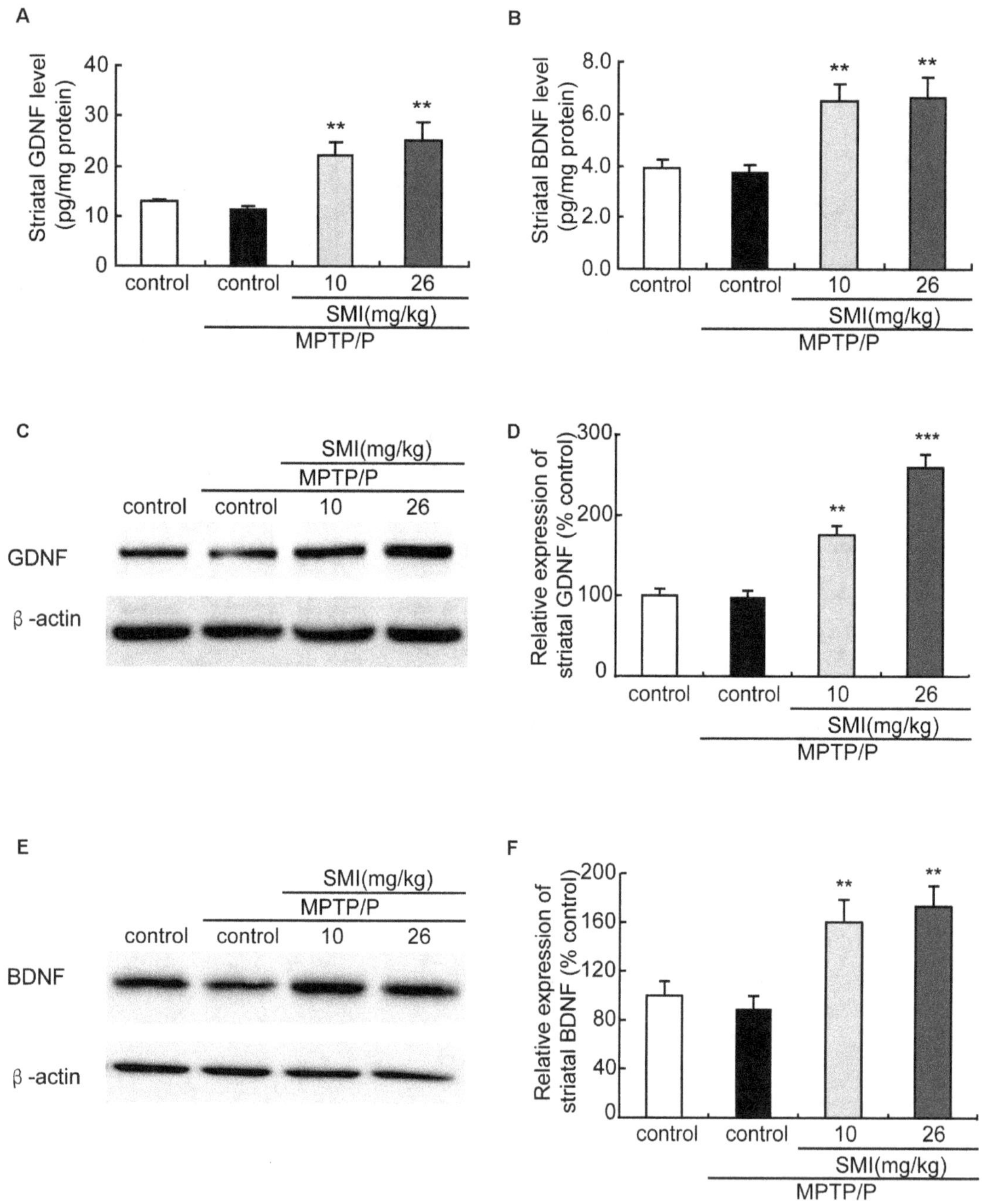

FIGURE 7 | Effect of SMI on striatal glial cell line-derived neurotrophic factor (GDNF) and brain-derived neurotrophic factor (BDNF) levels in chronic MPTP/probenecid-lesioned mice. **(A)** Striatal GDNF levels by ELISA. **(B)** Striatal BDNF levels by ELISA. Panels **(C,E)** show representative western blot bands of GDNF and BDNF. Panels **(D,F)** show relative protein expression levels were quantified by densitometry analysis using Image J software on GDNF and BDNF bands ($n = 4$). Statistical comparisons between groups, data are expressed as mean ± SEM, $^{**}P < 0.01$ and $^{***}P < 0.001$, respectively as compared with untreated model group, respectively.

with synaptic and neural plasticity. The phosphorylation of CREB (pCREB) was necessary for active transcription. CREB has been reported to up-regulate the expression of a set of genes including BDNF and GDNF (Cen et al., 2006; Wang et al., 2017). As shown in **Figure 8A**, Western blot revealed that the expression of pCREB/CREB was reduced in MPTP/probenecid-treated mice as compared with normal control mice ($P < 0.05$). We found SMI treatment elevated the level of CREB phosphorylation and the differences between SMI at dose of 26 mg/kg/day and MPTP control was highly significant ($P < 0.001$; **Figure 8B**). We speculated SMI up-regulated the expression of GDNF and BDNF by increasing the level of CREB phosphorylation. To test this possibility, we blocked CREB by CREB siRNA in MPP^+ treated SH-SY5Y cells and detected

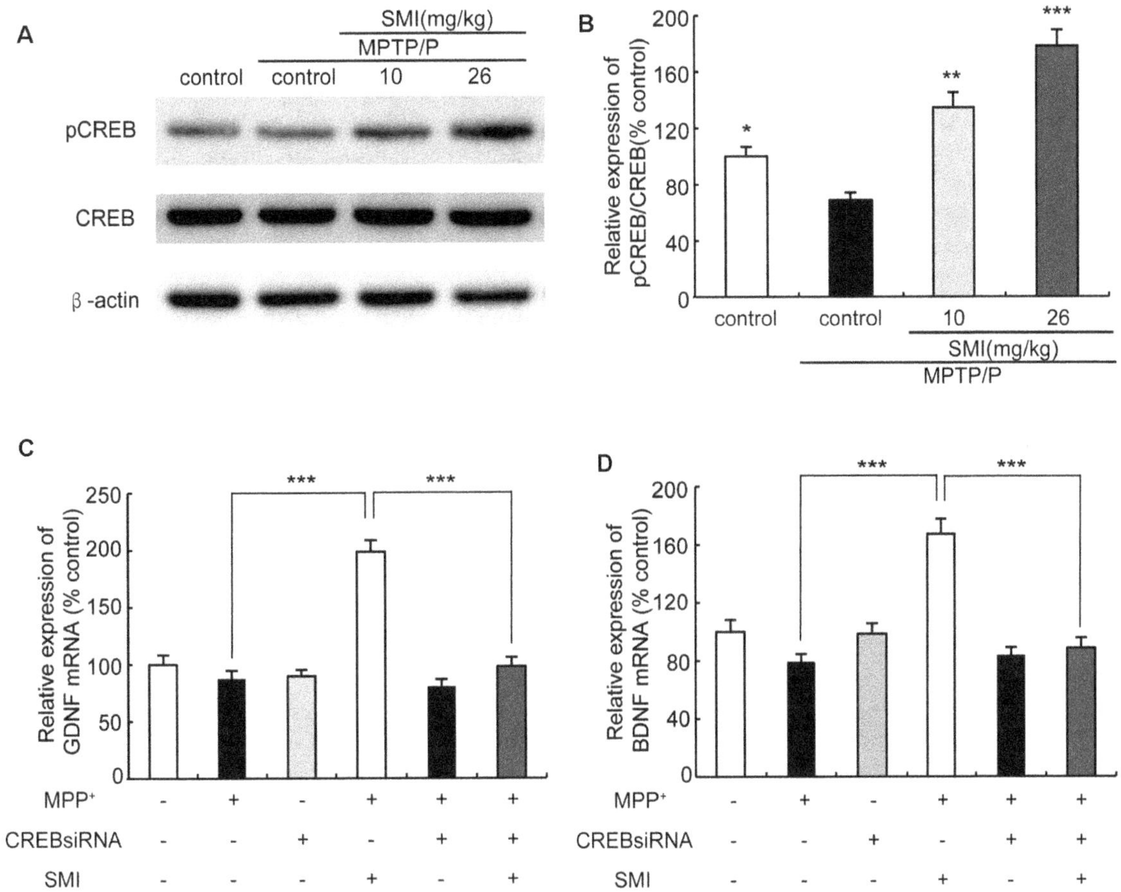

FIGURE 8 | Effect of SMI on cyclic AMP responsive element binding (CREB) phosphorylation in chronic MPTP/probenecid-lesioned mice and CREB siRNA on mRNA expression of GDNF and BDNF in MPP^+ treated SH-SY5Y cells. Panel **(A)** shows western blot bands of CREB and phosphorylation of CREB (pCREB). Panel **(B)** shows relative expression of pCREB/CREB were quantified by densitometry analysis using Image J software on CREB and pCREB bands (n = 4). Data are expressed as mean ± SEM, $^*P < 0.05$, $^{**}P < 0.01$ and $^{***}P < 0.001$, respectively as compared with untreated model group, respectively. Panels **(C,D)** show relative expression of GDNF and BDNF mRNA by real time PCR. Data are expressed as mean ± SEM, $^{***}P < 0.001$.

mRNA expression of GDNF and BDNF. We found that there was no significant difference in mRNA expression level of GDNF and BDNF between MPP^+ treated cells and normal control. However, SMI treatment significantly increased GDNF and BDNF transcription in MPP^+ treated cells ($P < 0.001$). After application of CREB siRNA, the elevation effect of SMI on mRNA expression of GDNF and BDNF was abolished. There was no significantly upregulation after SMI treatment ($P > 0.05$, **Figures 8C,D**).

DISCUSSION

It is for the first time that we have evaluated the neuroprotective effects of SMI as well as its effect on locomotor ability in chronic MPTP conjuncted with probenecid lesioned mice model of PD. Given SMI requiring long-term administration to exert well protective effects, the chronic MPTP/probenecid mice model which closely mimics the chronic and progressive neurodegeneration and behavioral deficits observed in human PD was more appropriate for investigating the drug's potent neuroprotective strategies (Peoples et al., 2012; Schildknecht et al., 2017; Nonnekes et al., 2018). Following 60 days' oral administration of SMI when the third dose of MPTP/probenecid injection afterwards.

It was demonstrated that MPTP/probenecid-intoxicated mice gave rise to impaired rotarod performance assessed by means of the rotarod test which is one of the most commonly utilized test to measure motor coordination in animals (Rozas et al., 1998; Petroske et al., 2001; Ayton et al., 2013). In the present study, we observed that rotarod performance was impaired in MPTP/probenecid-lesioned mice compared with the normal control and SMI administration improved MPTP/probenecid-induced motor deficits. The locomotor disorder is considered to be related to the injure of nigrostriatal dopaminergic system.

TH, DA, DAT and dopamine receptors are important hallmarks of the neurodegenerative alterations of nigro striatal dopaminergic neuron in PD (Peoples et al., 2012;

Naskar et al., 2015; Zhang et al., 2018). We observed in this article that TH-positive and Nissl positive neuron numbers in SNpc markedly reduced in MPTP-lesioned mice consistent with previous research reported (Alam et al., 2017; Peng et al., 2018), which can be elevated by administration of SMI starting at the early stage of the model production. TH is a marker of dopaminergic neurons and Nissl body is a marker of neurons. SMI increases the number of TH-positive neuron and Nissl staining cells in the substantia nigra of model mice, reflecting the increase in the number of dopaminergic neurons in the substantia nigra. In addition, the amount of TH in the substantia nigra is increased, which is beneficial to the synthesis of DA. Furthermore, SMI treatment increases striatal DA level of chronic PD mice model and does not change its metabolites concentration. We could speculate that SMI may protect striatal DA at a relatively constant level and does not affect the rate of DA renewal by protecting residual neurons (Xu et al., 2010; Sun et al., 2012). In the case of chronic PD mice model, striatal DAT density was lowered when compared with the vehicle-treated mice (Anandhan et al., 2012; Hong et al., 2015; Miville-Godbout et al., 2016). SMI treatment can reverse the decline of DAT density. This facilitates the ingestion of DA to prepare next release after its release into the synaptic cleft and exerting physiological effects. In addition, DAT is specifically expressed in dopaminergic neurons. Due to the protection of dopamine neurons by SMI, DA synthesis was not significantly reduced, thus avoiding the D1 receptor hypersensitivity and increase in number to some extent. In addition, the up-regulation of D2 receptor density by SMI suggests that SMI may be used in combination with levodopa to improve the down-regulation of D2 receptor density induced by the long-term use of levodopa (Morissette et al., 1996). Thus, we could speculate that SMI exerts effects of elevating nigral TH positive neurons and striatal DAT density in chronic MPTP-intoxicated mice, suggesting that it possesses action of improving dopaminergic neuron loss induced by MPTP and preventing or slowing the process of neuronal degeneration. We also found there was a recovery phenomenon appeared in MPTP/probenecid treated mice after 6 months which suggested us that we could observe the role of SMI in MPTP/probenecid treated mice for a longer period of time and get more information (Petroske et al., 2001).

Although there is undisputed about its significance of the potential neuroprotective effects of both BDNF and GDNF in preclinical studies and GDNF has been shown in some PD patients to have a positive effect (Gill et al., 2003; Love et al., 2005; Lu et al., 2013), unfortunately owing to large polypeptide structure and consequent poor oral bioavailability of exogenous BDNF, in clinical studies using BDNF as a therapeutic agent have been inconclusive (Thoenen and Sendtner, 2002). It is greatly urgent to execute potential strategy to stimulate the endogenous expression of neurotrophic factors after oral administration to slow down or reverse the progression of neuronal degeneration. Our previous study *in vitro* indicated that SMI relied on stimulating the intrinsic GDNF expression to exert neuroprotective effect on primary cultured mesencephalic dopaminergic neurons (Zhang et al., 2008). Hence, we evaluated whether SMI could have an impact on chronic MPTP/probenecid-induced mice *via* enhancing expression of BDNF and GDNF in striatum. In this article, we observed that there were no alterations in striatal BDNF and GDNF protein levels between chronic MPTP/probenecid lesioned mice alone and the vehicle treated mice. However, long-term administration of SMI greatly elevated GDNF and BDNF content in the striatum of MPTP/probenecid-lesioned mice. In addition, we used MPP^+-treated SH-SY5Y cells as an *in vitro* PD model to investigate the mechanism of SMI effect on GDNF and BDNF. We observed SMI treatment significantly increased GDNF and BDNF transcription in MPP^+ treated cells. We also found CREB siRNA abolished the elevation effect of SMI on mRNA expression of GDNF and BDNF in MPP^+-treated cells. We could speculate that SMI increased GDNF and BDNF protein level through promoting the phosphorylation of upstream transcription factor CREB and to increase mRNA expression of GDNF and BDNF. Presently there is a body of evidence revealing that BDNF and GDNF has strong neuroprotective effects on nigrostriatal dopaminergic neurons of animal PD models with 6-OHDA or MPTP, led to a substantial increase in the number of TH-positive neurons in SNpc as well as ameliorated behavioral disorders, stimulated TH positive fiber sprouting and elevated DA content (Biju et al., 2010; Ren et al., 2013). In the present research, it is reasonable to assume SMI protect and repair nigrostriatal dopaminergic system, at least in part, by promoting the phosphorylation of CREB to increase expression of endogenous GDNF and BDNF. GDNF and BDNF exert their neuroprotective effect to increase nigral TH positive neurons and striatal DAT density and subsequently ameliorate motor deficits in chronic MPTP/probenecid-intoxicated mice.

CONCLUSION

In summary, this study demonstrates that administration of the SMI to chronic MPTP/probenecid animals improved the pathological development of disease. The possible mechanism that SMI exerted neuroprotective effects may be partially related to up-regulating CREB phosphorylation which triggers endogenous neurotrophic factors, and ameliorating nigrostriatal dopaminergic system, which is likely to halt the ongoing progression.

AUTHOR CONTRIBUTIONS

YZ, HW and RX conceived the study. XH and SY performed the experiments and data analyses. RZ, LH and JX provided intellectual inputs. XH and SY wrote the manuscript. All authors edited and approved the manuscript.

FUNDING

This work was supported by The Chinese National Natural Science Foundation (Grant Nos: 81573401, 81373395, 81573415, 81503174, 81503044), Innovative research team of high-level local universities in Shanghai, Integration of traditional Chinese and western medicine, Construction Project of High Level Local Universities in Shanghai and Pharmacy, Construction Project of High Level Local Universities in Shanghai (XD18015).

ACKNOWLEDGMENTS

We would like to thank all individuals participating in the study.

REFERENCES

Alam, G., Edler, M., Burchfield, S., and Richardson, J. R. (2017). Single low doses of MPTP decrease tyrosine hydroxylase expression in the absence of overt neuron loss. *Neurotoxicology* 60, 99–106. doi: 10.1016/j.neuro.2017.03.008

Anandhan, A., Janakiraman, U., and Manivasagam, T. (2012). Theaflavin ameliorates behavioral deficits, biochemical indices and monoamine transporters expression against subacute 1-methyl-4-phenyl-1,2,3,6-tetrahydropyridine (MPTP)-induced mouse model of Parkinson's disease. *Neuroscience* 218, 257–267. doi: 10.1016/j.neuroscience.2012.05.039

Ayton, S., George, J. L., Adlard, P. A., Bush, A. I., Cherny, R. A., and Finkelstein, D. I. (2013). The effect of dopamine on MPTP-induced rotarod disability. *Neurosci. Lett.* 543, 105–109. doi: 10.1016/j.neulet.2013.02.066

Biju, K., Zhou, Q., Li, G., Imam, S. Z., Roberts, J. L., Morgan, W. W., et al. (2010). Macrophage-mediated GDNF delivery protects against dopaminergic neurodegeneration: a therapeutic strategy for Parkinson's disease. *Mol. Ther.* 18, 1536–1544. doi: 10.1038/mt.2010.107

Cass, W. A., Peters, L. E., Harned, M. E., and Seroogy, K. B. (2006). Protection by GDNF and other trophic factors against the dopamine-depleting effects of neurotoxic doses of methamphetamine. *Ann. N Y Acad. Sci.* 1074, 272–281. doi: 10.1196/annals.1369.024

Cen, X. B., Nitta, A., Ohya, S., Zhao, Y. L., Ozawa, N., Mouri, A., et al. (2006). An analog of a dipeptide-like structure of FK506 increases glial cell line-derived neurotrophic factor expression through cAMP response element-binding protein activated by heat shock protein 90/Akt signaling pathway. *J. Neurosci.* 26, 3335–3344. doi: 10.1523/JNEUROSCI.5010-05.2006

Fan, C. H., Ting, C. Y., Lin, C. Y., Chan, H. L., Chang, Y. C., Chen, Y. Y., et al. (2016). Noninvasive, targeted, and non-viral ultrasound-mediated GDNF-plasmid delivery for treatment of Parkinson's disease. *Sci. Rep.* 6:19579. doi: 10.1038/srep19579

Gill, S. S., Patel, N. K., Hotton, G. R., O'Sullivan, K., McCarter, R., Bunnage, M., et al. (2003). Direct brain infusion of glial cell line-derived neurotrophic factor in Parkinson disease. *Nat. Med.* 9, 589–595. doi: 10.1038/nm850

Hong, J., Sha, S., Zhou, L., Wang, C., Yin, J., and Chen, L. (2015). Sigma-1 receptor deficiency reduces MPTP-induced parkinsonism and death of dopaminergic neurons. *Cell Death Dis.* 6:e1832. doi: 10.1038/cddis.2015.194

Ibáñez, C. F., and Andressoo, J. O. (2017). Biology of GDNF and its receptors—relevance for disorders of the central nervous system. *Neurobiol. Dis.* 97, 80–89. doi: 10.1016/j.nbd.2016.01.021

Kramer, E. R., and Liss, B. (2015). GDNF-Ret signaling in midbrain dopaminergic neurons and its implication for Parkinson disease. *FEBS Lett.* 589, 3760–3772. doi: 10.1016/j.febslet.2015.11.006

Lang, A. E., Gill, S., Patel, N. K., Lozano, A., Nutt, J. G., Penn, R., et al. (2006). Randomized controlled trial of intraputamenal glial cell line-derived neurotrophic factor infusion in Parkinson disease. *Ann. Neurol.* 59, 459–466. doi: 10.1002/ana.20737

Li, J., Xia, Z., Sun, X., Zhang, R., Huang, G., Hickling, R., et al. (2013). Reversal of dopamine neurons and locomotor ability degeneration in aged rats with smilagenin. *Neuroscience* 245, 90–98. doi: 10.1016/j.neuroscience.2013.04.028

Liang, Y. Q., and Tang, X. C. (2006). Comparative studies of huperzine A, donepezil, and rivastigmine on brain acetylcholine, dopamine, norepinephrine and 5-hydroxytryptamine levels in freely-moving rats. *Acta Pharmacol. Sin.* 27, 1127–1136. doi: 10.1111/j.1745-7254.2006.00411.x

Love, S., Plaha, P., Patel, N. K., Hotton, G. R., Brooks, D. J., and Gill, S. S. (2005). Glial cell line-derived neurotrophic factor induces neuronal sprouting in human brain. *Nat. Med.* 11, 703–704. doi: 10.1038/nm0705-703

Lu, B., Nagappan, G. H., Guan, X. M., Nathan, P. J., and Wren, P. (2013). BDNF-based synaptic repair as a disease-modifying strategy for neurodegenerative diseases. *Nat. Rev. Neurosci.* 14, 401–416. doi: 10.1038/nrn3505

Miville-Godbout, E., Bourque, M., Morissette, M., Al-Sweidi, S., Smith, T., Mochizuki, A., et al. (2016). Plasmalogen augmentation reverses striatal dopamine loss in MPTP mice. *PLoS One* 11:e0151020. doi: 10.1371/journal.pone.0151020

Morissette, M., Goulet, M., Calon, F., Falardeau, P., Blanchet, P. J., Bedard, P. J., et al. (1996). Changes of D1 and D2 dopamine receptor mRNA in the brains of monkeys lesioned with 1-methyl-4-phenyl-1,2,3,6-tetrahydropyridine: correction with chronic administration of L-3,4-dihydroxyphenylalanine. *Mol. Pharmacol.* 50, 1073–1079.

Naskar, A., Prabhakar, V., Singh, R., Dutta, D., and Mohanakumar, K. P. (2015). Melatonin enhances L-DOPA therapeutic effects, helps to reduce its dose, and protects dopaminergic neurons in 1-methyl-4-phenyl-1,2,3,6-tetrahydropyridine-induced Parkinsonism in mice. *J. Pineal Res.* 58, 262–274. doi: 10.1111/jpi.12212

Nonnekes, J., Post, B., Tetrud, J. W., Langston, J. W., and Bloem, B. R. (2018). MPTP-induced parkinsonism: an historical case series. *Lancet Neurol.* 17, 300–301. doi: 10.1016/s1474-4422(18)30072-3

Peng, S., Wang, C. P., Ma, J. Y., Jiang, K. T., Jiang, Y. H., Gu, X. S., et al. (2018). Achyranthes bidentata polypeptide protects dopaminergic neurons from apoptosis in Parkinson's disease models both *in vitro* and *in vivo*. *Br. J. Pharmacol.* 175, 631–643. doi: 10.1111/bph.14110

Peoples, C., Shaw, V. E., Stone, J., Jeffery, G., Baker, G. E., and Mitrofanis, J. (2012). Survival of dopaminergic amacrine cells after near-infrared light treatment in MPTP-treated mice. *ISRN Neurol.* 2012:850150. doi: 10.5402/2012/850150

Petroske, E., Meredith, G. E., Callen, S., Totterdell, S., and Lau, Y. S. (2001). Mouse model of Parkinsonism: a comparison between subacute MPTP and chronic MPTP/probenecid treatment. *Neuroscience* 106, 589–601. doi: 10.1016/s0306-4522(01)00295-0

Pires, A. O., Teixeira, F. G., Mendes-Pinheiro, B., Serra, S. C., Sousa, N., and Salgado, A. J. (2017). Old and new challenges in Parkinson's disease therapeutics. *Prog. Neurobiol.* 156, 69–89. doi: 10.1016/j.pneurobio.2017.04.006

Popoli, P., Betto, P., Rimondini, R., Reggio, R., Pézzola, A., Ricciarello, G., et al. (1998). Age-related alteration of the adenosine/dopamine balance in the rat striatum. *Brain Res.* 795, 297–300. doi: 10.1016/s0006-8993(98)00356-4

Przedborski, S. (2017). The two-century journey of Parkinson disease research. *Nat. Rev. Neurosci.* 18, 251–259. doi: 10.1038/nrn.2017.25

Ren, Z., Wang, J., Wang, S., Zou, C., Li, X., Guan, Y., et al. (2013). Autologous transplantation of GDNF-expressing mesenchymal stem cells protects against MPTP-induced damage in cynomolgus monkeys. *Sci. Rep.* 3:2786. doi: 10.1038/srep02786

Rozas, G., López-Martín, E., Guerra, M. J., and Labandeira-García, J. L. (1998). The overall rod performance test in the MPTP-treated-mouse model of Parkinsonism. *J. Neurosci. Methods* 83, 165–175. doi: 10.1016/s0165-0270(98)00078-8

Schapira, A. H. V., Chaudhuri, K. R., and Jenner, P. (2017). Non-motor features of Parkinson disease. *Nat. Rev. Neurosci.* 18:509. doi: 10.1038/nrn.2017.91

Schildknecht, S., Di Monte, D. A., Pape, R., Tieu, K., and Leist, M. (2017). Tipping points and endogenous determinants of nigrostriatal degeneration by MPTP. *Trends Pharmacol. Sci.* 38, 541–555. doi: 10.1016/j.tips.2017.03.010

Sun, Z., Jia, J., Gong, X., Jia, Y., Deng, J., Wang, X., et al. (2012). Inhibition of glutamate and acetylcholine release in behavioral improvement induced by electroacupuncture in parkinsonian rats. *Neurosci. Lett.* 520, 32–37. doi: 10.1016/j.neulet.2012.05.021

Sun, M. K., Nelson, T. J., and Alkon, D. L. (2015). Towards universal therapeutics for memory disorders. *Trends Pharmacol. Sci.* 36, 384–394. doi: 10.1016/j.tips.2015.04.004

Sy, L. K., Lok, C. N., Wang, J. Y., Liu, Y., Cheng, L., Wan, P. K., et al. (2016). Identification of "sarsasapogenin-aglyconed" timosaponins as novel

Aβ-lowering modulators of amyloid precursor protein processing. *Chem. Sci.* 7, 3206–3214. doi: 10.1039/c5sc02377g

Tarazi, F. I., Sahli, Z. T., Wolny, M., and Mousa, S. A. (2014). Emerging therapies for Parkinson's disease: from bench to bedside. *Pharmacol. Ther.* 144, 123–133. doi: 10.1016/j.pharmthera.2014.05.010

Thoenen, H., and Sendtner, M. (2002). Neurotrophins: from enthusiastic expectations through sobering experiences to rational therapeutic approaches. *Nat. Neurosci.* 5, 1046–1050. doi: 10.1038/nn938

Visanji, N. P., Orsi, A., Johnston, T. H., Howson, P. A., Dixon, K., Callizot, N., et al. (2008). PYM50028, a novel, orally active, nonpeptide neurotrophic factor inducer, prevents and reverses neuronal damage induced by MPP^+ in mesencephalic neurons and by MPTP in a mouse model of Parkinson's disease. *FASEB J.* 22, 2488–2497. doi: 10.1096/fj.07-095398

Wang, L., Hu, X. H., Huang, Z. X., Nie, Q., Chen, Z. G., Xiang, J. W., et al. (2017). Regulation of CREB functions by phosphorylation and sumoylation in nervous and visual systems. *Curr. Mol. Med.* 16, 885–892. doi: 10.2174/1566524016666161223110106

Wong, Y. C., and Krainc, D. (2017). α-synuclein toxicity in neurodegeneration: mechanism and therapeutic strategies. *Nat. Med.* 23, 1–13. doi: 10.1038/nm.4269

Xu, G., Xiong, Z., Yong, Y., Wang, Z., Ke, Z., Xia, Z., et al. (2010). Catalpol attenuates MPTP induced neuronal degeneration of nigral-striatal dopaminergic pathway in mice through elevating glial cell derived neurotrophic factor in striatum. *Neuroscience* 167, 174–184. doi: 10.1016/j.neuroscience.2010.01.048

Zhang, Y., Xia, Z., Hu, Y., Orsi, A., and Rees, D. (2008). Role of glial cell derived neurotrophic factor in the protective effect of smilagenin on rat mesencephalic dopaminergic neurons damaged by MPP^+. *FEBS Lett.* 582, 956–960. doi: 10.1016/j.febslet.2008.02.039

Zhang, G. X., Xiong, N., Zhang, Z. T., Liu, L., Huang, J. S., Yang, J. L., et al. (2015). Effectiveness of traditional chinese medicine as an adjunct therapy for Parkinson's disease: a systematic review and meta-analysis. *PLoS One* 10:e0118498. doi: 10.1371/journal.pone.0118498

Zhang, N. S., Yan, F., Liang, X. L., Wu, M. X., Shen, Y. Y., Chen, M., et al. (2018). Localized delivery of curcumin into brain with polysorbate 80-modified cerasomes by ultrasound-targeted microbubble destruction for improved Parkinson's disease therapy. *Theranostics* 8, 2264–2277. doi: 10.7150/thno.23734

12

The Ischemic Immature Brain: Views on Current Experimental Models

Tânia Faustino-Mendes[1], *Marta Machado-Pereira*[1,2], *Miguel Castelo-Branco*[1,2,3] *and Raquel Ferreira*[1,2*]

[1] *Faculty of Health Sciences, University of Beira Interior, Covilhã, Portugal,* [2] *Health Sciences Research Centre (CICS-UBI), University of Beira Interior, Covilhã, Portugal,* [3] *Hospital Center of Cova da Beira, Covilhã, Portugal*

Keywords: perinatal, neonatal, stroke, experimental models, immature brain

Correspondence:
Raquel Ferreira
raquelmargarida@gmail.com

STROKE IN PRETERM AND TERM NEWBORNS

Perinatal stroke occurs between the 20th week of gestation and the 28th day after birth (Nelson, 2007). Brain injury within this period can also lead to conditions such as neonatal encephalopathy or to encephalopathy of prematurity. Considering the complex diagnosis and limited data available, the incidence of 1/2,300 live births is a likely underestimation (Nelson and Lynch, 2004; Lee et al., 2005). Nevertheless, these numbers are comparable to those in the elderly (Fernández-López et al., 2014). The most common subtypes are arterial ischemic stroke (Fernández-López et al., 2014), which induces a focal lesion similar to adult stroke, and cerebral sinovenous thrombosis (Govaert et al., 2009). Focal interruption of arterial or venous cerebral blood flow is usually secondary to thrombosis or embolism, with a multifactorial pathophysiology. Importantly, in the fetal circulatory system, placental or systemic venous emboli may pass through a patent *ductus arteriosus* or *foramen ovale* directly to the left carotid artery and subsequently to the left MCA, facilitating occlusion (Gunny and Lin, 2012). Confirmation by imaging or neuropathological studies is always mandatory (Govaert et al., 2009). Different risk factors have been recognized for perinatal stroke (**Supplementary Table 1**; Kurnik et al., 2003; Mirabelli-Badenier et al., 2012; Kasdorf and Perlman, 2013; Basu, 2014; Fernández-López et al., 2014; Kratzer et al., 2014; Machado et al., 2015; Buerki et al., 2016) but inflammation seems to be a prevalent underlying mechanism (Vexler and Yenari, 2009; Hagberg et al., 2015). For instance, chorioamnionitis, a bacterial infection of the amniochorionic membranes (Kasdorf and Perlman, 2013; Buerki et al., 2016) often leads to a longer labor period and worse prognosis (Vexler and Yenari, 2009). Nevertheless, although there is a substantial number of studies concerning neonatal encephalopathy (or hypoxic-ischemia encephalopathy), human data on perinatal stroke can be disparate; some authors found a positive correlation with pro-inflammatory polymorphisms, others did not (Hagberg et al., 2015).

Adult and perinatal stroke also cause distinct presenting symptoms: adults tend to present unilateral symptoms and only 3% have seizures; seizures are one of the most common presentations after perinatal stroke (Fernández-López et al., 2014). Hemiplegic cerebral palsy is also the most frequent long-term motor outcome of the latter (Nelson, 2007). However, several aspects delay the suspicion of diagnosis, since (i) newborns with seizures may appear clinically well-between episodes; (ii) initially, newborns may present discrete non-specific symptoms like lethargy, apnea, difficult feeding and impaired chewing; (iii) and some cases may be asymptomatic, presenting lateralized symptoms only around the 5th month. In fact, lateralized symptoms are rare in neonates (Nelson, 2007; Fernández-López et al., 2014). In 2011, Harbert and colleagues conducted the first human study demonstrating the positive effect of therapeutic hypothermia on perinatal stroke: active whole-body cooling *via* a blanket cooling device led to a significantly lower frequency of seizures (Harbert et al., 2011). Since these symptoms are associated to a worse prognosis, the risk of long-term neurologic disability is likely reduced. Given the complex pathophysiology and difficulty in obtaining an early and accurate diagnosis, new therapies are being tested, alone or in combination with hypothermia, to improve global outcome. Some include administration of growth factors, anticoagulant and antiplatelet agents, blood uric acid lowering medication, antioxidant and anti-inflammatory molecules, stem cells-based therapy and electrical stimulation (Cnossen et al., 2009; Gonzalez and Ferriero, 2009; Mirabelli-Badenier et al., 2012; Basu, 2014; Fernández-López et al., 2014; Kratzer et al., 2014).

IN VITRO APPROACHES

In vitro models resort to oxygen and glucose deprivation (OGD), followed by reoxygenation and nutrient replenishment. Since oxygen levels should be kept preferably under 2%, to represent the ischemic core, and around 7% if studying the ischemic penumbra (Tornabene and Brodin, 2016), these models can be very relatable while allowing easy assessment of cell activity, protein expression and release, and barrier properties of particular cell type(s). We have exposed either individualized cells or brain tissue, namely organotypic brain slice cultures (OSC), to very low O_2 rates (0.1%; Ferreira et al., 2016; Machado-Pereira et al., 2017). These tissue cultures provide unique characteristics and several advantages over cell models, since they preserve whole organ structure and maintain neuronal activity and synapse circuitry. OSC also maintain integrity *in vitro* for over 2 weeks allowing a series of pharmacological studies. Other advantages include the possibility of using younger animals if needed (e.g., 1–3-day-old mice), the refinement of experimental doses/conditions and the reduction of the number of animals for *in vivo* models. To the best of our knowledge only one group has used OSC, from P8-10 rats (Leonardo et al., 2009). A considerable drawback from OSC, and cell cultures, is the absence of blood flow and infiltrating immune cells. Nevertheless, they provide a snapshot of the neurovascular unit up to the time of brain isolation if a lesion and/or treatment is applied *a priori*. Younger animals such as 2-day-old mice still grant the ability to inject a therapeutic agent *via* the temporal vein, which is still visible at this age, to study its protective value (Machado-Pereira et al., 2018). Subsequently, therapeutic agents and stimuli can be further administered over tissue to evaluate their impact on neurovascular and glial activity.

ANIMAL MODELS OF PERINATAL STROKE

Experimental models are important to understand mechanisms of disease. Parameters like injury onset and duration, area of penumbra, reperfusion or therapeutic window are clearly defined, and symptoms can be easily identified and monitored. However, reproducing all the complex pathophysiological aspects of stroke in an otherwise healthy animal is challenging; typically, a stroke patient is elderly and has more than one health condition. One of the most frequently used adult models is induced by transient occlusion of the middle cerebral artery (MCA) with an intraluminal monofilament, blocking cerebral blood flow (usually 60 min) and causing reproducible infarcts in this territory (Carmichael, 2005; Sommer, 2017). A transient model allows the study of the significant effects of reperfusion. Regarding the perinatal period, the most common methodologies use unilateral ligation of the common carotid artery followed by hypoxia, or direct exposure to hypoxia alone. **Table 1** briefly describes procedures using rodents, rabbits, pigs and lambs. Animal models employing pigs, lambs or rabbits, are costly in terms of maintenance, in the sense that they have longer gestation periods and smaller litter size, while offering higher genetic dissimilarity with humans, comparing with mice (Leong et al., 2015). Importantly, most models use O_2 rates much higher (5–12%) than those believed to occur after an ischemic event. Only one group used a lower percentage (3.5–4%), albeit on rats of an age range comparable to a term and up to 2-years-old infant. In fact, normal brain tissue pO_2 is 33.8 ± 2.6 mmHg, which corresponds to $4.4 \pm 0.3\%$ O_2 in the microenvironment (Carreau et al., 2011). Three of the models used between 6 and 12% O_2: a fraction of inspired oxygen (FiO_2) of 0.06–0.12. Considering that atmospheric air is 21% O_2 or the equivalent to a FiO_2 of 0.21, these animals would be subjected to a third to a half O_2 available. Are lower O_2 rates fatal? Moreover, most models use 7-days-old or older animals, which offer a more reasonable size for surgery than younger pups. A week old rat, the most commonly used species, would represent a 2-months-old infant (well-beyond the 28th day post-birth) if considering peripheral organ systems (Sengupta, 2013; Titomanlio et al., 2015), and a term infant, if considering brain development (Titomanlio et al., 2015), raising further challenges on what age range to choose.

Age is very important, since the extent of ischemic injury is largely influenced by brain maturity (Sheldon et al., 1996; McQuillen et al., 2003; Webber et al., 2009). In preterm newborns, oligodendrocyte progenitor cells (OPC) are particularly more sensitive to ischemia (Back et al., 2002). Global ischemia, as in hypoxic-ischemia encephalopathy, disrupts OPC maturation, causing delayed or disrupted myelination, largely contributing to neuronal loss and periventricular white matter diffuse injury (periventricular leukomalacia; Back et al., 2007; Webber et al., 2009). Several experimental models have also been proposed to study this particular condition (Shen et al., 2010). For this reason, OPC constitute a potential target for the development of protective therapies focusing on the reduction of white matter loss in premature infants (Back et al., 2007). Subplate neurons, a transient neuronal population important for the formation of mature neuronal networks, are another vulnerable target. Additionally, interneuron migration to the neocortex is only completed at birth, in a process modulated by microglia activity (Leviton and Gressens, 2007; Xu et al., 2011). In term newborns, gray matter is focally affected, greatly impacting on motor function (Back et al., 2001; Fernández-López et al., 2014; Luhmann et al., 2016). The immature brain is also more susceptible to excitotoxicity and to free radicals considering the higher expression of receptors that signal for excitatory neurotransmitters and lower levels of anti-oxidant enzymes (Johnston, 2005; Lafemina et al., 2006). Overall, choosing the "right" age pertains to the fact that the perinatal period encompasses different stages of the circulatory and immune systems (Titomanlio et al., 2015; Lange et al., 2016). Accordingly, the therapeutic value of an agent directed at

TABLE 1 | Perinatal and neonatal animal models for ischemic injury, specifically rat, pig, mouse, rabbit, and lamb.

RAT		
P5-P17 Φ	Exposure to hypoxia (3.5–4% O_2 in N_2) until apnea or heart rate below 20% of baseline	Jensen, 1995
P10 Φ	Exposure to hypoxia (7, 5, 4% O_2 in N_2) for 8, 6, and 1 min, respectively	Dunn et al., 2017
P10 Φ	Left MCAO for 90 min by inserting a 6-0 nylon filament into the internal carotid artery; unilateral ligation of right CCA followed by hypoxia (8% O_2 in N_2) for 90 min	Ashwal et al., 2007
P7 ♀	MCAO for 180 min by inserting a 6-0 coated filament into the internal carotid artery	Fernández-López et al., 2013
P7 Φ	Unilateral ligation of right CCA followed by hypoxia (8% O_2 in N_2) for 60 min	Jantzie and Todd, 2010
P7 Φ	Unilateral ligation of CCA followed by hypoxia (8% O_2 in N_2) for 30, 60, 90, or 120 min	Silverstein and Johnston, 1984
P7 Φ	Unilateral ligation of left CCA followed by hypoxia (8% O_2 in 92% N_2) for 90 min	Bae et al., 2012
P7 Φ	Unilateral ligation of right CCA followed by hypoxia (8% O_2 in N_2) for 180 min	Jantzie et al., 2005
P7 Φ	Unilateral ligation of left CCA followed by hypoxia (8% O_2 in N_2) for 120 min	Lubics et al., 2005
P7 Φ	Unilateral ligation of CCA followed by hypoxia (8% O_2 in N_2) for 60–240 min	Vannucci and Vannucci, 2005
P4 ♂	Exposure to hypoxia (11% O_2 in N_2) for 360 min *per* day for 5 days	Schaeffer et al., 2013
P4 Φ	Exposure to hypoxia (11% O_2 in N_2) for 360 min *per* day for 5 days	Fendt et al., 2008
P2 Φ	Exposure to hypoxia (12% O_2 in N_2) for 14 days	Deruelle et al., 2006
P1 ♂	Exposure to hypoxia (12% FiO_2) for 10 days	Del Duca et al., 2009
P1 Φ	Unilateral ligation of right CCA followed by hypoxia (8% O_2 in N_2) for 210 min	Girard et al., 2009
P1 Φ	Exposure to hypoxia (5% O_2 in N_2) for 60 or 75 min	Slotkin et al., 1995
Newborn ♂/♀	Unilateral ligation of right CCA followed by hypoxia (8% O_2 in N_2) for 120 min	Kartal et al., 2016
PIG		
P3-P7 Φ	Exposure to a gas mixture (10% FiO_2) for 40 min, followed by 5 min of reoxygenation and 7 min of anoxia by clamping the endotracheal tube	Ni et al., 2011
P1-P4 ♂	Exposure to a gas mixture (FiO_2 6–8%) until hearth rate decreased to 60 beats/min (bradycardia) or mean arterial blood pressure decreased to 15 mmHg (severe hypotension)	Faa et al., 2012
P1-P3 Φ	Exposure to a gas mixture (12% O_2 in N_2) for 120 min to achieve a pO_2 of 30–40 mmHg	Stevens et al., 2008
Newborn Φ	Exposure to a gas mixture (8% O_2 in N_2) until the mean arterial blood pressure decreased to 20 mmHg or base excess reached −20 mmol/L	Garberg et al., 2017
MOUSE		
P9 Φ	Unilateral ligation of left CCA followed by hypoxia (10% O_2 in N_2) for 60 min	Kichev et al., 2014
P7 ♂	Exposure to hypoxia (10% O_2 in N_2) for 360 min *per* day (3 sessions of 120 min separated by 45 min intervals) for 6 days	Kameda et al., 2013
RABBIT		
E22 Φ	Uterine ischemia for 40 min, *via* arterial embolectomy catheter inserted through the maternal left femoral artery into the descending aorta	Yu et al., 2011
LAMB		
E126-141 Φ	Intrauterine hypoxia by induced maternal hypotension *via* infusion of trimetaphan camsylate glucose solution into a polyethylene catheter placed in the maternal femoral vein, for 60–90 min	Gersony et al., 1976

Rodent models usually resort to exposure to hypoxia alone (3.5–12% O_2) or to unilateral ligation of the common carotid artery, followed by hypoxia (8% O_2), in animals of varying ages. Pig models use exposure to a gas mixture ranging from 6 to 12% O_2 while lamb and rabbit models induce intrauterine ischemia. ♀, female; ♂, male; Φ undisclosed sex; CCA, common carotid artery E, embryonic days; MCAO, middle cerebral artery occlusion; min, minutes; P, post-natal days.

perinatal stroke would be better assessed using younger animals. Fundamentally, the brain vasculature during development is formed through two distinct processes: (i) vasculogenesis, in which angioblasts differentiate into endothelial cells forming the perineural vascular plexus, which in turn functions as a substrate for (ii) angiogenesis, the process of generating new vessels from pre-existing ones (Vasudevan and Bhide, 2008; Lee et al., 2009; Tam and Watts, 2010). These processes are consolidated by migrating mural cells, formation of an extracellular matrix and establishment of tight and adherens junctions that regulate permeability and transcellular transport (Lee et al., 2009; Tam and Watts, 2010). With increasing age, blood-brain barrier (BBB) functionality is less maintained after stroke since the expression of several of these proteins (e.g., occludin, claudins, zonula occludens proteins; Kratzer et al., 2014) that support the integrity of tight junctions is also changed. Another reason for a higher resistance of the BBB to ischemic injury in the early stages could be the maturation-dependent interplay between leukocytes and the endothelium and the less active pathophysiological role of the inflammatory process (Titomanlio et al., 2015). A restricted BBB opening may also account for limited neutrophil recruitment/infiltration. While regulatory T cells seem to play a neuroprotective role, microglia cells promote phagocytosis and tissue recovery, or white matter damage, depending on the adopted phenotype (Hagberg et al., 2015). In fact, microglia migrate to the brain even before blood vessel formation possibly impacting on the development of these structural elements (Rymo et al., 2011; Arnold and Betsholtz, 2013). Hence, in the perinatal period, the neuroinflammatory response has a preponderant role in stroke outcome (and to diffuse pattern of injury), relying more on the activation of microglia than on the extrinsic recruitment of inflammatory cells such as macrophages and neutrophils (Hagberg et al., 2015). A more mature brain offers a BBB more vulnerable to ischemic injury and to immune cell infiltration, and therefore, these cells assume a greater role and become associated to a focal pattern of injury. Consequently, several pro-/anti-inflammatory molecules and growth factors are released and have been studied as part of the impactful secretome unleashed by ischemia. Vascular endothelial growth factor (VEGF) is responsible for several processes upon ischemic stroke, including disruption of endothelial cell junctions and endothelial cell endocytosis, followed by increased BBB permeability, and consequently intracranial hemorrhage and intracranial hypertension (Angelo and Kurzrock, 2007; Lange et al., 2016; Suzuki et al., 2016). However, VEGF also promotes endothelial cell proliferation and migration, and enhances perfusion (reduced infarct volume and penumbra were associated to increased neuroprotection, including in neonatal stroke; Titomanlio et al., 2015; Lange et al., 2016; Suzuki et al., 2016). There are other cell types responsible for the development, regulation and maintenance of central nervous system angiogenesis and BBB integrity such as pericytes and astrocytes (Tam and Watts, 2010). These cells control the production and release of several factors that regulate the aforementioned processes (Lee et al., 2009; Tam and Watts, 2010; Arnold and Betsholtz, 2013). Therefore, diminished quantities of pericytes and astrocytes alongside blood vessels are associated to a higher susceptibility to ischemic injury (Fernández-López et al., 2014; Kratzer et al., 2014).

On a final note, rodent strains may display different levels of vulnerability to injury. For instance, CD1 mice are more vulnerable to damage induced by 30 min of hypoxia, than C57BL/6 and 129Sv mice, with the latter being the most resistant strain (Sheldon et al., 1998). Other murine strains (BDF, CFW, and BALB/C) display varying infarct volumes following 24 h of focal ischemia possibly because of differences in the anatomy of the posterior communicating arteries. BALB/C mice showed a more significant infarct volume and were proposed as the most suitable strain to conduct pharmacological studies in cerebral ischemia (Barone et al., 1993). In addition to differences in vascular anatomy, humans and other animals also display significantly different nutrient and oxygen metabolism, hemodynamics, and neural cell population density/activity (Dirnagl et al., 1999).

An interesting but poorly studied subject is the fact that perinatal stroke appears to be gender-dependent with male neonates and children being more commonly affected and with poorer outcomes (Turtzo and McCullough, 2010; Fernández-López et al., 2014). Turtzo and McCullough have extensively reviewed the role of gender and sex hormones in the perinatal, infant and adult periods. Although *in vitro* data from female pups suggest higher protection from OGD, and neuronal cells from males seem more susceptible to hypoxic injury (Heyer et al., 2005; Li et al., 2005), clinical studies and mechanisms of action remain inconclusive. Overall, ischemic cell death occurs *via* a caspase-independent pathway in males, while this process is caspase-dependent in females; ultimately, both pathways lead to mitochondrial dysfunction. The protection provided by female sex hormones, such as estrogen and progesterone, is a possible explanation. However, estrogen and progesterone administration to post-menopausal women were found to raise the risk of stroke (Turtzo and McCullough, 2010). To further investigate this issue in the perinatal period, it is possible to divide pups, even after birth, by a distinct physical trait: male mice have a visible pigment spot on the scrotum (Wolterink-Donselaar et al., 2009).

CONCLUSIONS

In vitro models are useful for assessing the potential of a therapeutic agent and constitute an inescapable stepping stone for *in vivo* models. However, current animal models still hold key limitations regarding the level of hypoxia and extent of focal injury, age and costs associated to the selected animal species/strain, as well as their basic anatomy. Importantly and understandably, all fail to reproduce the exact mechanisms of injury that occur specifically in perinatal stroke. Hence, it is urgent to continue advancing newer (and multifactorial) experimental models to attain more efficient therapies to treat this complex vascular condition and long-term sequela.

AUTHOR CONTRIBUTIONS

All authors listed have made a substantial, direct and intellectual contribution to the work, and approved it for publication.

FUNDING

Work supported by FEDER through POCI-COMPETE 2020 (POCI-01-0145-FEDER-007491, FCOMP-01-0124-FEDER-041099), and through CENTRO 2020 (CENTRO-01-0145-FEDER-000013), Foundation for Science and Technology (UID/Multi/00709/2013, IF/00178/2015/CP1300/CT0001), L'Oréal-UNESCO Portugal for Women in Science, BD Biosciences Immunology Grant.

REFERENCES

Angelo, L. S., and Kurzrock, R. (2007). Vascular endothelial growth factor and its relationship to inflammatory mediators. *Clin. Cancer Res.* 13, 2825–2830. doi: 10.1158/1078-0432.CCR-06-2416

Arnold, T., and Betsholtz, C. (2013). The importance of microglia in the development of the vasculature in the central nervous system. *Vasc. Cell* 5, 4. doi: 10.1186/2045-824X-5-4

Ashwal, S., Tone, B., Tian, H. R., Chong, S., and Obenaus, A. (2007). Comparison of two neonatal ischemic injury models using magnetic resonance imaging. *Pediatr. Res.* 61, 9–14. doi: 10.1203/01.pdr.0000251612.16069.4b

Back, S. A., Han, B. H., Luo, N. L., Chricton, C. A., Xanthoudakis, S., Tam, J., et al. (2002). Selective vulnerability of late oligodendrocyte progenitors to hypoxia–ischemia. *J. Neurosci.* 22, 455–463. doi: 10.1523/JNEUROSCI.22-02-00455.2002

Back, S. A., Luo, N. L., Borenstein, N. S., Levine, J. M., Volpe, J. J., and Kinney, H. C. (2001). Late oligodendrocyte progenitors coincide with the developmental window of vulnerability for human perinatal white matter injury. *J. Neurosci.* 21, 1302–1312. doi: 10.1523/JNEUROSCI.21-04-01302.2001

Back, S. A., Riddle, A., and McClure, M. M. (2007). Maturation-dependent vulnerability of perinatal white matter in premature birth. *Stroke* 38, 724–730. doi: 10.1161/01.STR.0000254729.27386.05

Bae, S. H., Kong, T. H., Lee, H. S., Kim, K. S., Hong, K. S., Chopp, M., et al. (2012). Long-lasting paracrine effects of human cord blood cells on damaged neocortex in an animal model of cerebral palsy. *Cell Transplant.* 21, 2497–2515. doi: 10.3727/096368912X640457

Barone, F. C., Knudsen, D. J., Nelson, A., Feuerstein, G., and Willette, R. N. (1993). Mouse strain differences in susceptibility to cerebral ischemia are related to cerebral vascular anatomy. *J. Cereb. Blood Flow Metab.* 13, 683–692. doi: 10.1038/jcbfm.1993.87

Basu, A. P. (2014). Early intervention after perinatal stroke: opportunities and challenges. *Dev. Med. Child. Neurol.* 56, 516–521. doi: 10.1111/dmcn.12407

Buerki, S. E., Grandgirard, D., Datta, A. N., Hackenberg, A., Martin, F., Schmitt-Mechelke, T., et al. (2016). Inflammatory markers in pediatric stroke: an attempt to better understanding the pathophysiology. *Eur. J. Paediatr. Neurol.* 20, 252–260. doi: 10.1016/j.ejpn.2015.12.006

Carmichael, S. T. (2005). Rodent models of focal stroke: size, mechanism, and purpose. *NeuroRx* 2, 396–409. doi: 10.1602/neurorx.2.3.396

Carreau, A., El Hafny-Rahbi, B., Matejuk, A., Grillon, C., and Kieda, C. (2011). Why is the partial oxygen pressure of human tissues a crucial parameter? Small molecules and hypoxia. *J. Cell. Mol. Med.* 15, 1239–1253. doi: 10.1111/j.1582-4934.2011.01258.x

Cnossen, M. H., van Ommen, C. H., and Appel, I. M. (2009). Etiology and treatment of perinatal stroke; a role for prothrombotic coagulation factors? *Semin. Fetal Neonatal Med.* 14, 311–317. doi: 10.1016/j.siny.2009.07.004

Del Duca, D., Wong, G., Trieu, P., Rodaros, D., Kouremenos, A., Tadevosyan, A., et al. (2009). Association of neonatal hypoxia with lasting changes in left ventricular gene expression: an animal model. *J. Thorac. Cardiovasc. Surg.* 138, 538–546.e1. doi: 10.1016/j.jtcvs.2009.04.042

Deruelle, P., Balasubramaniam, V., Kunig, A. M., Seedorf, G. J., Markham, N. E., and Abman, S. H. (2006). BAY 41-2272, a direct activator of soluble guanylate cyclase, reduces right ventricular hypertrophy and prevents pulmonary vascular remodeling during chronic hypoxia in neonatal rats. *Neonatology* 90, 135–144. doi: 10.1159/000092518

Dirnagl, U., Iadecola, C., and Moskowitz, M. A. (1999). Pathobiology of ischaemic stroke: an integrated view. *Trends Neurosci.* 22, 391–397. doi: 10.1016/S0166-2236(99)01401-0

Dunn, R., Queenan, B. N., Pak, D. T. S., and Forcelli, P. A. (2017). Divergent effects of levetiracetam and tiagabine against spontaneous seizures in adult rats following neonatal hypoxia. *Epilepsy Res.* 140, 1–7. doi: 10.1016/j.eplepsyres.2017.12.006

Faa, A., Iacovidou, N., Xanthos, T., Locci, A., Pampaloni, P., Aroni, F., et al. (2012). Hypoxia/reoxygenation-induced myocardial lesions in newborn piglets are related to interindividual variability and not to oxygen concentration. *Clinics* 67, 503–508. doi: 10.6061/clinics/2012(05)16

Fendt, M., Lex, A., Falkai, P., Henn, F., and Schmitt, A. (2008). Behavioural alterations in rats following neonatal hypoxia and effects of clozapine: implications for schizophrenia. *Pharmacopsychiatry* 41, 138–145. doi: 10.1055/s-2008-1058107

Fernández-López, D., Faustino, J., Derugin, N., and Vexler, Z. S. (2013). Acute and chronic vascular responses to experimental focal arterial stroke in the neonate rat. *Transl. Stroke Res.* 4, 179–188. doi: 10.1007/s12975-012-0214-5

Fernández-López, D., Natarajan, N., Ashwal, S., and Vexler, Z. S. (2014). Mechanisms of perinatal arterial ischemic stroke. *J. Cereb. Blood Flow Metab.* 34, 921–932. doi: 10.1038/jcbfm.2014.41

Ferreira, R., Fonseca, M. C., Santos, T., Sargento-Freitas, J., Tjeng, R., Paiva, F., et al. (2016). Retinoic acid-loaded polymeric nanoparticles enhance vascular regulation of neural stem cell survival and differentiation after ischaemia. *Nanoscale* 8, 8126–8137. doi: 10.1039/C5NR09077F

Garberg, H. T., Solberg, R., Barlinn, J., Martinez-Orgado, J., Løberg, E.-M., and Saugstad, O. D. (2017). High-dose cannabidiol-induced hypotension after global hypoxia-ischemia in piglets. *Neonatology* 112, 143–149. doi: 10.1159/000471786

Gersony, W. M., Morishima, H. O., Daniel, S. S., Kohl, S., Cohen, H., Brown, W., et al. (1976). The hemodynamic effects of intrauterine hypoxia: an experimental model in newborn lambs. *J. Pediatr.* 89, 631–635. doi: 10.1016/S0022-3476(76)80406-4

Girard, S., Kadhim, H., Beaudet, N., Sarret, P., and Sébire, G. (2009). Developmental motor deficits induced by combined fetal exposure to lipopolysaccharide and early neonatal hypoxia/ischemia: a novel animal model for cerebral palsy in very premature infants. *Neuroscience* 158, 673–682. doi: 10.1016/j.neuroscience.2008.10.032

Gonzalez, F. F., and Ferriero, D. M. (2009). Neuroprotection in the newborn infant. *Clin. Perinatol.* 36, 859–880, vii. doi: 10.1016/j.clp.2009.07.013

Govaert, P., Ramenghi, L., Taal, R., de Vries, L., and Deveber, G. (2009). Diagnosis of perinatal stroke I: definitions, differential diagnosis and registration. *Acta Paediatr.* 98, 1556–1567. doi: 10.1111/j.1651-2227.2009.01461.x

Gunny, R. S., and Lin, D. (2012). Imaging of perinatal stroke. *Magn. Reson. Imaging Clin. N. Am.* 20, 1–33. doi: 10.1016/j.mric.2011.10.001

Hagberg, H., Mallard, C., Ferriero, D. M., Vannucci, S. J., Levison, S. W., Vexler, Z. S., et al. (2015). The role of inflammation in perinatal brain injury. *Nat. Rev. Neurol.* 11, 192–208. doi: 10.1038/nrneurol.2015.13

Harbert, M. J., Tam, E. W., Glass, H. C., Bonifacio, S. L., Haeusslein, L. A., Barkovich, A. J., et al. (2011). Hypothermia is correlated with seizure absence in perinatal stroke. *J. Child. Neurol.* 26, 1126–1130. doi: 10.1177/0883073811408092

Heyer, A., Hasselblatt, M., von Ahsen, N., Häfner, H., Sirén, A. L., and Ehrenreich, H. (2005). *In vitro* gender differences in neuronal survival on hypoxia and in 17beta-estradiol-mediated neuroprotection. *J. Cereb. Blood Flow Metab.* 25, 427–430. doi: 10.1038/sj.jcbfm.9600056

Jantzie, L. L., Cheung, P. Y., and Todd, K. G. (2005). Doxycycline reduces cleaved caspase-3 and microglial activation in an animal model of neonatal hypoxia-ischemia. *J. Cereb. Blood Flow Metab.* 25, 314–324. doi: 10.1038/sj.jcbfm.9600025

Jantzie, L. L., and Todd, K. G. (2010). Doxycycline inhibits proinflammatory cytokines but not acute cerebral cytogenesis after hypoxia–ischemia in neonatal rats. *J. Psychiatry Neurosci.* 35, 20. doi: 10.1503/jpn.090061

Jensen, F. (1995). An animal model of hypoxia-induced perinatal seizures. *Ital. J. Neurol. Sci.* 16, 59–68. doi: 10.1007/BF02229075

Johnston, M. V. (2005). Excitotoxicity in perinatal brain injury. *Brain Pathol.* 15, 234–240. doi: 10.1111/j.1750-3639.2005.tb00526.x

Kameda, S. R., Fukushiro, D. F., Wuo-Silva, R., Trombin, T. F., Procópio-Souza, R., Brandão, L. C., et al. (2013). Opposite effects of neonatal hypoxia on acute amphetamine-induced hyperlocomotion in adult and adolescent mice. *Psychiatry Res.* 208, 74–77. doi: 10.1016/j.psychres.2013.03.021

Kartal, Ö., Aydinöz, S., Kartal, A. T., Kelestemur, T., Caglayan, A. B., Beker, M. C., et al. (2016). Time dependent impact of perinatal hypoxia on growth hormone, insulin-like growth factor 1 and insulin-like growth factor binding protein-3. *Metab. Brain Dis.* 31, 827–835. doi: 10.1007/s11011-016-9816-z

Kasdorf, E., and Perlman, J. M. (2013). Hyperthermia, inflammation, and perinatal brain injury. *Pediatr. Neurol.* 49, 8–14. doi: 10.1016/j.pediatrneurol.2012.12.026

Kichev, A., Rousset, C. I., Baburamani, A. A., Levison, S. W., Wood, T. L., Gressens, P., et al. (2014). Tumor necrosis factor-related apoptosis-inducing ligand (TRAIL) signaling and cell death in the immature central nervous system after hypoxia-ischemia and inflammation. *J. Biol. Chem.* 289, 9430–9439. doi: 10.1074/jbc.M113.512350

Kratzer, I., Chip, S., and Vexler, Z. S. (2014). Barrier mechanisms in neonatal stroke. *Front. Neurosci.* 8:359. doi: 10.3389/fnins.2014.00359

Kurnik, K., Kosch, A., Sträter, R., Schobess, R., Heller, C., Nowak-Göttl, U., et al. (2003). Recurrent thromboembolism in infants and children suffering from symptomatic neonatal arterial stroke: a prospective follow-up study. *Stroke* 34, 2887–2892. doi: 10.1161/01.STR.0000103745.03393.39

Lafemina, M. J., Sheldon, R. A., and Ferriero, D. M. (2006). Acute hypoxia-ischemia results in hydrogen peroxide accumulation in neonatal but not adult mouse brain. *Pediatr. Res.* 59, 680–683. doi: 10.1203/01.pdr.0000214891.35363.6a

Lange, C., Storkebaum, E., de Almodóvar, C. R., Dewerchin, M., and Carmeliet, P. (2016). Vascular endothelial growth factor: a neurovascular target in neurological diseases. *Nat. Rev. Neurol.* 12, 439–454. doi: 10.1038/nrneurol.2016.88

Lee, H. S., Han, J., Bai, H. J., and Kim, K. W. (2009). Brain angiogenesis in developmental and pathological processes: regulation, molecular and cellular communication at the neurovascular interface. *FEBS J.* 276, 4622–4635. doi: 10.1111/j.1742-4658.2009.07174.x

Lee, J., Croen, L. A., Backstrand, K. H., Yoshida, C. K., Henning, L. H., Lindan, C., et al. (2005). Maternal and infant characteristics associated with perinatal arterial stroke in the infant. *J. Am. Med. Assoc.* 293, 723–729. doi: 10.1001/jama.293.6.723

Leonardo, C. C., Hall, A. A., Collier, L. A., Gottschall, P. E., and Pennypacker, K. R. (2009). Inhibition of gelatinase activity reduces neural injury in an *ex vivo* model of hypoxia-ischemia. *Neuroscience* 160, 755–766. doi: 10.1016/j.neuroscience.2009.02.080

Leong, X. F., Ng, C. Y., and Jaarin, K. (2015). Animal models in cardiovascular research: hypertension and atherosclerosis. *BioMed Res. Int.* 2015, 528–757. doi: 10.1155/2015/528757

Leviton, A., and Gressens, P. (2007). Neuronal damage accompanies perinatal white-matter damage. *Trends Neurosci.* 30, 473–478. doi: 10.1016/j.tins.2007.05.009

Li, H., Pin, S., Zeng, Z., Wang, M. M., Andreasson, K. A., and McCullough, L. D. (2005). Sex differences in cell death. *Ann. Neurol.* 58, 317–321. doi: 10.1002/ana.20538

Lubics, A., Reglodi, D., Tamás, A., Kiss, P., Szalai, M., Szalontay, L., et al. (2005). Neurological reflexes and early motor behavior in rats subjected to neonatal hypoxic–ischemic injury. *Behav. Brain Res.* 157, 157–165. doi: 10.1016/j.bbr.2004.06.019

Luhmann, H. J., Sinning, A., Yang, J. W., Reyes-Puerta, V., Stüttgen, M. C., Kirischuk, S., et al. (2016). Spontaneous neuronal activity in developing neocortical networks: from single cells to large-scale interactions. *Front. Neural Circuits* 10:40. doi: 10.3389/fncir.2016.00040

Machado, V., Pimentel, S., Pinto, F., and Nona, J. (2015). Perinatal ischemic stroke: a five-year retrospective study in a level-III maternity. *Einstein* 13, 65–71. doi: 10.1590/S1679-45082015AO3056

Machado-Pereira, M., Santos, T., Ferreira, L., Bernardino, L., and Ferreira, R. (2017). Anti-inflammatory strategy for M2 microglial polarization using retinoic acid-loaded nanoparticles. *Mediators Inflamm.* 2017, 6742427. doi: 10.1155/2017/6742427

Machado-Pereira, M., Santos, T., Ferreira, L., Bernardino, L., and Ferreira, R. (2018). Intravenous administration of retinoic acid-loaded polymeric nanoparticles prevents ischemic injury in the immature brain. *Neurosci. Lett.* 673, 116–121. doi: 10.1016/j.neulet.2018.02.066

McQuillen, P. S., Sheldon, R. A., Shatz, C. J., and Ferriero, D. M. (2003). Selective vulnerability of subplate neurons after early neonatal hypoxia-ischemia. *J. Neurosci.* 23, 3308–3315. doi: 10.1523/JNEUROSCI.23-08-03308.2003

Mirabelli-Badenier, M., Braunersreuther, V., Lenglet, S., Galan, K., Veneselli, E., Viviani, G. L., et al. (2012). Pathophysiological role of inflammatory molecules in paediatric ischaemic brain injury. *Eur. J. Clin. Invest.* 42, 784–794. doi: 10.1111/j.1365-2362.2012.02640.x

Nelson, K. B. (2007). Perinatal ischemic stroke. *Stroke* 38, 742–745. doi: 10.1161/01.STR.0000247921.97794.5e

Nelson, K. B., and Lynch, J. K. (2004). Stroke in newborn infants. *Lancet Neurol.* 3, 150–158. doi: 10.1016/S1474-4422(04)00679-9

Ni, X., Yang, Z.-J., Carter, E. L., Martin, L. J., and Koehler, R. C. (2011). Striatal neuroprotection from neonatal hypoxia-ischemia in piglets by antioxidant treatment with EUK-134 or edaravone. *Dev. Neurosci.* 33, 299–311. doi: 10.1159/000327243

Rymo, S. F., Gerhardt, H., Sand, F. W., Lang, R., Uv, A., and Betsholtz, C. (2011). A two-way communication between microglial cells and angiogenic sprouts regulates angiogenesis in aortic ring cultures. *PLoS ONE* 6:e15846. doi: 10.1371/journal.pone.0015846

Schaeffer, E. L., Kühn, F., Schmitt, A., Gattaz, W. F., Gruber, O., Schneider-Axmann, T., et al. (2013). Increased cell proliferation in the rat anterior cingulate cortex following neonatal hypoxia: relevance to schizophrenia. *J. Neural Transm.* 120, 187–195. doi: 10.1007/s00702-012-0859-y

Sengupta, P. (2013). The laboratory rat: relating its age with human's. *Int. J. Prev. Med.* 4, 624–630.

Sheldon, R. A., Chuai, J., and Ferriero, D. M. (1996). A rat model for hypoxic-ischemic brain damage in very premature infants. *Neonatology* 69, 327–341. doi: 10.1159/000244327

Sheldon, R. A., Sedik, C., and Ferriero, D. M. (1998). Strain-related brain injury in neonatal mice subjected to hypoxia–ischemia. *Brain Res.* 810, 114–122. doi: 10.1016/S0006-8993(98)00892-0

Shen, Y., Plane, J. M., and Deng, W. (2010). Mouse models of periventricular leukomalacia. *J. Vis. Exp.* 39, 1951. doi: 10.3791/1951

Silverstein, F., and Johnston, M. V. (1984). Effects of hypoxia-ischemia on monoamine metabolism in the immature brain. *Ann. Neurol.* 15, 342–347. doi: 10.1002/ana.410150407

Slotkin, T. A., Lappi, S. E., McCook, E. C., Lorber, B. A., and Seidler, F. J. (1995). Loss of neonatal hypoxia tolerance after prenatal nicotine exposure: implications for sudden infant death syndrome. *Brain Res. Bull.* 38, 69–75. doi: 10.1016/0361-9230(95)00073-N

Sommer, C. J. (2017). Ischemic stroke: experimental models and reality. *Acta Neuropathol.* 133, 245–261. doi: 10.1007/s00401-017-1667-0

Stevens, J. P., Churchill, T., Fokkelman, K., Haase, E., Idikio, H., Korbutt, G., et al. (2008). Oxidative stress and matrix metalloproteinase-9 activity in the liver after hypoxia and reoxygenation with 21% or 100% oxygen in newborn piglets. *Eur. J. Pharmacol.* 580, 385–393. doi: 10.1016/j.ejphar.2007.11.019

Suzuki, Y., Nagai, N., and Umemura, K. (2016). A review of the mechanisms of blood-brain barrier permeability by tissue-type plasminogen activator treatment for cerebral ischemia. *Front. Cell Neurosci.* 10:2. doi: 10.3389/fncel.2016.00002

Tam, S. J., and Watts, R. J. (2010). Connecting vascular and nervous system development: angiogenesis and the blood-brain barrier. *Annu. Rev. Neurosci.* 33, 379–408. doi: 10.1146/annurev-neuro-060909-152829

Titomanlio, L., Fernández-López, D., Manganozzi, L., Moretti, R., Vexler, Z. S., and Gressens, P. (2015). Pathophysiology and neuroprotection of global and focal perinatal brain injury: lessons from animal models. *Pediatr. Neurol.* 52, 566–584. doi: 10.1016/j.pediatrneurol.2015.01.016

Tornabene, E., and Brodin, B. (2016). Stroke and drug delivery–*in vitro* models of the ischemic blood-brain barrier. *J. Pharma. Sci.* 105, 398–405. doi: 10.1016/j.xphs.2015.11.041

Turtzo, L. C., and McCullough, L. D. (2010). Sex-specific responses to stroke. *Fut. Neurol.* 5, 47–59. doi: 10.2217/fnl.09.66

Vannucci, R. C., and Vannucci, S. J. (2005). Perinatal hypoxic-ischemic brain damage: evolution of an animal model. *Dev. Neurosci.* 27, 81–86. doi: 10.1159/000085978

Vasudevan, A., and Bhide, P. G. (2008). Angiogenesis in the embryonic CNS: a new twist on an old tale. *Cell Adh. Migr.* 2, 167–169. doi: 10.4161/cam.2.3.6485

Vexler, Z. S., and Yenari, M. A. (2009). Does inflammation after stroke affect the developing brain differently than adult brain? *Dev. Neurosci.* 31, 378–393. doi: 10.1159/000232556

Webber, D. J., Van Blitterswijk, M., and Chandran, S. (2009). Neuroprotective effect of oligodendrocyte precursor cell transplantation in a long-term model of periventricular leukomalacia. *Am. J. Pathol.* 175, 2332–2342. doi: 10.2353/ajpath.2009.090051

Wolterink-Donselaar, I. G., Meerding, J. M., and Fernandes, C. (2009). A method for gender determination in newborn dark pigmented mice. *Lab. Anim.* 38, 35–38. doi: 10.1038/laban0109-35

Xu, G., Broadbelt, K. G., Haynes, R. L., Folkerth, R. D., Borenstein, N. S., Belliveau, R. A., et al. (2011). Late development of the GABAergic system in the human cerebral cortex and white matter. *J. Neuropathol. Exp. Neurol.* 70, 841–858. doi: 10.1097/NEN.0b013e31822f471c

Yu, L., Derrick, M., Ji, H., Silverman, R. B., Whitsett, J., Vásquez-Vivar, J., et al. (2011). Neuronal nitric oxide synthase inhibition prevents cerebral palsy following hypoxia-ischemia in fetal rabbits: comparison between JI-8 and 7-nitroindazole. *Dev. Neurosci.* 33, 312–319. doi: 10.1159/000327244

13

Mild Endoplasmic Reticulum Stress Protects Against Lipopolysaccharide-Induced Astrocytic Activation and Blood-Brain Barrier Hyperpermeability

*Yiwei Wang†, Yinan Chen†, Qin Zhou, Jiawen Xu, Qingqing Qian, Pengfei Ni and Yanning Qian**

Department of Anesthesiology, The First Affiliated Hospital of Nanjing Medical University, Nanjing, China

***Correspondence:**
Yanning Qian
yanning_qian@163.com

† These authors have contributed equally to this work.

Recent research has revealed that uncontrolled chronic neuroinflammation is closely associated with diverse neurodegenerative diseases, by impairing blood-brain barrier (BBB) function and astrocytic reaction. Endoplasmic reticulum (ER) stress is conventionally linked to the loss of neuronal structure and function and should be widely attenuated. This notion has been questioned by recent experimental studies, which have shown that non-harmful levels of ER stress had numerous beneficial roles against neurodegeneration, including neuroprotection and inhibition of cytokine production. Here, we investigated the mild ER stress-based regulation of LPS-induced inflammatory responses in astrocytes. Primary astrocytes were exposed to tunicamycin (TM), a compound that activates ER stress, with or without the ER-stress inhibitor sodium 4-phenylbutyrate (4-PBA) before LPS treatment. Astrocytic activation, proinflammatory factor production, and the extent of ER stress were assessed. In addition, the effect of mild ER stress on astrocytes and BBB function was determined *in vivo*. Male Sprague-Dawley rats received intracerebroventricular injections of TM with or without intraperitoneal 4-PBA before LPS administration. The levels of astrocytic activation and BBB permeability were measured after treatment. Our results showed that lower doses of TM resulted in a mild ER-stress response without inducing cytotoxicity and tissue toxicity. Non-toxic ER-stress preconditioning ameliorated LPS-induced overactivation and inflammatory responses in astrocytes. Moreover, pre-exposure to non-lethal doses of TM improved LPS-induced BBB impairment and cognitive ability dysfunction in rats. However, 4-PBA, reversed the protective effect of TM preconditioning *in vitro* and *in vivo*. We conclude that mild ER stress ("preconditioning") can alleviate LPS-induced astrocytic activation and BBB disruption. Our findings provide a better understanding for the regulatory role of ER stress in neuroinflammation and indicate that mild ER stress might have therapeutic value for the treatment of neurodegenerative diseases.

Keywords: endoplasmic reticulum stress, astrocytes, hormesis, blood-brain barrier, neuroinflammation, neurodegeneration

INTRODUCTION

Neurodegeneration is characterized by neuronal dysfunction and death in the central nervous system (CNS) (Estes and McAllister, 2016). Emerging evidence indicates that sustained inflammatory responses in the CNS associated with blood-brain barrier (BBB)-disruption contribute to neurodegenerative-disease progression (Glass et al., 2010; Broux et al., 2015). Systemic injection of lipopolysaccharide (LPS), a complex molecule containing both lipid and polysaccharide parts, can elicit neuroinflammation in the normal rat brain (Pintado et al., 2012). Animals with LPS-induced neuroinflammation are therefore frequently used as an experimental model for neurodegeneration and cognitive disorders (Qin et al., 2007).

Considering the many essential functions of astrocytes in the healthy CNS, astrocytic dysfunction might participate in the propagation and regulation of neuroinflammation. Astrocytes become activated in response to various stimuli, from subtle inflammatory changes in their microenvironment to massive neuronal damage (Sofroniew, 2015). Reactive astrocytes appear to play vital roles in mediating the production of proinflammatory effector molecules and amplifiers, such as chemokines, cytokines, and reactive oxygen species. These influence the state of surrounding cells (e.g., neurons, microglia, and other astrocytes), thereby triggering neuroinflammation leading to exacerbation of neurotoxicity and neurodegeneration (Gorina et al., 2011).

At least one-third of all proteins in the cell are first synthesized, folded, and structurally mature in the endoplasmic reticulum (ER); then, they are transported to the membrane compartment (Hetz and Mollereau, 2014). In astrocytes, the ER acquires a central role in sensing cellular stress after protein unfolding/misfolding in its lumen (known as ER stress), with the consequent activation of a cellular response termed the "unfolded protein response" (UPR). UPR is initiated by three principal stress sensors: the inositol-requiring protein 1α (IRE1α)-spliced X-box-binding protein 1 (XBP1s) pathway, the activating transcription factor (ATF)-6α pathway, and the protein kinase RNA-like ER kinase (PERK)-eukaryotic translation initiation factor 2α (EIF2α) pathway (Martin-Jiménez et al., 2017).

Endoplasmic reticulum stress in astrocytes has sometimes been viewed as a response mainly contributing to neurodegeneration, which should therefore be broadly attenuated (Martin-Jiménez et al., 2017). This notion is refuted by rapidly growing evidence, which shows that non-harmful levels of ER stress exert numerous beneficial functions that improve outcomes in CNS inflammation (Hetz and Mollereau, 2014; Matus et al., 2014). These findings have been reinforced by an array of related studies. A recent study showed that pretreatment with ER stressors protected against amyloid-β toxicity to reverse memory impairment in Alzheimer's disease (AD) (Casas-Tinto et al., 2011). Similarly, maintaining ER stress at a moderate level inhibits neuronal death in mouse and *Drosophila* Parkinson disease (PD) models (Fouillet et al., 2014). It is significant to emphasize that the roles of ER stress in neurodegenerative conditions are not stereotypically linear, but instead context-specific and complex, as determined by the type, severity, time, and duration of the insult. Specific mechanisms need to be identified and addressed.

In cardiac surgery, myocardial ischemic preconditioning is favorable for improving heart function. There is growing awareness that low perturbations of ER function also trigger a hormetic response, known as "ER hormesis," which involves a biologically-favorable response induced by exposing a cell/organism to non-lethal pharmacological ER stressors (Matus et al., 2014). However, there have so far been few scientific studies on the involvement of ER hormesis in astrocytes. Therefore, in the current study, we aimed to elucidate the effects of mild ER stress on LPS-induced inflammatory responses in astrocytes and to investigate whether mild ER stress exerts a protective effect against LPS-induced BBB hyperpermeability.

MATERIALS AND METHODS

Animals

One hundred and seventy-four male Sprague-Dawley (SD) rats (weight: 180–220 g) were used in the current study. All experiments were performed according to the ethical guidelines of the National Institutes of Health (NIH) guide for the Care and Use of Laboratory animals (NIH Publications No. 8023, revised 1978) and approved by the Nanjing Medical University Animal Care and Use Committee (IACUC-14030126). The rats were housed under standardized conditions (12-h light/dark cycle, 22.0 ± 1.0°C, and 40% humidity), and water and food were provided *ad libitum*. Based on the 3R principle for the ethical use of animals in research, all efforts were made to reduce animal use and suffering.

Intracerebroventricular Cannula Implantation

Rats were implanted with an indwelling lateral intracerebroventricular (icv) catheter for brain injection of drugs as previously described (Zhang et al., 2016). The animals were anesthetized (isoflurane, 2.1% inspired concentration in 0.3 FiO2) and placed on a stereotaxic apparatus. Stereotaxic coordinates for the placement of the icv cannulas were 0.8 mm rostral, 1.5 mm lateral to the bregma, and 3.7 mm ventral from the dorsal surface of the skull. Rats were individually housed after surgery and handled daily to familiarize the animals with the investigators and to check the guide catheter. Rats were allowed a minimum of 14 days to recover prior to icv administration of pharmacological agents and/or other experimental measurements.

Behavioral Tests

Trace fear conditioning, contextual assessment, and the Y-maze test were performed. The molecular-biology tests and the behavioral experiments were conducted using different animals. The behavioral test design is briefly illustrated in Supplementary Figure 1A. The specific methods can be found in the Supplementary Material.

Drug Administration

The well-known ER-stress inducer tunicamycin (TM) was diluted in sterile saline containing 10% dimethyl sulfoxide (DMSO) to create a stock concentration of 15 μg/μl. Then, 4-phenylbutyric acid (4-PBA), a common ER-stress inhibitor, was diluted with sterile saline to a concentration of 10 mg/ml and injected intraperitoneally (ip) at a dose of 100 mg/kg according to a previous study (Wang et al., 2017). LPS was dissolved in sterile saline to the concentration of 50 μg/ml. Each rat was ip-injected at a dose of 500 μg/kg, according to our previous study (Sun et al., 2015).

Experimental Protocol and Pharmacological Treatments

Experiment 1 (*In Vivo*)

Rats were divided into five groups (groups A–E), with 16 animals in each group. Empty treatments were administered to the rats in group A. Rats received either icv injections of 2 μl of vehicle (group B), 2 μl of 0.15 μg/μl TM (group C), 2 μl of 1.5 μg/μl TM (group D), or 2 μl of 15 μg/μl TM (group E). These concentrations were based on previous work from our laboratory (Wang et al., 2017). The study design is briefly illustrated in Supplementary Figures 1B,C.

Experiment 2 (*In Vivo*)

Rats were randomly divided into five groups (groups A–E), with 16 animals in each group. Rats in groups B, C, D, and E received icv cannula implantation, while empty treatments were administered to the rats in group A. Rats were administered an intraperitoneal injection of 100 mg/kg 4-PBA (group E) or an equivalent volume of sterile saline (groups B–D). Next, a dose of 2 μl of 1.5 μg/μl TM (groups D and E) or 2 μl of vehicle (10% DMSO in saline) (group B and C) was injected through the brain cannulas. One hour after 4-PBA/TM treatment, intraperitoneal injections were administered (group B: normal saline; groups C, D, and E: 500 μg/kg LPS). The experimental design is briefly illustrated in Supplementary Figures 1D,E.

According to the "3R" principle of ethical animal use, the same rats were used for group A in both experiments 1 and 2.

Experiment 1 (*In Vitro*)

Primary astrocytes were incubated for 24 h at different concentrations of TM (0.1, 1, and 10 ng/ml). The study design is briefly shown in Supplementary Figure 1F.

Experiment 2 (*In Vitro*)

Astrocytes were pretreated transiently with TM at 1 ng/ml with or without 4-PBA for 1 h, followed by thorough washing to remove the TM and 4-PBA, and incubated in fresh medium with or without LPS for 24 h. The experimental procedure is briefly illustrated in Supplementary Figure 1G.

Primary Astrocyte Cultures

Primary astrocyte cultures were prepared from neonatal (P1–P2) rat brains as previously described (Xu et al., 2018). Briefly, the cerebral cortices were isolated and digested at 37°C for 10 min in phosphate-buffered saline (PBS) containing 0.25% trypsin-EDTA. The dissociated cells were passed through a 100-μm pore mesh to remove debris. The cell suspension was seeded on poly-D-lysine-coated flasks in high-glucose Dulbecco's Modified Eagle's medium supplemented with 10% fetal bovine serum. The culture medium was changed for fresh solution every 3 days. After 10 days of cultivation, astrocytes were separated from the microglia by shaking for 5 h at 150 rpm. The purity of the astrocytes was >95% as confirmed by anti-GFAP immunochemical staining.

Cell Counting Kit-8 (CCK-8) Assay

Astrocytic viability was quantified using a CCK-8 assay based on the manufacturer's instructions (Beyotime, Shanghai, China). Briefly, 10 μl of the CCK-8 solution was added to each well of a 96-well plate containing 3×10^4 astrocytes following treatment with different concentrations of reagents and the absorbance was measured after a 1-h incubation at 37°C at 450 nm using a DTX-880 multimode microplate reader. Each experiment was repeated at least three times.

Enzyme-Linked Immunosorbent Assay (ELISA)

IL-6 and IL-1β levels in the astrocytic supernatant were measured using ELISA kits from R&D Systems (Minneapolis, MN, United States) according to the manufacturer's instructions. See the Supplementary Material for more information.

Western Blot Analysis

Hippocampal tissues and astrocytes were homogenized in RIPA lysis buffer, which contained 50 mM Tris, 150 mM NaCl, 1% Triton X-100, 2 mM EDTA, 1.5 μg/mL leupeptin, and 1 mM phenylmethylsulfonyl fluoride. The lysate was centrifuged for 20 min at 12,000 × *g* at 4°C. The protein content was determined by BCA assay (Thermo Scientific, Waltham, MA, United States), and 20 μg of protein was loaded per lane on a modified sodium dodecyl sulfate polyacrylamide gel electrophoresis. Separated proteins were transferred onto polyvinylidene difluoride membranes (Milipore, Bedford, MA, United States) and blocked for 1 h with 5% non-fat milk in Tris-buffered saline with Tween 20. Blocked membranes were probed overnight with specific primary antibodies diluted in 5% non-fat milk according to the recommendation of the manufacturer. After washing, membranes were incubated with anti-rabbit or anti-mouse IgG-HRP secondary antibodies, washed, and incubated with ECL reagent before exposure to film. Densitometry analysis was performed with the Image Lab software (Bio-Rad, Richmond, CA, United States) and quantified using the gel analysis plugin for Image J (NIH, Bethesda, MD, United States).

Immunohisto/Cytochemistry

The astrocyte culture medium was removed, and cells were fixed with 4% paraformaldehyde (PFA) for 30 min. The cells were then blocked with 5% bovine serum albumin containing 0.1% Triton X-100 for 1 h. Specific primary antibodies were added at an indicated concentration and incubated overnight at 4°C. Following washes with PBS, the secondary antibodies (Alexa-Fluor-conjugated) were added and incubated for 1 h at 37°C. The images were captured using a confocal microscope (Zeiss LSM 510; Zeiss, Oberkochen, Germany).

Immunohistochemistry was used to determine the activation of the astrocytes in the hippocampus. Briefly, rats were perfused transcardially with 37°C saline followed by ice-cold 4% PFA. The ipsilateral hippocampal tissue was removed and fixed for 1 h in 4% PFA at 4°C. The tissue was sectioned at 15 μm with a cryostat. Sections were incubated overnight with specific primary antibodies followed by the appropriate secondary antibodies. Confocal images were obtained with a confocal microscope (Zeiss LSM 510).

The confocal microscope parameters were maintained constant across all samples, and samples of different groups were always processed in parallel. Fluorescence intensity was quantified using ImageJ and normalized to the fluorescence levels observed in untreated samples as described.

Evan's Blue (EB) Extravasation

Two percent of EB dye (Sigma-Aldrich, St. Louis, MI, United States) in 0.9% saline (5 mL/kg) was injected intravenously (right femoral vein), and 30 min later, the rats were perfused transcardially with 0.9% saline to remove the intravascular blood and EB. Then, the brains were harvested and homogenized in 0.5 ml of 50% trichloroacetic acid and centrifuged at 10,000 × *g* for 10 min. EB concentrations in supernatants were measured using spectrophotometry at 620 nm.

Statistical Analysis

Data are expressed as mean ± SEM. Two-tailed unpaired *t*-tests were used for comparisons between two groups, and multiple comparisons were evaluated using an appropriate ANOVA. *Post hoc* comparisons were performed using Tukey's test when appropriate. The alpha level was set at $P < 0.05$.

RESULTS

Low Concentrations of TM Generated Non-toxic, Mild ER Stress in Astrocytes

Many studies have shown that astrocytes may be vulnerable to ER stress-induced cell apoptosis. Consequently, primary cultured astrocytes were first exposed to different concentrations of TM for 24 h and their activities were tested using the CCK8 reagent. Our results indicate that TM (<10 ng/ml) had no effects on the cell viability of astrocytes compared to the control group (**Figure 1A**). Therefore, doses of 0.1, 1, and 10 ng/ml were selected for the subsequent experiments. The next experiment was conducted to explore whether lower concentrations of TM could also cause mild ER stress in astrocytes.

IRE1α initiates the most conservative signaling pathway of ER stress that, upon phosphorylation, cuts the non-conventional splicing of XBP-1 (XBP1u) mRNA into spliced-XBP1 (XBP1s) mRNA, which encodes a transcription activator that regulates ER protein folding (Gardner et al., 2013). Thus, to further determine the extent of IRE1-signaling activation, we measured the protein levels of p-IRE1α, XBP1s, and XBP1u using western blot analysis with specific antibodies (**Figure 1B**). TM (0.1, 1, and 10 ng/ml) significantly increased the expression levels of p-IRE1α and XBP1s, while the same treatment reduced XBP1u expression (**Figures 1C,D**). As a crucial stress sensor of ER stress, PERK is a transmembrane kinase that phosphorylates EIF2α at Ser51(Gardner et al., 2013). However, persistent EIF2α phosphorylation paradoxically upregulates translation of ATF4 mRNA, which in turn activates pro-apoptotic components such as the transcription of CCAAT/enhancer binding protein (C/EBP) homologous protein (CHOP) (Hetz and Mollereau, 2014).

To characterize the activation kinetics of PERK signaling of ER stress, we examined the expression of p-PERK and its downstream products: p-EIF2α, ATF4, and CHOP using western blot analysis. Compared with the control group, p-PERK and p-EIF2α phosphorylation was modestly elevated at concentrations of 0.1, 1, and 10 ng/ml TM (**Figure 1C**). It is worth noting that lower doses of TM (0.1 and 1 ng/ml) were no longer effective at increasing ATF4 and CHOP expression levels but that high concentrations (10 ng/ml) did increase ATF4 and CHOP expression (**Figure 1E**).

Similar results were also observed in the immunofluorescence assay (**Figures 2A,B**). Consistent with the previous data, increases of IRE1α phosphorylation were observed following TM treatment (0.1, 1, and 10 ng/ml) in the primary cultured astrocytes (**Figure 2C**). CHOP levels, in contrast, were not changed in primary cultured astrocytes treated with TM at doses of 0.1 or 1 ng/ml. The CHOP expression was only elevated in response to the highest dose of TM (10 ng/ml) (**Figure 2D**). These findings showed that lower concentrations of TM (0.1 and 1 ng/ml) triggered benign and mild ER-stress responses in the astrocytes.

Mild ER Stress Attenuated LPS-Induced Astrocytic Inflammatory Responses and Overactivation

We observed that low concentrations of TM (0.1 and 1 ng/ml) caused mild ER stress in the astrocytes but did not induce cell death. In the following experiment, we therefore selected a dosage of TM (1 ng/ml) to generate mild ER stress in the astrocytes. Next, we investigated the effects of mild ER stress in LPS-stimulated astrocyte activation.

TM Inhibited IL-1β and IL-6 Production in Primary Cultured Astrocytes

Astrocytes were treated with LPS in the absence or presence of TM. Because astrocytes participate in neuroinflammation via the excessive secretion of proinflammatory factors, IL-6 and IL-1β were analyzed with ELISA. As the results shown in **Figure 3** illustrate, LPS enhanced the expression of IL-1β and IL-6. Additionally, 1 ng/ml TM did not enhance, but instead suppressed, LPS-induced proinflammatory factor expression.

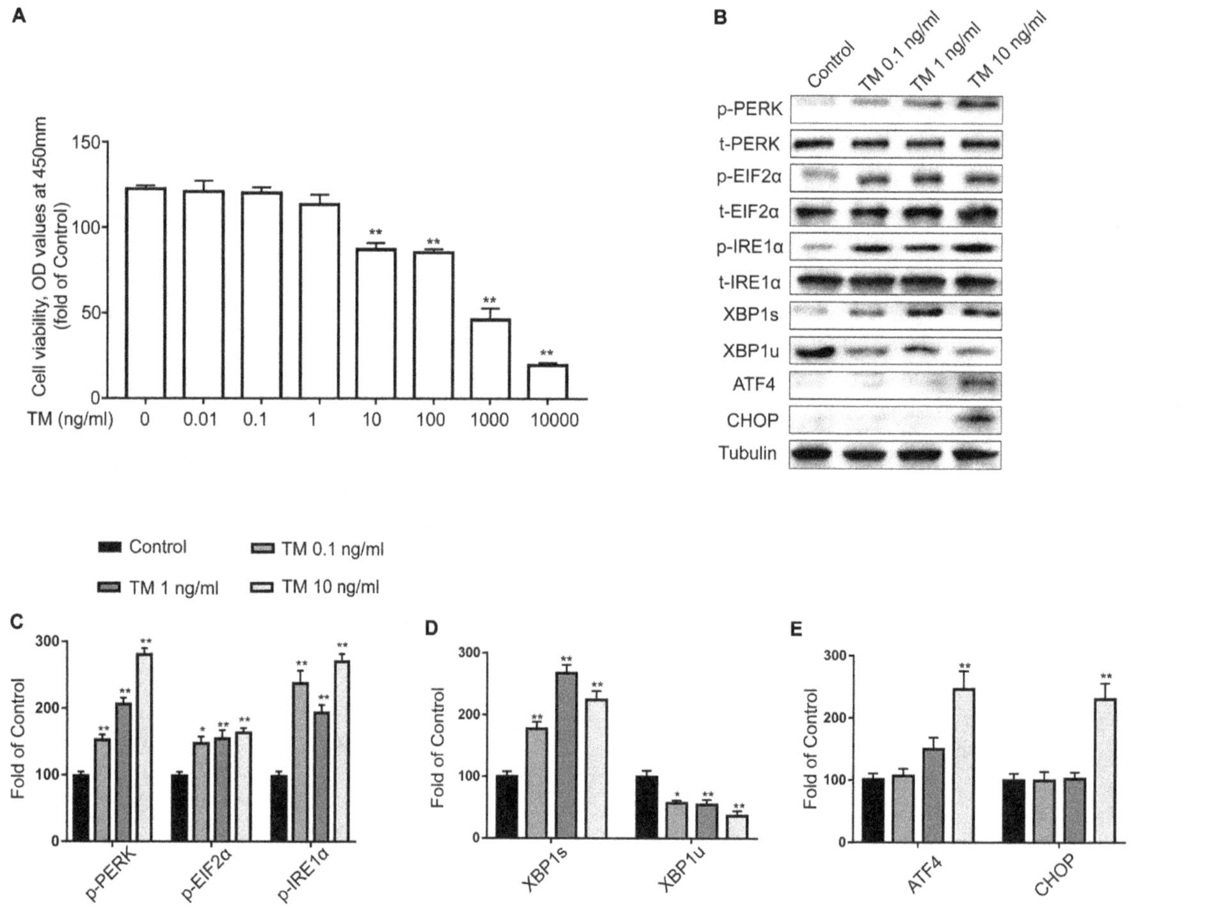

FIGURE 1 | Low doses of TM activated a non-toxic, mild ER stress in primary cultured astrocytes. **(A)** Primary astrocytes were treated with TM (0.01 to 10000 ng/ml) for 24 h followed by assessment of cell viability using the CCK-8 assay. **(B)** The expression levels of p-PERK, p-EIF2α, p-IRE1α, XBP1s, XBP1u, ATF4, and CHOP in primary cultured astrocytes were detected by Western blotting using specific antibodies. **(C)** Phosphorylated levels of PERK, EIF2α, and IRE1α were quantified and normalized to corresponding total levels. **(D)** Expression of XBP1s and XBP1u was quantified and normalized to Tubulin expression. **(E)** Expression of ATF4 and CHOP was quantified and normalized to Tubulin expression. Each value was then expressed relative to that of the control group, which was set to 100. All experiments were repeated three times. *$P < 0.05$, **$P < 0.01$ vs. control group. The data are presented as the mean ± SEM.

TM Reversed LPS-Induced Astrocyte Activation

To further confirm the protective effects of TM on primary astrocytes, GFAP expression levels corresponding to activated astrocytes were tested with western blot analysis. LPS significantly increased the expression of GFAP in primary cultured astrocytes compared with the levels observed in the control group, but these elevations were remarkably inhibited by TM pretreatment (**Figures 4A,B**). To validate these findings, astrocytes were labeled with GFAP by immunofluorescence (**Figures 4C,D**), which also confirmed that TM can inhibit LPS-induced astrocytic activation.

4-PBA Reversed TM-Induced Suppression of Astrocytic IL-1β, IL-6, and GFAP Production

Next, we examined whether mild ER-stress activation is responsible for TM-mediated inhibition of astrocytic activation and anti-inflammatory responses.

To test this hypothesis, we used a chemical chaperone, 4-PBA, to reduce ER stress. Astrocytes were first subjected to TM (1 ng/ml), individually or in the presence of 4-PBA at progressive concentrations for 1 h before treatment with LPS (100 ng/ml) for 24 h. Our results indicate that treatment of the primary cultured astrocytes with 1 ng/ml TM and 100 ng/ml LPS in the presence of T 4-PBA (<1,000 μM) had no significant cytotoxicity (**Figure 5**). We therefore selected a dose of 100 μM 4-PBA to ameliorate ER stress in the astrocytes. The primary cultured astrocytes were subjected to TM (1 ng/ml) and 4-PBA (100 μM) treatment for 1 h. Reperfusion was then performed by refreshing the astrocytes with normal medium, containing 100 ng/ml LPS. As shown in **Figure 6A**, there was a clear effect of 4-PBA against ER stress, as it obviously decreased p-PERK, p-EIF2α, p-IRE1α, and XBP1s protein levels and increased XBP1u protein levels compared to non-PBA treated cells (**Figures 6B–D**).

Importantly, 4-PBA partially blocked the TM-mediated inhibition of astrocytic activation and anti-inflammatory effects, as reflected by the increased expression of IL-1β, IL-6, and GFAP. We wondered whether this opposite effect was caused by the cytotoxic effects of 4-PBA.

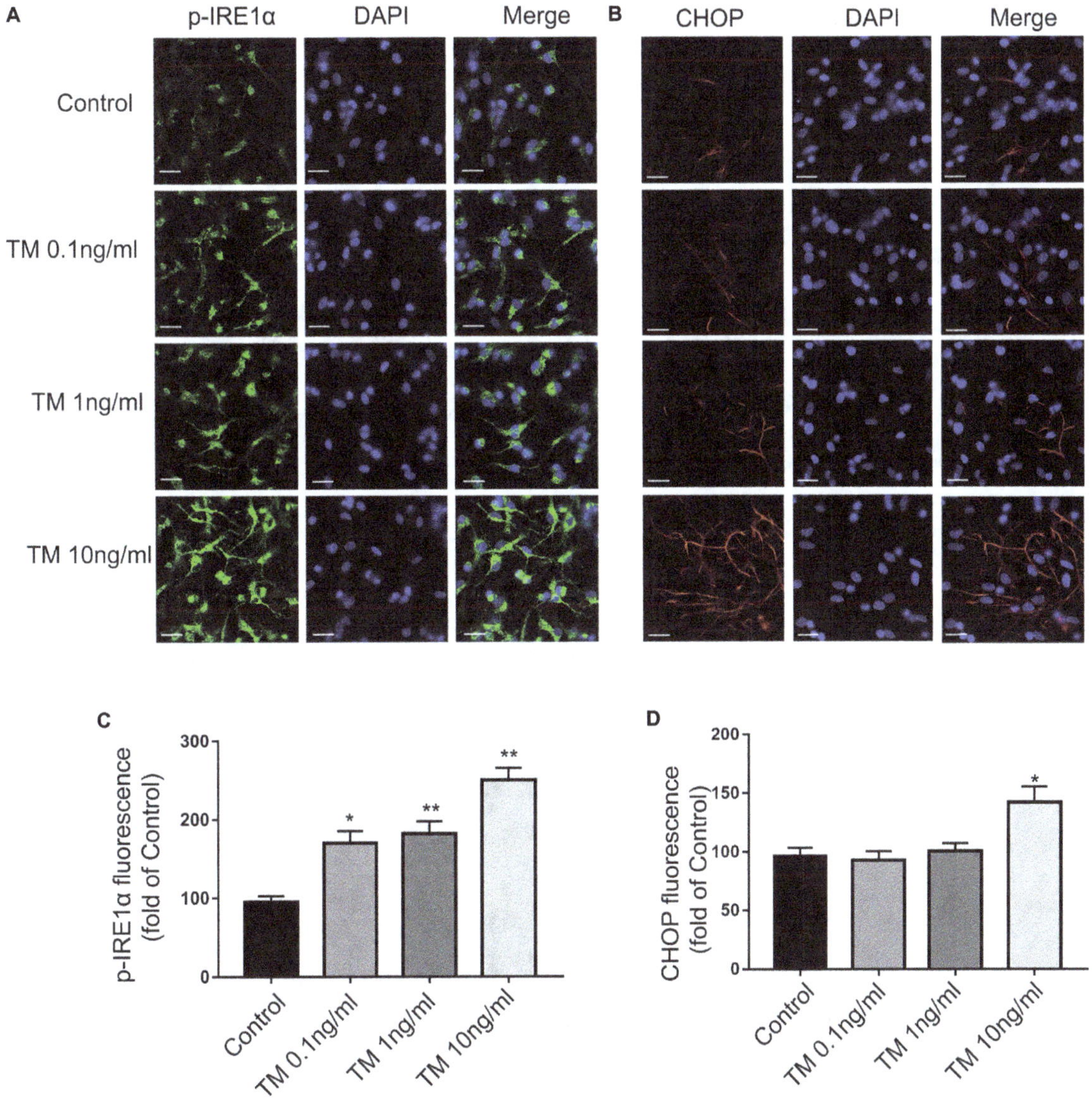

FIGURE 2 | Mild ER stress increased p-IRE1α expression but had no effect on CHOP expression in primary cultured astrocytes. **(A)** Astrocytes were stained with p-IRE1α antibody. p-IRE1α-immunopositivity in primary astrocytes was observed using confocal scanning. **(B)** Astrocytes were stained with CHOP antibody. CHOP-immunopositivity in primary astrocytes was observed using confocal scanning. Blue staining represents DAPI. Scale bar = 25 μm. **(C)** Quantitative data of the mean intensity of p-IRE1α fluorescence in primary astrocytes. **(D)** Quantitative data of the mean intensity of CHOP fluorescence in primary astrocytes. Each value was then expressed relative to that of the control group, which was set to 100. All experiments were repeated three times. $^{*}P < 0.05$, $^{**}P < 0.01$ vs. control group. The data are presented as the mean ± SEM.

Using the CCK-8 method, we excluded this possibility, as coincubation with LPS (100 ng/ml), TM (1 ng/ml), and 4-PBA (100 μM) for 24 h revealed no significant cytotoxicity and did not affect cell viability (**Figure 5**). Collectively, these data demonstrate that TM pretreatment protected astrocytes by, at least partly, inducing mild ER stress.

Mild ER Stress Ameliorated LPS-Induced Cognitive Decline

To confirm the *in vitro* findings, we also examined the effects of mild ER stress *in vivo*.

Our previous study showed that a 3-μg dose of TM triggered mild and benign perturbations of ER function in the rat hippocampus but did not induce drastic behavioral alterations or death (Wang et al., 2017). In the following experiment, rats were administered an icv injection of 3 μg TM to induce mild ER stress followed by systemic LPS administration.

Consistent with our previous experiment, LPS caused severe memory impairment in rats, as reflected by a significant reduction in freezing behavior and an improvement in the number of learning trials (Sun et al., 2015; Wang et al., 2017). Notably, TM pretreatment ameliorated

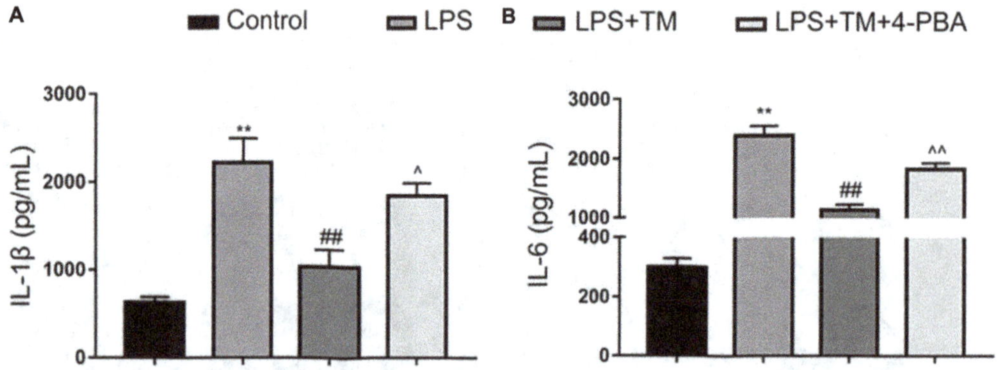

FIGURE 3 | Mild ER stress inhibits proinflammatory cytokine IL-1β and IL-6 production in primary cultured astrocytes. **(A)** The levels of the proinflammatory factors IL-1β were detected by ELISA. **(B)** The levels of the proinflammatory factors IL-6 were detected by ELISA. The data are representative of 3 independent experiments. $^{*}P < 0.05$, $^{**}P < 0.01$ vs. control group. $^{\#}P < 0.05$, $^{\#\#}P < 0.01$ vs. LPS treatment group. $^{\wedge}P < 0.05$, $^{\wedge\wedge}P < 0.01$ vs. TM treatment group. The data are presented as the mean ± SEM.

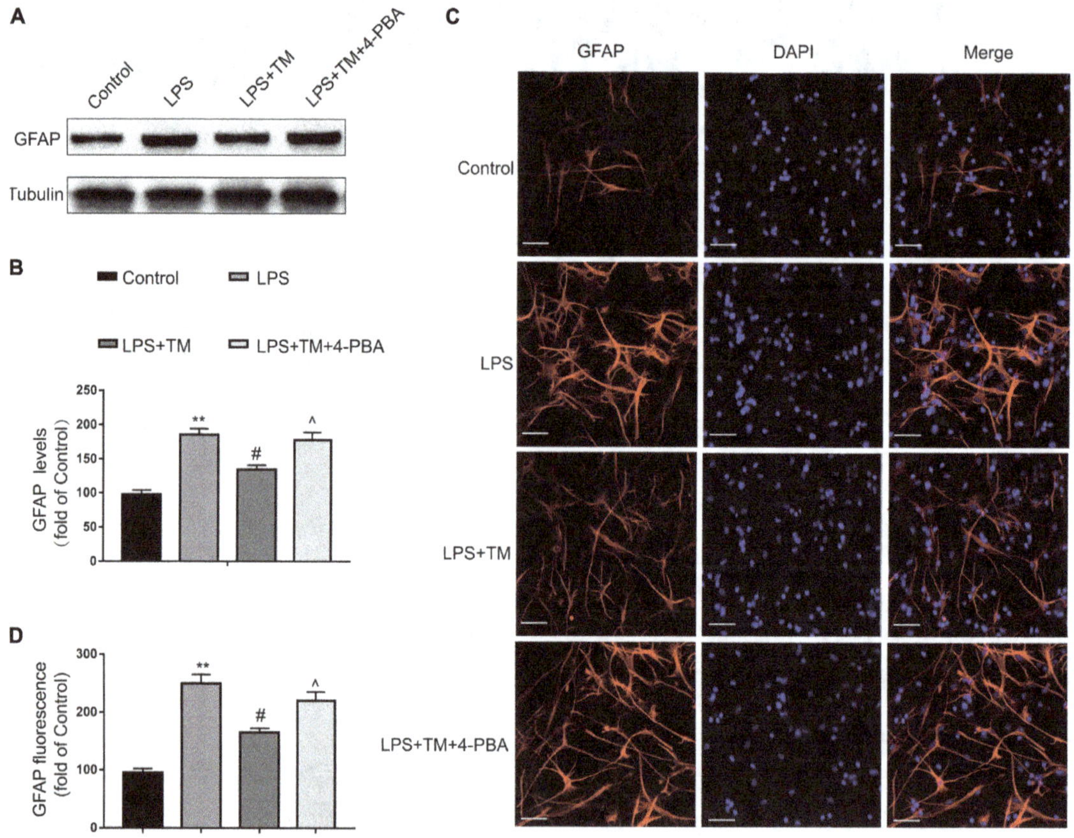

FIGURE 4 | Mild ER stress alleviated astrocyte activation. **(A)** The protein levels of GFAP were detected by Western blotting using specific antibody in the primary astrocytes. **(B)** Expression of GFAP was quantified and normalized to Tubulin levels. Each value is expressed relative to that in the control group, which was set to 100. **(C)** Astrocyte was stained with GFAP antibody as indicated. Blue staining represents DAPI. Scale bar = 25 μm. **(D)** Quantitative data of the mean intensity of GFAP fluorescence in primary astrocytes. Each value is expressed relative to that in the control group, which was set to 100. All experiments were repeated three times. $^{*}P < 0.05$, $^{**}P < 0.01$ vs. control group. $^{\#}P < 0.05$, $^{\#\#}P < 0.01$ vs. LPS treatment group. $^{\wedge}P < 0.05$, $^{\wedge\wedge}P < 0.01$ vs. TM treatment group. The data are presented as the mean ± SEM.

LPS-induced cognitive decline. However, concomitant administration of 4-PBA partially reversed the cognitive recovery conferred by TM (**Figure 7**). Therefore, these results further substantiate our previous findings that mild ER stress can protect against LPS-induced cognitive dysfunction.

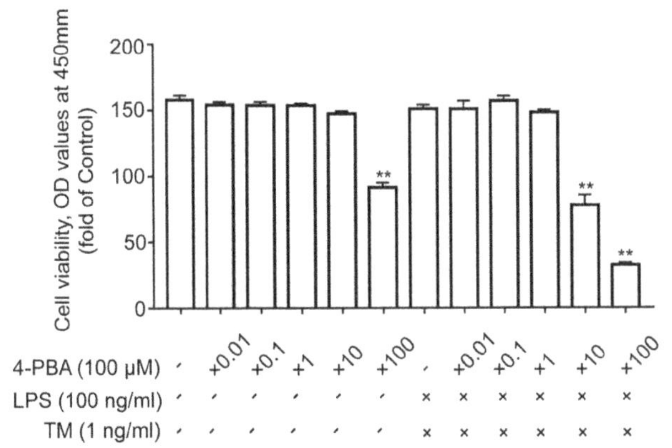

FIGURE 5 | The effects of 4-PBA on cell viability in primary astrocytes. Primary cultured astrocytes were subjected to LPS and TM and treated with the indicated dosage of 4-PBA. After 24 h of treatment, cell viability was determined using CCK-8. All experiments were repeated three times. $^{*}P < 0.05$, $^{**}P < 0.01$ vs. control group. The data are presented as the mean ± SEM.

Mild ER Stress Attenuated LPS-Induced Astrocytic Activation in the Hippocampus

The western blot analysis showed that systemic LPS administration enhanced the expression of GFAP in the hippocampi of rats, but these elevations were potently suppressed by TM pretreatment. Similar to the *in vitro* results, 4-PBA diminished the TM-mediated inhibition of astrocytic activation in the hippocampus (**Figures 8A,B**). These western blot findings were further validated by immunofluorescence (**Figures 8C,D**). Our results therefore further confirmed that mild ER stress was required for the TM-mediated protection.

Mild ER Stress Alleviated LPS-Induced BBB Hyperpermeability

Mild ER Stress Counteracted LPS-Induced Albumin Leakage in the Hippocampus

As BBB disruption leads to an extravasation of blood-borne proteins, we examined the leakage of albumin to confirm the integrity of the BBB. As shown in **Figure 9A**, LPS significantly increased albumin levels in the hippocampus of rats, compared with the naive group. Although TM administration induced a dramatic decrease in albumin expression, 4-PBA greatly diminished this effect (**Figure 9B**).

Mild ER Stress Inhibited the Decreases in Hippocampal Occludin and Claudin-5 Induced by LPS

Decreased tight-junction protein expressions are associated with alterations in BBB permeability. As occludin and claudin-5 are reportedly integral tight-junction membrane proteins (Qi et al., 2016), we examined the levels of occludin and claudin-5 in the hippocampus of rats with western blot analysis. LPS evoked significant decreases in occludin and claudin-5 protein expression compared with the naive group. Treatment with TM effectively negated the increases in hippocampal occludin and claudin-5 induced by LPS, while no elevated occludin and claudin-5 expression was detected after 4-PBA administration (**Figures 9C,D**).

Immunofluorescence staining was also used to analyze occludin and claudin-5 protein expression (**Figures 9E–H**), showing a marked decrease in occludin and claudin-5 protein levels in the LPS group compared with the naive group. Impressively, TM treatment significantly attenuated the occludin and claudin-5 protein expression decrease induced LPS, but 4-PBA cotreatment partially reversed the effect of TM. These results show that mild ER stress prevented BBB disruption by decreasing tight-junction protein levels.

Mild ER Stress Reversed the Increases in Hippocampal Matrix Metalloproteinase (MMP)-2 and MMP-9 Induced by LPS

Based on the recent observation that MMP activity is associated with the degradation of tight-junction proteins (Tasaki et al., 2014), we next monitored the expression of MMP-2 and MMP-9 upon mild ER stress induction. As expected, LPS treatment significantly increased MMP-2 and MMP-9 activity, while pretreatment with TM significantly attenuated LPS treatment-induced MMP-2 and MMP-9 activity. The expression levels of MMP-2 and MMP-9 were markedly increased after 4-PBA cotreatment, leading to significant reversal of these TM-evoked effects (**Figures 9I,J**). These results indicate that mild ER stress can inhibit LPS-induced MMP-2 and MMP-9 activation.

Mild ER Stress Reduced EB Extravasation in the LPS-Treated Rats

EB extravasation is a widely used marker for detecting breaches in the BBB. **Figure 10A** shows the EB extravasation in the extracted brains, indicating BBB disruption. As shown in **Figure 10B**, EB absorbance was increased in the LPS-treated rats compared with the naive group, which was apparently attenuated by TM treatment. Although TM alleviated LPS-induced BBB hyperpermeability, 4-PBA greatly diminished this effect as evidenced by increased EB content in the brain after 4-PBA administration.

DISCUSSION

Neurodegenerative diseases, exemplified by AD, PD, amyotrophic lateral sclerosis, and multiple sclerosis, pose the most pressing health and economic burden on developed societies with aging populations (Estes and McAllister, 2016). Neuroinflammation is an amplifier of neurodegenerative pathology, and thus, its influence is a subject of increasing interest (Glass et al., 2010).

In recent years, astrocytes have gained attention due to their pivotal role in brain homeostasis both in normal and pathological conditions (Haim and Rowitch, 2017). Long thought of as just supporting cells in the brain, astrocytes have in fact several

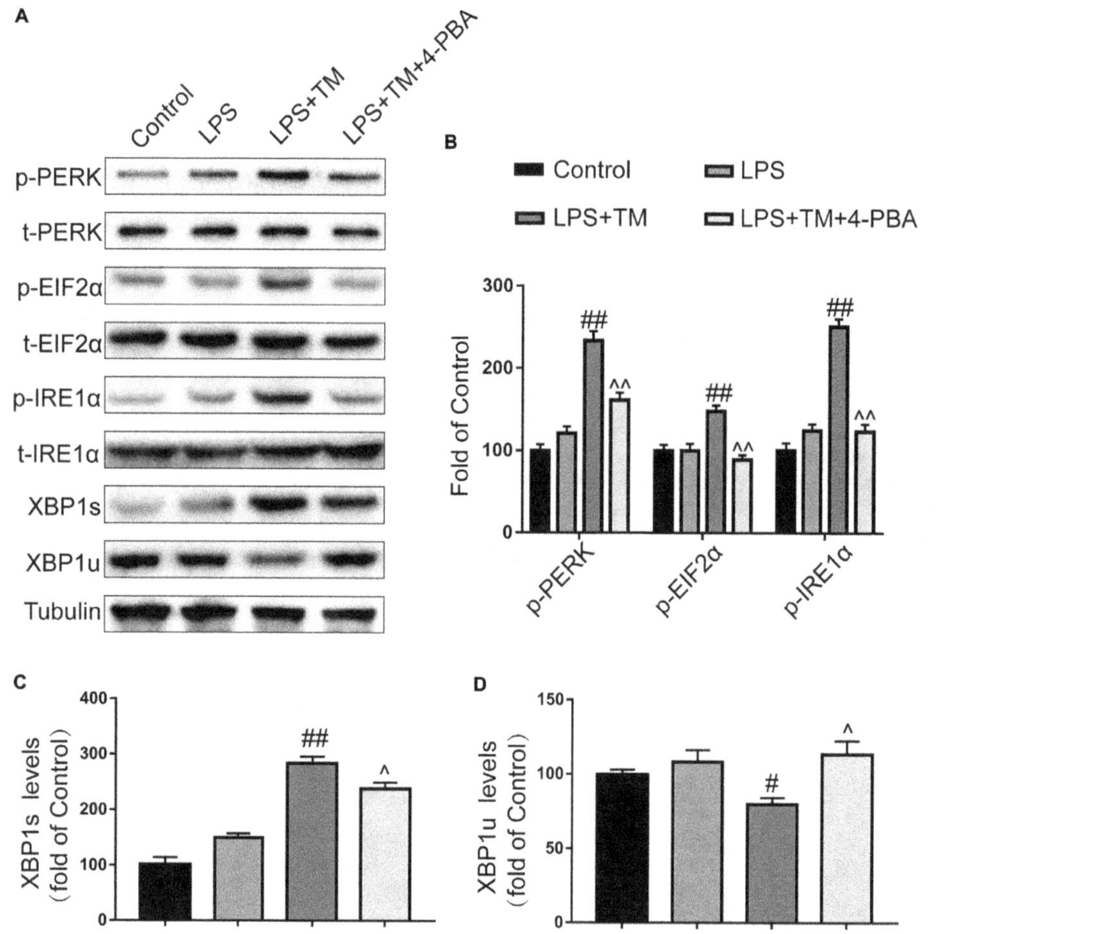

FIGURE 6 | 4-PBA partially inhibited mild ER stress in primary cultured astrocytes. **(A)** The expression levels of p-PERK, p-EIF2α, p-IRE1α, XBP1s, and XBP1u in primary cultured astrocytes were detected by Western blotting using specific antibodies. **(B)** Phosphorylated levels of PERK, EIF2α, and IRE1α were quantified and normalized to corresponding total levels. **(C)** Expression of XBP1s was quantified and normalized to Tubulin expression. **(D)** Expression of XBP1u was quantified and normalized to Tubulin expression. Each value is expressed relative to that in the control group, which was set to 100. All experiments were repeated three times. $^{\#}P < 0.05$, $^{\#\#}P < 0.01$ vs. LPS treatment group. $^{\wedge}P < 0.05$, $^{\wedge\wedge}P < 0.01$ vs. TM treatment group. The data are presented as the mean ± SEM.

housekeeping functions. Recently, astrocytes have become the focus of attention because of their metabolic coupling with neurons and the BBB (Cabezas et al., 2014).

The emerging evidence highlights the critical roles of astrocytes in regulating neuroinflammation through a process called "astrogliosis," (Sofroniew, 2015), which leads to an increase in the number, morphology, and motility of astrocytes and illustrates the role of the neuroinflammatory response in neurodegenerative diseases (Garwood et al., 2017). Astrogliosis is a well-characterized spectrum of cellular, molecular, and functional astrocytic changes in response to CNS damage. The cells in which astrogliosis occurs have the potential to be strongly reactive, thus contributing to the production of numerous proinflammatory molecules, such as cytokines, to exacerbate neuroinflammation (Khakh and Sofroniew, 2015; Bazargani and Attwell, 2016).

In recent years, numerous studies have shown that ER stress in astrocytes is associated with astrogliosis and the development of neuroinflammation (Cheng et al., 2013; Hong et al., 2016). However, these studies, which utilized high concentrations of pharmacological ER stressors to cause robust perturbation of ER function in experimental animals or cultured cells, failed to reproduce physiological and non-lethal levels of ER stress. ER stress activates the signaling events termed UPR. UPR is a heterogeneous and context-dependent cellular response, determined by the intensity or duration of the exposure to stress (Hetz and Mollereau, 2014). Under severe and robust ER stress, activation of the UPR operates as a pro-apoptotic program that reinforces the expression of pro-apoptotic components such as CHOP through ATF4; ER-related neurotoxicity consequently occurs. Under conditions of moderate and mild ER stress, ATF4 and CHOP are highly unstable at the mRNA and protein levels; these proteins are necessarily short-lived without a persistent and robust ER-stress signal transduction pathway (Matus et al., 2014). Therefore, mild perturbations of ER function may operate as an adaptive feedback mechanism of resistance against any possible further injuries.

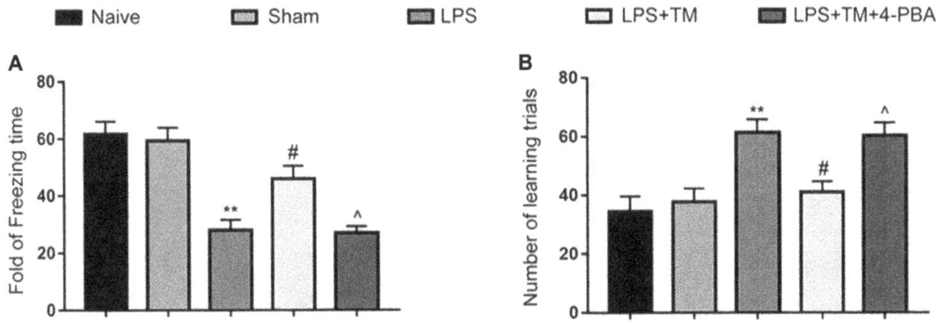

FIGURE 7 | Mild ER stress ameliorated LPS-induced cognitive impairment in the hippocampus. **(A)** Contextual fear response, as measured by freezing time, was determined in the rats (n = 12). **(B)** The number of learning trials was recorded to analyze the Y-maze test (n = 12). The data are presented as the mean ± SEM. $^{*}P < 0.05$, $^{**}P < 0.01$ vs. naïve group. $^{\#}P < 0.05$, $^{\#\#}P < 0.01$ vs. LPS treatment group. $^{\wedge}P < 0.05$, $^{\wedge\wedge}P < 0.01$ vs. TM treatment group. The data are representative of three independent experiments.

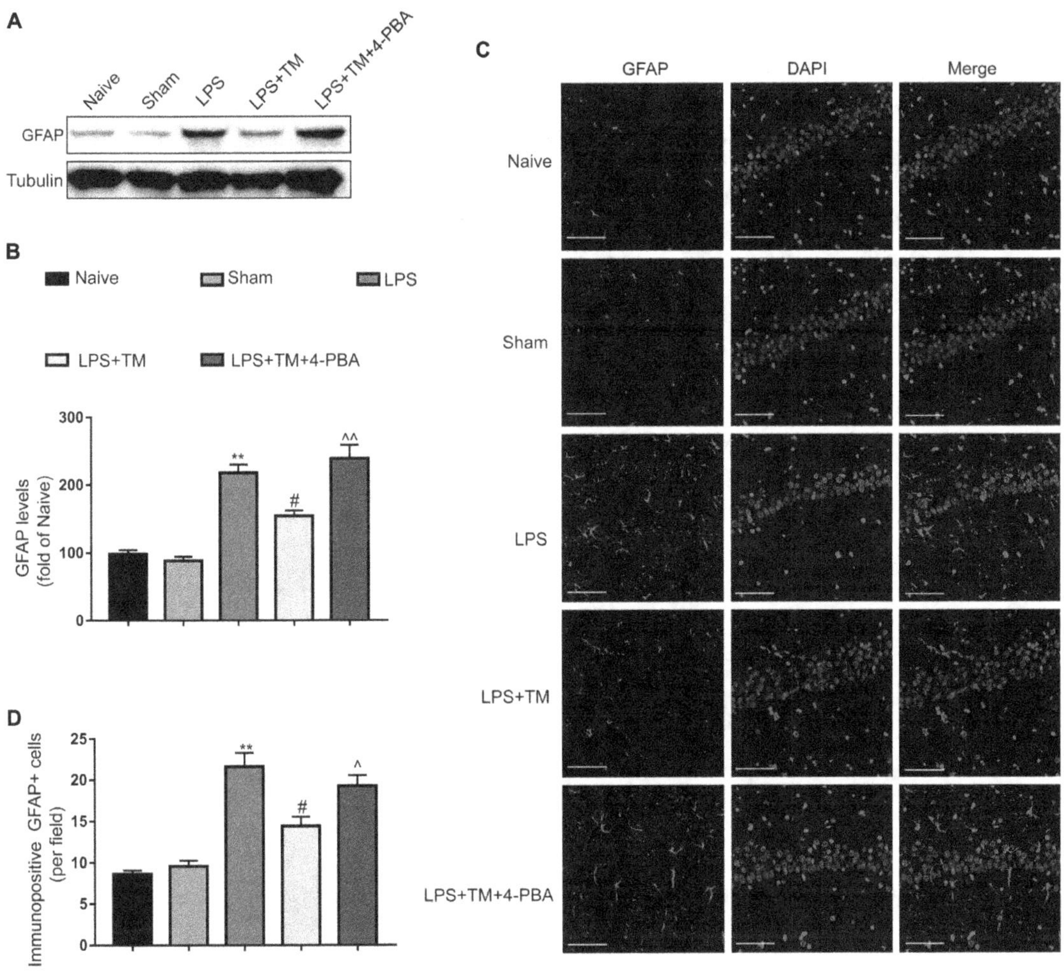

FIGURE 8 | Mild ER stress reduced the hippocampal astrocyte activation. **(A)** The protein levels of GFAP were detected by Western blotting using specific antibody in hippocampus. **(B)** Expression of GFAP was quantified and normalized to Tubulin levels. Each value was expressed relative to that of the naïve group, which was set to 100 (n = 6). **(C)** Immunofluorescent staining was used to detect GFAP, a maker of astrocytes, in hippocampal CA1 region. Blue staining represents DAPI. Scale bar = 200 μm. **(D)** Quantitative of GFAP-positive cells in the CA1 area of hippocampus. The data are representative of three independent experiments. $^{*}P < 0.05$, $^{**}P < 0.01$ vs. naïve group. $^{\#}P < 0.05$, $^{\#\#}P < 0.01$ vs. LPS treatment group. $^{\wedge}P < 0.05$, $^{\wedge\wedge}P < 0.01$ vs. TM treatment group. The data are presented as the mean ± SEM.

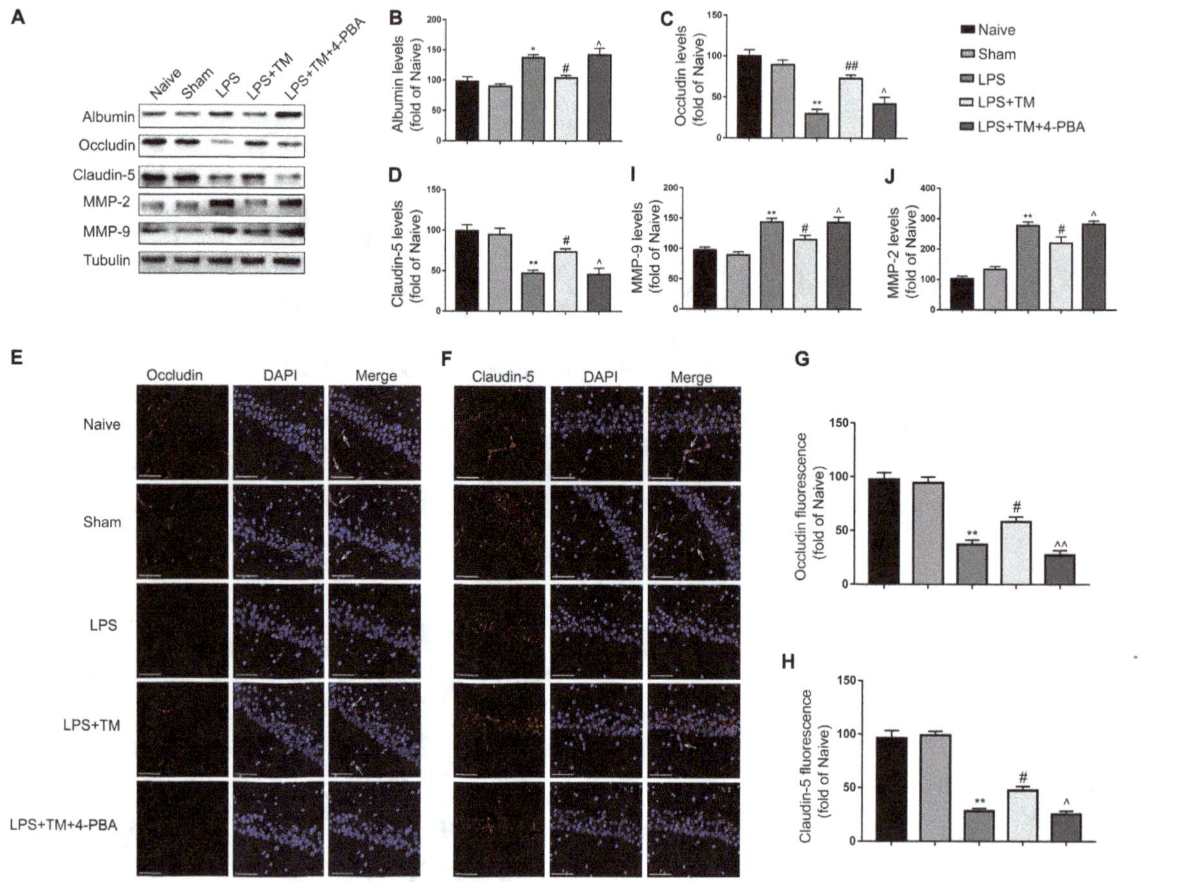

FIGURE 9 | Mild ER stress attenuated LPS-induced BBB hyperpermeability in hippocampus. **(A)** The expression levels of albumin, occludin, claudin-5, MMP-2, and MMP-9 were detected in the hippocampus of rats by Western blotting using specific antibodies. **(B–D)** Expression of albumin, occludin and claudin-5 was quantified and normalized to Tubulin levels. **(E,F)** Images acquired by confocal microscopy show the occludin and claudin-5 levels in the CA1 area of the hippocampus. The arrow in G points to an area in the CA1 area with high occludin immunoreactivity. The arrow in H points to an area in the CA1 area with high claudin-5 immunoreactivity. Scale bar, 100 μm. **(G,H)** Quantitative data of the mean intensities of occludin and claudin-5 fluorescence. **(I,J)** Expression of MMP-2 and MMP-9 was quantified and normalized to Tubulin levels. Each value was expressed relative to the values of the naïve group, which was set to 100 (*n* = 6). The data are representative of three independent experiments. $^{*}P < 0.05$, $^{**}P < 0.01$ vs. naïve group. $^{\#}P < 0.05$, $^{\#\#}P < 0.01$ vs. LPS treatment group. $^{\wedge}P < 0.05$, $^{\wedge\wedge}P < 0.01$ vs. TM treatment group. The data are presented as the mean ± SEM.

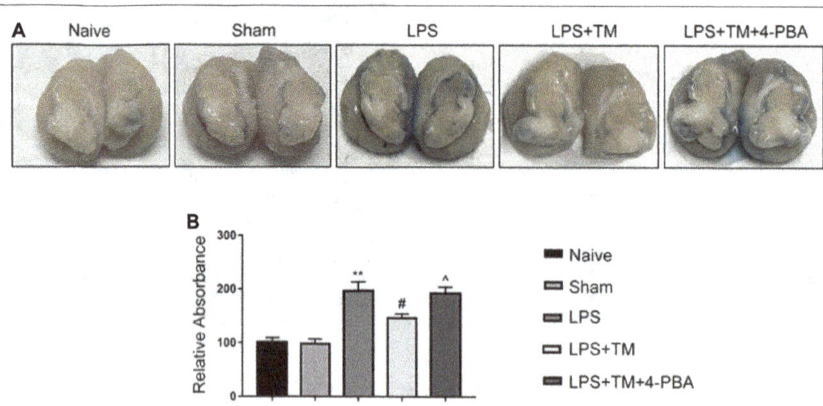

FIGURE 10 | Mild ER stress reduced EB extravasation in the LPS-treated rats. **(A)** Representative photographs of EB extravasation in the extracted brains of various groups. **(B)** The quantitative analysis of EB leakage. Each value was expressed relative to the values of the naïve group, which was set to 100 (*n* = 4). The data are presented as the mean ± SEM. $^{*}P < 0.05$, $^{**}P < 0.01$ vs. naïve group. $^{\#}P < 0.05$, $^{\#\#}P < 0.01$ vs. LPS treatment group. $^{\wedge}P < 0.05$, $^{\wedge\wedge}P < 0.01$ vs. TM treatment group.

We evaluated the levels of ATF4 and CHOP expression in astrocytes to further characterize the extent of ER stress in response to varying concentrations of TM. In the present investigation, activation of the PERK-EIF2α/IRE1-XBP1 pathway was detected at both high and low concentrations of TM. However, TM at the highest dose triggered a robust ER-stress response in astrocytes. Only at high concentrations (10 ng/ml) was TM able to trigger a robust ER-stress response in astrocytes, as evident by effective upregulation of ATF4 and CHOP, while lower doses of TM did not increase CHOP and ATF4 protein expression.

GFAP overexpression is a reliable marker for identifying reactive astrocytes under pathological conditions in the hypertrophic response of astrogliosis (Allaman et al., 2011). In this study, we observed that LPS altered the morphology of astrocytes, as demonstrated by terminal swelling filopodium-like processes, and induced the upregulation of GFAP expression. Additionally, LPS significantly induced the inflammatory cytokines, IL-1β, and IL-6, in cultured primary astrocytes. We defined *in vitro* and *in vivo* experimental conditions in which mild ER stress did not induce astrocytic lethality but rather suppressed LPS-induced overactivation and inflammatory responses in astrocytes. We demonstrated that astrocyte protection occurred as an intrinsic consequence of non-toxic, mild activation of ER stress.

It was reported that the heterogeneity between mild ER stress and robust ER stress pertains to differences in the expression of downstream proteins. Although less is known about this non-toxic ER stress in various models, current information points toward a concept that describes this adaptive reaction, which we refer to as "hormesis" (Matus et al., 2014). For instance, TM at a low dosage orchestrated neuroprotection in *Drosophila* and mouse models of PD (Fouillet et al., 2014), AD (Casas-Tinto et al., 2011), brain inflammation (Hosoi et al., 2014), and brain ischemia/reperfusion (Ibuki et al., 2012).

Our previous study revealed that preconditioning with the ER stress-inducer, TM, at a low dosage protected against LPS-induced cognitive decline and neuroinflammation, while 4-PBA partly counteracted this protective effect (Wang et al., 2017). We have proposed that ER-mediated hormesis (or ER hormesis) is responsible for protection after LPS challenge. This hypothesis is also supported by our current results that showed that mild doses of TM relieved LPS-stimulated BBB hyperpermeability.

Albumin is a vascular marker that crosses the BBB very slowly and is therefore often used to measure the loss of BBB integrity (Xaio et al., 2001). Using the albumin quota, we confirmed the role of mild ER stress in BBB function. We found more albumin leakage in the hippocampus following LPS injection, which was inhibited by pretreatment with TM. Furthermore, our study showed that TM treatment alleviated BBB dysfunction and hyperpermeability, evident by the increased levels of tight-junction proteins claudin-5 and occludin along with reduced expression of MMP-2 and MMP-9. It is becoming clear that, on one hand, astrocytes can exert proinflammatory effects by releasing molecules that enhance BBB permeability; on the other hand, however, astrocytes can promote BBB-structure repair by releasing trophic factors (Cabezas et al., 2014). It is difficult to determine the specific mechanism underlying the astrocytic influence on the BBB in our experiment. Further detailed work is required to address this issue in the future.

In summary, our results support a potential protective role of mild ER stress in alleviating LPS-induced astrocytic overactivation and BBB disruption. The central feature of this protective mild ER stress appears to be the triggering and maintenance of ER stress at a moderate level that facilitates survival, without increasing the levels of pro-apoptotic proteins such as CHOP and ATF4. While many crucial questions remain to be answered, our study findings provide not only a better understanding of the role of ER stress in neurodegeneration but also the basis for a prospective cure for neurodegeneration in the future.

AUTHOR CONTRIBUTIONS

YC, QZ, JX, QQ, and PN performed the experiments. YW and YQ designed the study. YW wrote the manuscript. All authors read and approved the final manuscript.

FUNDING

This project was funded by the National Natural Science Foundation of China (No. 81671387) and Postgraduate Research & Practice Innovation Program of Jiangsu Province (KYCX17_1250).

ACKNOWLEDGMENTS

We would like to thank Dr. Le-ting Zhou from Southeast University for his kind help of revising our manuscript.

REFERENCES

Allaman, I., Bélanger, M., and Magistretti, P. J. (2011). Astrocyte–neuron metabolic relationships: for better and for worse. *Trends Neurosci.* 34, 76–87. doi: 10.1016/j.tins.2010.12.001

Bazargani, N., and Attwell, D. (2016). Astrocyte calcium signaling: the third wave. *Nat. Neurosci.* 19, 182–189. doi: 10.1038/nn.4201

Broux, B., Gowing, E., and Prat, A. (2015). Glial regulation of the blood-brain barrier in health and disease. *Semin. Immunopathol.* 37, 577–590. doi: 10.1007/s00281-015-0516-2

Cabezas, R., Avila, M., Gonzalez, J., El-Bachã, R. S., Bãez, E., Garciã-Segura, L. M., et al. (2014). Astrocytic modulation of blood brain barrier: perspectives on Parkinson's disease. *Front. Cell. Neurosci.* 8:211. doi: 10.3389/fncel.2014.00211

Casas-Tinto, S., Zhang, Y., Sanchez-Garcia, J., Gomez-Velazquez, M., Rincon-Limas, D. E., and Fernandez-Funez, P. (2011). The ER stress factor XBP1s prevents amyloid-beta neurotoxicity. *Hum. Mol. Genet.* 20, 2144–2160. doi: 10.1093/hmg/ddr100

Cheng, L., Zhao, H., Zhang, W., Liu, B., Liu, Y., Guo, Y., et al. (2013). Overexpression of conserved dopamine neurotrophic factor (CDNF) in astrocytes alleviates endoplasmic reticulum stress-induced cell damage and inflammatory cytokine secretion. *Biochem. Biophys. Res. Commun.* 435, 34–39. doi: 10.1016/j.bbrc.2013.04.029

Estes, M. L., and McAllister, A. K. (2016). Maternal immune activation: implications for neuropsychiatric disorders. *Science* 353, 772–777. doi: 10.1126/science.aag3194

Fouillet, A., Levet, C., Virgone, A., Robin, M., Dourlen, P., Rieusset, J., et al. (2014). ER stress inhibits neuronal death by promoting autophagy. *Autophagy* 8, 915–926. doi: 10.4161/auto.19716

Gardner, B. M., Pincus, D., Gotthardt, K., Gallagher, C. M., and Walter, P. (2013). Endoplasmic reticulum stress sensing in the unfolded protein response. *Cold Spring Harb. Perspect. Biol.* 5:a13169. doi: 10.1101/cshperspect.a013169

Garwood, C. J., Ratcliffe, L. E., Simpson, J. E., Heath, P. R., Ince, P. G., and Wharton, S. B. (2017). Review: astrocytes in Alzheimer's disease and other age-associated dementias: a supporting player with a central role. *Neuropathol. Appl. Neurobiol.* 43, 281–298. doi: 10.1111/nan.12338

Glass, C. K., Saijo, K., Winner, B., Marchetto, M. C., and Gage, F. H. (2010). Mechanisms underlying inflammation in neurodegeneration. *Cell* 140, 918–934. doi: 10.1016/j.cell.2010.02.016

Gorina, R., Font-Nieves, M., Márquez-Kisinousky, L., Santalucia, T., and Planas, A. M. (2011). Astrocyte TLR4 activation induces a proinflammatory environment through the interplay between MyD88-dependent NFκB signaling, MAPK, and Jak1/Stat1 pathways. *Glia* 59, 242–255. doi: 10.1002/glia.21094

Haim, L. B., and Rowitch, D. H. (2017). Functional diversity of astrocytes in neural circuit regulation. *Nat. Rev. Neurosci.* 18, 31–41. doi: 10.1038/nrn.2016.159

Hetz, C., and Mollereau, B. (2014). Disturbance of endoplasmic reticulum proteostasis in neurodegenerative diseases. *Nat. Rev. Neurosci.* 15, 233–249. doi: 10.1038/nrn3689

Hong, Y., Wang, X., Sun, S., Xue, G., Li, J., and Hou, Y. (2016). Progesterone exerts neuroprotective effects against abeta-induced neuroinflammation by attenuating ER stress in astrocytes. *Int. Immunopharmacol.* 33, 83–89. doi: 10.1016/j.intimp.2016.02.002

Hosoi, T., Noguchi, J., Takakuwa, M., Honda, M., Okuma, Y., Nomura, Y., et al. (2014). Inhibition of inducible nitric oxide synthase and interleukin-1β expression by tunicamycin in cultured glial cells exposed to lipopolysaccharide. *Brain Res.* 1558, 11–17. doi: 10.1016/j.brainres.2014.02.035

Ibuki, T., Yamasaki, Y., Mizuguchi, H., and Sokabe, M. (2012). Protective effects of XBP1 against oxygen and glucose deprivation/reoxygenation injury in rat primary hippocampal neurons. *Neurosci. Lett.* 518, 45–48. doi: 10.1016/j.neulet.2012.04.053

Khakh, B. S., and Sofroniew, M. V. (2015). Diversity of astrocyte functions and phenotypes in neural circuits. *Nat. Neurosci.* 18, 942–952. doi: 10.1038/nn.4043

Martin-Jiménez, C. A., García-Vega, Á., Cabezas, R., Aliev, G., Echeverria, V., González, J., et al. (2017). Astrocytes and endoplasmic reticulum stress: a bridge between obesity and neurodegenerative diseases. *Prog. Neurobiol.* 158, 45–68. doi: 10.1016/j.pneurobio.2017.08.001

Matus, S., Castillo, K., and Hetz, C. (2014). Hormesis: protecting neurons against cellular stress in Parkinson disease. *Autophagy* 8, 997–1001. doi: 10.4161/auto.20748

Pintado, C., Gavilan, M. P., Gavilan, E., Garcia-Cuervo, L., Gutierrez, A., Vitorica, J., et al. (2012). Lipopolysaccharide-induced neuroinflammation leads to the accumulation of ubiquitinated proteins and increases susceptibility to neurodegeneration induced by proteasome inhibition in rat hippocampus. *J. Neuroinflammation* 9:87. doi: 10.1186/1742-2094-9-87

Qi, Z., Liang, J., Pan, R., Dong, W., Shen, J., Yang, Y., et al. (2016). Zinc contributes to acute cerebral ischemia-induced blood–brain barrier disruption. *Neurobiol. Dis.* 95, 12–21. doi: 10.1016/j.nbd.2016.07.003

Qin, L., Wu, X., Block, M. L., Liu, Y., Breese, G. R., Hong, J., et al. (2007). Systemic LPS causes chronic neuroinflammation and progressive neurodegeneration. *Glia* 55, 453–462. doi: 10.1002/glia.20467

Sofroniew, M. V. (2015). Astrocyte barriers to neurotoxic inflammation. *Nat. Rev. Neurosci.* 16, 249–263. doi: 10.1038/nrn3898

Sun, J., Zhang, S., Zhang, X., Zhang, X., Dong, H., and Qian, Y. (2015). IL-17A is implicated in lipopolysaccharide-induced neuroinflammation and cognitive impairment in aged rats via microglial activation. *J. Neuroinflammation* 12:165. doi: 10.1186/s12974-015-0394-5

Tasaki, A., Shimizu, F., Sano, Y., Fujisawa, M., Takahashi, T., Haruki, H., et al. (2014). Autocrine MMP-2/9 secretion increases the BBB permeability in neuromyelitis optica. *J. Neurol. Neurosurg. Psychiatry* 85, 419–430. doi: 10.1136/jnnp-2013-305907

Wang, Y., Zhou, Q., Zhang, X., Qian, Q., Xu, J., Ni, P., et al. (2017). Mild endoplasmic reticulum stress ameliorates lipopolysaccharide-induced neuroinflammation and cognitive impairment via regulation of microglial polarization. *J. Neuroinflammation* 14:223. doi: 10.1186/s12974-017-1002-7

Xaio, H., Banks, W. A., Niehoff, M. L., and Morley, J. E. (2001). Effect of LPS on the permeability of the blood-brain barrier to insulin. *Brain Res.* 896, 36–42.

Xu, J., Zhang, X., Qian, Q., Wang, Y., Dong, H., Li, N., et al. (2018). Histamine upregulates the expression of histamine receptors and increases the neuroprotective effect of astrocytes. *J. Neuroinflammation* 15:41. doi: 10.1186/s12974-018-1068-x

Zhang, X., Dong, H., Li, N., Zhang, S., Sun, J., Zhang, S., et al. (2016). Activated brain mast cells contribute to postoperative cognitive dysfunction by evoking microglia activation and neuronal apoptosis. *J. Neuroinflammation* 13:127. doi: 10.1186/s12974-016-0592-9

14

There is Selective Increase in Pro-thrombotic Circulating Extracellular Vesicles in Acute Ischemic Stroke and Transient Ischemic Attack: A Study of Patients from the Middle East and Southeast Asia

Abdelali Agouni[1†], Aijaz S. Parray[2†], Naveed Akhtar[2], Fayaz A. Mir[3], Paula J. Bourke[2], Sujata Joseph[2], Deborah M. Morgan[2], Mark D. Santos[2], Muhammad F. Wadiwala[2], Saadat Kamran[2], Siveen K. Sivaraman[3] and Ashfaq Shuaib[2,4]*

[1] Department of Pharmaceutical Sciences, College of Pharmacy, Qatar University, Doha, Qatar, [2] The Stroke Program, The Neuroscience Institute, Academic Health System, Hamad Medical Corporation, Doha, Qatar, [3] Interim Translational Institute, Academic Health System, Hamad Medical Corporation, Doha, Qatar, [4] Department of Medicine (Neurology), University of Alberta, Edmonton, AB, Canada

***Correspondence:**
Abdelali Agouni
aagouni@qu.edu.qa

† These authors have contributed equally to this work

Stroke attacks were found to be present at a younger age in patients from Southeast Asia (SE) and the Middle East (ME) resident in the state of Qatar. Extracellular vesicles (EVs), which are small membrane vesicles with pro-thrombotic properties, may contribute to the high risk of stroke in this population. Thus, total and cell-specific medium size EVs were counted by flow cytometry in platelet-free plasma from healthy volunteers and patients with transient ischemic attacks (TIA) and acute ischemic stroke (AIS) from SE and ME. Acutely, within 48 h of attacks, there was an increase in total endothelial EVs in TIA (6.73 ± 1.77; $P = 0.0156$; $n = 21$) and AIS (11.23 ± 1.95; $P = 0.0007$; $n = 66$) patients compared to controls (2.04 ± 0.78; $n = 24$). Similar increases were also evident in EVs originating from platelets, erythrocytes, granulocytes, and leukocytes. Compared to controls, there was also an increase in EVs derived from activated endothelial cells, platelets, granulocytes, leukocytes, and pro-coagulant EVs (Annexin V^{+}) at 5 and 30-days following the acute events, while a decrease was observed in erythrocyte-derived EVs. This is the first study characterizing EVs in TIA and AIS patients from ME and SE showing an increase in EVs associated with endothelial and platelet cell activation, which may contribute to the elevated risk of stroke at a younger age in this population.

Keywords: extracellular vesicles (EVs), acute ischemic stroke (AIS), transient ischemic attacks (TIA), thrombosis, biomarkers

INTRODUCTION

Acute ischemic stroke (AIS) is the leading cause of disability and the second most common cause of death and dementia worldwide. The incidence of AIS is particularly high in Southeast Asia (SE) and the Middle East (ME) where the prevalence of hypertension and diabetes is high and an increasing proportion of the population are obese and suffer from metabolic syndrome (1–3).

Enhanced platelet aggregation and cell activation are important contributors to the pathophysiology and progression of AIS and are closely associated with stroke risk factors such as hypertension and diabetes. In addition, loss of vascular homeostasis and low-grade inflammation can further contribute to endothelial dysfunction and atherogenesis, a primary factor in the pathogenesis of AIS (4). In this context, circulating extracellular vesicles (EVs), particularly the endoplasmic membrane-derived microparticles or microvesicles, owing to their crucial pro-coagulant role may contribute to the onset and development of AIS (5).

EVs are membrane-containing vesicles that are released from activated or apoptotic cells of any type. EVs are classified into three main categories based on their size and their mechanism of cellular release: exosomes (30–130 nm), microparticles or microvesicles (100–1,000 nm), and the larger apoptotic bodies (>1,000 nm) (6). Based on the most recent position statement of the International Society for Extracellular Vesicles (ISEV), the term EVs was adopted throughout this article as a generic term to refer to lipid membrane-delineated, replication-defective, and not carrying a functional nucleus, naturally cell-shed vesicles (7). Elevated circulating levels of EVs, particularly those of medium size (microparticles), were reported in many cardiovascular diseases associated with inflammation and thrombotic alterations including stroke and coronary artery disease (8, 9). Total numbers of circulating EVs or those deriving from specific cell populations were found to correlate with the presence and severity of multiple disorders and are thus considered as biomarkers for the monitoring of disease progression. For instance, EVs originating from platelets were found to correlate with atypical carotid intima/media thickness in obese patients (10). In addition, high plasma numbers of pro-coagulant EVs were reported in patients suffering from metabolic syndrome (11, 12). Levels of EVs shed from endothelial cells (13) and platelets (14) were reported to increase in AIS. In another study, circulating EVs from platelets, endothelial cells, erythrocytes, leukocytes, lymphocytes, monocytes, and smooth muscle cells increased at the onset, and at 7 and 90 days in patients suspected with AIS compared to controls (15). Recently, however, Landers-Ramos et al. (16) reported that EVs levels of endothelial origin were not increased in chronic stroke patients compared to young and old healthy volunteers. Nonetheless, chronic stroke patients also suffering from diabetes had higher plasma levels of endothelial-derived EVs in comparison to those free of diabetes (16).

Studies that have investigated EVs in stroke were mostly conducted in small numbers of patients and in homogenous ethnic populations. There are currently no reports available of EVs in stroke patients from ME and SE. Furthermore, none of the available studies has investigated the levels of circulating EVs in patients with TIA, a major precursor and risk factor for AIS. Another crucial point, is that most previous studies only looked at the expression of select sub-populations of EVs in stroke patients.

The aim of the present study was therefore to count the number of circulating medium size EVs and phenotype them according to their cellular origins in patients with TIA and AIS patients from SE and ME origins resident the state of Qatar, at onset (within 48 h of attacks), 5 and 30-days following the initiation of appropriate pharmacotherapy.

MATERIALS AND METHODS

Patients

The study was reviewed and approved by the Institutional Ethical Board (IRB) of Hamad Medical Corporation (#15304/15) and fully adhered to the principles of the declaration of Helsinki. All participants of the study gave written informed consent prior to their enrolment in the investigation. Patients were enrolled in the study within 48 h of stroke onset. Individuals aged 18 years and older and who gave written informed consent were included. Stroke was defined according to World Health Organization (WHO) criteria as "rapidly developing clinical signs of focal (or global) disturbance of cerebral function, with symptoms lasting 24 h or longer or leading to death, with no apparent cause other than vascular origin." TIA was defined as a brief episode of neurologic dysfunction resulting from transient cerebral ischemia but that is not accompanied by cerebral infarction. All AIS and TIA patients received at Hamad General hospital were eligible for inclusion.

Data Collection

The baseline medical history includes age, gender, ethnicity, nationality, marital status, household income, employment status, smoking status, alcohol intake, medical comorbidities (including a history of diabetes, dyslipidemia, coronary artery disease, peripheral vascular disease, chronic kidney disease, heart failure, and sleep apnea), and all current prescription and over-the-counter medications (including dosage, frequency and timing of administration). The cerebrovascular event type (AIS vs. TIA) was documented using the Trial of Org 10,172 in Acute Stroke Treatment (TOAST) classification and the date of stroke was recorded. This information is currently recorded routinely in the stroke database. We also recorded the type of work, duration of time since they moved to Qatar (for expatriate subjects) and the circumstances when the stroke occurred.

Physical examination included automated office blood pressure (BP) [taken with a BPTru® automated monitor by measuring six readings in the arm with the higher BP, discarding the first reading and averaging the latter two], height, weight, and waist circumference.

Laboratory tests included a complete blood count, electrolytes (sodium, potassium, chloride, total carbon dioxide), creatinine, fasting glucose, glycated hemoglobin (A1c), fasting lipid profile, c-reactive protein, and urine microalbumin. Computerized tomography (CT) head scan, echocardiogram, and standard (not

3D) carotid ultrasound results were performed as part of routine clinical care at the time of stroke were recorded in the case record forms (CRF). These tests are performed as part of routine clinical care.

Isolation of Platelet-Free Plasma (PFP) From Whole Blood

Peripheral venous blood (10 mL) from control subjects, AIS, and TIA patients was obtained in ethylenediaminetetraacetic acid tubes (Vacutainers; Becton Dickinson) by using a 21-gauge needle to reduce platelet stimulation. Samples were assayed within 2 h of collection at room temperature. Blood samples were then subjected low speed centrifugation (270 $\times$ *g*) for 20 min to separate platelet-rich plasma from whole blood. Following this, platelet-rich plasma was centrifuged for further 20 min at a speed of 1,500 $\times$ *g* to collect PFP, which was then frozen and stored at -80°C until subsequent analysis for EVs content (11, 12, 17, 18).

Count and Identification of Cellular Origins of EVs

Specific cellular subpopulations of medium size EVs were identified in PFP according the expression of surface-specific proteins as previously done by us (11, 12, 17, 18). Specific fluorescent antibodies targeting the following surface antigens were used in this study: PE-CD146 (endothelial cells), PE-CD41 (platelets), PC7-CD45 (leukocytes), PC7-CD235a (erythrocytes), PE-CD62E (E-Selectin$^+$ EVs), and PE-CD62P (P-Selectin$^+$ EVs) (Beckman Coulter through Sedeer Medical, Doha, Qatar). Irrelevant human IgG were used as isotype-matched negative controls for each sample (Beckman Coulter). To count medium size EVs and determine plasma concentrations for each cell origin, separate assays for each surface marker were conducted. Briefly, 10 μL of PFP from healthy controls or patients were incubated with 5 μL of each specific antibody for 45 min protected from light. Then, samples were suspended in 300 μL of 0.9% saline solution and 10 μL Flowcount microbeads (Beckman Coulter), a mix of fluorescent beads with known concentration used to calculate absolute counts, were mixed before samples were analyzed by flow cytometry using a BD LSRFortessa analyzer (BD Biosciences, USA) as previously shown by us (11, 12, 17, 18).

For the identification of the number of pro-coagulant EVs (expressing phosphatidylserine), separate assays were conducted to determine Annexin V binding. Briefly, 2 μL of Annexin V (Beckman Coulter) were incubated with 5 μL PFP from each participant for 30 min protected from light. Then, samples were suspended in 300 μL of Annexin-V labeling buffer, and 5 μL (equal volume to sample) of Flowcount microbeads (Beckman Coulter) were added before the analysis of samples by flow cytometry using a BD LSRFortessa analyzer (BD Biosciences) as previously shown by us (11, 12, 17, 18).

Statistical Data Analysis

Data are expressed as mean $\pm$ SEM or mean $\pm$ SD; *n* indicates the number of subjects included in each experimental group. Statistical analyses were performed by Mann-Whitney *U* or analysis of one-way variance (ANOVA) for repeated measures and subsequent Tukey's *post-hoc* test. $P < 0.05$ was accepted as statistically significant. Analyses were performed using GraphPad Prism 7 software (GraphPad Software Inc., San Diego, USA).

RESULTS

Patients Baseline Characteristics

Between September 2016 and May 2018, we recruited 24 healthy controls and a total of 119 patients with suspected acute stroke, of whom 87 patients (66 [76%] AIS and 21 [24%] TIA) were eventually included in the study after exclusion of stroke mimics.

The baseline characteristics of the 24 healthy volunteers and the 87 patients included in the study are shown in **Table 1**. Similar to previous experience, the average age in both TIA (48.6 $\pm$ 9.5) and AIS patients (50.5 $\pm$ 11.1) was young (3). The patient population was predominantly male in AIS patients (95.5%). In terms of disease classification, most AIS patients suffered from a small vessel disease (59.1%), followed by cardio-embolic attacks (16.7%) and large vessel disease (15.2%) (**Table 1**).

Total Number of Circulating of EVs and Their Cellular Origins at Onset of Attacks

The count of total EVs regardless of their cellular origin did not differ between controls, TIA and AIS patients (**Figure 1**) within 48 h of onset of attacks. TIA and AIS patients had significantly higher percentage of circulating EVs derived from endothelial cells (CD146$^+$; **Figure 2A**) and activated endothelial cells that express E-selectin (CD62E$^+$; **Figure 2B**) compared to healthy volunteers. Furthermore, there was a trend for AIS patients to express more of total and activated endothelial-derived EVs compared to TIA patients (**Figures 2A,B**).

Whereas, platelet-derived EVs (CD41$^+$) were not significantly different between controls, TIA, or AIS patients (**Figure 2C**), the number of EVs derived from activated platelets expressing P-selectin (CD62P$^+$) was significantly higher in TIA and AIS patients compared to controls (**Figure 2D**). Interestingly, AIS patients exhibited a significantly higher percentage of activated platelets-derived EVs compared to TIA patients (**Figure 2D**).

EVs derived from erythrocytes (CD235a$^+$) were found to be significantly higher in the blood from both TIA and AIS patients compared to healthy volunteers (**Figure 2E**). Similarly, EVs derived from circulating immune cells, granulocytes (CD66$^+$; **Figure 2F**) and leukocytes (CD45$^+$; **Figure 2G**), were also significantly higher in TIA and AIS patients compared to controls although there was a non-significant trend for AIS patients to express more of these two EV subtypes compared to TIA patients (**Figures 2F,G**). Finally, the percentage of pro-coagulant EVs expressing Annexin V at their surface was not significantly different between the three groups within 48 h of onset of attacks (**Figure 2H**).

The Total Number of EVs Increased Over Time in AIS and TIA Patients as a Percentage of Onset Levels

To investigate the impact of disease progression and the initiation of treatment on the expression of EVs, we assessed the

TABLE 1 | Baseline Characteristics of subjects enrolled in the study.

	Controls ($n = 24$)	Transient Ischemic Attack ($n = 21$)	Acute Ischemic Stroke ($n = 66$)	*P* value
Age (years)	47.7 ± 7.4	48.6 ± 9.5	50.5 ± 11.1	0.485
GENDER				
Male	18 (75)	17 (81.0)	63 (95.5)	0.033
Female	6 (25)	4 (19.0)	3 (4.5)	
ETHNICITY				
ME	6 (29)	12 (57.1)	22 (33.3)	0.013
SE	18 (71)	9 (42.9)	44 (66.7)	
Prior use of statins	0	7 (33.3)	8 (12.1)	0.025
Prior use of anti-hypertensive	0	6 (28.6)	12 (18.2)	0.306
Prior use of anti-diabetic medications	0	3 (14.3)	10 (15.2)	0.923
Diabetic on admission	0	7 (33.3)	27 (40.9)	0.535
Hypertensive on admission	0	13 (61.9)	45 (68.2)	0.595
Dyslipidemia on admission	0	15 (71.4)	38 (57.6)	0.257
Previous stroke	0	1 (4.8)	2 (3.0)	0.705
Coronary artery disease	0	2 (9.5)	6 (9.1)	0.952
Atrial fibrillation	0	1 (4.8)	3 (4.5)	0.967
Smoking history	0	6 (28.6)	29 (43.9)	0.211
IV thrombolysis received	0	2 (9.5)	12 (18.2)	0.347
PROGNOSIS AT DISCHARGE				
Good (mRS 0–2)		21 (100.0)	48 (72.7)	0.007
Poor (mRS 3–6)		0.0	18 (27.3)	
PROGNOSIS AT 90-DAYS				
Good (mRS 0–2)		20 (95.2)	57 (86.4)	0.267
Poor (mRS 3–6)		1 (4.8)	9 (13.6)	
TOAST CLASSIFICATION				
Small vessel disease			39 (59.1)	
Large vessel disease			10 (15.2)	
Cardio-embolic			11 (16.7)	
Stroke of determined origin			3 (4.5)	
Stroke of undetermined origin			3 (4.5)	
OTHER				
Small vessel disease present		11 (52.4)	39 (59.1)	0.588
Silent infarct present		4 (19.0)	25 (37.9)	0.111
White matter ischemia present		14 (66.7)	52 (78.0)	0.258
Cerebral micro-bleeds present		4 (19.0)	20 (30.3)	0.315
Admission NIHSS		1.67 ± 2.1	3.35 ± 3.4	0.035
Systolic blood pressure		162.4 ± 26.1	157.4 ± 33.1	0.522
Diastolic blood pressure		94.7 ± 17.1	93.9 ± 21.0	0.883
Body Mass Index		27.6 ± 3.1	27.1 ± 3.9	0.634
HbA1c levels		6.4 ± 1.4	6.7 ± 2.1	0.545
Cholesterol levels		4.9 ± 1.3	5.2 ± 1.2	0.557
Triglyceride levels		1.9 ± 1.0	1.6 ± 0.9	0.353
HDL levels		1.1 ± 0.7	0.9 ± 0.2	0.031
LDL levels		3.1 ± 1.0	3.5 ± 1.0	0.086

Results are presented as mean ± SD or number (%) as appropriate. P-value from one-way ANOVA for quantitative variables and from Chi-square analysis for qualitative variables. mRS, modified Rankin scale; NIHSS, national institutes of health stroke scale.

progression of numbers of total EVs over time at 5- and 30-days post-attacks (**Figure 3**). The counts of EVs are expressed either as absolute numbers or as percentage of increase compared to the levels observed at onset of attacks for every patient. As shown in **Figure 3A**, the absolute number of total EVs continued to increase over time in both TIA and AIS patients, with the levels

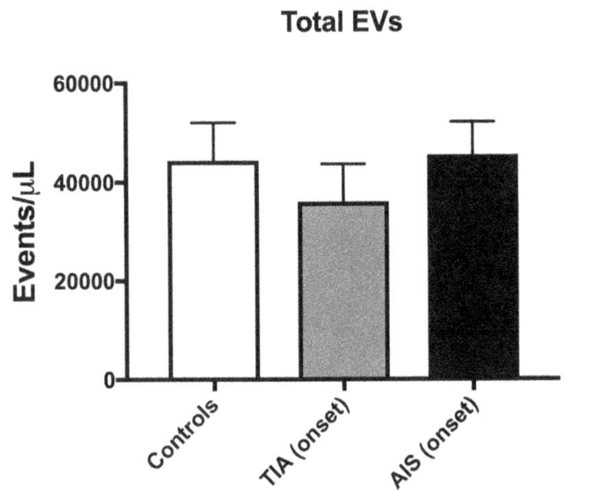

FIGURE 1 | Circulating total EV levels, at onset of attacks, in patients with TIA and AIS compared to healthy controls. Histograms represent events/μL in plasma poor in platelets (PFP) expressed as mean ± SEM. Controls, $n = 24$; TIA, $n = 21$; AIS, $n = 66$.

at the 30-days' time point being the most significant increase. As observed in **Figure 3B**, the number of total EVs, expressed as percentage of onset levels, also steadily increased over time at 5- and 30-days post-attacks both in TIA and AIS patients.

EVs From Selected Cellular Origins Increased Over Time Compared to Onset Levels

The increase in EVs at 5- and 30-days post-attacks varied depending on their cells of origin. TIA and AIS patients had higher levels of EVs derived from endothelial ($CD146^+$; **Figure 4A**) and activated endothelial cells ($CD62E^+$; **Figure 4B**) at 5- and 30-days compared to onset levels. The increase in EVs from activated endothelial cells ($CD62E^+$; **Figure 4B**) was highest in AIS patients, indicating a stronger activation of endothelial cells as the disease progresses in AIS patients compared to TIA patients. Similarly, EVs derived from both platelets ($CD41^+$; **Figure 4C**) and activated platelets ($CD62P^+$; **Figure 4D**) also significantly increased over time at 5- and 30-days in both TIA and AIS patients, indicating a sustained activation of platelets despite appropriate treatment being started. The expression of EVs derived from immune cells, granulocytes ($CD66b^+$; **Figure 4F**) and leukocytes ($CD45^+$; **Figure 4G**), also increased over time in both TIA and AIS patients, indicating a sustained activation of these cell types on the short-term following the start of pharmacotherapy. However, the levels of erythrocyte-derived EVs ($CD235a^+$; **Figure 4E**) decreased significantly over time at 5- and 30-days post-attacks in both TIA and AIS patients, suggesting a reduction in the activation of these cells over time following the initiation of therapy.

Although at onset of attacks, circulating levels of pro-coagulant EVs (Annexin V^+) were not different between controls, TIA and AIS (**Figure 2**), the numbers of Annexin V^+ EVs, expressed as a proportion of onset levels, increased with time in both TIA and AIS patients at 5- and 30-days post-attacks (**Figure 4H**), indicating that the shedding of pro-coagulant EVs increased over time.

As a Proportion of Total EVs at Each Time Point, the Initiation of Treatment Did Not Affect the Short-Term Expression of EVs Both in TIA and AIS Patients

As shown in **Figure 5**, the levels of circulating EVs, expressed as a percentage of total EVs at each time point, from all the cell origins investigated did not change in AIS patients over the monitored period (5- and 30-days post-attacks). Similar pattern was observed with TIA patients, where circulating levels of EVs from all cell origins studied did not vary, as a percentage of total EVs for each time point, after 5- and 30-days following the initiation of the pharmacotherapy (**Figure 6**). These data demonstrate that, as a percentage of total EVs at each time point, circulating levels of EVs from various cellular origins were constant over time (at 5- and 30-days) although their numbers have increased compared to onset time point. The increased number of total EVs over time drives the increase of specific populations of EVs without affecting their overall proportion in blood. Together, these findings further indicate that in both TIA and AIS patients, cellular activation continued to be elevated on the short-term despite the management of risk factors and the administration of appropriate pharmacotherapy to the patients.

DISCUSSION

For many decades, EVs were considered as inert cell debris or platelet dust derived from platelets which are rich in phospholipids and endowed of pro-coagulant capacity (8). Later, it was found that EVs could transport cargo content including secretable and non-secretable biological molecules such as active lipids, nucleic acids (microRNA and mRNA) in addition to membrane and cytosolic proteins to target cells (8, 19, 20). Circulating EVs derive from platelets, red and white blood cells, endothelial cells, and monocytes; however, most EVs found in the blood are from platelet origin (8, 9). EVs regulate inflammation and have pro-coagulant properties (21). Plasma numbers of EVs are elevated in cardiovascular disorders associated with thrombotic alterations including stroke and coronary artery disease (8, 9). Plasma levels of total EVs or those deriving from specific cell populations were found to correlate with the presence and severity of multiple disorders and are thus considered as biomarkers for the monitoring of disease progression and hence can provide a signature for changes occurring inside the body (11, 12, 22).

We report in the current study that although the total number of EVs did not differ between TIA and AIS patients compared to controls within 48 h of attacks onset, both TIA and AIS patients had higher circulating levels of EVs derived from endothelial cells ($CD146^+$), activated endothelial cells ($CD62E^+$), activated platelets ($CD62P^+$), granulocytes ($CD66b^+$), and leukocytes ($CD45^+$) compared to controls; however, AIS patients had higher

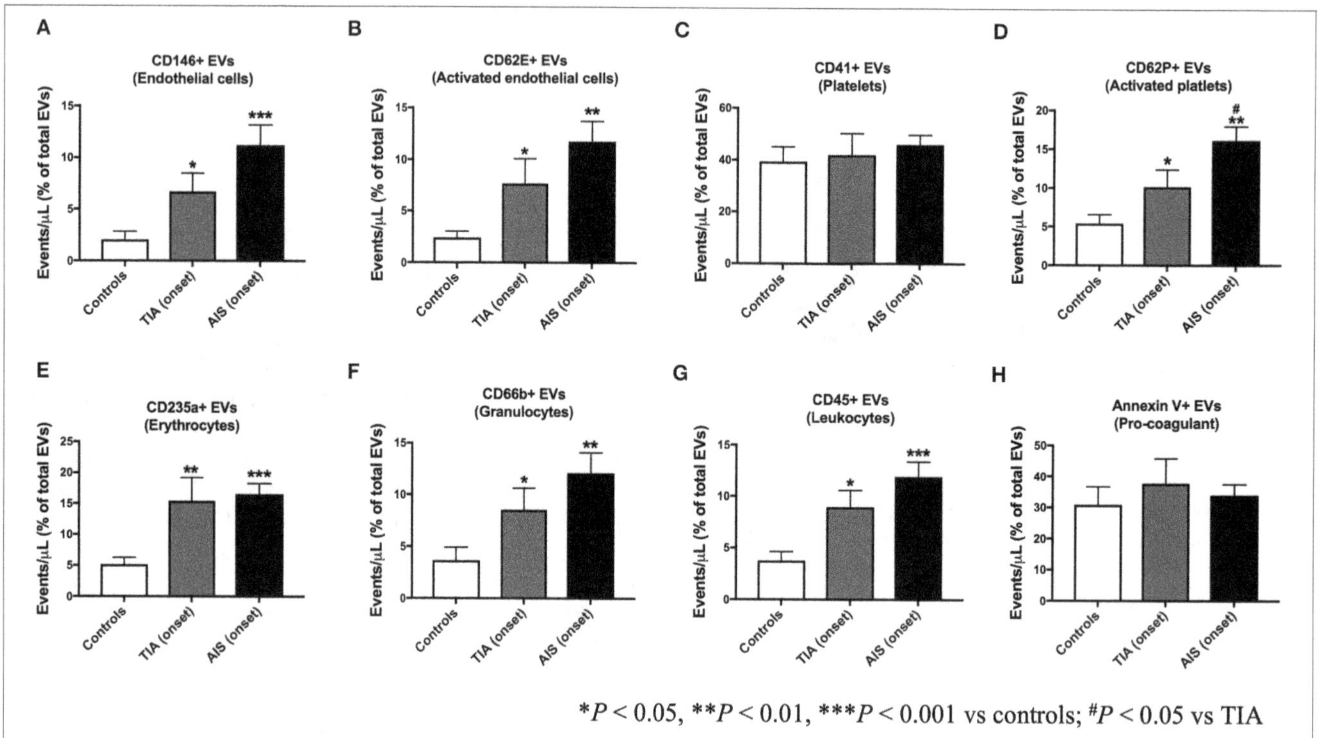

FIGURE 2 | Circulating EV levels, expressed as percentage of total EVs, at onset of attacks, in patients with TIA and AIS compared to healthy controls. Histograms represent circulating levels of EVs derived from: **(A)** endothelial cells ($CD146^+$), **(B)** activated endothelial cells ($CD62E^+$), **(C)** platelets (CD41), **(D)** activated platelets ($CD62P^+$), **(E)** erythrocytes ($CD235a^+$), **(F)** granulocytes ($CD66b^+$), **(G)** leukocytes ($CD45^+$), **(H)** and pro-coagulant (Annexin V^+) origins. Histograms represent events/μL (% of total EVs) in PFP expressed as mean ± SEM. Controls, $n = 24$; TIA, $n = 21$; AIS, $n = 66$. $^*P < 0.05$, $^{**}P < 0.01$, $^{***}P < 0.001$ vs. controls; $^\#P < 0.05$ vs. TIA.

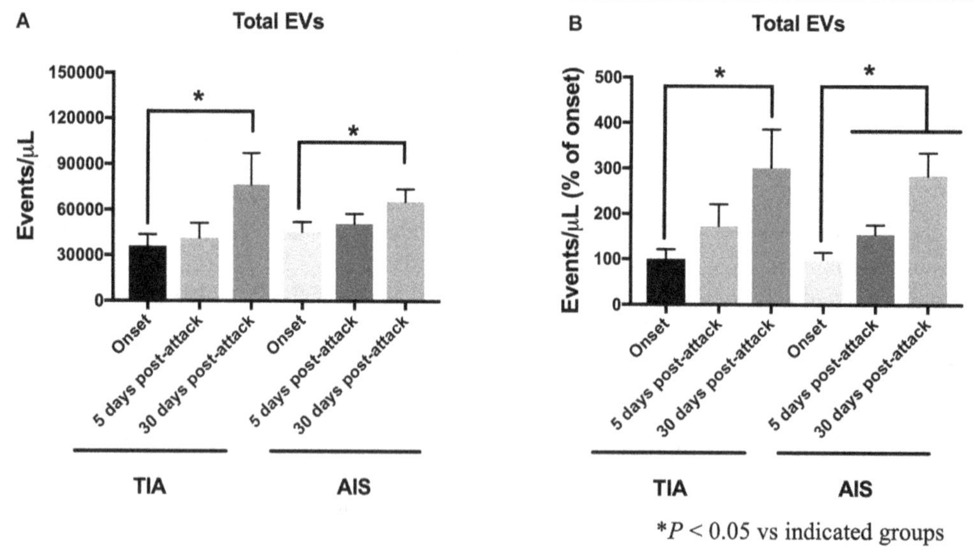

FIGURE 3 | Circulating total EV levels, at onset, 5-days and 30-days post-attacks in patients with TIA and AIS patients. **(A)** Histograms represent total EVs expressed as events/μL in PFP. **(B)** Histograms represent total EVs expressed as events/μL (% of onset levels) in PFP. Data are expressed as mean ± SEM. Controls, $n = 24$; TIA, $n = 21$; AIS, $n = 66$. $^*P < 0.05$ vs. indicated groups.

numbers compared to TIA patients. While there are few reports regarding the phenotype of expression of circulating EVs in AIS, there is a severe paucity of information regarding EVs numbers in blood from TIA patients and how they differ compared to AIS patients. To the best of our knowledge, this is the first report to determine circulating levels of EVs from various cell origins

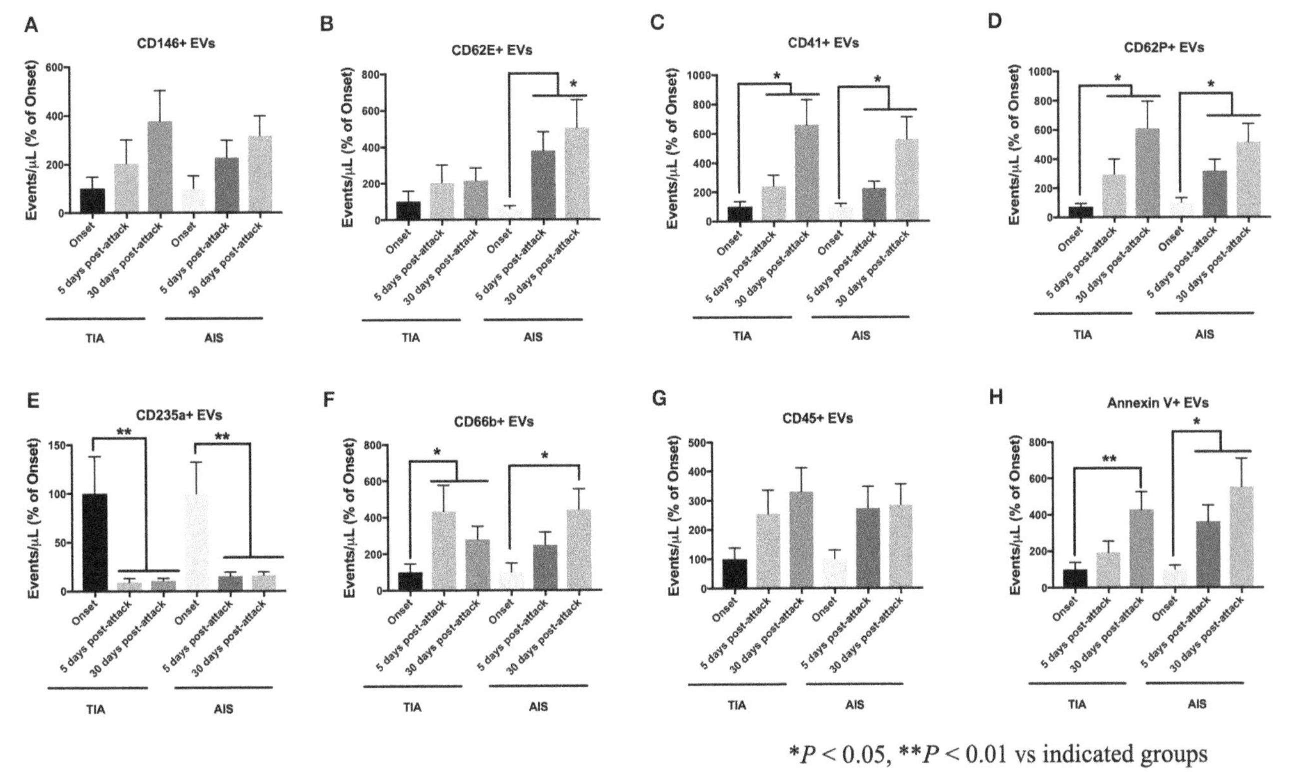

FIGURE 4 | Circulating EV levels, expressed as events/μL (% of onset levels), at onset, 5-days and 30-days post attacks, in PFP from patients with TIA and AIS. Histograms represent circulating levels of EVs derived from: **(A)** endothelial cells ($CD146^+$), **(B)** activated endothelial cells ($CD62E^+$), **(C)** platelets (CD41), **(D)** activated platelets ($CD62P^+$), **(E)** erythrocytes ($CD235a^+$), **(F)** granulocytes ($CD66b^+$), **(G)** leukocytes ($CD45^+$), **(H)** and pro-coagulant (Annexin V^+) origins. Data are expressed as mean ± SEM. Controls, $n = 24$; TIA, $n = 21$; AIS, $n = 66$. $^*P < 0.05$, $^{**}P < 0.01$ vs. indicated groups.

in TIA patients and compare them to AIS patients and healthy controls. Only one previous publication could be found reporting increased levels of platelet-derived EVs in TIA compared to controls (23).

In relation to AIS, our findings are partly in agreement with the few previous studies which investigated EVs levels in AIS patients. Li et al. (13) have studied EVs in a cohort composed of patients with AIS and gender-matched healthy volunteers. In accordance with our data, authors reported that patients had higher levels of endothelial-derived EVs and EVs carrying markers of cell activation ($CD62E^+$); however, no differences in platelet-derived EVs were noted (13). Another study, reported in a cohort of AIS patients that platelet-derived EVs were, however, increased compared to control subjects (14). Recently, it was observed that plasma levels of endothelial-derived EVs were not increased in chronic stroke patients compared to younger and old healthy volunteers (16). These findings are in contrast with our observations and the discrepancy may be attributable to the ethnic differences between the study cohorts [Chinese in Chen et al. (14) vs. SE and ME in our study]. In addition, the study by Chen et al. (14), determined the levels of platelet-derived EVs using anti-CD61 antibody, while in our study we have used an anti-CD41 antibody. Both CD41 and CD61 are platelet-specific glycoproteins, which were widely used as surface markers for the detection of EVs from platelet origin (24, 25). However, in our hands, we have observed similar results to those observed with CD41 when CD61 was used as a surface marker to detect platelet-derived EVs (data not shown for CD61) and hence the discrepancy between the **two** studies may be more related to the ethnic differences in study populations.

More recently, circulating EVs from platelets, endothelial cells, erythrocytes, leukocytes, lymphocytes, monocytes, and smooth muscle cells were analyzed in patients with suspected AIS at the onset of attacks, and then at 7 and 90 days. In line with our observations reported here, authors observed that EVs from all these cell origins were increased in stroke patients compared to controls at onset of attacks and that their levels remained high at 7 and 90 days following the acute events (15). In our hands, we observed that, by contrast to Chiva-Blanch et al. (15), the number of EVs from endothelial cells, activated endothelial cells, platelets, activated platelets, granulocytes, leukocytes, and pro-coagulant origin, expressed as percentage of onset levels, all increased in both TIA and AIS patients after 5 and 30 days post-attacks and the initiation of treatment and the management of risk factors (e.g., diabetes or hypertension). These data, show an escalated cell activation, particularly in endothelial cells and platelets, acutely after the attacks in both

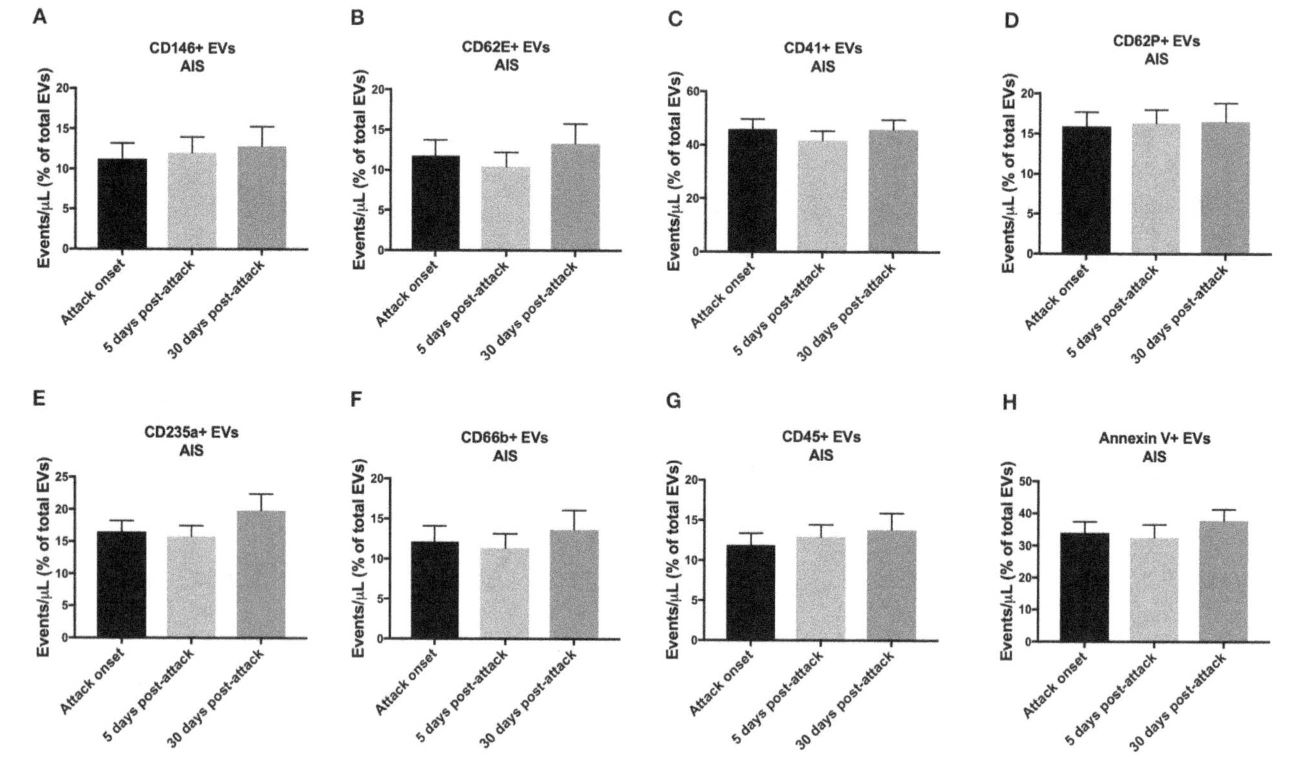

FIGURE 5 | Circulating EV levels, expressed as events/μL (% of total EVs), at onset, 5-days and 30-days post-attacks in PFP from patients with AIS. Histograms represent circulating levels of EVs derived from: **(A)** endothelial cells ($CD146^+$), **(B)** activated endothelial cells ($CD62E^+$), **(C)** platelets (CD41), **(D)** activated platelets ($CD62P^+$), **(E)** erythrocytes ($CD235a^+$), **(F)** granulocytes ($CD66b^+$), **(G)** leukocytes ($CD45^+$), **(H)** and pro-coagulant (Annexin V^+) origins. Data are expressed as mean ± SEM. AIS, $n = 66$.

TIA and AIS patients, which may contribute to heightened endothelial and pro-thrombotic activities contributing thus to an elevated risk of stroke recurrence. However, we cannot rule out that the elevation of EVs levels following the attacks and the start of pharmacotherapy might be related to the resolution of thrombi and the secondary consequences of ischemic episodes. Thus, a longer follow-up of these patients is warranted to determine the long-term changes of EVs and further ascertain the prognostic value of circulating EVs levels in TIA and AIS patients with regards to the risk of recurrence.

Of particular interest, in our study, plasma levels of EVs from platelets ($CD41^+$), activated platelets ($CD62P^+$), and pro-coagulant (Annexin V^+) origins increased, as a percentage of onset numbers, on the short-term (at 5- and 30-days after acute attacks), indicating a higher number of EVs with pro-thrombotic activity, which may contribute to the increased risk of recurrence of stroke in these patients, including those with no major consequences (TIA). EVs from platelet origin are indeed strongly pro-thrombotic (21). It has been reported that one single platelet-derived EV had nearly the same pro-coagulant activity as one activated platelet despite the surface area was 2 orders of magnitude smaller, suggesting that the surface of platelet-derived EVs is 50 to 100–fold more pro-coagulant than that of activated platelets (26). Furthermore, though not directly assessed in this study, EVs expressing tissue factor (TF) may also enhance the coagulation process in stroke patients. EVs carrying TF were found to be highly expressed in several ischemic conditions such as atherosclerosis and acute coronary syndromes (27). It was reported that the expression of TF at the surface of EVs enhanced their pro-coagulant response (28). Higher circulating levels of EVs expressing TF were observed in AIS patients compared to healthy controls. Moreover, 1 week after the diagnosis, the activity of EVs was found to be more elevated in stroke patients not treated with tissue plasminogen activator compared to their basal activity at the onset of attacks (29).

While we have observed that erythrocyte-derided EVs ($CD235a^+$) were increased to the same extent in both TIA and AIS compared to controls within 48 h of onset of attacks, we found that their levels, expressed as a proportion of onset levels, decreased in both TIA and AIS patients at 5- and 30-days following the initiation of pharmacotherapy. In contrast with our observation, Chiva-Blanch et al. (15), found that erythrocyte-derived EVs were higher in AIS patients compared to controls and continued to be high at 7 and 90 days post-stroke attacks (15). Our data suggest that the administration of treatment to patients led to a decrease in the expression of erythrocyte-derided EVs, which were previously linked to hypercoagulable states. Consistent with our observations, Tan et al. (30), observed that high circulating levels of phosphatidylserine-positive erythrocyte-derived EVs, which were highly pro-coagulant, in patients suffering from

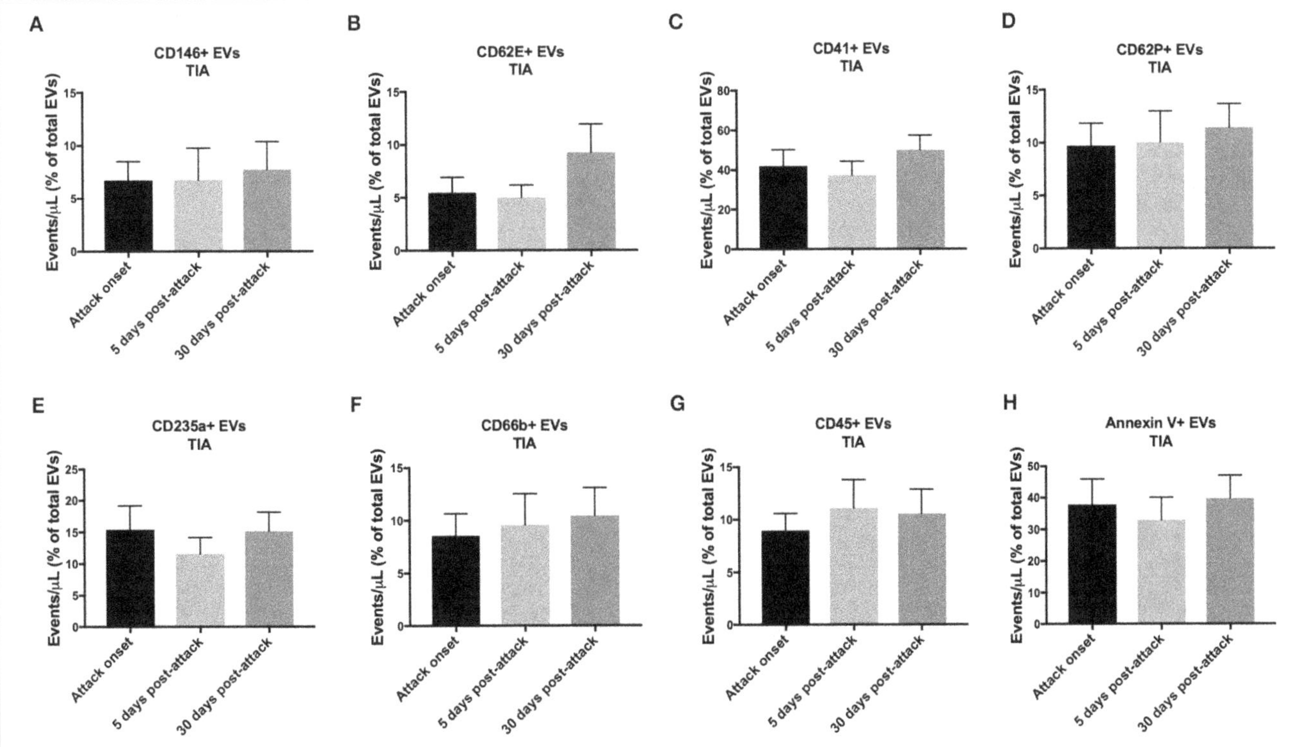

FIGURE 6 | Circulating EV levels, expressed as events/µL (% of total EVs), at onset, 5-days and 30-days post-attacks in PFP from patients with TIA. Histograms represent circulating levels of EVs derived from: **(A)** endothelial cells ($CD146^+$), **(B)** activated endothelial cells ($CD62E^+$), **(C)** platelets (CD41), **(D)** activated platelets ($CD62P^+$), **(E)** erythrocytes ($CD235a^+$), **(F)** granulocytes ($CD66b^+$), **(G)** leukocytes ($CD45^+$), **(H)** and pro-coagulant (Annexin V^+) origins. Data are expressed as mean ± SEM. TIA, $n = 21$.

the hypercoagulable status of polycythemia vera and that the treatment of patients with hydroxyurea was associated with a decrease in the shedding of EVs from erythrocytes (30).

Our data characterized for the **first** time circulating EVs in patients with AIS and compared them to TIA in a multiethnic population from SE and ME origins. We provided here, a very comprehensive analysis of most circulating EVs from vascular wall, blood, and immune cells. We found here that EVs of various origins, especially those associated with endothelial cell injury and platelet activation, are increased in TIA and AIS patients and that their levels persist to be high on the short-term up to 30-days post-attacks, indicating a sustained cellular activation, which may be associated with a heightened risk of recurrence of acute events. Therefore, longer follow-up studies are required to ascertain the value of EVs as biomarkers for the risk of stroke recurrence, especially in a population presenting with stroke at young age like this one.

AUTHOR CONTRIBUTIONS

AA and AS wrote the article and all authors contributed to the drafting of the manuscript and its critical revision for intellectual content. AA, AS, and ASP were involved in the study conception and design and in the interpretation of data. AA and AS acquired funding and supervised the experiments. AA, ASP, FM, and SS conducted sample analysis, and data acquisition, processing, statistical analysis, and interpretation. AS oversaw the whole clinical process and contributed to the analysis and interpretation of data. NA, PB, SJ, DM, MS, MW, and SK collected clinical data, refined diagnosis, and collected clinical samples for the study. NA contributed to the interpretation of clinical data.

ACKNOWLEDGMENTS

This work was supported by a Qatar University high collaborative grant (QUCG-CPH-2018\2019-2) to AA. The publication of this article was funded by Qatar National Library. The statements made herein are solely the responsibility of the authors.

REFERENCES

Brainin M, Teuschl Y, Kalra L. Acute treatment and long-term management of stroke in developing countries. *Lancet Neurol.* (2007) 6:553–61. doi: 10.1016/S1474-4422(07)70005-4

Feigin VL, Roth GA, Naghavi M, Parmar P, Krishnamurthi R, Chugh S, et al. Global burden of stroke and risk factors in 188 countries, during 1990–2013: a systematic analysis for the Global Burden of Disease Study 2013. *Lancet Neurol.* (2016) 15:913–24. doi: 10.1016/S1474-4422(16)30 073-4

Akhtar N, Salam A, Kamran S, D'Souza A, Imam Y, Own A, et al. Pre- existing Small vessel disease in patients with acute stroke from the Middle East, Southeast Asia, and Philippines. *Transl Stroke Res.* (2018) 9:274–82. doi: 10.1007/s12975-017-0578-7

Jensen HA, Mehta JL. Endothelial cell dysfunction as a novel therapeutic target in atherosclerosis. *Expert Rev Cardiovasc Ther.* (2016) 14:1021–33. doi: 10.1080/14779072.2016.1207527

Wang B, Cai W, Zhang Z, Zhang H, Tang K, Zhang Q, et al. Circulating microparticles in patients after ischemic stroke: a systematic review and meta- analysis. *Rev Neurosci.* (2018). doi: 10.1515/revneuro-2017-0105. [Epub of print].

Chiang CY, Chen C. Toward characterizing extracellular vesicles at a single-particle level. *J Biomed Sci.* (2019) 26:9. doi: 10.1186/s12929-019-0502-4

Thery C, Witwer KW, Aikawa E, Alcaraz MJ, Anderson JD, Andriantsitohaina R, et al. Minimal information for studies of extracellular vesicles 2018 (MISEV2018): a position statement of the International Society for Extracellular Vesicles and update of the MISEV2014 guidelines. *J Extracell Vesicles.* (2018) 7:1535750. doi: 10.1080/20013078.2018.1535750

Agouni A, Andriantsitohaina R, Martinez MC. Microparticles as biomarkers of vascular dysfunction in metabolic syndrome and its individual components. *Curr Vasc Pharmacol.* (2014) 12:483–92. doi: 10.2174/1 570161112666140423223148

Chen Y, Li G, Liu ML. Microvesicles as Emerging biomarkers and therapeutic targets in cardiometabolic diseases. *Genomics Proteomics Bioinformatics.* (2018) 16:50–62. doi: 10.1016/j.gpb.2017.03.006

Csongradi E, Nagy B Jr, Fulop T, Varga Z, Karanyi Z, Magyar MT, et al. Increased levels of platelet activation markers are positively associated with carotid wall thickness and other atherosclerotic risk factors in obese patients. *Thromb Haemost.* (2011) 106:683–92. doi: 10.1160/TH11-01-0030

Agouni A, Lagrue-Lak-Hal AH, Ducluzeau PH, Mostefai HA, Draunet- Busson C, Leftheriotis G, et al. Endothelial dysfunction caused by circulating microparticles from patients with metabolic syndrome. *Am J Pathol.* (2008) 173:1210–9. doi: 10.2353/ajpath.2008.080228

Agouni A, Ducluzeau PH, Benameur T, Faure S, Sladkova M, Duluc L, et al. Microparticles from patients with metabolic syndrome induce vascular hypo- reactivity via Fas/Fas-ligand pathway in mice. *PLoS ONE.* (2011) 6:e27809. doi: 10.1371/journal.pone.0027809 (2018) 103:1560–70. doi: 10.1113/EP087116

Mostefai HA, Meziani F, Mastronardi ML, Agouni A, Heymes C, Sargentini C, et al. Circulating microparticles from patients with septic shock exert protective role in vascular function. *Am J Respir Crit Care Med.* (2008) 178:1148–55. doi: 10.1164/rccm.200712-1835OC

Priou P, Gagnadoux F, Tesse A, Mastronardi ML, Agouni A, Meslier N, et al. Endothelial dysfunction and circulating microparticles from patients with obstructive sleep apnea. *Am J Pathol.* (2010) 177:974–83. doi: 10.2353/ajpath.2010.091252

Tual-Chalot S, Leonetti D, Andriantsitohaina R, Martinez MC. Microvesicles: intercellular vectors of biological messages. *Mol Interv.* (2011) 11:88–94. doi: 10.1124/mi.11.2.5

Zaborowski MP, Balaj L, Breakefield XO, Lai CP. Extracellular vesicles: composition, biological relevance, and methods of study. *Bioscience.* (2015) 65:783–97. doi: 10.1093/biosci/biv084

Morel O, Jesel L, Freyssinet JM, Toti F. Cellular mechanisms underlying the formation of circulating microparticles. *Arterioscler Thromb Vasc Biol.* (2011) 31:15–26. doi: 10.1161/ATVBAHA.109.200956

Sinning JM, Jansen F, Hammerstingl C, Meier A, Losch J, Rohwer K, et al. Circulating microparticles decrease after cardiac stress in patients with significant coronary artery stenosis. *Clin Cardiol.* (2016) 39:570–7. doi: 10.1002/clc.22566

Lee YJ, Jy W, Horstman LL, Janania J, Reyes Y, Kelley RE, et al. Elevated platelet microparticles in transient ischemic attacks, lacunar infarcts, and multiinfarct dementias. *Thromb Res.* (1993) 72:295–304.

Bennett JS, Berger BW, Billings PC. The structure and function of platelet integrins. *J Thromb Haemost.* (2009) 7(Suppl. 1):200–5. doi: 10.1111/j.1538-7836.2009.03378.x

Nolan JP, Jones JC. Detection of platelet vesicles by flow cytometry. *Platelets.* (2017) 28:256–62. doi: 10.1080/09537104.2017.1280602

Sinauridze EI, Kireev DA, Popenko NY, Pichugin AV, Panteleev MA, Krymskaya OV, et al. Platelet microparticle membranes have 50- to 100- fold higher specific procoagulant activity than activated platelets. *Thromb Haemost.* (2007) 97:425–34. doi: 10.1160/TH06-06-0313

Morel O, Toti F, Hugel B, Bakouboula B, Camoin-Jau L, Dignat- George F, et al. Procoagulant microparticles: disrupting the vascular homeostasis equation? *Arterioscler Thromb Vasc Biol.* (2006) 26:2594–604. doi: 10.1161/01.ATV.0000246775.14471.26

Owens APIII, Mackman N. Microparticles in hemostasis and thrombosis. *Circ Res.* (2011) 108:1284–97. doi: 10.1161/CIRCRESAHA.110.233056

Switonska M, Slomka A, Sinkiewicz W, Zekanowska E. Tissue-factor-bearing microparticles (MPs-TF) in patients with acute ischaemic stroke: the influence of stroke treatment on MPs-TF generation. *Eur J Neurol.* (2015) 22:e328–99. doi: 10.1111/ene.12591

Tan X, Shi J, Fu Y, Gao C, Yang X, Li J, et al. Role of erythrocytes and platelets in the hypercoagulable status in polycythemia vera through phosphatidylserine exposure and microparticle generation. *Thromb Haemost.* (2013) 109:1025–+ +Li P, Qin C. Elevated circulating VE-cadherin CD144 endothelial microparticles in ischemic cerebrovascular disease. *Thromb Res.* (2015) 135:375–81. doi: 10.1016/j.thromres.2014.12.006

Chen Y, Xiao Y, Lin Z, Xiao X, He C, Bihl JC, et al. The role of circulating platelets microparticles and platelet parameters in acute ischemic stroke patients. *J Stroke Cerebrovasc Dis.* (2015) 24:2313–20. doi: 10.1016/j.jstrokecerebrovasdis.2015.06.018

Chiva-Blanch G, Suades R, Crespo J, Pena E, Padro T, Jimenez-Xarrie E, et al. Microparticle shedding from neural progenitor cells and vascular compartment cells is increased in ischemic stroke. *PLoS ONE.* (2016) 11:e0148176. doi: 10.1371/journal.pone.0148176

Landers-Ramos RQ, Serra MC, Blumenthal JB, Ryan AS, Hafer-Macko CE, Prior SJ. Type 2 diabetes and older age contribute to elevated plasma microparticle concentrations independent of chronic stroke. *Exp. Physiol.* 32. doi: 10.1160/TH12-11-0811

15

Expression of *Tmem119/Sall1* and *Ccr2/CD69* in FACS-Sorted Microglia- and Monocyte/ Macrophage-Enriched Cell Populations After Intracerebral Hemorrhage

Qian Li[†‡], *Xi Lan*[‡], *Xiaoning Han and Jian Wang**

Department of Anesthesiology and Critical Care Medicine, The Johns Hopkins University School of Medicine, Baltimore, MD, United States

***Correspondence:**
Jian Wang
jwang79@jhmi.edu

[†]Present address:
Qian Li,
Department of Biochemistry and Molecular Biology, Beijing Key Laboratory of Neural Regeneration and Repair, School of Basic Medical Sciences, Capital Medical University, Beijing, China;
Advanced Innovation Center for Human Brain Protection, Beijing, China

[‡]*These authors have contributed equally to this work*

Activation and polarization of microglia and macrophages are critical events in neuroinflammation and hematoma resolution after intracerebral hemorrhage (ICH). However, distinguishing microglia and monocyte-derived macrophages histologically can be difficult. Although they share most cell surface markers, evidence indicates that the gene regulation and function of these two cell types might be different. Flow cytometry is the gold standard for discriminating between the two cell populations, but it is rarely used in the ICH research field. We developed a flow cytometry protocol to identify and sort microglia and monocyte-derived macrophages from mice that have undergone well-established ICH models induced by collagenase or blood injection. In addition, we combined a recently established magnetic-activated cell separation system that allows eight tissue samples to be assessed together. This protocol can be completed within 5–8 h. Sorted cells are fully preserved and maintain expression of microglia-specific (*Tmem119/Sall1*) and macrophage-specific (*Ccr2/CD69*) markers. They retain phagocytic ability, respond to lipopolysaccharide stimulation, and engulf fluorescent latex beads. Thus, this protocol represents a very important tool for researching microglial and monocyte-derived macrophage biologic function after ICH and other brain diseases.

Keywords: fluorescent-activated cell sorting, intracerebral hemorrhage, monocyte-derived macrophage, magnetic-activated cell separation, microglia

INTRODUCTION

Intracerebral hemorrhage (ICH), the second most common type of stroke, affects more than 1 million people each year (Kim and Bae, 2017; Thabet et al., 2017). As the most important innate immune cell types, microglia and infiltrating monocyte-derived macrophages play critical roles in neuroinflammation (Wang and Tsirka, 2005; Wang, 2010; Wu et al., 2010; Lan et al., 2017a),

---

Abbreviations: FACS, fluorescence-activated cell sorting; ICH, intracerebral hemorrhage; MACS, magnetic-activated cell separation; MMϕ, microglia/macrophages; PI, propidium iodide.

hematoma resolution (Flores et al., 2016; Chang et al., 2017; Lan et al., 2018), white matter injury (Li et al., 2017d, 2018), and neuronal toxicity (Wu et al., 2011; Yang J. et al., 2016; Zhang et al., 2017) after ICH. Recent studies have indicated that microglia and macrophages may have opposing functions after ICH: macrophage depletion exacerbates brain damage after experimental ICH (Min et al., 2016), whereas elimination of microglia improves ICH outcomes in the same animal model (Li et al., 2017a). Therefore, distinguishing microglial and macrophage function, activation, and polarization is critical to understanding ICH pathophysiology (Lan et al., 2017c, 2018).

Magnetic-activated cell separation (MACS) has been used to isolate microglia and monocyte-derived macrophages (MMϕ) in mouse models of Alzheimer's disease (Kronenberg et al., 2017), glioma (Szulzewsky et al., 2015), ischemic stroke (Yang B. et al., 2016), and ICH (Lan et al., 2017a). However, to our knowledge, no protocol exists for separating the two cell types after ICH. Here, we used a MACS tissue dissociation system to dissociate the brains of mice after collagenase-induced or blood-induced ICH. Then, after removing myelin and red blood cells (RBCs), we counted live cells and used fluorescence-activated cell sorting (FACS).

Flow cytometry can provide highly sensitive detection and accurate analysis of different cell populations. In our optimized procedure, we used fluorescent antibodies Ly6g, CD11b, and CD45 together with propidium iodide (PI) to stain brain cells, and subsequently sorted the cells by flow cytometry. The populations of $Ly6g^-/CD45^{high}/CD11b^+$ and $Ly6g^-/CD45^{Int}/CD11b^+$, which encompass infiltrating monocytes/macrophages and resident microglia, were sorted separately (Hellstrom Erkenstam et al., 2016; Varvel et al., 2016; Vinet et al., 2016). We confirmed that the expression of *Tmem119/Sall1* and *Ccr2/CD69* differed in FACS-sorted microglia- and monocyte/macrophage-enriched cell populations, respectively. These isolated cells had maximally preserved biologic characteristics after ICH, including inflammatory responses, phagocytosis, and dynamic polarization. They also can be applied to real-time PCR, RNA nanostring, mass spectrometry/proteomics, and *in vitro* cell culture.

This MACS and FACS-based method allows us to distinguish microglia and infiltrating monocytes/macrophages after ICH using MMϕ cell surface markers. This method is fast, efficient, simple, and accurate. Therefore, our optimized protocol provides an important tool for studying MMϕ function after ICH and other brain diseases.

MATERIALS AND EQUIPMENT

Animals

All animal experiments were conducted in accordance with guidelines from the National Institutes of Health and were approved by the Institutional Animal Care and Use Committee at The Johns Hopkins University School of Medicine. Adult male C57BL/6 mice (8–10 weeks old) were purchased from Charles River Laboratories (Frederick, MD).

ICH Mouse Models

- Collagenase VII-S, cat #C2399, Sigma-Aldrich
- 50-μL Hamilton syringe, cat #80100
- 1-μL Hamilton syringe, cat #80908
- Motorized microinjector,
- DC Temperature Controller 40-90-8D, FHC Inc., ME

Tissue Dissociation

- Neural Tissue Dissociation kit (P), cat #130-092-628, Miltenyi Biotec
- C Tubes, cat #130-096-334, Miltenyi Biotec
- gentleMACS Dissociator, cat #130-093-235, Miltenyi Biotec
- MACSmix Tube Rotator, cat #130-090-753, Miltenyi Biotec
- Myelin Removal Beads, cat #130-096-731, Miltenyi Biotec
- Myelin removal buffer: PBS solution containing 0.5% bovine serum albumin (BSA)
- Red Blood Cell Lysis Solution, cat #130-094-183, Miltenyi Biotec
- LS columns, cat #130-042-401, Miltenyi Biotec
- QuadroMACS Separator, cat #130-091-051, Miltenyi Biotec
- HBSS with Ca^{2+}/Mg^{2+}, cat #14025134, Thermo Fisher Scientific
- HBSS without Ca^{2+}/Mg^{2+}, cat #14170161, Thermo Fisher Scientific
- 70-micron cell strainer, cat #352350, Corning Inc.

Flow Cytometry and Fluorescence-Activated Cell Sorting (FACS)

- FITC-CD11b, cat #130-081-201, Miltenyi Biotec
- PE-CD45, cat #130-102-596, Miltenyi Biotec
- APC-Ly6g, cat #560599, BD Pharmingen
- BV421-CD45, cat #103133, Biolegend
- Flow buffer (HBSS without Ca^{2+}/Mg^{2+}, 10 mM HEPES, 1% BSA)
- Blocking buffer (1% goat serum, 0.5% BSA, and 2 mM EDTA in PBS)
- MoFlo cytometer, Beckman Coulter

Real-Time PCR and Cell Culture

- TRIzol reagent, cat #15596018, Thermo Fisher Scientific
- NanoDrop 2000 spectrophotometer, Thermo Fisher Scientific
- SuperScript VILO cDNA Synthesis kit, cat #11754250, Thermo Fisher Scientific
- TaqMan Universal Master Mix II, cat #4440038, Thermo Fisher Scientific
- Real-time PCR primers, TaqMan® Gene Expression Assay, Thermo Fisher Scientific
- QuantStudio™ 3 Real-Time PCR System, 96-well, 0.1 mL
- DMEM/F-12, cat #11330057, Thermo Fisher Scientific
- Fetal bovine serum (FBS), cat #10438026, Thermo Fisher Scientific
- Penicillin-streptomycin, cat #15140148, Thermo Fisher Scientific
- M-CSF, cat #315-02, PeproTech

- Culture medium: DMEM/F-12 with 10% FBS, 100 U/mL penicillin-streptomycin and 20 ng/μL M-CSF
- pHrodo Red Zymosan Bioparticles Conjugate for Phagocytosis, cat #P35364, Thermo Fisher Scientific

Step-By-Step Procedure

ICH Mouse Models: 20 min to 50 min/Each Mouse

Mice were anesthetized with 1–3% isoflurane and ventilated with oxygen-enriched air (20%:80%) via a nose cone. We used two well-established ICH mouse models - the collagenase-induced model and the blood-induced model - for this protocol (Li and Wang, 2017). For the collagenase-induced ICH model, we injected collagenase VII-S (0.0525 U in 0.35 μL sterile saline) into the striatum (0.1 μL/min) at the following coordinates relative to the bregma: 0.8 mm anterior, 2 mm lateral, and 2.8 mm deep (Li et al., 2017b; Yang et al., 2017; Zhu et al., 2018). For the blood-induced ICH model, we injected 20 μL of autologous whole blood at a rate of 1 μL/min at those the same coordinates (Zhu et al., 2014; Meng et al., 2017; Wu et al., 2017). We chose the injection volumes based on preliminary experiments in which we matched hematoma volume in the two models on day 1 post-ICH, when hematoma reaches its maximum (Wang et al., 2015), to ensure a fair comparison. Our results showed that the hematoma size induced by 0.0525 U collagenase (6.86 ± 1.11 mm^3, $n = 5$) was similar to that induced by 20 μL blood injection (6.92 ± 1.27 mm^3, $n = 5$) at 1 day post-ICH (**Figure 1**). Therefore, we used those dosages for our subsequent experiments.

Animal core body temperature was maintained at 37.0 ± 0.5°C throughout the surgery and recovery periods with a DC Temperature Controller 40-90-8D. Sham control mice underwent the same procedure, including needle insertion, but without collagenase or whole blood injection.

NOTE: Completion of the procedure requires 20 min per mouse for the collagenase-induced ICH model and 50 min per mouse for the blood-induced ICH model.

Brain Tissue Preparation: 10 min/Each Mouse

At 24 h after ICH induction, mice were sacrificed and perfused with ice-cold phosphate-buffered saline (PBS; Thermo Fisher Scientific, Waltham, MA). Based on our pre-calculated injury volume, we collected a 4 mm-thick sample from the ipsilateral caudate putamen (~80 mg/sample) that included all of the injured area (Chang et al., 2015). Each sample was quickly transferred to 1 mL of cold Hanks' buffered salt solution (HBSS; without Ca^{2+}/Mg^{2+}) for the dissociation steps.

NOTE: Sacrifice the mice as soon as possible to keep brain tissue fresh and maximally maintain the live cell status. Delay may result in fewer live cells.

Tissue Dissociation With the gentleMACS™ Dissociator: 40 min/up to 8 Mice

The automated dissociation system (Lee and Lufkin, 2012) was purchased from Miltenyi Biotec (Auburn, CA). The manufacturer's instructions were followed for reagent preparation and major steps (**Figure 2**).

(1) Transfer tissues into the C tubes containing 37°C pre-warmed enzyme mix 1 (50 μL Enzyme P and 1900 μL Buffer X).
(2) Run the gentleMACS program "m_brain_01" when C-tubes are attached onto the gentleMACS Dissociator.
(3) Incubate the samples for 15 min at 37°C, and then run on program "m_brain_02."
(4) Add 30 μL of enzyme mix 2 (20 μL Buffer Y and 10 μL Enzyme A) into each sample and re-incubate them for 10 min at 37°C.
(5) Run on program "m_brain_03" with another incubation for 10 min at 37°C; then spin down quickly (4000 rpm for 10–15 s at room temperature) and collect the cells.
(6) Resuspend the cells gently in 10 mL of HBSS (with Ca^{2+}/Mg^{2+}) and pass them through a 70-micron cell strainer to a new 50 mL tube.
(7) After washing the cells in 10 mL HBSS (with Ca^{2+}/Mg^{2+}), centrifuge them at 300 × g for 10 min at 4°C and then collect them for myelin and RBC removal.

NOTE:

(a) The gentleMACS™ Dissociator can hold up to eight C tubes at once. Thus, more samples may take more than 40 min.
(b) Before attaching the C tubes to the dissociator, make sure they have been tightened.

Sample Clearing: 80 min

All procedures were carried out according to the manufacture's protocol.

Myelin removal:

- Incubate cells with Myelin Removal Beads (200 μL beads and 1800 μL buffer per sample) for 15 min at 4°C.
- Wash cells in 5 mL of myelin removal buffer and centrifuge at 300 × g for 10 min at 4°C.
- Suspend pellets in 1 mL buffer and apply them onto the LS column (3 columns for each 200 μL beads).
- Collect the unlabeled cells in a 15 mL tube.
- Centrifuge at 300 × g for 10 min at 4°C and collect cell pellets for the next steps.

RBC removal:

- Collect the cell pellets and suspend them in 20 times volume of 1 × Red Blood Cell Lysis Solution (~1 mL per sample).
- After incubating the samples at 4°C for 10 min, add 10 mL of 0.5% BSA buffer and centrifuge them at 300 × g for 5 min. Cell pellets proceed to the FACS step.

NOTE:

(a) The volume of Myelin Removal Beads used depends on the tissue weight. If the mouse brain is greater than 500 mg, more beads may be needed to remove myelin debris.
(b) The LS column should be rinsed with 3 mL of buffer before the suspended cells are applied to it.

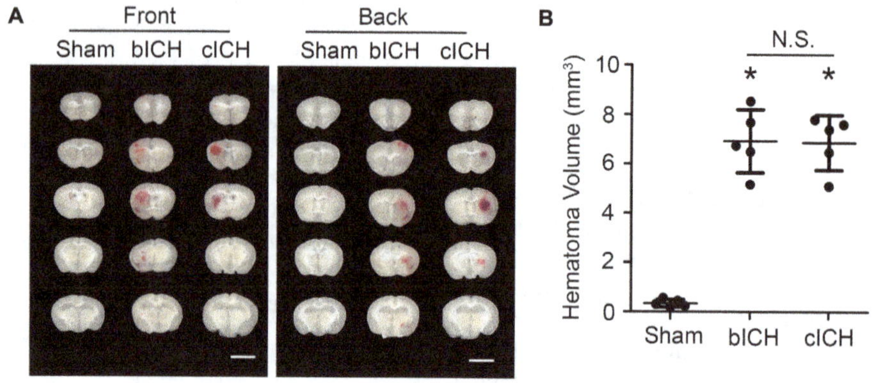

FIGURE 1 | Hematomas on day 1 after blood-induced intracerebral hemorrhage (bICH) and collagenase-induced ICH (cICH) were matched for size. Eight- to ten-week-old male C57BL/6 mice underwent collagenase injection, blood injection, or sham procedure. Mice were sacrificed at day 1 post-ICH. **(A)** Representative images from fresh brain coronal sections. **(B)** Quantification of hematoma volume. $*p < 0.05$ vs. Sham; N.S., not significant; $n = 5$. Results are presented as scatter plots (mean ± SD). One-way ANOVA followed by Dunn's multiple comparison post-test. Scale bars: 1 mm.

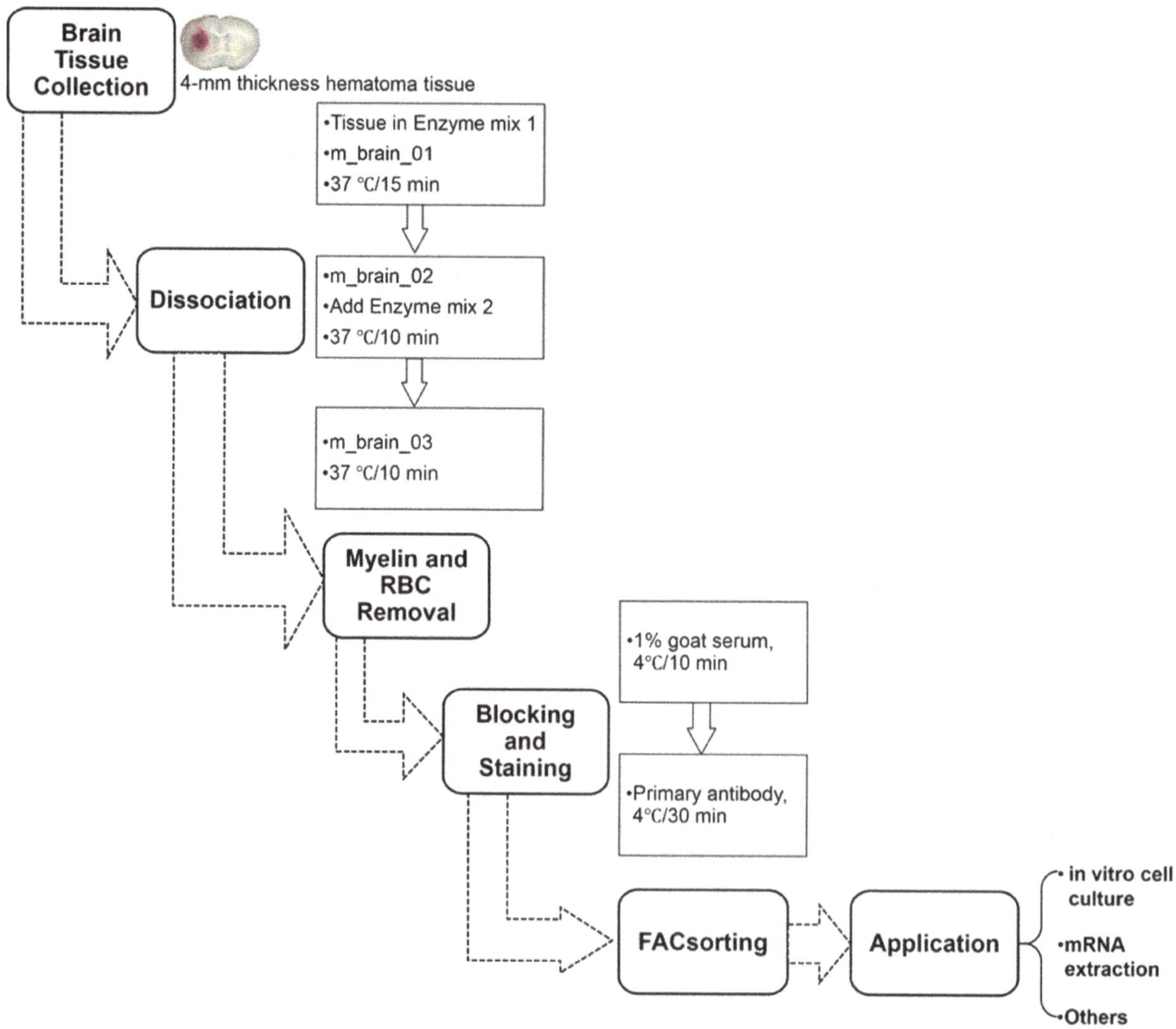

FIGURE 2 | Procedure for isolating mouse microglia and monocyte-derived macrophages after ICH. RBC, red blood cells.

(c) Carefully avoid air bubbles when eluting cells, as they may block columns.

Tissue Dissociation With Percoll

The manual Percoll dissociation procedure was performed based on a published protocol (Lelios and Greter, 2014). Briefly, fresh brain tissue was collected, cut, and digested in 0.4 mg/mL collagenase IV (Sigma-Aldrich) for 45 min at 37°C. Tissue was homogenized by passing it through a syringe with an 18G, 1½ inch needle. The cell suspension was then passed through a 70-micron cell strainer. Cells were washed in PBS, mixed with Percoll (Cat #17089102, GE Healthcare Life Sciences), and then centrifuged at 15,000 × *g* for 30 min. After the topmost layer was discarded, the remainder was filtered through a 70-micron cell strainer. Finally, the cell suspension was centrifuged at 450 × *g* for 5 min at 4°C and the cell pellet collected for the FACS step.

FACS

Cell surface staining: 50–60 min

- Incubate the cells in blocking buffer for 10 min at 4°C.
- Incubate cells with the primary antibodies for 30 min at 4°C.
    - To observe cell morphology and measure pro-inflammatory cytokines and mRNA, we used FITC-CD11b (1:10), PE-CD45 (1:10), and APC-Ly6g (1:10).
    - For evaluation of cell phagocytic function, we used FITC-CD11b (1:10) and BV421-CD45 (1:10).
- Use the corresponding isotype antibodies as negative controls (**Supplementary Figure 1**).
- Stained samples are washed three times and centrifuged at 300 × *g* for 5 min at 4°C. Resuspend cells in 0.5–1 mL filtered flow buffer. Add PI to distinguish dead cells.

NOTE:

(a) Cells should be kept on ice until being sorted on a MoFlo cytometer (Beckman Coulter).
(b) The volume of blocking buffer depends on the total cell number counted before staining. We recommend 1 × 10^6 cells/200 μL buffer for blocking.
(c) Antibodies can be added directly into blocking buffer at the ratio we suggested.
(d) Alternatives:
For *ex vivo* cell culture, cells can be sorted into culture medium.
For mRNA extraction and real-time PCR, cells can be sorted into TRIzol reagent.
(e) Cell sorting time depends on the live cell numbers; it usually takes 20–30 min to run each mouse sample.

Other Methods

mRNA Extraction and Real-Time PCR

TRIzol reagent was added to the pellets, which were triturated and incubated for 5 min at room temperature. Then, after 100 μL of chloroform was added to the lysate (200 μL/1 mL TRIzol), the samples were incubated for 2 min and centrifuged at 12,000 × *g* for 15 min at 4°C. We transferred the aqueous phase, which contained the RNA, to a new RNase/DNase-free tube and added 5 μg glycogen as a carrier and 250 μL isopropanol to each sample. The samples were incubated for 10 min and then centrifuged at 12,000 × *g* for 10 min at 4°C. We then discarded the supernatants, washed the pellets with 500 μL of 75% ethanol (1 mL/1 mL TRIzol), and centrifuged them again at 7,500 × *g* for 5 min at 4°C. Supernatants were discarded and the RNA pellets air dried. We used 10–15 μL warm (55°C) RNase/DNase-free water to dissolve the pellets. The RNA concentration was measured on a NanoDrop 2000 spectrophotometer.

For the real-time PCR assay, we followed the protocol provided by the manufacturer. Briefly, for the reverse transcription (RT) reaction, reaction mix (4 μL), enzyme mix (2 μL), RNA (500 ng), and DEPC-treated water were mixed to a total volume of 20 μL. We used the RT reaction program provided by the manufacturer. To measure mRNA, we prepared the reaction mix by combining 7.5 μL TaqMan Universal Master Mix II (2×), 1 μL primers, 50 ng cDNA template, and RNase/DNase-free water to a total volume of 15 μL. Mixtures were transferred to MicroAmp Fast Optical 96-Well Reaction Plates (cat #4346907) for use in the Applied Biosystems 7500 Fast Real-time PCR system (Thermo Fisher Scientific) (Li et al., 2017c). Reactions were incubated at 50°C for 2 min, 95°C for 10 min, and for 40 cycles of 95°C for 15 s and 60°C for 1 min. Relative mRNA expression was calculated by $2^{-\Delta\Delta Ct}$, and GAPDH was used as an internal control. The following TaqMan Gene Expression Assay Mixes (Applied Biosystems) were used: *IL-1β* (Mm00434228_m1), *CD32* (Mm004388875_m1), *IL-10* (Mm00439614_m1), *YM-1* (Mm00657889_m1), *Temel19* (Mm00525305_m1), *Sall1* (Mn00491266_m1), *Ccr2* (Mm00438270_m1), *CD69* (Mm01183378_m1), and *GAPDH* (Mm99999915_g1).

Microglial and Macrophage Culture

CD11b$^+$/CD45^{Int} (microglia) and CD11b$^+$/CD45^{high} (monocytes/macrophages) were sorted in DMEM/F-12 with FBS and penicillin-streptomycin at 4°C. Cell supernatants were centrifuged at 300 × *g* for 10 min and resuspended in culture medium. Cells were seeded at 5,000 per well on poly-l-lysine-coated Nunc Lab-Tek II Chamber Slides (Thermo Fisher Scientific, cat #154534) and cultured at 37°C in 5% CO_2. The medium was changed after 24 h. To detect the specific gene expression in cultured microglia and macrophages, we photographed cell morphology under a microscope and then collected cells for mRNA measurement on day 3. At the same time point, lipopolysaccharide (LPS; 25 ng/mL, Sigma-Aldrich, cat #L2630) was added to another set of microglia or monocytes/macrophages for 12 h (Lan et al., 2011). Cell supernatants were collected for ELISA (R&D Systems, Minneapolis, MN), and cells were fixed in 4% paraformaldehyde for immunofluorescence microscopy (Nikon Eclipse 90i fluorescence microscope) (Lan et al., 2017b).

TABLE 1 | Cell numbers by gentleMACS and Percoll methods.

	GentleMACS with Myelin Removal Beads (n = 6)		Tissue dissociation with Percoll (n = 3)	
	Sham	**ICH day 1**	**Sham**	**ICH day 1**
Cell counts before FACS	$(2.13 \pm 0.23) \times 10^6$	$(1.67 \pm 0.12) \times 10^6$	$(1.92 \pm 0.41) \times 10^6$	$(1.32 \pm 0.33) \times 10^6$
Total events collected by FACS (per mouse)	$(1.56 \pm 0.19) \times 10^6$	$(1.02 \pm 0.22) \times 10^6$	$(1.01 \pm 0.21) \times 10^6$	$(0.6 \pm 0.11) \times 10^6$
(FSC-H+SSC-H) subtype (% of total events)	27.9%	22.5%	31.2%	25.8%
No. of microglia	$(13.2 \pm 2.13) \times 10^3$	$(16.4 \pm 3.52) \times 10^3$	$(12.8 \pm 2.11) \times 10^3$	$(12.1 \pm 3.33) \times 10^3$
No. of monocytes/macrophages	$(2.12 \pm 0.52) \times 10^3$	$(6.8 \pm 1.52) \times 10^3$	$(2.91 \pm 0.24) \times 10^3$	$(4.13 \pm 0.92) \times 10^3$

ICH, intracerebral hemorrhage; FACS, fluorescent-activated cell sorting; FSC-H, forward scatter height; SSC-H, side scatter height.

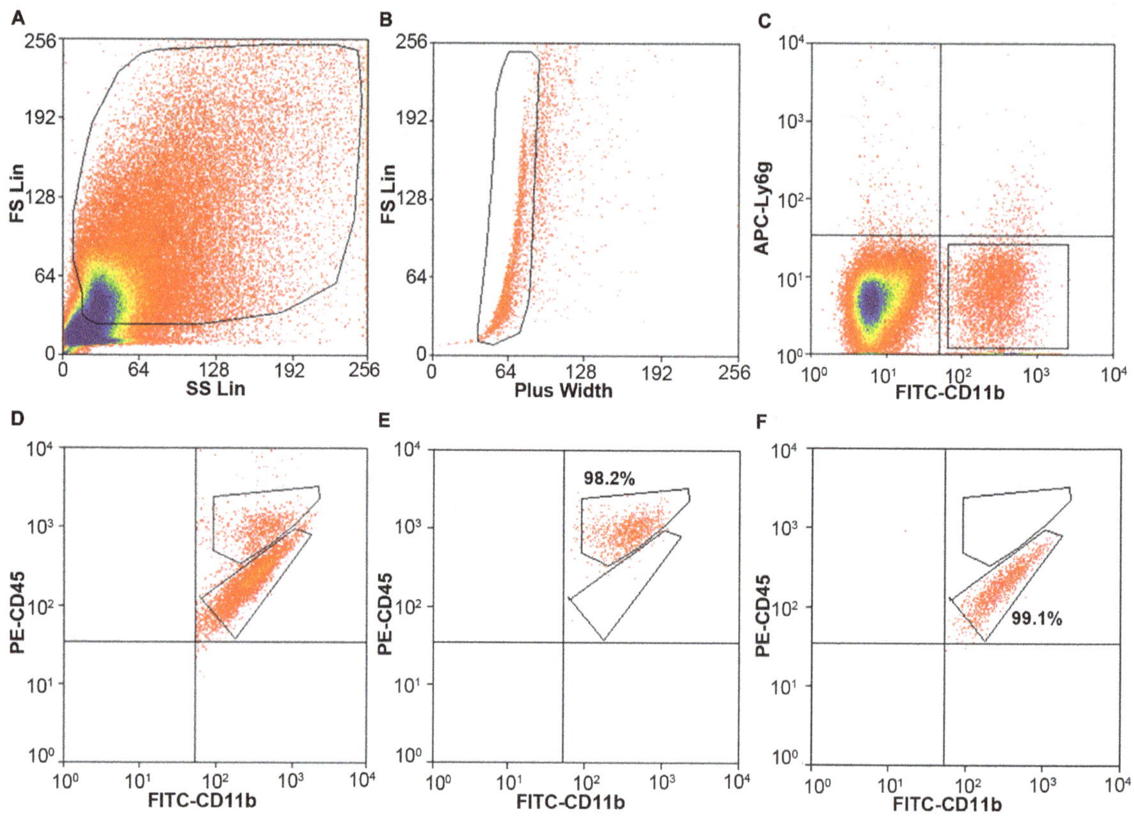

FIGURE 3 | Cell gating by flow cytometry. Eight- to ten-week-old male C57BL/6 mice underwent collagenase injection. Mice were sacrificed on day 1 post-ICH. Mouse brain was perfused with phosphate-buffered saline and dissociated into single cells. Cells were stained with APC-Ly6g, FITC-CD11b, PE-CD45, and propidium iodide (PI). **(A)** Representative gating of all cells. **(B)** Representative gating of singlets. **(C)** Representative gating of $Ly6g^{-}CD11b^{+}$ PI^{-} cells. **(D)** Representative gating of $CD11b^{+}CD45^{high}$ and $CD11b^{+}CD45^{int}$ after gating from **(C)**. **(E,F)** the post-sort purity of monocytes/macrophages **(E)** and microglia **(F)**.

Phagocytosis Assay

pHrodo Red Zymosan Bioparticles Conjugates were dissolved in DMEM/F-12 at 100 μg/mL. Then each well of cells was incubated with 100 μL of the beads for 4–6 h at 37°C. Cells were then washed three times in PBS and fixed in 4% paraformaldehyde for immunofluorescence microscopy.

Statistics

Data are presented as bar graphs (mean ± SD) or dot plots. We made two-group comparisons with a two-tailed Student's t-test followed by Welch's correction. One-way ANOVA was used for comparisons among multiple groups; Dunn's *post hoc* analysis was used to determine where those differences occurred. All analyses were carried out with GraphPad Software (GraphPad Prism 5.0; GraphPad Software, Inc., La Jolla, CA). The criterion for statistical significance was $p < 0.05$.

RESULTS

Cell Counts After Brain Dissociation

After tissue dissociation and removal of myelin debris and red blood cells, we counted live cells in each group at the 24-h time point. Using our method (**Table 1**), we collected approximately

$2.13 \pm 0.23 \times 10^6$ cells from each sham mouse (n = 6), $1.51 \pm 0.22 \times 10^6$ cells from each mouse in the blood-induced ICH group (n = 6), and $1.67 \pm 0.12 \times 10^6$ cells from each mouse in the collagenase-induced ICH group (n = 6). Using the Percoll protocol (**Table 1**), we collected $1.92 \pm 0.41 \times 10^6$ cells from each sham mouse (n = 3) and $1.32 \pm 0.33 \times 10^6$ cells from each mouse in the collagenase-induced ICH group (n = 3).

Flow Cytometry and FACS

Cells stained for cell surface markers and with PI were analyzed by flow cytometry. We gated $Ly6g^-CD11b^+PI^-$ cells (**Figure 3**) and sorted the two populations of microglia and monocytes/macrophages into the culture medium. The post-sort purity was 98.2% for monocyte/macrophages (**Figure 3E**) and 99.1% for microglia (**Figure 3F**). $APC\text{-}Ly6g^-FITC\text{-}CD11b^+BV421\text{-}CD45^{Int}PI^-$ and $APC\text{-}Ly6g^-FITC\text{-}CD11b^+BV421\text{-}CD45^{high}PI^-$ cell populations were sorted for cell phagocytosis measurement; $APC\text{-}Ly6g^-FITC\text{-}CD11b^+PE\text{-}CD45^{Int}PI^-$ and $APC\text{-}Ly6g^-FITC\text{-}CD11b^+PE\text{-}CD45^{high}PI^-$ cell populations were sorted for other experiments. Our results showed that the $Ly6g^-CD11b^+CD45^{Int}$ population, which comprises microglia, and the $Ly6g^-CD11b^+CD45^{high}$ population, which comprises infiltrating monocytes/macrophages (Greter et al., 2015; Varvel et al., 2016), were clearly separated by CD11b and CD45 staining at 24 h post-ICH in both mouse models (**Figure 4**). Limited blood-brain barrier damage caused by needle insertion

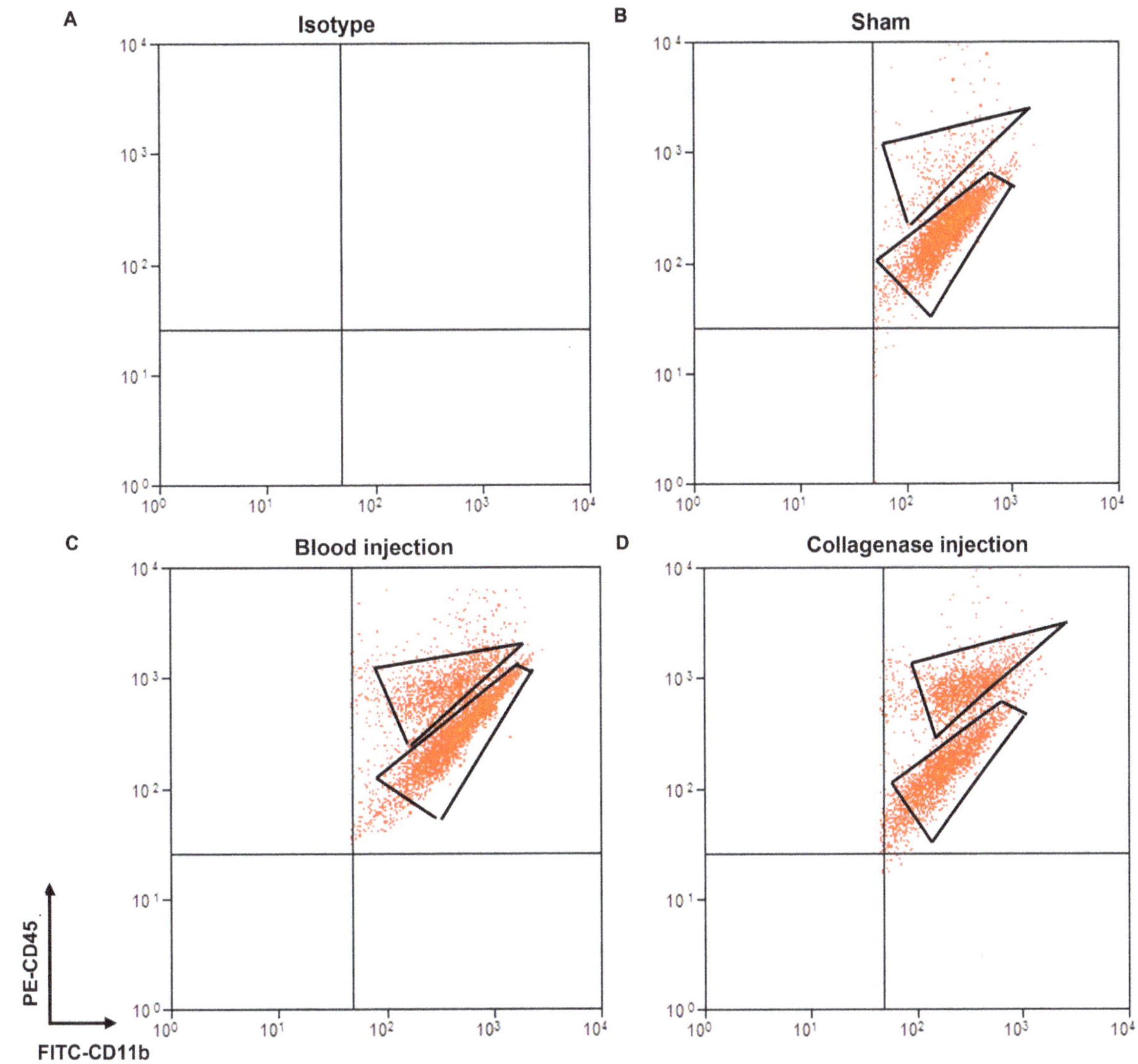

FIGURE 4 | Separation of microglia and monocytes/macrophages by flow cytometry on day 1 after blood-induced or collagenase-induced ICH. Eight- to ten-week-old male C57BL/6 mice underwent collagenase injection, blood injection, or sham procedure. Mice were sacrificed at day 1 post-ICH. Mouse brain was perfused with phosphate-buffered saline and dissociated into single cells. Cells were stained with propidium iodide (PI) and isotype **(A)** or APC-Ly6g, FITC-CD11b, and PE-CD45 **(B–D)** for flow cytometry. Representative images show cell populations in each group, and gates show cells sorted into $Ly6g^-CD11b^+CD45^{high}PI^-$ and $Ly6g^-CD11b^+CD45^{Int}PI^-$ populations.

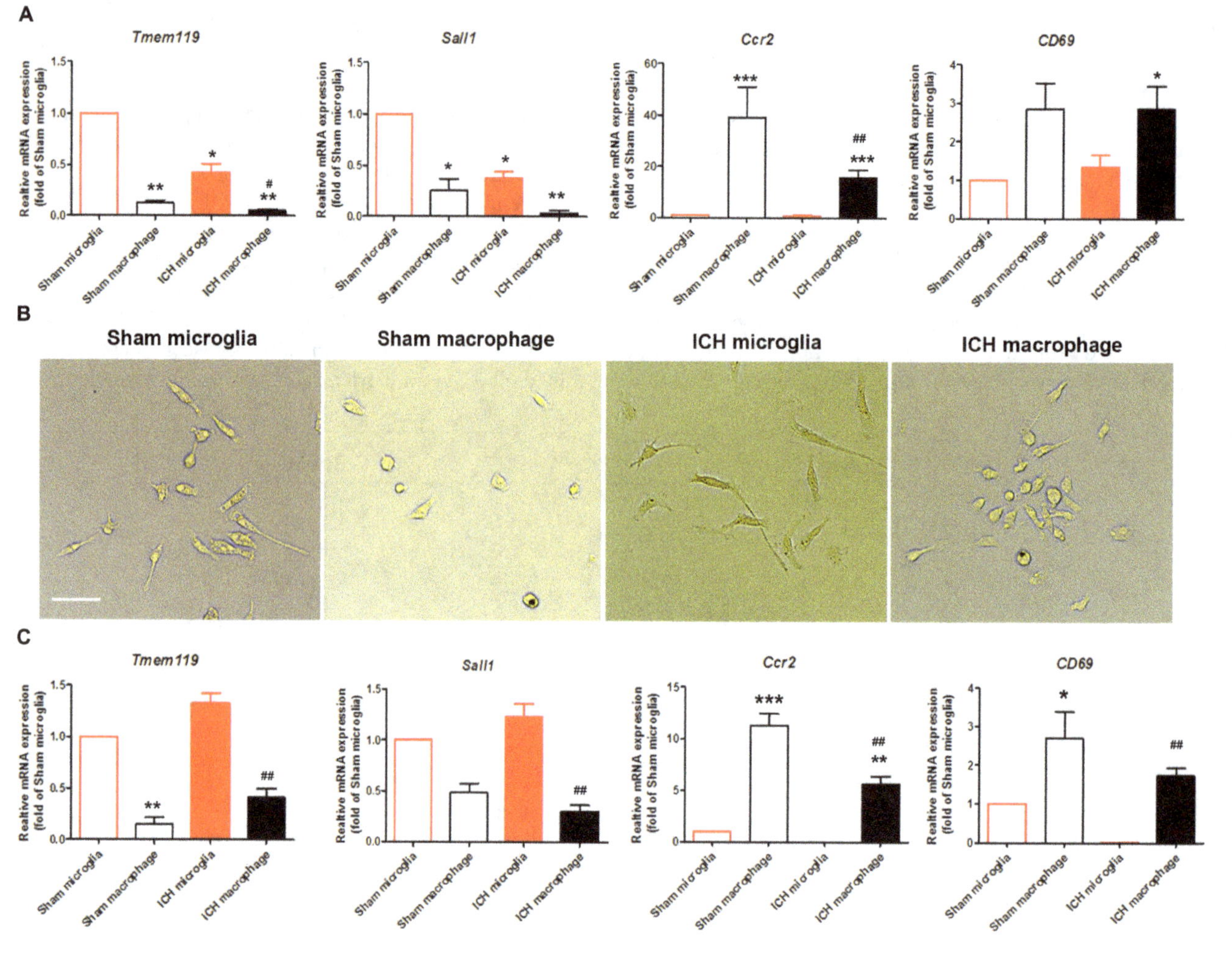

FIGURE 5 | Expression of microglia- and monocyte/macrophage-specific markers in sorted and cultured cells after ICH. Eight- to ten-week-old male C57BL/6 mice underwent collagenase injection or sham procedure. Mice were sacrificed at day 1 post-ICH. Mouse brain was perfused with phosphate-buffered saline and dissociated into single cells. Microglia (Ly6g$^-$CD11b$^+$CD45^{Int}PI$^-$) and monocytes/macrophages (Ly6g$^-$CD11b$^+$CD45^{high}PI$^-$) were isolated and sorted. **(A)** mRNA from cells was extracted and real-time PCR carried out with different primers. *GAPDH* was used as an internal control, and results are shown as fold of control. **(B)** Sorted cells were seeded and bright field images were taken after 3 days in culture. Representative images are shown. **(C)** mRNA was extracted after sorted cells were cultured for 3 days. Real-time PCR was carried out with different primers. *GAPDH* was used as an internal control, and results are shown as fold of sham microglia. *$p < 0.05$, **$p < 0.01$, ***$p < 0.001$ vs. corresponding control; #$p < 0.05$, ##$p < 0.01$ vs. corresponding group in sham animals; $n = 3$. Results are presented as mean ± SD. One-way ANOVA followed by Dunn's multiple comparison post-test. Scale bars: **(B)** 20 μm.

accounts for the small number of CD11b$^+$CD45^{high} cells in the sham group (**Figure 4B**). No positive staining was observed in the isotype group (**Figure 4A**). Cells were then used for *in vitro* culture and mRNA measurement.

We also compared our method with the classic Percoll method. With our method (**Table 1**), 1.02 × 10^6 events were counted by flow cytometry for each collagenase-induced ICH mouse brain, and the (FSC height + SSC height) subtype, gated as live cells, was 22.5% of total counts (**Figure 3**). With the Percoll method (**Table 1**), the total number of events for each collagenase-induced ICH mouse brain was 0.6 × 10^6, and the (FSC height + SSC height) subtype was 25.8% (**Supplementary Figure 2**). After gentleMACS dissociation and cell sorting, 6.8 ± 1.52 × 10^3 Ly6g$^-$CD11b$^+$CD45^{high}PI$^-$ monocytes/macrophages and 16.4 ± 3.52 × 10^3 Ly6g$^-$CD11b$^+$CD45^{Int}PI$^-$ microglia were collected, respectively, from collagenase-induced ICH mouse brain (n = 6). By the Percoll method, 4.13 ± 0.92 × 10^3 monocytes/macrophages and 12.1 ± 3.33 × 10^3 microglia were sorted from the ICH mice (n = 3).

Purity of Microglia and Monocyte-Derived Macrophages in Sorted and Cultured Cells

The literature has reported that Tmem119 and Sall1 are microglia-specific markers (Bennett et al., 2016; Buttgereit et al., 2016), that Ccr2 is a monocyte/macrophage-specific marker (Gu et al., 2016), and that CD69 is enriched in monocytes/macrophages but does not change in activated

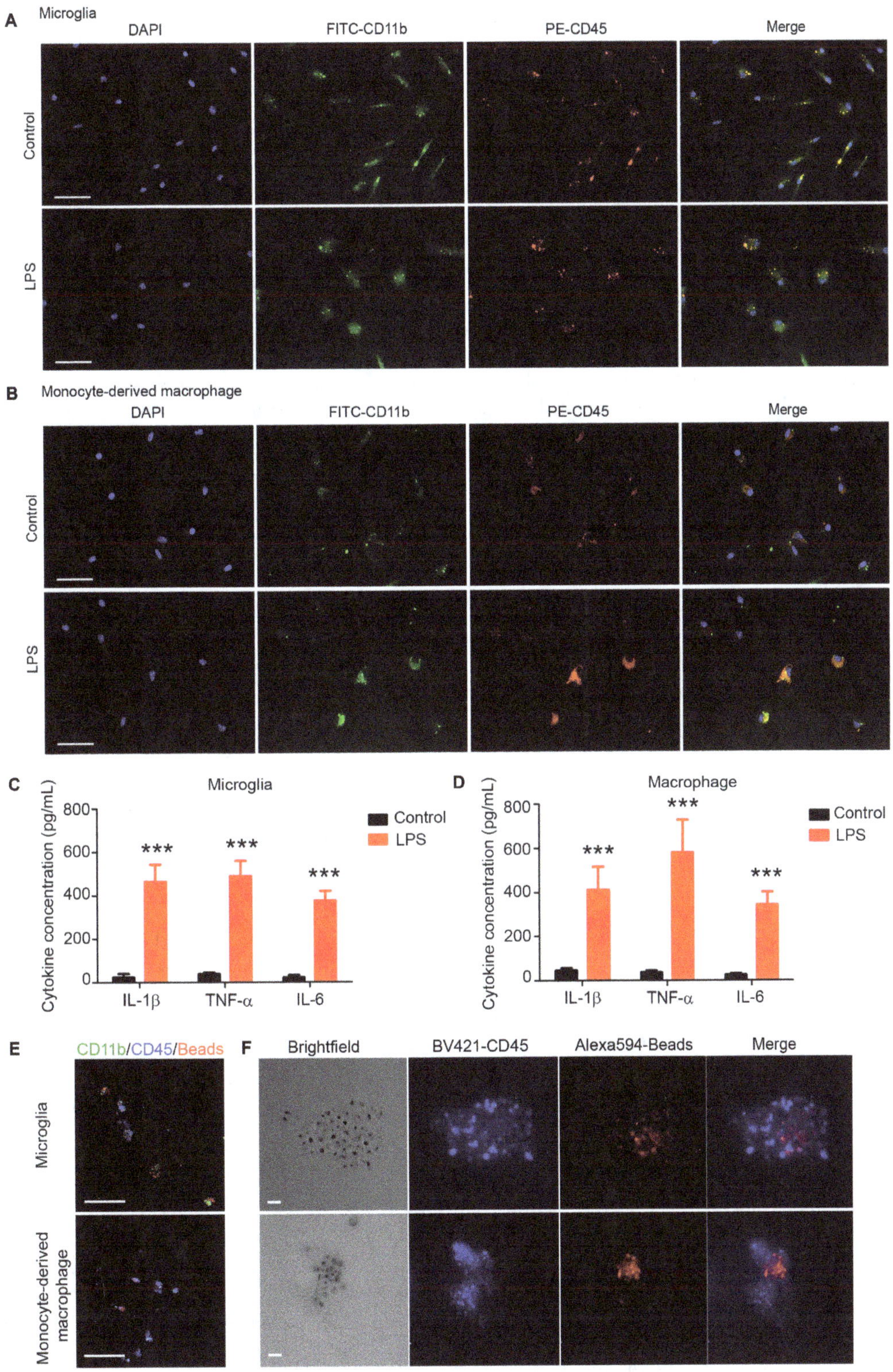

FIGURE 6 | Sorted microglia and monocytes/macrophages respond to lipopolysaccharide (LPS) stimulation and phagocytose beads *ex vivo*. At 1 day after mice were injected with collagenase, microglia (Ly6g$^-$CD11b$^+$CD45^{Int}PI$^-$) and macrophages (Ly6g$^-$CD11b$^+$CD45^{high}PI$^-$) were isolated, sorted, and seeded onto slides. Cells recovered briefly and were incubated with LPS or vehicle for 12 h. Representative images of **(A)** microglia and **(B)** monocyte-derived macrophages are shown. **(C,D)** Conditioned medium was collected and ELISA assays were performed. ***$p < 0.001$ vs. corresponding control; $n = 3$. Results are presented as mean ± SD. Two tailed Student's t-test followed by Welch's correction. **(E,F)** Cells were incubated with fluorescence-conjugated latex beads for 4–6 h and fixed before imaging. Representative images are shown. Scale bars: **(A,B)** 50 μm; **(E)** 100 μm; and **(F)** 10 μm.

microglia (Lewis et al., 2014). To confirm the purity of the two sorted populations, we extracted mRNA and performed real-time PCR with sorted Ly6g$^-$CD11b$^+$CD45^{Int} and Ly6g$^-$CD11b$^+$CD45^{high} cells. As expected, *Tmem119* and *Sall1* were more highly expressed in the microglial cell population, whereas *Ccr2* and *CD69* were more highly expressed in the monocyte/macrophage cell population (**Figure 5A**). The expression levels of *Tmem119*, *Sall1*, and *Ccr2* were decreased at 1-day post-ICH compared with those in sham animals (**Figure 5A**). After the sorted cells had been cultured for 3 days, we observed morphologic differences between microglia and macrophages, and microglia from the ICH group exhibited morphology typical of activated microglia (**Figure 5B**). Subsequently, we performed real-time RT PCR and verified the specific markers of these two cell populations. As expected, *Tmem119* and *Sall1* were still expressed mainly in microglia, and *Ccr2* and *CD69* were expressed mainly in monocytes/macrophages (**Figure 5C**). However, the expression level of *Tmem119* and *Sall1* was higher in the ICH group than in the sham group, whereas the expression levels of *Ccr2* and *CD69* remained lower in the ICH group than in the sham group (**Figure 5C**). These results indicate that the expression of those genes is differentially regulated by ICH and by *in vitro* culturing.

LPS Response and Phagocytosis by Sorted Microglia and Macrophages *in vitro*

Microglia and monocyte-derived macrophages showed healthy morphology with FITC-CD11b, PE-CD45, and DAPI staining (**Figures 6A,B**, first row). After LPS stimulation (**Figures 6A,B**, second row), microglia (**Figure 6A**) and monocytes/macrophages (**Figure 6B**) exhibited reactivated morphologies, with larger cell bodies and more dendrite branches than the control group.

ELISA assays showed that levels of proinflammatory cytokines (IL-1β, TNF-α, and IL-6) were significantly higher in the LPS-induced microglia (**Figure 6C**) and macrophages (**Figure 6D**) than in the control groups. Furthermore, we used APC-Ly6g, FITC-CD11b, and BV421-CD45 to sort microglia and monocytes/macrophages in a parallel experiment. We found that sorted cells were able to phagocytose fluorescent latex beads *in vitro* (**Figures 6E,F**). These results indicate that the sorted microglia and monocytes/macrophages maintained their inflammatory reactivity to LPS and their phagocytic function.

M1 and M2 Marker mRNA Expression in Microglia and Monocytes/Macrophages

To evaluate whether our method can be used to observe MMϕ polarization after ICH, we extracted mRNA and performed real-time PCR with sorted Ly6g$^-$CD11b$^+$CD45^{Int}PI$^-$ and Ly6g$^-$CD11b$^+$CD45^{high}PI$^-$ cells. Our results showed that M1 markers, *IL-1β* and *CD32*, and M2 markers, *IL-10* and *YM-1*, were increased in both microglia and monocytes/macrophages (**Figure 7**). Notably, *YM-1* was significantly elevated in the monocyte/macrophage population on day 1 post-ICH (**Figure 7**).

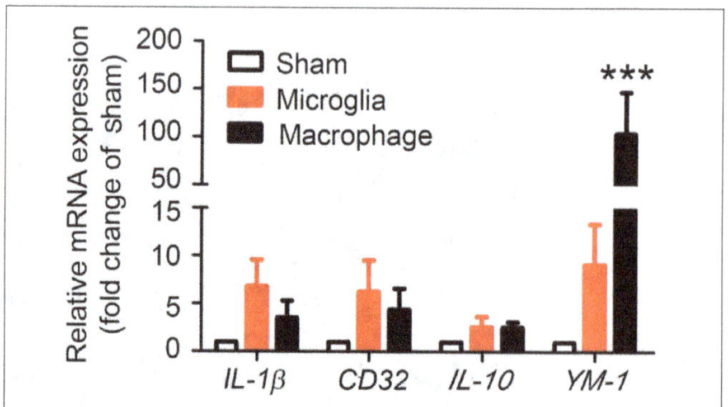

FIGURE 7 | Sorted microglia and monocytes/macrophages express M1 and M2 markers *ex vivo*. At 1 day after mice underwent collagenase injection or sham procedure, microglia (Ly6g$^-$CD11b$^+$CD45^{Int}PI$^-$) and monocytes/macrophages (Ly6g$^-$CD11b$^+$CD45^{high}PI$^-$) were isolated and sorted. mRNA from cells was extracted and real-time PCR carried out with different primers. *GAPDH* was used as an internal control, and results are shown as fold of sham. ***$p < 0.001$ vs. corresponding control; $n = 3$. Results are presented as mean ± SD. One-way ANOVA followed by Dunn's multiple comparison post-test.

Potential Pitfalls and Troubleshooting

Isolate Microglia/Macrophages at Different Time Points Post-ICH and From Sham-Operated Group

The number of infiltrating MMϕ differs at different time points after ICH. Therefore, sorted MMϕ may not be sufficient for mRNA extraction or cell culture. To isolate MMϕ more than 5 days after ICH, we recommend pooling two or more mouse brains together to collect enough cells. To collect enough macrophages from sham-operated mice, we suggest pooling at least three mouse brains together.

Maintain Cell Viability Before/During FACS

Brain cells are more vulnerable than other cells (tumor cells or blood cells), and hemorrhagic brain contains more debris than non-traumatic brain tissue. Thus, tissues/cells need to be kept on ice at all times except during enzyme incubation. All procedures require quick (perfusion) and gentle (incubation and resuspension) techniques. If the FACSorting takes more than 3 h, we suggest that cells be resuspended in Neurobasal medium (cat. 21103049, Thermo Fisher Scientific) with 1% BSA to maximally maintain cell viability.

Cell Collection After FACS

In some cases, the number of sorted cells may be small. To maximally preserve the viability and number of sorted cells, we recommend seeding cells directly onto poly-l-lysine–coated cover slips or 6- or 12-well plates. Cells can be sorted directly into TRIzol reagent and stored at -80°C for up to 6 months before mRNA is extracted.

DISCUSSION

Microglia and monocyte-derived macrophage activation and polarization play an important role in hematoma resolution after ICH (Mracsko and Veltkamp, 2014; Zhou et al., 2014; Lan et al., 2017c; Zhang et al., 2017). In preclinical studies, upregulation of M2-like MMϕ has been shown to ameliorate outcomes after ICH (Wan et al., 2016; Yang J. et al., 2016; Chang et al., 2017; Pascual et al., 2017; Yu et al., 2017; Zhou et al., 2017). However, the concept of MMϕ phenotypes in these studies was unclear. Most evaluations of MMϕ polarization use whole brain homogenates in Western blotting, ELISA, or real-time PCR to detect changes in protein or mRNA expression. However, owing to the global expression of most proinflammatory and anti-inflammatory cell markers on neurons, astrocytes, MMϕ, and even oligodendrocytes (Ren and Dubner, 2008), these methods cannot be used to precisely determine the dynamic changes in MMϕ after ICH. Furthermore, recent studies indicated that the roles of microglia and monocyte-derived macrophages might differ after ICH: the infiltrating $CCR2^{+}Ly6c^{high}$ cells accelerated neurologic deficits in the acute phase after ICH (Hammond et al., 2014), and the activity of $CD11b^{+}/CD45^{high}$ cells was similar to that of monocytes, which contribute to brain injury post-ICH (Min et al., 2016). However, microglial depletion was beneficial for brain recovery on day 3 post-ICH (Li et al., 2017a). These results indicate that evaluating the functions of microglia and monocyte-derived macrophages separately is critical in preclinical and clinical studies of ICH (Lan et al., 2018). Therefore, a protocol is needed that can reliably sort microglia and monocyte-derived macrophages from the ICH brain.

Several methods have been developed to separate microglia and monocytes/macrophages in the mouse ICH brain. The traditional method for distinguishing resident microglia from infiltrating monocytes/macrophages is based on cell morphology (amoeboid, ramified or reactivated (Jeong et al., 2013; Li et al., 2018)) and CD45 staining (Perego et al., 2011). However, this method can only identify cellular location (in the hematoma core or perihematoma regions) and marker expression (by immunostaining other cell markers); the ability to assess cellular function is very limited. Another method is to generate bone marrow chimeras using $Cx3cr1^{gfp/+}$ transgenic (Ajami et al., 2007; Tashima et al., 2016) or other transgenic mice. This approach allows researchers to separate the infiltrating bone marrow-derived monocytes/macrophages ($Cx3cr1^{gfp/+}$) from resident microglia ($Cx3cr1^{-/-}$). Unfortunately, bone marrow transplantation has the potential to cause acute and chronic inflammatory responses (Mildner et al., 2007), which may affect the MMϕ function and even alter the expression of some cell surface markers (Moravan et al., 2016). Recently, researchers developed new tools based on cell surface markers to distinguish microglia and infiltrating monocytes/macrophages. The $CX3CR1^{CreER/+}$:$R26^{IDTR/+}$ transgenic mouse was developed to enable microglia and monocytes/macrophages to be observed separately (Parkhurst et al., 2013). Moreover, a new anti-TMEM119 antibody, which can specifically identify microglia in the brain, was applied to study microglia and monocyte-derived macrophage differences (Bennett et al., 2016). Nevertheless, even as new approaches and tools are developed to study MMϕ, flow cytometry-based FACS remains the gold standard to separate microglia and monocytes/macrophages for *ex vivo* and *in vitro* ICH study, as this method allows maximal retention of cell properties after brain damage.

In the present study, we used Ly6g, CD11b, and CD45 antibodies to label microglia and monocytes/macrophages, as these are classical cell markers of these two populations. As an alternative, CD44 is also a good marker to distinguish microglia, monocytes, and monocyte-derived macrophages after brain injury. Studies showed that the $CD11b^{high}CD44^{low}$ population was also $CD45^{Int}$ and $Ly6c^{low}$, and that the $CD11b^{high}CD44^{high}$ population was $CD45^{high}$ and $Ly6c^{high}$ in an experimental autoimmune encephalomyelitis (EAE) model (Lewis et al., 2014). Therefore, the combination of cell markers CD44, CD11b, CD45, and Ly6g could potentially be more reliable for separating microglia, monocytes, and macrophages. It will be valuable in the future to perform another series of experiments to show that this combination of markers is also useful after ICH.

The tissue dissociation efficiency is a key factor that affects the activity of sorted cells. In our optimized protocol, we chose the gentleMACS dissociation system, which is flexible and fast and allows the preparation of eight samples simultaneously. To isolate live cells from adult mouse brain, we used Myelin Removal Beads to decrease the debris content and maintain cell viability. Furthermore, because of the substantial bleeding in a hemorrhagic brain, we also added double volume of Red Blood Cell Lysis Solution to maximally eliminate the effect of autofluorescence. The dissociation process can be completed in approximately 2 h and is not affected by the sample number (up to 8); the whole procedure, including sorting, can be finished in 8 h. More importantly, the cell viability and status are not heavily dependent on the proficiency of the operator. Thus, variability between groups within and between experiments, even those carried out by different individuals, is minimal, making data reliable and reproducible. Additionally, the process produces approximately 1.5–3.0 × 10^6 live cells that can be collected for subsequent FACS. This number should be sufficient for follow-up experiments (e.g., immunostaining, real-time PCR, and nanostring) without needing to pool several brains together in most cases, which could potentially increase variability. Compared to the classic Percoll-based dissociation protocol, we found no significant differences in the percentage of FSC height + SSC height subtype or microglia/macrophage cell numbers by FACS. However, the total number of events collected for each sample was less with the Percoll method than with our method on day 1 post-ICH.

After flow cytometry, two populations of $CD11b^{+}CD45^{Int}$ (microglia) and $CD11b^{+}CD45^{high}$ (monocytes/macrophages) can be clearly separated from mice with ICH. However, we did observe a small macrophage population in sham mice. We also used Ly6g antibody to distinguish neutrophils from monocytes. We gated $Ly6g^{-}/CD11b^{+}$ and sorted microglia and monocytes/macrophages separately. One alternative approach is to use $Cx3cr1^{GFP/+}CCR2^{RFP/+}$ mice (Mizutani et al., 2012) and gate $Cx3cr1^{+}CCR2^{-}$ to separate monocytes from MMϕ. To confirm the purity of the gated cells, we performed real-time RT PCR to examine specific markers: *Tmem119* and *Sall1* for microglia, *Ccr2* and *CD69* for monocyte/macrophages. As expected, *Tmem119* and *Sall1* were expressed mainly in the microglial ($CD11b^{+}CD45^{Int}$) population, and *Ccr2* and *CD69* were expressed mainly in the monocyte/macrophage population ($CD11b^{+}CD45^{high}$). Importantly, cultured cells retained the specific marker expression for days post-sorting.

We also found that the expression level of those markers changes after acute ICH. *Tmem119* is a recently discovered specific microglial marker in the brain (Bennett et al., 2016). However, its biologic function is unknown. *Tmem119* expression was shown to be elevated in the brains of patients with Alzheimer's disease, but not in those with amyotrophic lateral sclerosis or Parkinson's disease (Satoh et al., 2016). Interestingly, *Tmem119* is a target gene of TGFβ1 in postnatal microglia but cannot be regulated by TGFβ1 in mature microglia (Attaai et al., 2018). Our results showed that *Tmem119* expression significantly decreased on day 1 post-ICH, suggesting that it may participate in microglial function after acute brain injury. *Sall1* is another important transcriptional regulator that is required for microglia to retain a healthy phenotype and characteristics (Buttgereit et al., 2016). Similar to *Tmem119*, *Sall1* was significantly suppressed on day 1 post-ICH; however, after 3 days of culture, this reduction disappeared in ICH microglia, perhaps suggesting self-recovery. Therefore, whether the reduction of *Sall1* expression can be used as a biomarker for ICH diagnosis needs further investigation.

It has been reported that in an EAE animal model, Ccr2 was rarely expressed in microglia but highly expressed in monocyte-derived macrophages. Moreover, Ccr2 expression decreased in macrophages of mice with EAE scores of 0 and 3 compared with that of naïve mice (Lewis et al., 2014). Our data indicated that Ccr2 is a specific monocyte/monocyte-derived macrophage marker after ICH, and its expression was downregulated after ICH. Unlike Ccr2, CD69 was highly expressed in macrophages, but we did not observe a significant change in *CD69* expression on day 1 post-ICH. Therefore, a time-course experiment is needed to study the dynamic expression changes and function of CD69 after ICH.

For *in vitro* studies, researchers commonly use primary microglia from p0 mouse pups to investigate microglial function. However, these cells are not completely mature (Moussaud and Draheim, 2010). Moreover, astrocyte-contaminated microglia may have altered cytokine production after stimulation (Bohlen et al., 2017). With our protocol, the sorted cells are mature, can be cultured *in vitro*, retain a healthy morphology, and can be reactivated by stimulation with LPS for proinflammatory cytokine upregulation. Furthermore, the microglia we collected maintained the ability to engulf beads by phagocytosis. These results provide evidence that the sorted MMϕ have excellent viability, activity, and function. When we measured levels of extracted mRNA by real-time PCR, we were able to examine the changes in microglial activation and polarization more precisely, accurately, and efficiently than is possible with immunostaining. In a future study, we will apply nanostring technology and proteomics to further investigate the changes in microglia and monocyte-derived macrophages after ICH.

This protocol has several limitations. First, the MACS sorter, dissociation kit, and C tubes are relatively more expensive than components needed for the traditional method. Second, to achieve the best results, different dissociation kits need to be used for neonatal and adult mice. In addition, because massive bleeding is induced in the ICH model, it is difficult to completely remove red blood cells. Third, gating of the monocyte-derived macrophages would be different from gating of the monocytes because transformation of monocytes into macrophages alters cell size and changes surface marker expression in the ICH animals at different time points. Thus, to investigate the transformation of monocytes into macrophages after ICH, we will sort $Ly6c^{+}Ly6g^{-}CD11b^{+}CD45^{high}$ monocytes and $Ly6c^{-/-and+/-}Ly6g^{-}CD11b^{+}CD45^{high}$ macrophages separately in our future research.

CONCLUSION

In conclusion, we established a method based on MACS dissociation and sorting by FACS flow cytometry to separate microglia and monocyte-derived macrophages after ICH. The whole process can be achieved within 5–8 h, and the sorted microglia and monocyte-derived macrophages maintain their post-ICH characteristics, an attribute that is critical for ICH research. This fast, efficient, and precise protocol will be valuable for multiple applications and an important means by which to study the role of microglia and monocyte-derived macrophages after ICH and other brain diseases.

AUTHOR CONTRIBUTIONS

QL, XL, and JW designed the experiments and wrote the manuscript. QL, XL, XH, and JW analyzed the data.

FUNDING

The author(s) disclosed receipt of the following financial support for the research, authorship, and/or publication of this article: This research was supported by the National Institutes of Health (R01NS078026, R01AT007317, R56NS096549, and R01NS102583 to JW) and the American Heart Association (Grant-in-Aid, 17GRNT33660766 to JW; Postdoctoral Fellowship Awards 16POST29640010 to QL; Scientist

Development Grant, 16SDG30980031 to XH), Award from the American Heart Association and the DC Women's Board 17POST3366019 to XL, and a Stimulating and Advancing ACCM Research (StAAR) grant from the Department of Anesthesiology and Critical Care Medicine, Johns Hopkins University.

ACKNOWLEDGMENTS

We thank Dr. Hao Zhang from Johns Hopkins Bloomberg School of Public Health for flow cytometry assistance and Claire Levine, MS, ELS, for editing the manuscript in draft form.

REFERENCES

Ajami, B., Bennett, J. L., Krieger, C., Tetzlaff, W., and Rossi, F. M. (2007). Local self-renewal can sustain CNS microglia maintenance and function throughout adult life. *Nat. Neurosci.* 10, 1538–1543. doi: 10.1038/nn2014

Attaai, A., Neidert, N., Von Ehr, A., Potru, P. S., Zoller, T., and Spittau, B. (2018). Postnatal maturation of microglia is associated with alternative activation and activated TGFbeta signaling. *Glia* doi: 10.1002/glia.23332 [Epub ahead of print].

Bennett, M. L., Bennett, F. C., Liddelow, S. A., Ajami, B., Zamanian, J. L., Fernhoff, N. B., et al. (2016). New tools for studying microglia in the mouse and human CNS. *Proc. Natl. Acad. Sci. U.S.A.* 113, E1738–E1746. doi: 10.1073/pnas.1525528113

Bohlen, C. J., Bennett, F. C., Tucker, A. F., Collins, H. Y., Mulinyawe, S. B., and Barres, B. A. (2017). Diverse requirements for microglial survival, specification, and function revealed by defined-medium cultures. *Neuron* 94, 759.e8–773.e8. doi: 10.1016/j.neuron.2017.04.043

Buttgereit, A., Lelios, I., Yu, X., Vrohlings, M., Krakoski, N. R., Gautier, E. L., et al. (2016). Sall1 is a transcriptional regulator defining microglia identity and function. *Nat. Immunol.* 17, 1397–1406. doi: 10.1038/ni.3585

Chang, C. F., Cai, L., and Wang, J. (2015). Translational intracerebral hemorrhage: a need for transparent descriptions of fresh tissue sampling and preclinical model quality. *Transl. Stroke Res.* 6, 384–389. doi: 10.1007/s12975-015-0399-5

Chang, C. F., Wan, J., Li, Q., Renfroe, S. C., Heller, N. M., and Wang, J. (2017). Alternative activation-skewed microglia/macrophages promote hematoma resolution in experimental intracerebral hemorrhage. *Neurobiol. Dis.* 103, 54–69. doi: 10.1016/j.nbd.2017.03.016

Flores, J. J., Klebe, D., Rolland, W. B., Lekic, T., Krafft, P. R., and Zhang, J. H. (2016). PPARgamma-induced upregulation of CD36 enhances hematoma resolution and attenuates long-term neurological deficits after germinal matrix hemorrhage in neonatal rats. *Neurobiol. Dis.* 87, 124–133. doi: 10.1016/j.nbd.2015.12.015

Greter, M., Lelios, I., and Croxford, A. L. (2015). Microglia versus myeloid cell nomenclature during brain inflammation. *Front. Immunol.* 6:249. doi: 10.3389/fimmu.2015.00249

Gu, N., Peng, J., Murugan, M., Wang, X., Eyo, U. B., Sun, D., et al. (2016). Spinal microgliosis due to resident microglial proliferation is required for pain hypersensitivity after peripheral nerve injury. *Cell Rep.* 16, 605–614. doi: 10.1016/j.celrep.2016.06.018

Hammond, M. D., Taylor, R. A., Mullen, M. T., Ai, Y., Aguila, H. L., Mack, M., et al. (2014). CCR2+ Ly6C(hi) inflammatory monocyte recruitment exacerbates acute disability following intracerebral hemorrhage. *J. Neurosci.* 34, 3901–3909. doi: 10.1523/JNEUROSCI.4070-13.2014

Hellstrom Erkenstam, N., Smith, P. L., Fleiss, B., Nair, S., Svedin, P., Wang, W., et al. (2016). Temporal characterization of microglia/macrophage phenotypes in a mouse model of neonatal hypoxic-ischemic brain injury. *Front. Cell. Neurosci.* 10:286. doi: 10.3389/fncel.2016.00286

Jeong, H. K., Ji, K., Min, K., and Joe, E. H. (2013). Brain inflammation and microglia: facts and misconceptions. *Exp. Neurobiol.* 22, 59–67. doi: 10.5607/en.2013.22.2.59

Kim, J. Y., and Bae, H. J. (2017). Spontaneous intracerebral hemorrhage: management. *J. Stroke* 19, 28–39. doi: 10.5853/jos.2016.01935

Kronenberg, G., Uhlemann, R., Schoner, J., Wegner, S., Boujon, V., Deigendesch, N., et al. (2017). Repression of telomere-associated genes by microglia activation in neuropsychiatric disease. *Eur. Arch. Psychiatry Clin. Neurosci.* 267, 473–477. doi: 10.1007/s00406-016-0750-1

Lan, X., Han, X., Li, Q., Li, Q., Gao, Y., Cheng, T., et al. (2017a). Pinocembrin protects hemorrhagic brain primarily by inhibiting toll-like receptor 4 and reducing M1 phenotype microglia. *Brain Behav. Immun.* 61, 326–339. doi: 10.1016/j.bbi.2016.12.012

Lan, X., Han, X., Li, Q., and Wang, J. (2017b). (-)-Epicatechin, a natural flavonoid compound, protects astrocytes against hemoglobin toxicity via Nrf2 and AP-1 signaling pathways. *Mol. Neurobiol.* 54, 7898–7907. doi: 10.1007/s12035-016-0271-y

Lan, X., Han, X., Li, Q., Yang, Q. W., and Wang, J. (2017c). Modulators of microglial activation and polarization after intracerebral haemorrhage. *Nat. Rev. Neurol.* 13, 420–433. doi: 10.1038/nrneurol.2017.69

Lan, X., Han, X., Liu, X., and Wang, J. (2018). Inflammatory responses after intracerebral hemorrhage: from cellular function to therapeutic targets. *J. Cereb. Blood Flow Metab.* doi: 10.1177/0271678X18805675 [Epub ahead of print].

Lan, X., Liu, R., Sun, L., Zhang, T., and Du, G. (2011). Methyl salicylate 2-O-beta-D-lactoside, a novel salicylic acid analogue, acts as an anti-inflammatory agent on microglia and astrocytes. *J. Neuroinflammation* 8:98. doi: 10.1186/1742-2094-8-98

Lee, M. Y., and Lufkin, T. (2012). Development of the "Three-step MACS": a novel strategy for isolating rare cell populations in the absence of known cell surface markers from complex animal tissue. *J. Biomol. Tech.* 23, 69–77. doi: 10.7171/jbt.12-2302-003

Lelios, I., and Greter, M. (2014). Isolation of leukocytes from mouse central nervous system. *Methods Mol. Biol.* 1193, 15–19. doi: 10.1007/978-1-4939-1212-4_2

Lewis, N. D., Hill, J. D., Juchem, K. W., Stefanopoulos, D. E., and Modis, L. K. (2014). RNA sequencing of microglia and monocyte-derived macrophages from mice with experimental autoimmune encephalomyelitis illustrates a changing phenotype with disease course. *J. Neuroimmunol.* 277, 26–38. doi: 10.1016/j.jneuroim.2014.09.014

Li, M., Li, Z., Ren, H., Jin, W. N., Wood, K., Liu, Q., et al. (2017a). Colony stimulating factor 1 receptor inhibition eliminates microglia and attenuates brain injury after intracerebral hemorrhage. *J. Cereb. Blood Flow Metab.* 37, 2383–2395. doi: 10.1177/0271678X16666551

Li, Q., Han, X., Lan, X., Gao, Y., Wan, J., Durham, F., et al. (2017b). Inhibition of neuronal ferroptosis protects hemorrhagic brain. *JCI Insight* 2, e90777. doi: 10.1172/jci.insight.90777

Li, Q., Han, X., Lan, X., Hong, X., Li, Q., Gao, Y., et al. (2017c). Inhibition of tPA-induced hemorrhagic transformation involves adenosine A2b receptor activation after cerebral ischemia. *Neurobiol. Dis.* 108, 173–182. doi: 10.1016/j.nbd.2017.08.011

Li, Q., Wan, J., Lan, X., Han, X., Wang, Z., and Wang, J. (2017d). Neuroprotection of brain-permeable iron chelator VK-28 against intracerebral hemorrhage in mice. *J. Cereb. Blood Flow Metab.* 37, 3110–3123. doi: 10.1177/0271678X17709186

Li, Q., and Wang, J. (2017). "Animal models: cerebral hemorrhage," in *Primer on Cerebrovascular Diseases*, eds K. M. Welch, L. R. Caplan, B. K. Siesjo, B. Weir, and D. J. Reis (Cambridge, MA: Academic Press), 306–311.

Li, Q., Weiland, A., Chen, X., Lan, X., Han, X., Durham, F., et al. (2018). Ultrastructural characteristics of neuronal death and white matter injury in mouse brain tissues after intracerebral hemorrhage: coexistence of ferroptosis. Autophagy, and Necrosis. *Front. Neurol.* 9:581. doi: 10.3389/fneur.2018.00581

Meng, Z., Zhao, T., Zhou, K., Zhong, Q., Wang, Y., Xiong, X., et al. (2017). A20 ameliorates intracerebral hemorrhage-induced inflammatory injury by regulating TRAF6 polyubiquitination. *J. Immunol.* 198, 820–831. doi: 10.4049/jimmunol.1600334

Mildner, A., Schmidt, H., Nitsche, M., Merkler, D., Hanisch, U. K., Mack, M., et al. (2007). Microglia in the adult brain arise from Ly-6ChiCCR2+ monocytes only under defined host conditions. *Nat. Neurosci.* 10, 1544–1553. doi: 10.1038/nn2015

Min, H., Jang, Y. H., Cho, I. H., Yu, S. W., and Lee, S. J. (2016). Alternatively activated brain-infiltrating macrophages facilitate recovery from collagenase-induced intracerebral hemorrhage. *Mol. Brain* 9:42. doi: 10.1186/s13041-016-0225-3

Mizutani, M., Pino, P. A., Saederup, N., Charo, I. F., Ransohoff, R. M., and Cardona, A. E. (2012). The fractalkine receptor but not CCR2 is present on microglia from embryonic development throughout adulthood. *J. Immunol.* 188, 29–36. doi: 10.4049/jimmunol.1100421

Moravan, M. J., Olschowka, J. A., Williams, J. P., and O'banion, M. K. (2016). Brain radiation injury leads to a dose- and time-dependent recruitment of peripheral myeloid cells that depends on CCR2 signaling. *J. Neuroinflammation* 13:30. doi: 10.1186/s12974-016-0496-8

Moussaud, S., and Draheim, H. J. (2010). A new method to isolate microglia from adult mice and culture them for an extended period of time. *J. Neurosci. Methods* 187, 243–253. doi: 10.1016/j.jneumeth.2010.01.017

Mracsko, E., and Veltkamp, R. (2014). Neuroinflammation after intracerebral hemorrhage. *Front. Cell. Neurosci.* 8:388. doi: 10.3389/fncel.2014.00388

Parkhurst, C. N., Yang, G., Ninan, I., Savas, J. N., Yates, J. R. III, Lafaille, J. J., et al. (2013). Microglia promote learning-dependent synapse formation through brain-derived neurotrophic factor. *Cell* 155, 1596–1609. doi: 10.1016/j.cell.2013.11.030

Pascual, G., Avgustinova, A., Mejetta, S., Martin, M., Castellanos, A., Attolini, C. S., et al. (2017). Targeting metastasis-initiating cells through the fatty acid receptor CD36. *Nature* 541, 41–45. doi: 10.1038/nature20791

Perego, C., Fumagalli, S., and De Simoni, M. G. (2011). Temporal pattern of expression and colocalization of microglia/macrophage phenotype markers following brain ischemic injury in mice. *J. Neuroinflammation* 8:174. doi: 10.1186/1742-2094-8-174

Ren, K., and Dubner, R. (2008). Neuron-glia crosstalk gets serious: role in pain hypersensitivity. *Curr. Opin. Anaesthesiol.* 21, 570–579. doi: 10.1097/ACO.0b013e32830edbdf

Satoh, J., Kino, Y., Asahina, N., Takitani, M., Miyoshi, J., Ishida, T., et al. (2016). TMEM119 marks a subset of microglia in the human brain. *Neuropathology* 36, 39–49. doi: 10.1111/neup.12235

Szulzewsky, F., Pelz, A., Feng, X., Synowitz, M., Markovic, D., Langmann, T., et al. (2015). Glioma-associated microglia/macrophages display an expression profile different from M1 and M2 polarization and highly express Gpnmb and Spp1. *PLoS One* 10:e0116644. doi: 10.1371/journal.pone.0116644

Tashima, R., Mikuriya, S., Tomiyama, D., Shiratori-Hayashi, M., Yamashita, T., Kohro, Y., et al. (2016). Bone marrow-derived cells in the population of spinal microglia after peripheral nerve injury. *Sci. Rep.* 6:23701. doi: 10.1038/srep23701

Thabet, A. M., Kottapally, M., and Hemphill, J. C. III (2017). Management of intracerebral hemorrhage. *Handb. Clin. Neurol.* 140, 177–194. doi: 10.1016/B978-0-444-63600-3.00011-8

Varvel, N. H., Neher, J. J., Bosch, A., Wang, W., Ransohoff, R. M., Miller, R. J., et al. (2016). Infiltrating monocytes promote brain inflammation and exacerbate neuronal damage after status epilepticus. *Proc. Natl. Acad. Sci. U.S.A.* 113, E5665–E5674. doi: 10.1073/pnas.1604263113

Vinet, J., Vainchtein, I. D., Spano, C., Giordano, C., Bordini, D., Curia, G., et al. (2016). Microglia are less pro-inflammatory than myeloid infiltrates in the hippocampus of mice exposed to status epilepticus. *Glia* 64, 1350–1362. doi: 10.1002/glia.23008

Wan, S., Cheng, Y., Jin, H., Guo, D., Hua, Y., Keep, R. F., et al. (2016). Microglia activation and polarization after intracerebral hemorrhage in mice: the role of protease-activated receptor-1. *Transl. Stroke Res.* 7, 478–487. doi: 10.1007/s12975-016-0472-8

Wang, J. (2010). Preclinical and clinical research on inflammation after intracerebral hemorrhage. *Prog. Neurobiol.* 92, 463–477. doi: 10.1016/j.pneurobio.2010.08.001

Wang, J., and Tsirka, S. E. (2005). Contribution of extracellular proteolysis and microglia to intracerebral hemorrhage. *Neurocrit. Care* 3, 77–85. doi: 10.1385/NCC:3:1:077

Wang, M., Hong, X., Chang, C. F., Li, Q., Ma, B., Zhang, H., et al. (2015). Simultaneous detection and separation of hyperacute intracerebral hemorrhage and cerebral ischemia using amide proton transfer MRI. *Magn. Reson. Med.* 74, 42–50. doi: 10.1002/mrm.25690

Wu, H., Wu, T., Han, X., Wan, J., Jiang, C., Chen, W., et al. (2017). Cerebroprotection by the neuronal PGE2 receptor EP2 after intracerebral hemorrhage in middle-aged mice. *J. Cereb. Blood Flow Metab.* 37, 39–51. doi: 10.1177/0271678X15625351

Wu, H., Wu, T., Xu, X., Wang, J., and Wang, J. (2011). Iron toxicity in mice with collagenase-induced intracerebral hemorrhage. *J. Cereb. Blood Flow Metab.* 31, 1243–1250. doi: 10.1038/jcbfm.2010.209

Wu, H., Zhang, Z., Hu, X., Zhao, R., Song, Y., Ban, X., et al. (2010). Dynamic changes of inflammatory markers in brain after hemorrhagic stroke in humans: a postmortem study. *Brain Res.* 1342, 111–117. doi: 10.1016/j.brainres.2010.04.033

Yang, B., Parsha, K., Schaar, K., Xi, X., Aronowski, J., and Savitz, S. I. (2016). Various cell populations within the mononuclear fraction of bone marrow contribute to the beneficial effects of autologous bone marrow cell therapy in a rodent stroke model. *Transl. Stroke Res.* 7, 322–330. doi: 10.1007/s12975-016-0462-x

Yang, J., Ding, S., Huang, W., Hu, J., Huang, S., Zhang, Y., et al. (2016). Interleukin-4 ameliorates the functional recovery of intracerebral hemorrhage through the alternative activation of microglia/macrophage. *Front. Neurosci.* 10:61. doi: 10.3389/fnins.2016.00061

Yang, J., Li, Q., Wang, Z., Qi, C., Han, X., Lan, X., et al. (2017). Multimodality MRI assessment of grey and white matter injury and blood-brain barrier disruption after intracerebral haemorrhage in mice. *Sci. Rep.* 7:40358. doi: 10.1038/srep40358

Yu, A., Zhang, T., Duan, H., Pan, Y., Zhang, X., Yang, G., et al. (2017). MiR-124 contributes to M2 polarization of microglia and confers brain inflammatory protection via the C/EBP-alpha pathway in intracerebral hemorrhage. *Immunol. Lett.* 182, 1–11. doi: 10.1016/j.imlet.2016.12.003

Zhang, Z., Zhang, Z., Lu, H., Yang, Q., Wu, H., and Wang, J. (2017). Microglial polarization and inflammatory mediators after intracerebral hemorrhage. *Mol. Neurobiol.* 54, 1874–1886. doi: 10.1007/s12035-016-9785-6

Zhou, K., Zhong, Q., Wang, Y. C., Xiong, X. Y., Meng, Z. Y., Zhao, T., et al. (2017). Regulatory T cells ameliorate intracerebral hemorrhage-induced inflammatory injury by modulating microglia/macrophage polarization through the IL-10/GSK3beta/PTEN axis. *J. Cereb. Blood Flow Metab.* 37, 967–979. doi: 10.1177/0271678X16648712

Zhou, Y., Wang, Y., Wang, J., Anne Stetler, R., and Yang, Q. W. (2014). Inflammation in intracerebral hemorrhage: from mechanisms to clinical translation. *Prog. Neurobiol.* 115, 25–44. doi: 10.1016/j.pneurobio.2013.11.003

Zhu, W., Gao, Y., Chang, C. F., Wan, J. R., Zhu, S. S., and Wang, J. (2014). Mouse models of intracerebral hemorrhage in ventricle, cortex, and hippocampus by injections of autologous blood or collagenase. *PLoS One* 9:e97423. doi: 10.1371/journal.pone.0097423

Zhu, W., Gao, Y., Wan, J., Lan, X., Han, X., Zhu, S., et al. (2018). Changes in motor function, cognition, and emotion-related behavior after right hemispheric intracerebral hemorrhage in various brain regions of mouse. *Brain Behav. Immun.* 69, 568–581. doi: 10.1016/j.bbi.2018.02.004

16

Activin Receptor-Like Kinase 1 Combined with VEGF-A Affects Migration and Proliferation of Endothelial Cells from Sporadic Human Cerebral AVMs

*Qiang Hao[1,2], Hao Wang[1], Jun-Lin Lu[1,2], Li Ma[1,2], Xiao-Lin Chen[1,2], Xun Ye[1,2], Ya-Hui Zhao[1,2], Ming-Tao Li[1,2], Yu Chen[1,2] and Yuan-Li Zhao[1,2,3,4,5,6]**

[1] Department of Neurosurgery, Beijing Tiantan Hospital, Capital Medical University, Beijing, China, [2] Department of Neurosurgery, Peking University International Hospital, Peking University, Beijing, China, [3] China National Clinical Research Center for Neurological Diseases, Beijing, China, [4] Stroke Center, Beijing Institute for Brain Disorders, Beijing, China, [5] Beijing Key Laboratory of Translational Medicine for Cerebrovascular Disease, Beijing, China, [6] Basic Medical Science Department, Capital Medical University, Beijing, China

***Correspondence:**
Yuan-Li Zhao
zhaoyuanli@126.com

Heterozygous loss of activin receptor-like kinase 1 (Alk1) can lead to hereditary hemorrhagic telangiectasia (HHT), which is a kind of vascular disease characterized by direct connections between arteries and veins with the lacking of capillaries, and develops into arteriovenous malformations (AVMs) in later stage. However, the changes of Alk1 in human sporadic cerebral AVMs (cAVMs) remain unknown. In the present study, we used endothelial cells (ECs) derived from human cAVMs (cAVM-ECs) specimens, to explore the characteristics of cAVM-ECs and the relationship between Alk1 and human sporadic cAVMs. Our data showed that there were obvious morphological changes in cAVM-ECs, and they could trans-differentiate into mesenchyme-like cells easily in a short period. In addition, the abilities of migration of cAVM-ECs were poorer than that in human aortic endothelial cells (HA-ECs). The abilities of proliferation of cAVM-ECs in patients with different ages were lower than HA-ECs. Immunofluorescent staining and Western blot showed that the levels of Alk1 mRNA and protein in the HA-ECs were both higher than that in cAVM-ECs. In addition, the levels of Alk1 mRNA had no significant differences between different ages in cAVM-ECs groups. The levels of VEGF-A mRNA in the cAVM were higher than HA-ECs. Besides, levels of VEGF-A mRNA expression were lower in older cAVM patients. Therefore, we conclude that Alk1 might induce the formation of sporadic human cAVMs through affecting migration and proliferation of endothelial cells combined with VEGF-A.

Keywords: cerebral arteriovenous malformation, endothelial cells, morphology, migration, proliferation, activin receptor like kinase 1, VEGF-A

INTRODUCTION

Cerebral arteriovenous malformations are vascular disorders characterized by an anomalous tangle of nidus in vessels, which are characterized by direct connections between arteries and veins with the lacking of capillaries. Hemorrhage is one of the most serious complications (da Costa et al., 2009; Lawton et al., 2015). Therefore, the most important therapeutic strategy is to prevent the rupture of cAVMs. Current clinical treatments include surgical resection, radiotherapy, and embolization. However, all of these treatments may bring high risks of morbidity, leading to serious complications (da Costa et al., 2009). For example, surgical resection may induce neural functional deficits when cAVMs are located in the functional areas; the intervention of radiosurgery may be restricted by sizes of cAVMs (Wang et al., 2016). However, embolization is a minimally invasive treatment, which may be restricted when cAVMs are scattered and/or feeded by small feeding arteries (Sammons et al., 2011). Therefore, biological therapeutic method may be a promising option for cAVMs. Before biological therapies are developed, we should fully understand the pathophysiology and molecular mechanisms of cAVMs. As an important component of vessels in cAVMs, the endothelium has great theoretical potential as a therapeutic target.

Based on the researches of histological properties of cAVMs in patients with hereditary hemorrhagic telangiectasia (HHT), we speculate that the development of cAVMs originate from a focal dilation of a post capillary venues, leading to arteriole dilation progression and subsequent loss of intervening capillaries (Braverman et al., 1990). In previous studies, sub-dermal arteriovenous malformations (AVMs) are induced in wounds of activin receptor-like kinase 1 (Alk1)-mutant mice, which appeared in the form of both arteries and veins elongation followed by arterial-venous connections *de novo* (Kim et al., 2011; Laux et al., 2013; Garrido-Martin et al., 2014). Although these solid findings are confirmed by the longitudinal imaging of vascular growth, they still remained unclear in cellular level. Therefore, abnormal behaviors of endothelial cells (ECs) may cause AVMs and need to be elucidated in the sporadic patients with cAVMs. Considering the possible relationship between Alk1 function and cAVMs development, we hypothesized that Alk1 may play an important role in the formation of cAVMs by trans-differentiation and changes of ability of migration and proliferation in ECs derived from cAVMs.

Therefore, in this study, we isolated ECs from sporadic human cAVMs patients, to explore the potential mechanisms of occurrence and development of cAVMs in sporadic patients and get a better understanding *in vitro*.

MATERIALS AND METHODS

Isolation of ECs

Human surgical specimens were obtained in accordance with The Human Subject Review Committee of Tian Tan Hospital. cAVM-ECs were obtained from four males and four females, aged from 8 to 51 years old (average of 29.6 ± 14.55). Patients who involved in this study had not adopted gamma knife irradiation or embolization, and information was described in the **Table 1**. cAVM-ECs were isolated and selected by Flow cytometer, and identified by detecting ECs special markers (CD31 and CD34). In addition, their functional properties were detected by LDL-uptake and tube formation. All of cAVM-ECs used in this experiment were passaged to the forth generation at most. Human aortic endothelial cells (HA-ECs) were gained from ScienCell Company (ScienCell, Cat No. 6100, United States) and used as control ECs.

Immunocytochemistry

cAVM-ECs and HA-ECs were fixed in 4% paraformaldehyde for 20 min at RT, then blocked in 5% goat serum and incubated at 4°C with the following primary antibody: Rabbit polyclonal anti-human Alk1 (1:200, Cat No. ab68703, Abcam, United States). The slides were then incubated with the appropriate secondary antibody: Anti-Rabbit IgG H&L (Alexa Fluor®488) (1:200, Cat No. ab150077, Abcam, United States) for 1 h. Coverslips with immunostained cells were mounted on glass slides in Vectashield mounting medium containing DAPI (Vector Laboratories, Cat No. H1200, United States). Immunostained cells were counted randomly from five fields under a Nikon Eclipse microscope.

Cell Migration Assay

The ability of ECs migration was detected by scratch test. cAVM-ECs and HA-ECs were seeded into a 12-well plate at the concentration of 0.5×10^5 cells per well, respectively. When cells contacted with each other, they were scratched vertically with a 100 μl-pipette tip. Then, cells were washed twice with PBS and placed in serum-free culture medium. After 6 and 12 h, distances between the two sides of cells were measured under an invert phase-contrast microscope in five random fields, respectively. Each migration test was run in triplicate.

Cell Proliferation Assay

cAVM-ECs from eight patients were successfully passaged to the forth generation. To detect the proliferative ability of these cells, we seeded different patients' cAVM-ECs at the density of 0.1×10^5 per well, and the cells were cultured for 8 days. Then the cAVM-ECs were digested and counted. HA-ECs were used as control.

Western Blot

For preparation of total protein lysates, cells were lysed in cold RIPA buffer and centrifuged at 13,000 × *g* for 5 min at 4°C. Protein lysates were subjected to 10% SDS-PAGE gels, and then were transferred onto PVDF membranes. After blocking with 5% non-fat dried milk for 2 h at RT, membranes were incubated with the primary antibodies overnight at 4°C: Primary antibodies against Alk1 (1:1,000, Cell Signaling Technology, Cat No. 31278, United States) and GAPDH (1:5,000, Cell Signaling Technology, Cat No. 51332, United States), each primary antibody was diluted in blocking buffer and then incubated overnight at 4°C. The membranes were washed three times and incubated with horseradish peroxidase (HRP)-linked secondary antibody at RT

TABLE 1 | Clinical data of cerebral arteriovenous malformations patients who underwent microsurgical cAVMs resection.

Patient No.	Age (years)	Sex	Hemorrhage	cAVM size (cm)	Spetzler-Martin grade	Radiosurgery
1	14	Female	Yes	3	3	No
2	32	Male	No	4	4	No
3	51	Female	No	4	4	No
4	29	Female	Yes	5	5	No
5	17	Female	No	4	4	No
6	44	Male	Yes	6	5	No
7	8	Male	Yes	3	3	No
8	42	Male	No	5	4	No

The cAVMs endothelial cells (cAVMs-ECs) used in this experiment were derived from them.

for 1 h. Membranes were washed three times with TBST at RT. Protein bands were visualized on X-ray film. GAPDH was used as a loading control.

Quantitative Real-Time PCR

According to the manufacturer's protocol, total RNAs were isolated from EC using TRIzol reagent (Invitrogen). cDNAs were synthesized by reverse transcription using SuperScript III First-Strand Synthesis System kit (Invitrogen). TaqMan Gene Expression Assays (Applied Biosystems) was used for qPCR to quantify relative expression of each gene using Mx3000P QPCR System (Agilent Technologies). Predesigned qPCR primers: Alk1 (forward): 5′-CCACTCATTCCTCCTGGGTA-3′, Alk1 (reverse): 5′-ACTTCCTGACTAGGGGAGGAGTAG-3′; VEGF (forward): 5′-CCCACGAAGTGGTGAAGTTCA-3′, VEGF (reverse): 5′-CCACCAGGGTCTCGATGG-3′; GAPDH (forward): 5′-GATGGTGAAGGTCGGAGTGAAC-3′, GAPDH (reverse): 5′-GTCATTGATGGCGACGATGT-3′. RNase free dH_2O was used as the negative control reaction.

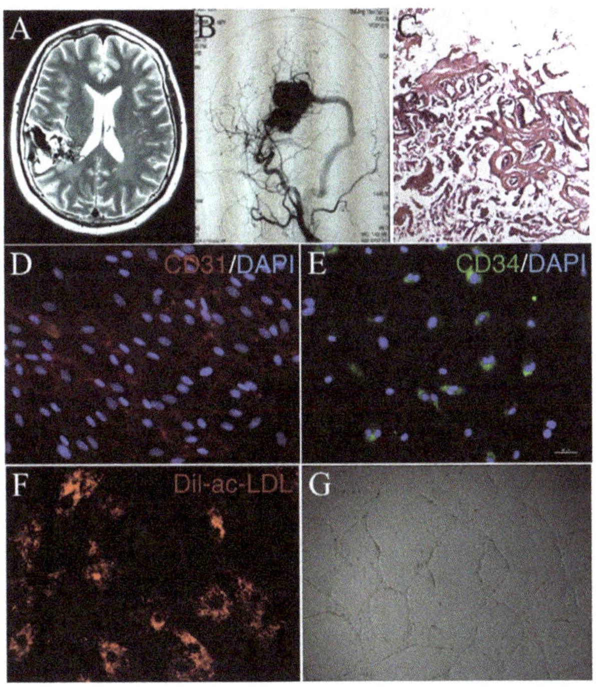

FIGURE 1 | The general characteristics of cAVM and cAVM-ECs. **(A)** T2WI of MRI imaging; **(B)** Digital subtraction angiography (DSA) showed cerebral middle artery provided blood for the cAVM nidus as a feeder artery, which connected to the sigmoid sinus through thick draining vessel; **(C)** Photomicrograph of cAVM with deformed vascular wall, and the nidus of the cAVM had many collagen fibers, lacking of smooth muscle and elastic fibers; **(D,E)** Immunostaining of ECs showed special markers CD31 and CD34 expressed in cAVM-ECs; **(F)** LDL uptake assay of cAVM-ECs; **(G)** Tube formation of cAVM-ECs. Scale bar = 200 μm.

Statistical Analysis

All data were presented as Mean ± SD and subjected to statistical analysis using GraphPad Prism software 6.0 (United States). Student's t-test was used for group comparisons between two groups. When there were more than two groups, the one-factor ANOVA (ANOVA) followed by Tukey's *post-hoc* test was used for comparisons between groups. Statistical significance was defined at $p < 0.05$.

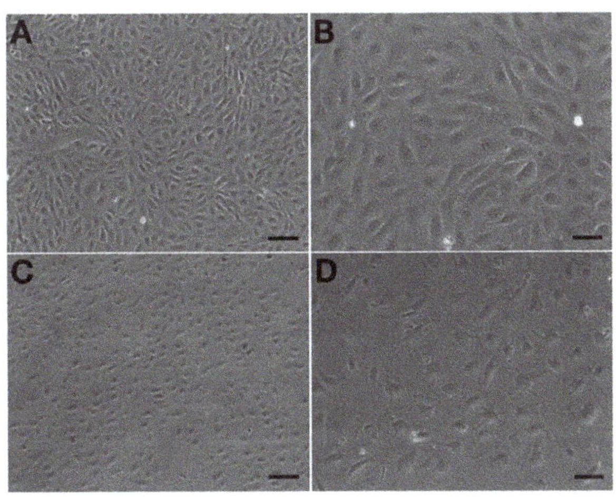

FIGURE 2 | Morphology of human aortic endothelial cells (HA-ECs) and cAVM-ECs. **(A,B)** Morphology of HA-ECs under microscope in **(A)** 40×, Scale bar = 100 μm; **(B)** 100×, Scale bar = 50 μm, showed classical round borders and cobblestone appearance; **(C,D)** showed irregular borders and flatty bodies with smaller nuclei, **(C)** 40×, Scale bar = 100 μm; **(D)** 100×, Scale bar = 50 μm.

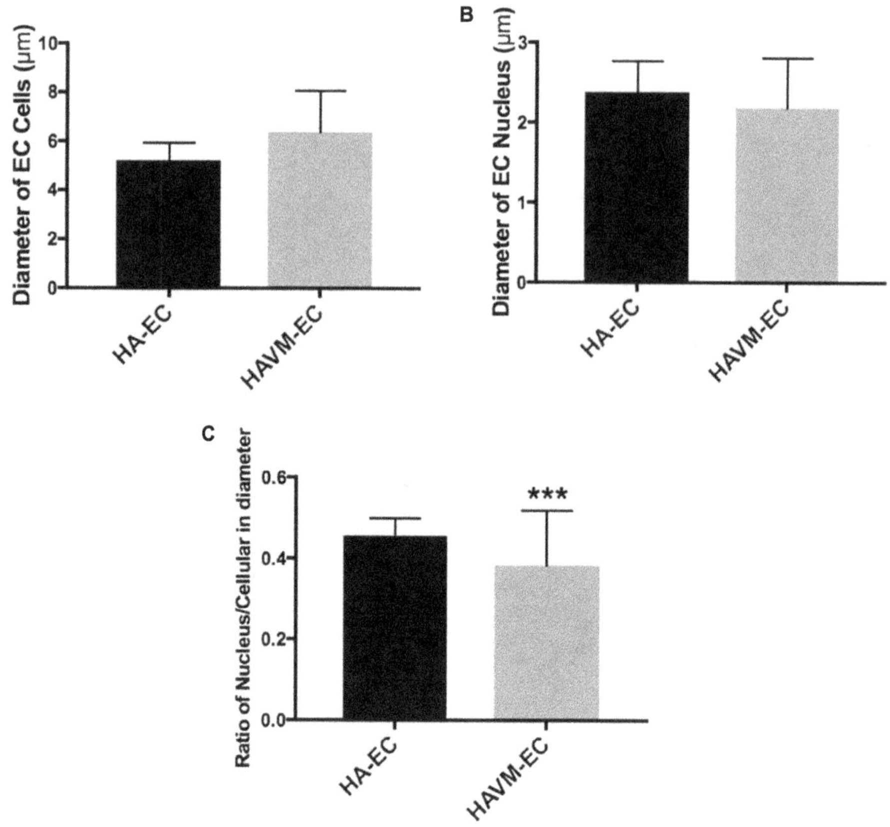

FIGURE 3 | Changes of morphology in cAVM-ECs. **(A)** Average diameters of body in cAVM-ECs and HA-ECs, (6.391 ± 0.5283) μm in cAVM-ECs, were larger than that (5.222 ± 0.2224) μm in HA-ECs ($p > 0.05$); **(B)** The average diameters of nucleus in cAVM-ECs (2.183 ± 0.1981) μm, were smaller than that (2.377 ± 0.1226) μm in HA-ECs ($p > 0.05$); **(C)** Ratios of nucleus to cellular in cAVM-ECs was (0.3437 ± 0.02426), and that in HA-ECs was (0.4557 ± 0.01356), and there was a significant difference between them ($p < 0.05$).

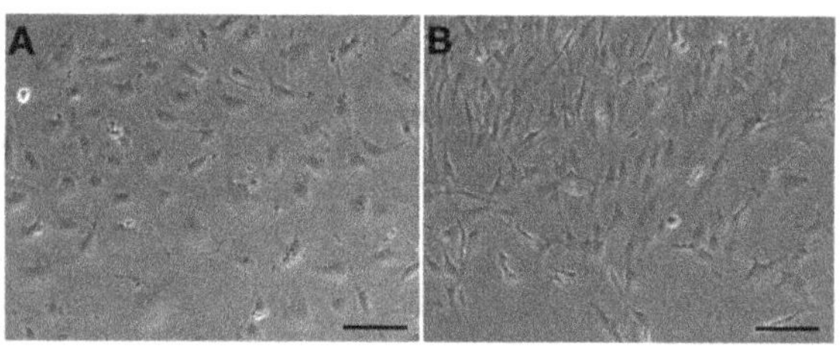

FIGURE 4 | cAVM-ECs trans-differentiated into mesenchyme-like cells in a short period. **(A)** HA-ECs kept the general morphology of ECs when passaged to 7th–8th population without morphological change; **(B)** The morphology of cultured cAVM-ECs changed into spindle-like cells after passaged to the forth generation.

RESULTS

Isolated ECs From Human cAVM (cAVM-ECs)

cAVMs were characterized by conglomerate of tortuous vessels, including feeding arteries and draining veins. We found cluttered vessels flow void in the right temporal-parental area in T2WI of MRI imaging (**Figure 1A**). Digital subtraction angiography (DSA) results showed that cerebral middle artery provided blood for the cAVM nidus as feeder artery, which was connected with the sigmoid sinus through thick draining vessel (**Figure 1B**). Under the operational microscope (Carl Zeiss, Pentero 800, United States), we found abnormal vessels nidus occupied on the brain surface scrabbly (**Figure 1C**). In addition, immunostaining results demonstrated that cAVM-ECs expressed typical EC markers, such as CD31 and CD34 (**Figures 1D,E**). These cells derived from cAVMs also possessed the functional properties of general ECs, including the ability of Dil-Ac-LDL uptake and tube formation on 3D matrigel (**Figures 1F,G**). Therefore, the isolated cAVM-ECs not only have the cellular characteristics in morphology and special markers of ECs, but also have the common functional properties of ECs (Hao et al., 2018).

Morphological Characteristics of cAVM-ECs

Observed under a phase-contrast microscope, the HA-ECs had classical round borders and cobblestone appearances (**Figures 2A,B**). When cAVM-ECs contacted with each other, they showed irregular borders and flatty bodies (**Figures 2C,D**). Compared to HA-ECs, these isolated cells showed rough edges

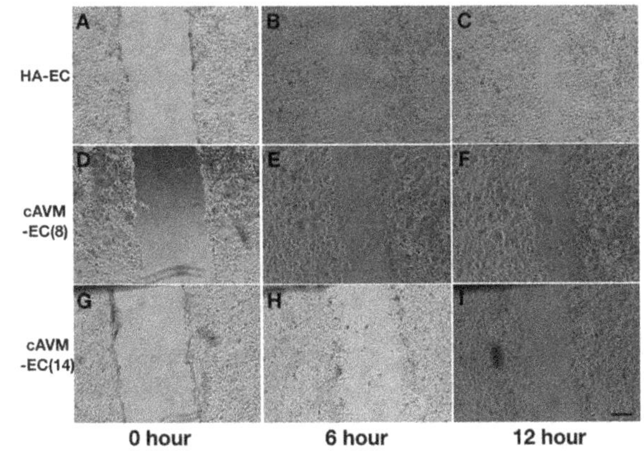

FIGURE 5 | Scratch assay in cAVM-ECs and HA-ECs. When HA-ECs and cAVM-ECs (derived from 8- and 14-year-old patients) were seeded in the 24-well plate, we detected the ability of migration among three groups at 6 and 12 h after seeding, respectively. **(A–C)** Scratch assay in HA-ECs, **(A)** 0 h after Scratched, **(B)** 6 h after Scratched, **(C)** 12 h after Scratched; **(D–F)** Scratch assay in cAVM-ECs (derived from 8-year-old patient), **(D)** 0 h after Scratched, **(E)** 6 h after Scratched, **(F)** 12 h after Scratched; **(G–I)** Scratch assay in cAVM-ECs (derived from 14-year-old patient), **(G)** 0 h after Scratched, **(H)** 6 h after Scratched, **(I)** 12 h after Scratched; Scale bar = 100 μm.

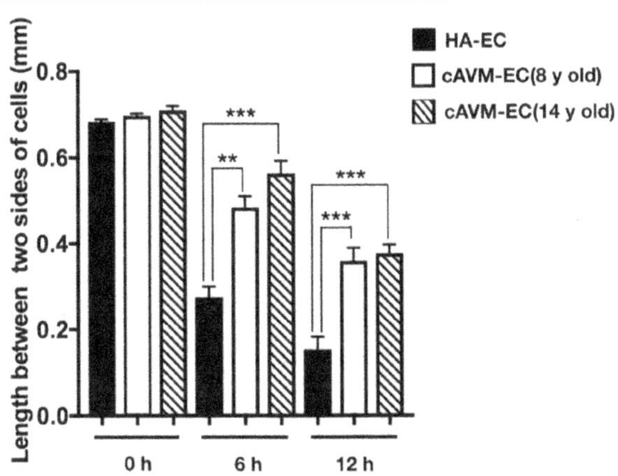

FIGURE 6 | Statistical analysis of scratch assay in cAVM-ECs and HA-ECs. After 6 h, the distances between two sides of scratch in HA-ECs were (0.276 ± 0.024) mm, (0.483 ± 0.026) mm in cAVM-ECs of 8-year-old, and (0.563 ± 0.030) mm in cAVM-ECs of 14-year-old (all *$p < 0.05$). After 12 h, the distances between two sides of scratch in HA-ECs were (0.153 ± 0.029) mm, (0.359 ± 0.030) mm in cAVM-ECs of 8-year-old, (0.376 ± 0.021) mm in and cAVM-ECs of 14-year-old (all *$p < 0.05$). Besides, the distances between two sides of scratch in cAVM of 8- and 14-year-old patients had no significant difference.

and had no obvious gloss. In addition, the average diameter of cAVM-ECs body was 6.391 ± 0.5283 μm, which was larger than that in HA-ECs (5.222 ± 0.2224 μm) ($p > 0.05$); the average diameter of nucleus of cAVM-ECs was 2.183 ± 0.1981 μm, which was smaller than that in HA-ECs (2.377 ± 0.1226 μm) ($p > 0.05$). There was no significant difference between cAVM-ECs and HA-ECs. However, the ratio of nucleus to cellular in diameter of

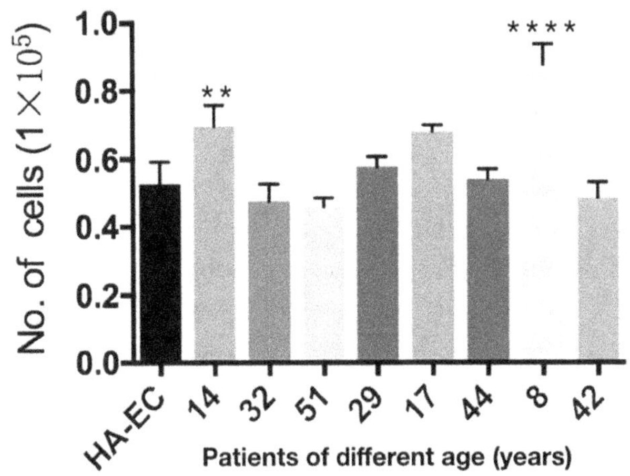

FIGURE 7 | Proliferative ability of HA-ECs and cAVM-ECs with different ages. HA-ECs and cAVM-ECs derived from eight patients were successfully passaged to the forth generation. The results showed that the number of HA-ECs was (0.527 ± 0.065) million, which was less than that in cAVM-ECs from (patient 8-year-old) (0.877 ± 0.06) million and cAVM-ECs from (patient 14-year-old) (0.697 ± 0.061) (all *$p < 0.05$).

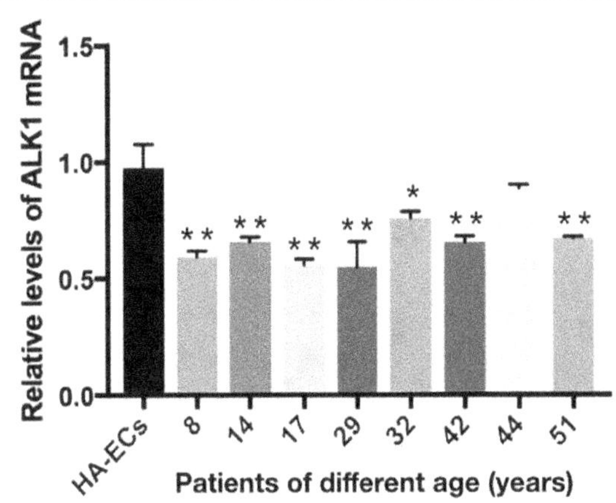

FIGURE 8 | mRNA expression of gene Alk1 in HA-ECs and cAVM-ECs in patients with different ages. Levels of VEGF-A mRNA expression (0.986 ± 0.134) in the HA-ECs were lower than that in cAVM-ECs (8 years) (4.183 ± 0.238) and cAVM-ECs (14 years) (3.834 ± 0.451) (all *$p < 0.05$). In addition, the levels of VEGF-A mRNA expression were (2.92 ± 0.58) in cAVM-ECs (17 years), (3.04 ± 0.79) in cAVM-ECs (29 years), (3.08 ± 0.37) in cAVM-ECs (32 years), (2.08 ± 0.28) in cAVM-ECs (42 years), (1.97 ± 0.24) in cAVM-ECs (44 years), and (1.97 ± 0.25) in cAVM-ECs (51 years), all of that were higher than that (0.986 ± 0.134) in HA-ECs (all *$p < 0.05$).

cAVM-ECs (0.3437 ± 0.02426) was smaller than that in HA-ECs (0.4557 ± 0.01356), and there was significant difference ($p < 0.05$) (**Figure 3**). These results showed that obvious changes existed in the morphology of cAVM-ECs.

Trans-Differentiation Into Mesenchyme-Like Cells in a Short Period

Human aortic endothelial cells could be passaged to seventh or eighth population without morphological changes (**Figure 4A**).

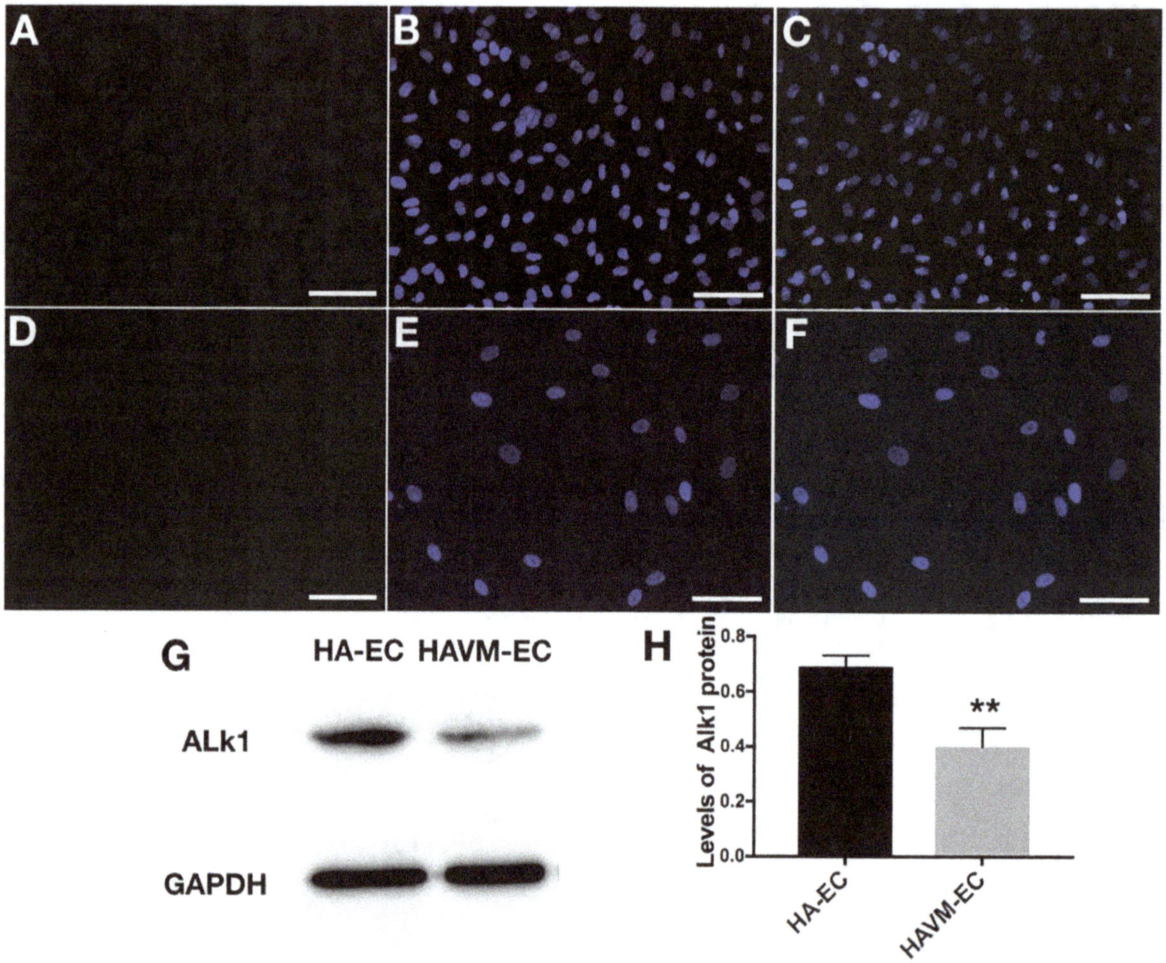

FIGURE 9 | Expression of Alk1 proteins in HA-ECs and cAVM-ECs. **(A–D)** Immunofluorescent staining to detect the Alk1 protein expressed in HA-ECs and cAVM-ECs. **(A–C)** In HA-ECs, **(A)** Alk1 protein was stained by Green fluorescent, **(B)** nuclei was stained by DAPI in Green fluorescent; **(C)** merge; **(D–F)** In cAVM-ECs, **(D)** Alk1 protein was stained by Green fluorescent, **(E)** nuclei was stained by DAPI in Green fluorescent; the fluorescence intensity in cAVM-ECs was obviously lower than in HA-ECs; **(F)** merge. Scale bar = 200 μm; **(G)** Detect the expression of Alk1 by Western blot, **(H)** expression of Alk1 proteins in the HA-ECs cultures were significantly higher than that in cAVM-ECs *in vitro* (*$p < 0.05$).

However, compared to HA-ECs, the morphology of cAVM-ECs changed into spindle-like cells after passaged to the forth generation (**Figure 4B**). These results demonstrate that the cAVM-ECs can not maintain the characteristics of morphology for a long time, and easily trans-differentiate into mesenchyme-like cells in a short period.

Poor Ability of Migration in cAVM-ECs

After HA-ECs and cAVM-ECs (derived from 8- and 14-year-old patients) were seeded in the 24-well plate, we analyzed the ability of migration among three groups in 6 and 12 h, respectively. Because of limitation of cAVM-ECs sources, we just detected cAVM-ECs from 8- to 14-year-old patients. The distances between two sides of scratch in HA-ECs were shorter than that in the other two cAVM-ECs groups, measured, respectively, at 6 and 12 h after seeded. 6 h later, the distances between two sides of scratch in HA-ECs were 0.276 ± 0.024 and 0.483 ± 0.026 mm in cAVM-ECs of 8-year-olds, and 0.563 ± 0.030 mm in cAVM-ECs of 14-year-olds (all*$p < 0.05$). 12 h later, the distances between two sides of scratch in HA-ECs were 0.153 ± 0.029 mm, 0.359 ± 0.030 mm in cAVM-ECs of 8-year-old, and 0.376 ± 0.021 mm in cAVM-ECs of 14-year-old (all *$p < 0.05$). In addition, the distances in cAVM of 8- and 14-year-old patients had no significant difference (**Figures 5, 6**). These results demonstrate that ability of migration in the cAVM-ECs groups decreases significantly compared to HA-ECs group.

Proliferative Ability of cAVM-ECs Derived From Different Age Patients

Human aortic endothelia cells and cAVM-ECs from eight patients were successfully passaged to the forth generation. To detect the proliferative ability of these cells, we seeded HA-ECs and cAVM-ECs derived from different age patients at the density of 0.1×10^5 per well. Cultured for 8 days later, all of the ECs were digested and counted. The results showed that the number of HA-ECs was 0.527 ± 0.065 million and less than that in cAVM-ECs (0.877 ± 0.06 million in 8-year-old patient and 0.697 ± 0.061 million in 14-year-old patient) (all $^*p < 0.05$). In addition, there were no significant differences in other patients groups. Besides, the number of cAVM-ECs in 8-year-old patient was higher than that in all the other groups ($^*p < 0.05$) (**Figure 7**).

Lower Expression of Alk1 in cAVM-ECs

The levels of Alk1 mRNA were tested by qRT-PCR. Results showed that the levels of expression of Alk1 mRNA were 0.59 ± 0.03 in cAVM-ECs (8 years), 0.66 ± 0.02 in cAVM-ECs (14 years), 0.66 ± 0.02 in cAVM-ECs (17 years), 0.55 ± 0.1 in cAVM-ECs (29 years), 0.76 ± 0.03 in cAVM-ECs (32 years), 0.66 ± 0.02 in cAVM-ECs (42 years), and 0.67 ± 0.01 in cAVM-ECs (51 years), and all of them were lower than that in HA-ECs (0.98 ± 0.1) (all $^*p < 0.05$). In addition, there were no significant differences between the different cAVM-ECs groups. The levels of Alk1 mRNA in cAVM-ECs (44 years) (0.89 ± 0.01) was lower than that in HA-ECs (0.96 ± 0.1), however, there was no significant difference between them (**Figure 8**). In addition, immunofluorescent staining showed that HA-ECs and cAVM-ECs were Alk1-positive in Cytoplasm. However, the fluorescence intensity in cAVM-ECs was obviously lower than that in HA-ECs (**Figures 9A–F**). Besides, due to the limitation of the cAVM-ECs sources, we combined all of the cAVM-ECs groups to detect the average levels of Alk1 expression. Western blot results also confirmed that the levels of Alk1 proteins in the HA-ECs were higher than that in cAVM-ECs ($^*p < 0.05$) (**Figures 9G,H**).

Increasing Expression of VEGF-A in cAVM-ECs

The levels of VEGF-A gene expression were examined by qRT-PCR analysis. Results showed the levels of VEGF-A mRNA were 0.98 ± 0.13 in the HA-ECs, which was lower than that in cAVM-ECs (8 years) (4.183 ± 0.238) and cAVM-ECs (14 years) (3.834 ± 0.451) (all $^*p < 0.05$). In addition, the levels of VEGF-A mRNA were 2.92 ± 0.58 in cAVM-ECs (17 years), 3.04 ± 0.79 in cAVM-ECs (29 years), 3.08 ± 0.37 in cAVM-ECs (32 years), 2.08 ± 0.28 in cAVM-ECs (42 years), 1.97 ± 0.24 in cAVM-ECs (44 years), and 1.97 ± 0.25 in cAVM-ECs (51 years), which all of those were higher than that in the HA-ECs (0.98 ± 0.13) (all $^*p < 0.05$). These results showed that the levels of VEGF-A in cAVM-ECs were higher than that in HA-ECs. In addition, the levels of VEGF-A in the older patients with cAVM were lower than that in the younger patients (**Figure 10**).

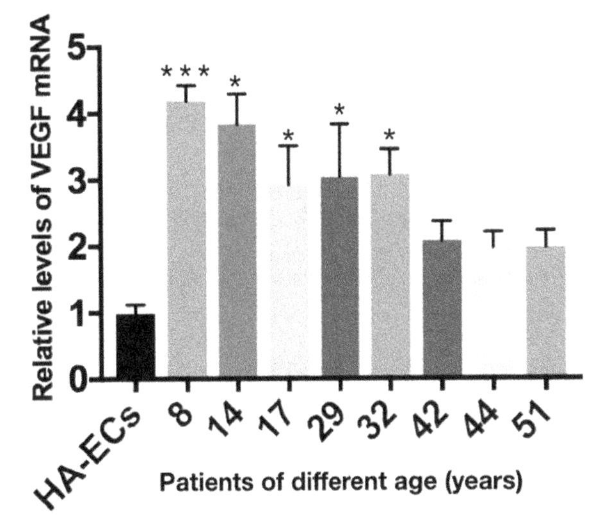

FIGURE 10 | mRNA expression of gene VEGF in HA-ECs and cAVM-ECs with different ages. Level of VEGF-A mRNA expression in the HA-ECs (0.98 ± 0.13) was lower than that in cAVM-ECs (8 years) (4.183 ± 0.238) and cAVM-ECs (14 years) (3.834 ± 0.451) (all $^*p < 0.05$). Level of VEGF-A mRNA expression in cAVM-ECs (17 years) was (2.92 ± 0.58), in cAVM-ECs (29 years) was (3.04 ± 0.79), in cAVM-ECs (32 years) was (3.08 ± 0.37), in cAVM-ECs (42 years) was (2.08 ± 0.28), in cAVM-ECs (44 years) was (1.97 ± 0.24), and in cAVM-ECs (51 years) was (1.97 ± 0.25), all of that were higher than that in the HA-ECs (0.98 ± 0.13) (all $^*p < 0.05$).

DISCUSSION

The isolated human cAVM-ECs owned the general characteristics of ECs, such as cobblestone-like morphology, the special markers of ECs (CD31 and CD34), and the functional properties of LDL intake and tube formation. However, compared with normal HA-ECs, we found some changes of AVM-ECs in morphology, such as irregular borders, smaller nucleus and bigger cell bodies, all of which might induce functional changes of these cells. For instance, in our experiment, we found that AVM-ECs could differentiate into mesenchyme-like cells when passaged into forth generation. In addition, cAVM-ECs proliferated faster and migrated more slowly than that in HA-ECs. These results demonstrate that ECs play an important role in the occurrence and development in sporadic human cAVMs.

In the scratch assay, we found that the speeds of migration in cAVM-ECs were obviously lower than that in HA-ECs. In addition, we detected the levels of Alk1 expression in cAVM-ECs and HA-ECs, using immunofluorescent staining and qRT-PCR, respectively. The results showed that the density of fluorescent of Alk1 positive cells in cAVM-ECs was lower than that in HA-ECs. In addition, levels of Alk1 proteins expression in HA-ECs were higher than that in cAVM-ECs, detected by Western blot assay. Besides, qRT-PCR results were in accordance with Western blot, and there were no significant differences between the different cAVM-ECs groups. Lower levels of Alk1 expression might inhibit the ability of cAVM-ECs migration. Rochon et al. reported, the main role of Alk1-mutant could not alter the arterial EC proliferation, but could alter the movement of arterial ECs in vessels. In Alk1-mutant ECs, directed migration of ECs could be impaired (Rochon et al., 2016). Therefore we speculate that decreased Alk1 expression results in poorer ability of migration in sporadic cAVM-ECs, and Alk1 plays an important role in the formation of cAVMs.

In the proliferation assay, we compared the proliferative ability between the HA-ECs group and cAVM-ECs with different ages groups. The results showed that cAVM-ECs proliferated faster than HA-ECs. We also detected the levels of

VEGF-A expression in HA-ECs and cAVM-ECs with different ages using qRT-PCR. We found that levels of VEGF-A expression in cAVM-ECs were higher than that in HA-ECs. VEGF-A did not only stimulate endothelial migration, but also enhanced the ability of proliferation (Eichmann and Simons, 2012). This conclusion was partly in accordance with our results. However, Pro Gerhardt pointed that neighboring cells contributed to elongation and stability of the new vessel (stalk cells), when some of ECs formed polarized filopodia protrusions and acquire the leading tip position in the nascent sprout (tip cells) (Gerhardt et al., 2003).

In our previous research, we found that the Alk1-mutant mice would not form cAVMs without local VEGF over-expression. Hence, we thought that down-regulation of Alk1 expression combined with the up-regulation of VEGF, could accurately reflect the formation development of cAVMs in the sporadic patients. Actually, we found that the levels of VEGF expression were higher in the sporadic patients than that in normal control in another experiment, detected by ELISA Testing blood samples. The down-regulation of Alk1 expression might influent the ability of migration in ECs, while over-expression of VEGF might enhance the proliferative ability. Both of which could induce the formation of an abnormal vessel nidus. In addition, high doses of VEGF injected in the selected cerebral area of the Alk1-mutant mice could lead to cerebral hemorrhage. Professor Park and Martin reported previously, regional or tissue-specific conditional gene deletion of either Eng or Alk1 could produce AVMs when *de novo* angiogenesis was stimulated by VEGF in mice (Park et al., 2009; Garrido-Martin et al., 2014).

In addition to the above-mentioned, products of ENG and MADH4 were also the receptors or signaling molecules of the TGFβ/BMPs pathway (Urness et al., 2000; Sorensen et al., 2003). They might affect proliferation, differentiation, migration and extracellular matrix formations of ECs, which all played a critical role in the proper development of the blood vessels. Alk1 might promote cell migration and proliferations collaborated with ENG.

In order to further explore the further mechanism of cAVMs formation and development in sporadic patients, we should optimize the methods of isolation and culturing to increase the yield of cAVM-ECs. And the anti-VEGF treatment may be a promising option to treat AVMs. In the future, VEGF might be neutralized to reduce their levels, and to detect whether it could repair the morphology and reduce the rate of hemorrhage induced by cAVMs.

CONCLUSION

Alk1 might induce the formation of sporadic human cAVMs through affecting migration and proliferation of ECs, combined with VEGF-A.

AUTHOR CONTRIBUTIONS

Y-LZ designed the whole experiments and QH participated in the whole proceed. J-LL, HW, X-LC, LM, XY, M-TL, Y-HZ, and YC took part in the collection of AVM tissues and discussion.

FUNDING

This study was supported by grant nos. 81571110, 81271313, and 81500995 to Y-LZ, from The National Natural Science Fund, China, Grant nos. 2017A07 to Y-LZ, from Beijing Bai Qian Wan Talent Engineering Fund, Beijing, China, Grant nos. PX2016034 to HW from Beijing Municipal Administration of Hospitals Incubating Program.

REFERENCES

Braverman, I. M., Keh, A., and Jacobson, B. S. (1990). Ultrastructure and three-dimensional organization of the telangiectases of hereditary hemorrhagic telangiectasia. *J. Invest. Dermatol.* 95, 422–427. doi: 10.1111/1523-1747.ep12555569

da Costa, L., Wallace, M. C., Ter Brugge, K. G., O'Kelly, C., Willinsky, R. A., and Tymianski, M. (2009). The natural history and predictive features of hemorrhage from brain arteriovenous malformations. *Stroke* 40, 100–105. doi: 10.1161/STROKEAHA.108.524678

Eichmann, A., and Simons, M. (2012). VEGF signaling inside vascular endothelial cells and beyond. *Curr. Opin. Cell. Biol.* 24, 188–193. doi: 10.1016/j.ceb.2012.02.002

Garrido-Martin, E. M., Nguyen, H. L., Cunningham, T. A., Choe, S. W., Jiang, Z., Arthur, H. M., et al. (2014). Common and distinctive pathogenetic features of arteriovenous malformations in hereditary hemorrhagic telangiectasia 1 and hereditary hemorrhagic telangiectasia 2 animal models–brief report. *Arterioscler. Thromb Vasc. Biol.* 34, 2232–2236. doi: 10.1161/ATVBAHA.114.303984

Gerhardt, H., Golding, M., Fruttiger, M., Ruhrberg, C., Lundkvist, A., Abramsson, A., et al. (2003). VEGF guides angiogenic sprouting utilizing endothelial tip cell filopodia. *J. Cell Biol.* 161, 1163–1177. doi: 10.1083/jcb.200302047

Hao, Q., Chen, X., Ma, L., Wang, T., Hu, Y., and Zhao, Y. (2018). Procedure for the isolation of isolation of endothelial cells from human cerebral arteriovenous malformation(cAVM) tissues. *Front. Cell. Neurosci.* 12:30. doi: 10.3389/fncel.2018.00030

Kim, H., Su, H., Weinsheimer, S., Pawlikowska, L., and Young, W. L. (2011). Brain arteriovenous malformation pathogenesis: a response-to-injury paradigm. *Acta. Neurochir. Suppl.* 111, 83–92. doi: 10.1007/978-3-7091-0693-8_14

Laux, D. W., Young, S., Donovan, J. P., Mansfield, C. J., Upton, P. D., and Roman, B. L. (2013). Circulating Bmp10 acts through endothelial Alk1 to mediate flow-dependent arterial quiescence. *Development* 140, 3403–3412. doi: 10.1242/dev.095307

Lawton, M. T., Rutledge, W. C., Kim, H., Stapf, C., Whitehead, K. J., Li, D. Y., et al. (2015). Brain arteriovenous malformations. *Nat. Rev. Dis. Primers* 1:15008. doi: 10.1038/nrdp.2015.8

Park, S. O., Wankhede, M., Lee, Y. J., Choi, E. J., Fliess, N., Choe, S. W., et al. (2009). Real-time imaging of de novo arteriovenous malformation in a mouse

doi: 10.1172/JCI39482

Rochon, E. R., Menon, P. G., and Roman, B. L. (2016). Alk1 controls arterial endothelial cell migration in lumenized vessels. *Development* 143, 2593–2602. doi: 10.1242/dev.135392

Sammons, V., Davidson, A., Tu, J., and Stoodley, M. A. (2011). Endothelial cells in the context of brain arteriovenous malformations. *J. Clin. Neurosci.* 18, 165–170. doi: 10.1016/j.jocn.2010.04.045

Sorensen, L. K., Brooke, B. S., Li, D. Y., and Urness, L. D. (2003). Loss of distinct arterial and venous boundaries in mice lacking endoglin, a vascular-specific TGFbeta coreceptor. *Dev. Biol.* 261, 235–250. doi: 10.1016/S0012-1606(03)00158-1

Urness, L. D., Sorensen, L. K., and Li, D. Y. (2000). Arteriovenous malformations in mice lacking activin receptor-like kinase-1. *Nat. Genet.* 26, 328–331. doi: 10.1038/81634

mor function and surgical outcomes in patients with cerebral arterivenous malformation involving primary motor area: insight from fMRI and DTI. *Chin. Neurosurg. J.* 12, 1–9.

17

Dose-Dependent Influences of Ethanol on Ischemic Stroke: Role of Inflammation

*Guodong Xu[1,2], Chun Li[1], Anne L. Parsiola[1], Jiyu Li[1], Kimberly D. McCarter[1], Runhua Shi[3], William G. Mayhan[4] and Hong Sun[1]**

[1]Department of Cellular Biology & Anatomy, Louisiana State University Health Sciences Center-Shreveport, Shreveport, LA, United States, [2]Department of Neurology, Hebei General Hospital, Shijiazhuang, China, [3]Department of Medicine/Feist-Weiller Cancer Center, Louisiana State University Health Sciences Center-Shreveport, Shreveport, LA, United States, [4]Basic Biomedical Sciences, Sanford School of Medicine, The University of South Dakota, Vermillion, SD, United States

***Correspondence:**
Hong Sun
hsun1@lsuhsc.edu

Chronic ethanol consumption dose-dependently affects both incidence and prognosis of ischemic stroke. Our goal was to determine whether the influence of chronic ethanol consumption on ischemic stroke is related to an altered inflammatory profile in the brain. Male C57BL/6J mice were divided into six groups and gavage fed with 0.175, 0.35, 0.7, 1.4, 2.8 g/kg/day ethanol or volume-matched water once a day for 8 weeks. Adhesion molecules, microglial activation, neutrophil infiltration, pro- and anti-inflammatory cytokines/chemokines, blood-brain barrier (BBB) permeability, and matrix metallopeptidases (MMPs) in the cerebral cortex before and following a 90-min unilateral middle cerebral artery occlusion (MCAO)/24-h reperfusion were evaluated. Brain ischemia/reperfusion (I/R) injury was significantly reduced in 0.7 g/kg/day ethanol group (peak blood ethanol concentration: 9 mM) and worsened in 2.8 g/kg/day ethanol group (peak blood ethanol concentration: 37 mM). Baseline E-selectin was downregulated in all ethanol groups, whereas baseline intercellular adhesion molecule-1 (ICAM-1) was only downregulated in 0.35 and 0.7 g/kg/day ethanol groups. Interestingly, baseline vascular cell adhesion molecule-1 (VCAM-1) was upregulated in 0.35, 0.7, and 1.4 g/kg/day ethanol groups. Post-ischemic upregulation of ICAM-1 and E-selectin were suppressed in all ethanol groups. Post-ischemic neutrophil infiltration and microglial activation were significantly less in the low-moderate (0.175–1.4 g/kg/day) ethanol groups but greater in the 2.8 g/kg/day ethanol group compared to the vehicle group. At basal conditions, ethanol increased one pro- and two anti-inflammatory cytokines/chemokines at the 0.7 g/kg/day dose, and 13 pro- and eight anti-inflammatory cytokines/chemokines at the 2.8 g/kg/day dose. After ischemia, 0.7 g/kg/day ethanol suppressed post-ischemic pro-inflammatory cytokines/chemokines and enhanced post-ischemic anti-inflammatory cytokines/chemokines. Moreover, 0.7 g/kg/day ethanol significantly reduced baseline MMP-9 activity and alleviated post-ischemic BBB breakdown. On the other hand,

2.8 g/kg/day ethanol worsened post-ischemic BBB breakdown. Our findings suggest that low-moderate ethanol consumption may prevent ischemic stroke and reduce brain I/R injury by suppressing inflammation, whereas heavy alcohol consumption may induce ischemic stroke and worsen brain I/R injury by aggravating inflammation.

Keywords: ethanol, ischemic stroke, adhesion molecule, microglia, neutrophil infiltration, cytokine/chemokine, matrix metalloproteinase

INTRODUCTION

Ischemic stroke continues to be one of the leading causes of mortality and permanent disability worldwide (Favate and Younger, 2016; Benjamin et al., 2017). Intravenous recombinant tissue plasminogen activator (tPA) and endovascular therapy are currently used to treat acute ischemic stroke. Both treatments result in recanalization/reperfusion. Although recanalization/reperfusion is critical for restoring normal function, it paradoxically induces and worsens brain injury, called brain ischemia/reperfusion (I/R) injury (Jean et al., 1998). The mechanisms underlying brain I/R injury are complex and involve several interacting elements, including oxidative/nitrosative stress, activation of apoptotic and autophagic pathways, and increased inflammatory response (Jean et al., 1998; Kalogeris et al., 2012; Chen et al., 2014).

Post-ischemic inflammatory responses are characterized by the accumulation of inflammatory cells and mediators in the ischemic brain. The recruitment of leukocytes (including neutrophils) to the ischemic area appears to be a central feature after transient focal cerebral ischemia (Gronberg et al., 2013). When neutrophils are depleted from the circulation the infarct volume is reduced and cerebral blood flow (CBF) is improved during the reperfusion period (Jean et al., 1998; Herz et al., 2015). The recruitment of leukocytes into the ischemic area is facilitated by upregulation of adhesion molecules on endothelial cells prior to and during reperfusion (Supanc et al., 2011). In addition, the recruitment of leukocytes is associated with inflammatory activation of microglia and subsequent production of matrix metallopeptidases (MMPs), chemokines, and cytokines. Microglia are key modulators of the immune response in the brain. After ischemia, microglia rapidly proliferate, transform their morphology and migrate toward injured neurons (Weinstein et al., 2010). Activated microglia directly contribute to brain I/R injury by phagocytosis and producing inflammatory and cytotoxic mediators (Shukla et al., 2017). MMPs are responsible for remodeling extracellular matrix (Bonnans et al., 2014). In addition to microglia, neurons, astrocytes, and endothelial cells also express MMPs (Turner and Sharp, 2016). After transient focal cerebral ischemia, MMPs are upregulated and activated under the influence of inflammatory mediators (Ceulemans et al., 2010). Activated MMPs stimulate leukocyte adherence and transmigration and promote blood-brain barrier (BBB) breakdown and hemorrhagic transformation (Lakhan et al., 2009; Ceulemans et al., 2010). Cytokines are among the principal mediators of the inflammatory response and are involved in virtually every facet of stroke (Kim et al., 2014). Cytokines can be elaborated by leukocytes, macrophages, endothelial cells and resident cells within the brain (Kim et al., 2014). After transient focal cerebral ischemia, pro-inflammatory cytokines, such as interleukin-1 (IL-1), tumor necrosis factor-α (TNF-α), and IL-6, stimulate and aggravate the inflammatory response (Shukla et al., 2017).

Ethanol is one of the most commonly and regularly used chemical substances. Epidemiological studies suggest that low-moderate ethanol intake lowers the incidence of ischemic stroke and reduces mortality and infarct volume from ischemic stroke, whereas heavy ethanol consumption increases the incidence of ischemic stroke and worsens the prognosis of ischemic stroke (Hansagi et al., 1995; Ikehara et al., 2008; Patra et al., 2010; Ronksley et al., 2011; Ducroquet et al., 2013; Zhang et al., 2014). Ischemic stroke is most often caused by atherosclerosis, which has been well recognized as a chronic inflammatory process (Bruno et al., 2008). The relationship between regular ethanol intake and incidence of atherosclerosis appears to be U-shaped (Kiechl et al., 1998). Thus, our goal was to determine whether the influence of ethanol on ischemic stroke is related to an altered inflammatory profile in the brain.

MATERIALS AND METHODS

Animal Models of Ethanol Preconditioning

This study was carried out in accordance with the recommendations of the National Institutes of Health Guide for the Care and Use Laboratory Animals. The protocol was approved by the Institutional Animal Care and Use Committee at the Louisiana State University Health Science Center-Shreveport. One hundred twenty male C57BL/6J mice (20–25 g) were randomly divided into six groups: vehicle (n = 24), 0.175 g/kg/day ethanol (n = 16), 0.35 g/kg/day ethanol (n = 16), 0.7 g/kg/day ethanol (n = 24), 1.4 g/kg/day ethanol (n = 16), and 2.8 g/kg/day ethanol (n = 24). Ethanol groups were gavage fed with 10 ml/kg 1.75% (0.175 g/kg/day ethanol group), 3.5% (0.35 g/kg/day ethanol group), 7% (0.7 g/kg/day ethanol group), 14% (1.4 g/kg/day ethanol group) or 28% (2.8 g/kg/day ethanol group) ethanol once a day for 8 weeks. The vehicle group was gavage fed with 10 ml/kg water. Fasting blood glucose was measured by Bayer Breeze2 Blood Glucose Meter (Bayer HealthCare, Mishawaka, IN, USA). Prior to the measurement, mice were fasted for 12 h during the daytime. To determine whether 8-week feeding changes the peak concentration of blood ethanol, time courses of plasma ethanol concentration in the 0.7 and 2.8 g/kg/day groups were measured using an Ethanol Assay Kit (ab65343, Abcam) at the beginning and end of 8-week feeding period. The measurement was performed according to the manufacturer's instructions. Same mice were used for same time point in each group. Blood pressure and heart rate were measured using a CODA mouse tail-cuff system (Kent Scientific, Torrington, CT, USA). Prior to the actual measurement, mice were trained for three consecutive days to acclimate to being restrained and to also having the tail cuff placed on them. At the end of 8 weeks of feeding, all mice were subjected to transient focal cerebral ischemia.

Transient Focal Cerebral Ischemia

To avoid a possible effect of acute ethanol, alcohol was not given on the day before the experiment. Transient focal cerebral ischemia was induced by unilateral middle cerebral artery occlusion (MCAO). Since disability-free outcome is better when reperfusion is established less than 90 min after the onset of ischemic stroke (Meretoja et al., 2014), 90-min was selected as the MCAO period. Prior to the procedure, mice were anesthetized with isoflurane (induction at 5% and maintenance at 1.5%) in a gas mixture containing 30% O_2/70% N_2 *via* a facemask. Body temperature was maintained with a temperature controlled heating pad (Harvard Apparatus, March, Germany). A laser-Doppler flow probe (PERIMED, PF 5010 LDPM Unit, Sweden) was attached to the right side of the dorsal surface of the skull to monitor regional CBF (rCBF). The right common and external carotid arteries were exposed and ligated. The MCA was occluded by inserting a silicon rubber-coated monofilament (Doccol Corporation, Sharon, MA, USA) from the basal part of the external carotid artery and advanced cranially into the internal carotid artery to the point where the MCA branched off from the internal artery. The onset of the MCAO was indicated by an immediate drop in rCBF. After the occlusion of the right MCA for 90 min, reperfusion was achieved by withdrawing the suture and reopening the common carotid artery. Animals were allowed to recover for 24 h.

Assessment of Neurological Deficits, Infarct Volume and Edema

A 24-point scoring system was used to evaluate sensorimotor deficits at 24 h of reperfusion (Sun et al., 2008). Sensorimotor testing was graded on a scale of 0–3 each on spontaneous activity, symmetry of movement, response to vibrissae touch, floor walking, beam walking, symmetry of forelimbs, climbing wall of wire cage, reaction to touch on either side of trunk. Neurological scores were assigned as follows: 0, complete deficit; 1, definite deficit with some function; 2, decreased response or mild deficit; 3, no evidence of deficit/symmetrical responses. After neurological evaluation, 30 mice (n = 5 for each group) were euthanized and exsanguinated. The brains were quickly removed and placed in ice-cold saline for 5 min, and cut into six 1.75 mm-thick coronal sections. Sections were stained with 2% 2,3,5-triphenyltetrazolium chloride (TTC; Sigma) for 15 min at 37°C. Sliced images were digitalized, the volumes of infarct lesion, ipsilateral hemisphere and contralateral hemisphere were measured using ImageJ. Total infarct volume was expressed as a percentage of the contralateral hemisphere. Edema was determined by the volume ratio of the ipsilateral hemisphere to the contralateral hemisphere and expressed as a percentage increase of the contralateral hemisphere. All researchers involved in assessing brain injury were blinded to the experimental groups.

Western Blot Analysis

Thirty mice (n = 5 for each group) were euthanized and exsanguinated. Cortical tissues were isolated from the peri-infarct area and contralateral corresponding area to measure protein expression of intercellular adhesion molecule-1 (ICAM-1), vascular cell adhesion molecule-1 (VCAM-1), E-selectin and P-selectin. The brains were cut into six 1.75 mm-thick coronal sections. Under the microscope, the infarct core was identified as an opaque area, and the area bordering 2 mm the infarct core was considered as the peri-infarct area (Choi et al., 2015; McCarter et al., 2017). A researcher who was blinded to the experimental groups collected cortical tissues from the peri-infarct area. The samples were homogenized in ice-cold lysis buffer (150 mmol/l NaCl, 50 mmol/l Tris-HCl, 10 mmol/l EDTA, 0.1% Tween-20, 1% Triton, 0.1% mercaptoethanol, 0.1 mmol/l phenylmethyl sulfonyl fluorides, 5 μg/ml leupeptin, and 5 μg/ml aprotinin, pH 7.4). Lysates were then centrifuged at 12,000× g for 20 min at 4°C, and the supernatants were collected. Protein concentration of the supernatants was determined by the Bradford protein assay (Bio-Rad). SDS-PAGE was performed on a 10% gel on which 20 μg of total protein per well was loaded. After SDS-PAGE, the proteins were transferred to a polyvinylidene difluoride membrane. Immunoblotting was performed using mouse anti-ICAM-1 (sc-8439, Santa Cruz Biotechnology), rabbit anti-VCAM-1 (ab134047, Abcam), rabbit anti-E-selectin (ab18981, Abcam) and goat anti-P-selectin (AF737, R&D systems) as primary antibodies and peroxidase conjugated goat anti-mouse, mouse anti-rabbit, and mouse anti-goat IgG as the secondary antibody. The bound antibody was detected using enhanced chemiluminescence (ECL) detection (Genesee Scientific for ICAM-1, VCAM-1; Thermo Scientific for E-selectin, P-selectin), and the bands were analyzed using ChemiDoc^{TM} MP Imaging System (Bio-Rad). To quantify, protein expression of ICAM-1, VCAM-1, E-selectin and P-selectin was normalized to GAPDH and expressed as percentage changes to the vehicle without I/R.

Immunohistochemistry Staining

Thirty mice (n = 5 for each group) were anesthetized and perfused transcardially with 1× phosphate-buffered saline (PBS), followed by 4% paraformaldehyde in 0.1 mmol/L PBS. The brains were removed, fixed overnight in 4% paraformaldehyde in 0.1 M PBS, dehydrated in a graded series of sugar solutions over the course of 72 h, then embedded in O.C.T. compound (Fisher Scientific) and quick frozen for 5 min in liquid nitrogen. The frozen brains were then cut into 14 μm sections and placed on frost-free slides. The sections were washed with 1× PBS, blocked with 10% bovine serum albumin (BSA) for at least 1 h, and then incubated overnight at 4°C with 1:100 rabbit anti-myeloperoxidase (anti-MPO; Abcam) for visualization of neutrophils or 1:100 rabbit anti-ionized calcium binding adaptor molecule 1 (anti-Iba1; Wako Chemicals Inc., Richmond, VA, USA) for visualization of microglia as primary antibodies. The sections were then incubated with 1:200 AlexaFluor 555 donkey anti-rabbit (Santa Cruz Technology) for 1 h at room temperature. Sections were mounted with DAPI mounting medium with Vector shield and visualized using a fluorescence microscope. Cells positive for MPO represented infiltrating neutrophils. For quantitative analysis, positive cells were counted in three separate areas per section surrounding the infarct area in at least three slides per mouse in each group. To quantify microglia, cells positive for Iba1 were observed and counted. Resting microglia present with long processes extending from their cell body. Resting microglia present with long processes extending from their cell body. Upon activation, microglia change form from highly ramified to completely lacking processes. In addition, activated microglia show increased Iba1 expression (Taylor and Sansing, 2013; Yang et al., 2015). Thus, microglia with increased Iba1 expression and three processes or less were deemed to be activated (Ahmad et al., 2014; Yang et al., 2015).

Cytokine Array

Expression of cytokines in the right cerebral hemisphere was measured using the Proteome Profiler Mouse Cytokine Array Kit, Panel A (ARY006, R&D Systems) in 24 mice (n = 4 for vehicle, vehicle + I/R, 0.7 g/kg/day ethanol, 0.7 g/kg/day ethanol + I/R, 2.8 g/kg/day ethanol, and 2.8 g/kg/day ethanol + I/R). The array was performed according to the manufacturer's instructions. Results were analyzed using ImageJ software and expressed as percentage change relative to vehicle without I/R.

IgG Staining

Three sections (Bregma 1.21 mm, −0.23 mm and −1.31 mm) per mouse (n = 5 for each group) were blocked with 10% BSA for 1 h. Subsequently, the sections were incubated overnight at 4°C with 1:200 goat anti-mouse IgG (BA-9200, Vector), followed by incubating with 1:200 AlexaFluor 555 (Invitrogen) for 1 h at room temperature. Staining was analyzed with a fluorescence microscope and an image analysis system (NIS-Elements, Nikon). The mean fluorescence intensity of equal size around the infarct core and contralateral corresponding area was measured. IgG staining was normalized to contralateral corresponding area and expressed as percentage changes to the vehicle group.

Gelatin Zymography

MMP activity in the cortical tissues prepared for Western Blot analysis was measured using gelatin zymography. Gelatin zymography was carried out using SDS-polyacrylamide gels containing 0.8% gelatin (Sigma, St. Louis, MO, USA). After electrophoresis, the gels were washed with a buffer (pH 7.5) containing 50 mM Tris-HCl, 5 mM $CaCl_2$, 1 μM $ZnCl_2$, 0.02% NaN_3, and 2.5% Triton X-100 to remove the SDS and renature the gelatinases. Gels were then developed in a buffer (pH 7.5) containing 50 mM Tris-HCl, 5 mM $CaCl_2$, 1 μM $ZnCl_2$, 0.02% NaN_3 for 7 days at 37°C. Enzymatic activity was visualized as negative staining with 0.25% Coomassie Brilliant Blue R-250 (Sigma, St. Louis, MO, USA). The molecular sizes of gelatinolytic activity were determined by comparison to Molecular Weight Markers (Bio-Rad, Hercules, CA, USA). The gel was photographed and analyzed using ChemiDoc^{TM} MP Imaging System (Bio-Rad).

Statistical Analysis

Data are presented as means ± SE. Differences in physiological parameters, cerebral I/R injury, microglia activation, neutrophil infiltration, brain edema, and IgG staining between groups were evaluated by one-way analysis of variance (ANOVA) followed by Dunnett's test for multiple comparisons to the control group. Differences in protein expression of adhesion molecules, cytokines and chemokines, and MMP activity between groups were evaluated by two-way ANOVA followed by Bonferroni's test for multiple within and between group comparisons. All analyses were done using statistical analysis software SAS9.4 for windows (SAS Institute, Cary, NC, USA). $P \leq 0.05$ was considered as statistical significant.

RESULTS

Physiological Parameters

After 8-weeks of gavage feeding there was no significant difference in body weight among six groups (**Table 1**). Since cerebral I/R injury was significantly altered in the 0.7 g/kg/day and 2.8 g/kg/day ethanol groups, mean arterial blood pressure (MABP), heart rate, and fasting blood glucose were measured in the vehicle, 0.7 g/kg/day, and 2.8 g/kg/day ethanol groups. There was no significant difference in MABP, heart rate, or fasting blood glucose among three groups (**Table 1**).

Cerebral I/R Injury

Ethanol altered the total infarct volume at 24 h of reperfusion as indicated by a significant main effect of gavage feeding ($F_{(5,27)}$ = 8.9; p = 0.000043, n = 6). *Post hoc* analysis revealed that 0.7 g/kg/day ethanol reduced infarct volume compared to vehicle (p = 0.010214; **Figures 1A,B**). On the other hand, 2.8 g/kg/day ethanol increased infarct volume

TABLE 1 | Effect of ethanol consumption on body weight, blood pressure, heart rate and fasting blood glucose.

	Vehicle	0.175 g/kg/day	0.35 g/kg/day	0.7 g/kg/day	1.4 g/kg/day	2.8 g/kg/day
Body weight (g)	29.4 ± 0.4	28.6 ± 0.6	27.7 ± 0.6	29.1 ± 0.3	27.9 ± 0.5	28.7 ± 0.5
MABP (mmHg)	81.0 ± 3.8	ND	ND	82.3 ± 2.8	ND	90.6 ± 4.5
Heart rate (bpm)	637 ± 40	ND	ND	564 ± 57	ND	644 ± 17
Fasting blood glucose (mg/dl)	139 ± 8	ND	ND	118 ± 12	ND	156 ± 10

Values are means ± SE for five rats in each group. ND stands for Not Determined.

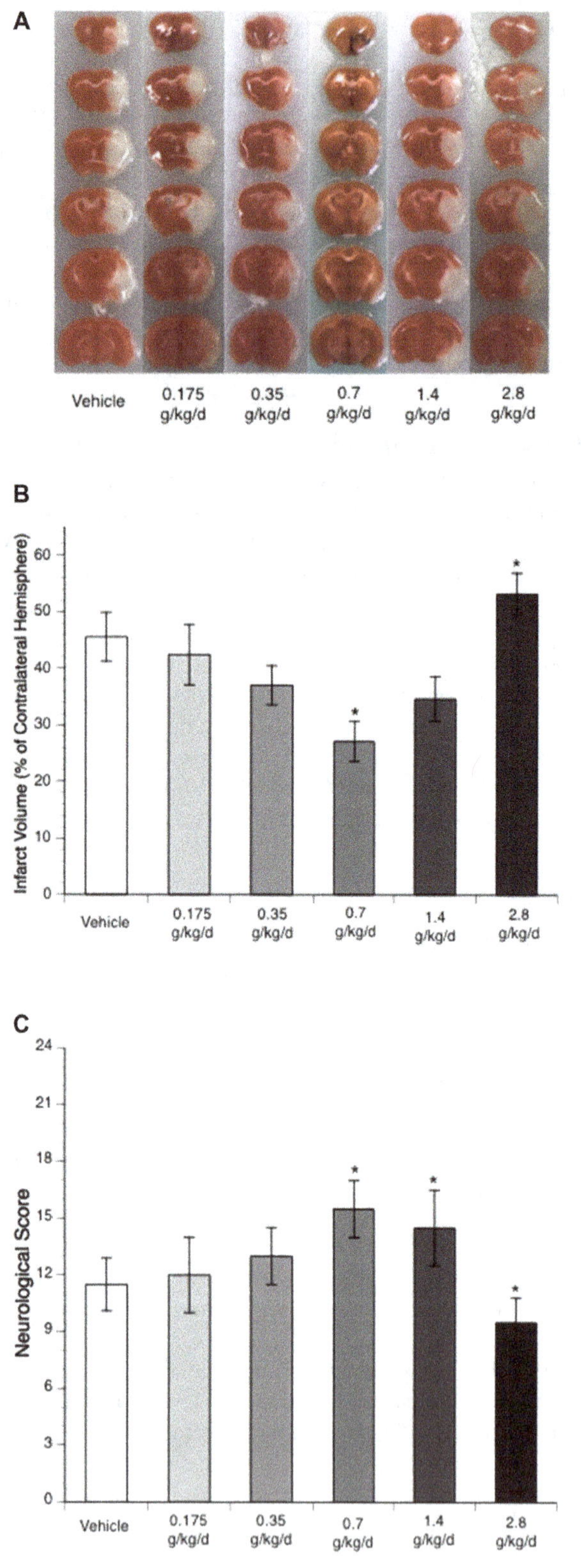

FIGURE 1 | Influence of ethanol on brain injury following a 90-min middle cerebral artery occlusion (MCAO)/24-h reperfusion. **(A)** Representative brain sections stained with 2,3,5-triphenyltetrazolium chloride (TTC). **(B)** Total infarct volume (n = 6). **(C)** Neurological score (n = 15). Values are means ± SE. *$P < 0.05$ vs. Vehicle.

compared to vehicle (p = 0.036302; **Figure 1B**). Consistently, ethanol altered the neurological deficits at 24 h of reperfusion as indicated by a significant main effect of gavage feeding ($F_{(5,84)}$ = 10.92; $p < 0.000001$, n = 15). *Post hoc* analysis showed that 0.7 g/kg/day ethanol significantly improved neurological deficits (p = 0.001570), whereas 2.8 g/kg/day ethanol significantly worsened neurological deficits compared to vehicle (p = 0.041920; **Figure 1C**). Interestingly, although the total infarct volume was not significantly reduced (p = 0.193254), neurological deficits significantly improved in the 1.4 g/kg/day ethanol group (p = 0.006; **Figure 1C**). Since both infarct volume and neurological deficits were significantly altered in the 0.7 g/kg/day and 2.8 g/kg/day ethanol groups, plasma ethanol concentration was measured at 15 min, 30 min, 1 h and 2 h after gavage feeding in these two groups. At the beginning of an 8-week feeding period, the peak concentrations (0.7 g/kg/day ethanol group: 9.0 ± 0.4 mM; 2.8 g/kg/day ethanol group: 37.0 ± 1.5 mM) appeared at 15 min in the 0.7 g/kg/day ethanol group and 30 min in the 2.8 g/kg/day ethanol group (**Figure 2**). The ethanol concentration reduced rapidly and approached to zero at 2 h in the 0.7 g/kg/day ethanol group. In contrast, plasma ethanol concentration declined slowly in the 2.8 g/kg/day ethanol group. Eight-week feeding produced a significant decrease and a significant increase in plasma ethanol concentration at 15 min (p = 0.013) and 1 h (p = 0.049), respectively, in the 2.8 g/kg/day ethanol group. However, 8-week feeding did not affect the peak concentration and its time point in both the 0.7 g/kg/day and 2.8 g/kg/day ethanol groups (**Figure 2**).

Protein Expression of Adhesion Molecules

Ethanol altered baseline expression of ICAM-1 as indicated by a significant main effect of gavage feeding ($F_{(5,24)}$ = 4.48; p = 0.005020, n = 5). *Post hoc* analysis showed that 0.35 and 0.7 g/kg/day ethanol significantly downregulated baseline ICAM-1 (p = 0.031723 and p = 0.020119, respectively; **Figure 3A**). A 90-min MCAO significantly upregulated ICAM-1 at 24 h of reperfusion in all groups (Vehicle group: $F_{(1,8)}$ = 81.90; p = 0.000018, n = 5; 0.175 g/kg/day group: $F_{(1,8)}$ = 12.23; p = 0.008117, n = 5; 0.35 g/kg/day group: $F_{(1,8)}$ = 14.85; p = 0.004856, n = 5; 0.7 g/kg/day group: $F_{(1,8)}$ = 15.75; p = 0.004127, n = 5; 1.4 g/kg/day group: $F_{(1,8)}$ = 6.77; p = 0.031492, n = 5; 2.8 g/kg/day group: $F_{(1,8)}$ = 31.23; p = 0.000517, n = 5; **Figure 3A**). There was a significant interaction of ethanol and ischemic stroke on ICAM-1 expression at 24 h of reperfusion ($F_{(11,48)}$ = 15.53; $p < 0.000001$, n = 5). Mice fed with ethanol had significantly less upregulation in ICAM-1 at 24 h of reperfusion ($F_{(5,24)}$ = 31.54; $p < 0.000001$, n = 5). *Post hoc* analysis showed that 0.175, 0.35, 0.7, 1.4, and 2.8 g/kg/day ethanol significantly reduced post-ischemic ICAM-1 (p = 0.000223, $p < 0.000001$, $p < 0.000001$, $p < 0.000001$, and $p < 0.000001$, respectively; **Figure 3A**). In addition to ICAM-1, ethanol also reduced baseline expression of E-selectin as indicated by a significant main effect of gavage feeding ($F_{(5,24)}$ = 32.53; $p < 0.000001$, n = 5). *Post hoc* analysis showed that 0.175, 0.35, 0.7, 1.4, and

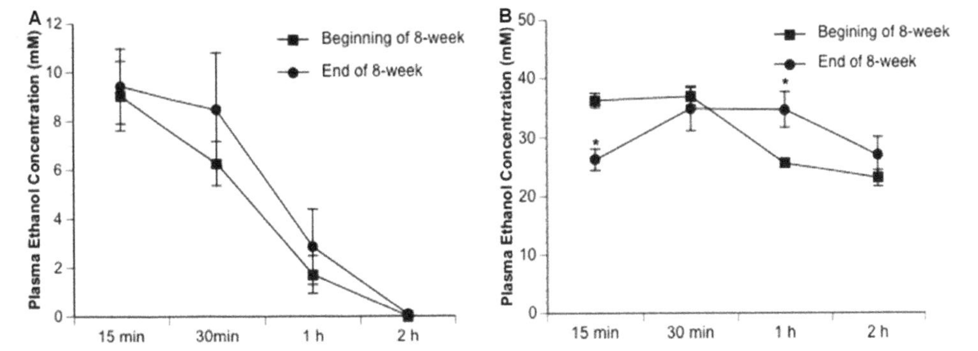

FIGURE 2 | Dynamic change of plasma ethanol concentration in the 0.7 g/kg/day **(A)** and 2.8 g/kg/day **(B)** ethanol groups at the beginning and end of an 8-week feeding period. Values are means ± SE for four mice in each group. *$P < 0.05$ vs. Beginning of 8-week.

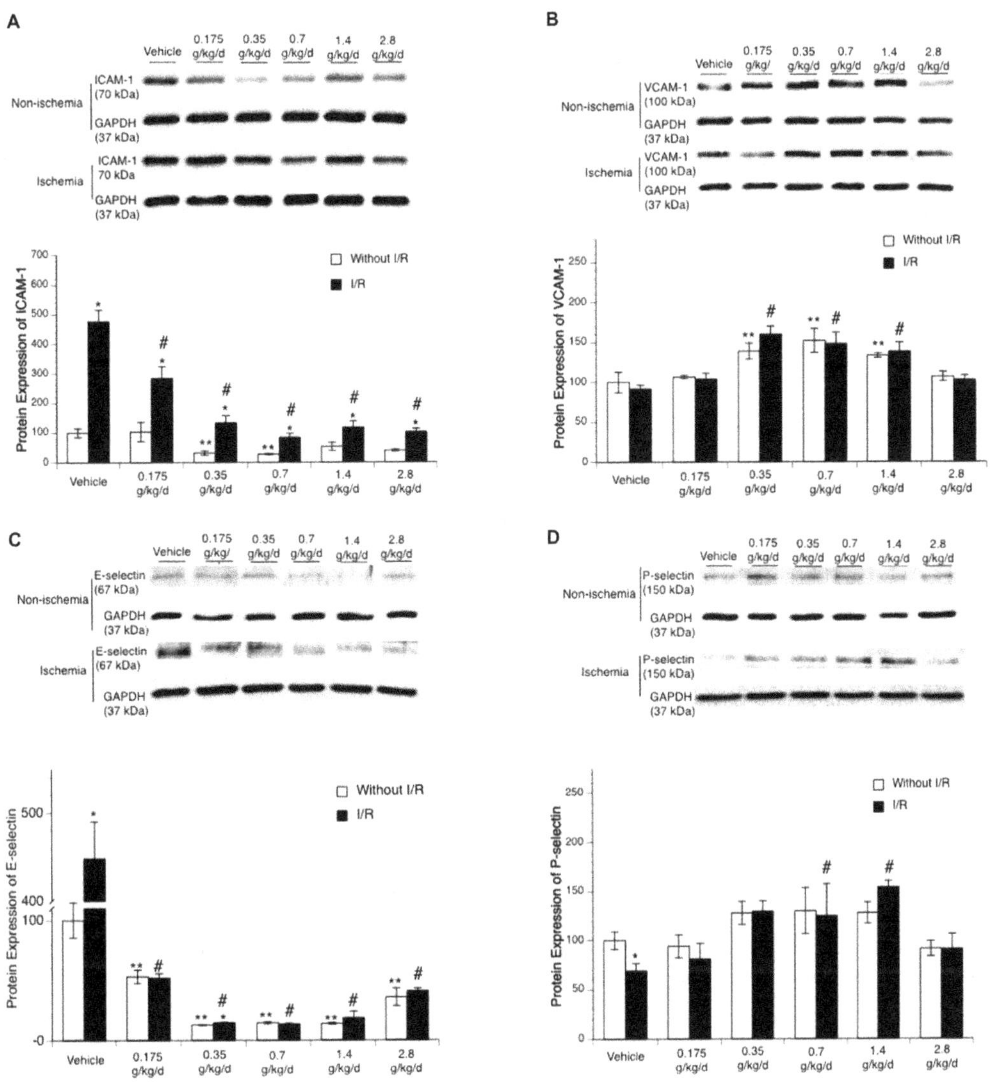

FIGURE 3 | Influence of ethanol on expression of intercellular adhesion molecule-1 (ICAM-1; **A**), vascular cell adhesion molecule-1 (VCAM-1; **B**), E-selectin **(C)** and P-selectin **(D)** following a 90-min MCAO/24-h reperfusion. Values are means ± SE for five mice in each group. Data shown are representative blots for each group. Ischemic side and contralateral side were run on separate gels with two samples from the vehicle group as internal control. **$P < 0.05$ vs. Vehicle without ischemia/reperfusion (I/R). *$P < 0.05$ vs. Without I/R. $^{\#}P < 0.05$ vs. Vehicle with I/R.

2.8 g/kg/day ethanol significantly downregulated baseline E-selectin ($p < 0.00001$, $p < 0.000001$, $p = 0.000163$, $p < 0.000001$, and $p < 0.000001$, respectively; **Figure 3C**). A 90-min MCAO significantly upregulated E-selectin at 24 h of reperfusion in the vehicle group ($F_{(1,8)} = 65.21$; $p = 0.000041$, $n = 5$). There was a significant interaction of ethanol and ischemic stroke on E-selectin expression ($F_{(11,48)} = 62.58$; $p < 0.000001$, $n = 5$). Mice fed with ethanol had significantly less upregulation in E-selectin at 24 h of reperfusion ($F_{(5,24)} = 100.17$; $p < 0.000001$, $n = 5$). *Post hoc* analysis revealed that only 0.35 g/kg/day ethanol significantly upregulated E-selectin at 24 h of reperfusion ($F_{(1,8)} = 10.10$; $p = 0.013023$, $n = 5$; **Figure 3C**). In contrast to ICAM-1 and E-selectin, ethanol upregulated baseline expression of VCAM-1 ($F_{(5,24)} = 23.20$; $p < 0.000001$, $n = 5$). *Post hoc* analysis showed that 0.35, 0.7, and 1.4 g/kg/day ethanol significantly upregulated baseline VCAM-1 ($p = 0.000045$, $p < 0.000001$, and $p = 0.005964$, respectively; **Figure 3B**). Ethanol did not significantly alter baseline expression of P-selectin (**Figure 3D**). In addition, 90-min MCAO did not significantly upregulate either VCAM-1 or P-selectin at 24 h of reperfusion in any group. Interestingly, P-selectin was slightly but significantly downregulated at 24 h of reperfusion in the vehicle group ($F_{(1,8)} = 6.46$; $p = 0.034622$, $n = 5$; **Figure 3D**). Ethanol altered post-ischemic VCAM-1 ($F_{(5,24)} = 11.84$; $p = 0.000008$, $n = 5$) and P-selectin ($F_{(5,24)} = 5.16$; $p = 0.002354$, $n = 5$). *Post hoc* analysis revealed that 0.35, 0.7, and 1.4 g/kg/day ethanol significantly increased post-ischemic VCAM-1 ($p = 0.000171$, $p = 0.000028$, and $p = 0.010020$, respectively; **Figure 3B**). *Post hoc* analysis also revealed that 0.35 and 0.7 g/kg/day ethanol significantly increased post-ischemic P-selectin ($p = 0.001953$ and $p = 0.022819$, respectively; **Figure 3D**). However, there was no significant interaction of ethanol and ischemic stroke on either VCAM-1 ($F_{(11,48)} = 0.40$; $p = 0.846695$, $n = 5$) or P-selectin ($F_{(11,48)} = 0.89$; $p = 0.495995$, $n = 5$).

Microglial Activation

To assess microglial activation, immunofluorescence staining with Iba1 was analyzed. No activated microglia were detected at 24 h of reperfusion in the contralateral hemisphere of ischemic brain. Ethanol altered post-ischemic microglial activation at 24 h of reperfusion in the ipsilateral hemisphere of the ischemic brain as indicated by a significant main effect of gavage feeding ($F_{(5,56)} = 52.23$; $p < 0.000001$, $n = 5$). *Post hoc* analysis showed that 0.175, 0.35, 0.7, and 1.4 g/kg/day ethanol significantly inhibited post-ischemic microglial activation ($p = 0.00004$, $p < 0.000001$, $p < 0.000001$ and $p = 0.000001$, respectively; **Figures 4A,B**). In contrast, 2.8 g/kg/day ethanol significantly promoted post-ischemic microglial activation compared to vehicle ($p = 0.000613$; **Figures 4A,B**).

Neutrophil Infiltration

Immunofluorescence staining with MPO was counted to examine neutrophil infiltration. No neutrophil infiltration was detected at 24 h of reperfusion in the contralateral hemisphere. Ethanol altered post-ischemic neutrophil infiltration at 24 h of reperfusion in the ipsilateral hemisphere of the ischemic

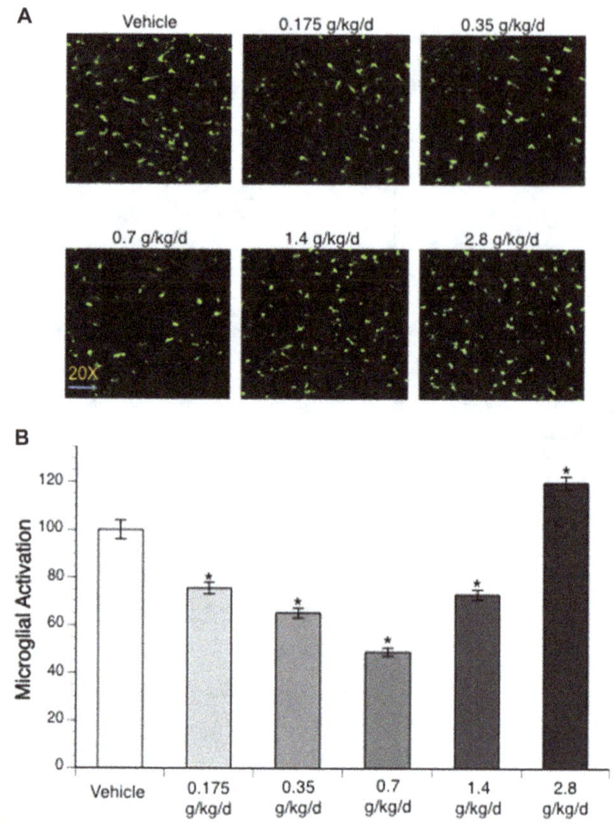

FIGURE 4 | Influence of ethanol on microglial activation following a 90-min MCAO/24-h reperfusion. **(A)** Representative Iba1 staining. **(B)** Values are mean ± SE for five mice in each group. $^*P < 0.05$ vs. Vehicle.

brain as indicated by a significant main effect of gavage feeding ($F_{(5,52)} = 53.92$; $p < 0.000001$, $n = 5$). *Post hoc* analysis revealed that 0.175, 0.35, 0.7, and 1.4 g/kg/day ethanol significantly attenuated post-ischemic neutrophil infiltration ($p = 0.022635$, $p = 0.000818$, $p = 0.000002$ and $p = 0.001079$, respectively; **Figures 5A,B**). On the other hand, 2.8 g/kg/day ethanol significantly exacerbated post-ischemic neutrophil infiltration compared to vehicle ($p < 0.000001$; **Figures 5A,B**).

Cytokines and Chemokines

Since cerebral I/R injury was significantly altered in the 0.7 g/kg/day and 2.8 g/kg/day ethanol groups, cytokines and chemokines were only measured in the vehicle, 0.7 g/kg/day, and 2.8 g/kg/day ethanol groups. Thirty-three cytokines/chemokines were detected using the cytokine array (**Figure 6** and **Table 2**). Ethanol altered 13 baseline pro-inflammatory cytokines/chemokines (IL-1β, IL-3, IL-7, IL-17, IL-23, sICAM, TREM-1, CCL3, CCL12, CXCL2, CXCL9, CXCL10, CXCL11) as indicated by significant main effects of gavage feeding (IL-1β: $F_{(2,9)} = 99.16$; $p < 0.000001$, $n = 4$; IL-3: $F_{(2,9)} = 194.83$; $p < 0.000001$, $n = 4$; IL-7: $F_{(2,9)} = 31.09$; $p = 0.000091$, $n = 4$; IL-17: $F_{(2,9)} = 8.77$; $p = 0.007697$, $n = 4$; IL-23: $F_{(2,9)} = 4.15$; $p = 0.052952$, $n = 4$; sICAM: $F_{(2,9)} = 4.19$; $p = 0.051810$, $n = 4$; TREM-1: $F_{(2,9)} = 4.91$; $p = 0.036217$, $n = 4$; CCL3: $F_{(2,9)} = 20.07$;

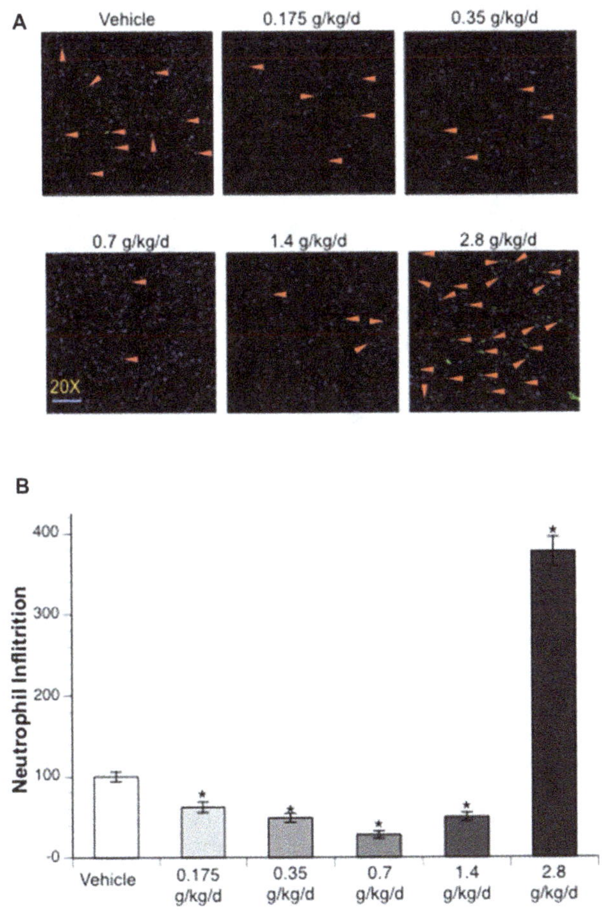

FIGURE 5 | Influence of ethanol on neutrophil infiltration following a 90-min MCAO/24-h reperfusion. **(A)** Representative MPO staining. **(B)** Values are mean ± SE for five mice in each group. *$P < 0.05$ vs. Vehicle.

$p = 0.000481$, $n = 4$; CCL12: $F_{(2,9)} = 15.38$; $p = 0.001249$, $n = 4$; CXCL2: $F_{(2,9)} = 5.37$; $p = 0.029185$, $n = 4$; CXCL9: $F_{(2,9)} = 13.43$; $p = 0.001988$, $n = 4$; CXCL10: $F_{(2,9)} = 4.79$; $p = 0.038350$, $n = 4$; CXCL11: $F_{(2,9)} = 6.41$; $p = 0.018620$, $n = 4$). *Post hoc* analysis revealed that 0.7 g/kg/day ethanol only significantly increased baseline CCL12 ($p = 0.006008$; **Figure 6C**), whereas 2.8 g/kg/day ethanol significantly increased baseline IL-1β ($p < 0.000001$), IL-3 ($p < 0.000001$), IL-7 ($p = 0.000116$), IL-17 ($p = 0.010393$), IL-23 ($p = 0.037578$), sICAM ($p = 0.036577$), TREM-1 ($p = 0.026932$), CCL3 ($p = 0.000472$), CCL12 ($p = 0.000965$), CXCL2 ($p = 0.024882$), CXCL9 ($p = 0.001251$), CXCL10 ($p = 0.038815$), and CXCL11 ($p = 0.013630$) compare to vehicle (**Figure 6** and **Table 2**). On the other hand, ethanol altered all eight detected anti-inflammatory cytokines/chemokines (IL-1ra, IL-4, IL-13, IL-27, G-CSF, M-CSF, TIMP-1, and CXCL13) as indicated by significant main effects of gavage feeding (IL-1ra: $F_{(2,9)} = 21.21$; $p = 0.000393$, $n = 4$; IL-4: $F_{(2,9)} = 4.97$; $p = 0.035154$, $n = 4$; IL-13: $F_{(2,9)} = 14.60$; $p = 0.001494$, $n = 4$; IL-27: $F_{(2,9)} = 43.65$; $p = 0.000023$, $n = 4$; G-CSF: $F_{(2,9)} = 41.27$; $p = 0.000029$, $n = 4$; M-CSF: $F_{(2,9)} = 5.93$; $p = 0.022740$, $n = 4$; TIMP-1: $F_{(2,9)} = 65.65$; $p = 0.000004$, $n = 4$; CXCL13: $F_{(2,9)} = 31.68$; $p = 0.000084$, $n = 4$). *Post hoc* analysis revealed that 0.7 g/kg/day ethanol significantly increased baseline IL-27 ($p = 0.010523$) and TIMP-1 ($p = 0.039746$; **Figure 6C**), whereas 2.8 g/kg/day ethanol significantly increased baseline IL-1ra ($p = 0.000234$), IL-4 ($p = 0.023458$), IL-13 ($p = 0.001525$), IL-27 ($p = 0.000013$), G-CSF ($p = 0.000026$), M-CSF ($p = 0.021383$), TIMP-1 ($p = 0.019979$) and CXCL13 ($p = 0.000056$) compare to vehicle (**Figure 6** and **Table 2**). A 90-min MCAO increased nearly all pro- [IL-1α ($p = 0.004446$), IL-1β ($p = 0.000049$), IL-3 ($p = 0.003363$), IL-6 ($p = 0.000427$), IL-7 ($p = 0.001322$), IL-16 ($p = 0.006295$), IL-17 ($p = 0.002063$), IL-23 ($p = 0.008776$), TNFα ($p = 0.008415$), sICAM ($p = 0.005868$), C5a ($p = 0.002926$), TREM-1 ($p = 0.000090$), IFNγ ($p = 0.015976$), CCL2 ($p < 0.000001$), CCL3 ($p = 0.000165$), CCL4 ($p = 0.000002$), CCL5 ($p = 0.000333$), CCL12 ($p < 0.000001$), CXCL1 ($p < 0.000001$), CXCL2 ($p = 0.000002$), CXCL9 ($p = 0.001983$), CXCL10 ($p = 0.003656$), CXCL11 ($p = 0.017108$), CXCL12 ($p = 0.003795$), and CXCL13 ($p = 0.004357$)] and anti-(IL-1ra ($p = 0.000022$), IL-4 ($p = 0.006545$), IL-13 ($p = 0.006153$), IL-27 ($p < 0.000001$), G-CSF ($p = 0.000538$), M-CSF ($p = 0.004005$), TIMP-1 ($p < 0.000001$) and CXCL13 ($p = 0.000056$) inflammatory cytokines/chemokines at 24 h of reperfusion in the vehicle group. The number of upregulated pro- and anti-inflammatory cytokines/chemokines at 24 h of reperfusion was less in two ethanol groups. Twelve pro-[IL-1β ($p = 0.000325$), IL-3 ($p = 0.016041$), IL-6 ($p = 0.012197$), IL-16 ($p = 0.022580$), IL-17 ($p = 0.042719$), C5a ($p = 0.010869$), TREM-1 ($p = 0.003024$), CCL2 ($p = 0.000093$), CCL3 ($p = 0.000472$), CCL12 ($p < 0.000001$), CXCL1 ($p = 0.000006$), and CXCL2 ($p = 0.001563$)] and four anti-[IL-1ra ($p = 0.000008$), IL-27 ($p = 0.000154$), G-CSF ($p = 0.008262$), and TIMP-1 ($p = 0.000185$)] inflammatory cytokines/chemokines were increased in the 0.7 g/kg/day ethanol group. Only ten pro- [IL-1β ($p = 0.003581$), IL-3 ($p = 0.009448$), IL-6 ($p = 0.005024$), TREM-1 ($p = 0.008930$), CCL2 ($p = 0.000002$), CCL3 ($p = 0.040100$), CCL4 ($p = 0.002640$), CCL12 ($p < 0.000001$), CXCL1 ($p = 0.000001$), and CXCL2 ($p = 0.000067$)] and three anti-[IL-1ra ($p = 0.013861$), IL-27 ($p = 0.02689$), and TIMP-1 ($p = 0.000008$)] inflammatory cytokines/chemokines were increased in the 2.8 g/kg/day ethanol group (**Figure 6** and **Table 2**). There were significant interactions of ethanol and ischemic stroke on IL-1β ($F_{(5,18)} = 25.71$; $p = 0.000005$, $n = 4$), IL-3 ($F_{(5,18)} = 6.00$; $p = 0.010051$, $n = 4$), CCL12 ($F_{(5,18)} = 30.40$; $p = 0.000002$, $n = 4$), IL-1a ($F_{(5,18)} = 5.86$; $p = 0.010941$, $n = 4$). *Post hoc* analysis revealed that 0.7 g/kg/day ethanol significantly reduced post-ischemic IL-1β ($p = 0.020488$) and increased IL-1ra ($p = 0.047886$) at 24 h of reperfusion. *Post hoc* analysis also revealed that 2.8 g/kg/day ethanol significantly increased post-ischemic IL-3 ($p = 0.006474$), IL-23 ($p = 0.034201$), and CCL12 ($p = 0.000689$) at 24 h of reperfusion (**Figure 6** and **Table 2**).

BBB Breakdown

Again, since cerebral I/R injury was significantly altered in the 0.7 g/kg/day and 2.8 g/kg/day ethanol groups, BBB breakdown-related measurements were only conducted in the vehicle, 0.7 g/kg/day, and 2.8 g/kg/day ethanol groups. No IgG leakage

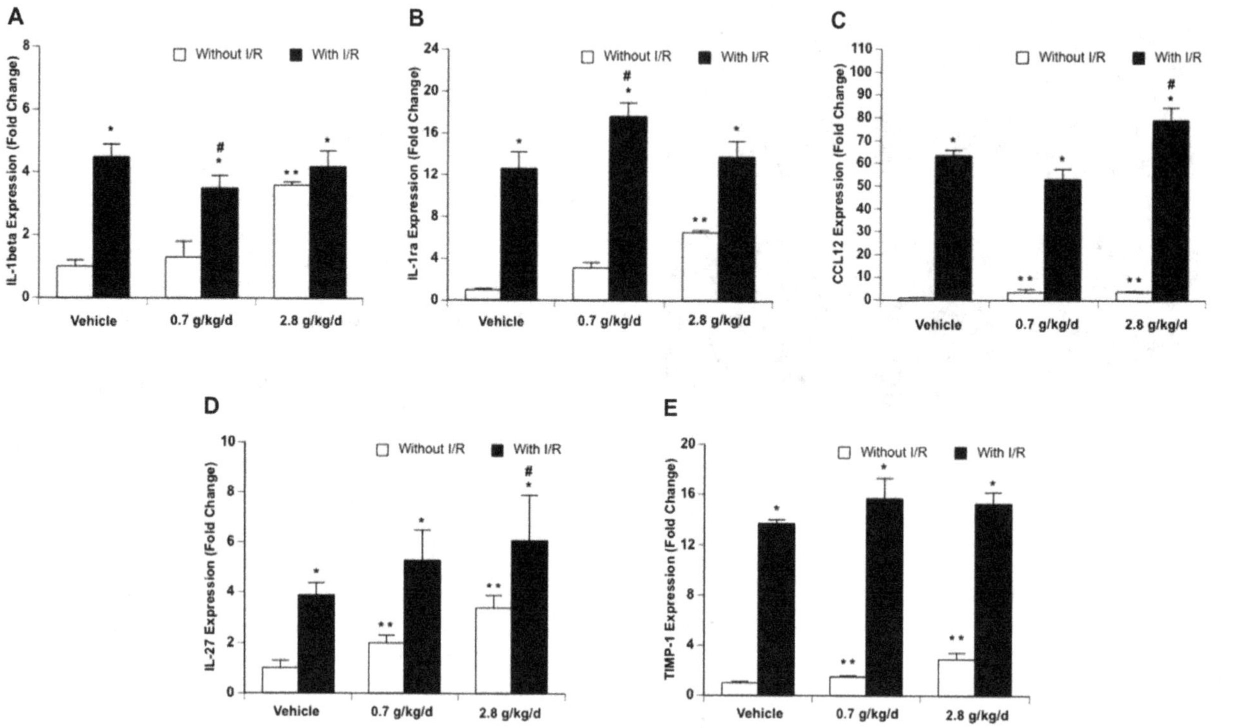

FIGURE 6 | Influence of ethanol on expression of interleukin-1β (IL-1β; **A**), IL-1ra **(B)**, CCL-12 **(C)**, IL-27 **(D)** and TIMP-1 **(E)** following a 90-min MCAO/24-h reperfusion. Values are means ± SE for four mice in each group. $^{**}P < 0.05$ vs. Vehicle without I/R. $^{*}P < 0.05$ vs. Without I/R. $^{\#}P < 0.05$ vs. Vehicle with I/R.

TABLE 2 | Effect of ethanol consumption on cytokines and chemokines in the cerebrum before and following a 90-min middle cerebral artery occlusion (MCAO)/24-h reperfusion.

Cytokines/Chemokines	Vehicle	0.7 g/kg/day	2.8 g/kg/day	Vehicle + I/R	0.7 g/kg/day + I/R	2.8 g/kg/day + I/R
IL-1α	1.0 ± 0.1	1.0 ± 0.2	1.1 ± 0.3	1.8 ± 0.2*	1.6 ± 0.3	1.4 ± 0.5
IL-2	1.0 ± 0.2	2.1 ± 0.5	2.3 ± 0.4	1.2 ± 0.1	1.8 ± 1.2	4.1 ± 2.0
IL-3	1.0 ± 0.2	1.1 ± 0.2	5.1 ± 0.2**	6.0 ± 1.1*	4.0 ± 0.9*	17.8 ± 3.4*#
IL-4	1.0 ± 0.3	2.4 ± 1.1	4.5 ± 1.0**	3.2 ± 0.5*	2.6 ± 0.9	9.8 ± 2.6#
IL-6	ND	ND	ND	1.0 ± 0.1*	1.2 ± 0.3*	0.4 ± 0.1*
IL-7	1.0 ± 0.1	1.2 ± 0.4	3.5 ± 0.2**	2.9 ± 0.3*	2.6 ± 0.7	3.4 ± 0.5
IL-13	1.0 ± 0.1	1.2 ± 0.1	2.5 ± 0.4**	2.0 ± 0.2*	1.7 ± 0.3	1.5 ± 0.8
IL-16	1.0 ± 0.1	1.1 ± 0.2	1.1 ± 0.3	1.8 ± 0.2*	2.1 ± 0.3*	0.8 ± 0.5
IL-17	1.0 ± 0.3	1.0 ± 0.5	3.4 ± 0.5**	2.8 ± 0.2*	2.8 ± 0.4*	2.1 ± 0.5
IL-23	1.0 ± 0.2	2.4 ± 1.1	4.5 ± 1.0**	3.2 ± 0.5*	2.6 ± 0.9	9.8 ± 2.6#
TNFα	1.0 ± 0.6	2.4 ± 1.6	4.7 ± 0.5	12.2 ± 2.8*	16.9 ± 6.9	11.4 ± 6.9
G-CSF	1.0 ± 0.4	1.6 ± 0.4	4.6 ± 0.1**	4.9 ± 0.5*	6.3 ± 1.2*	4.7 ± 1.8
M-CSF	1.0 ± 0.2	1.2 ± 0.3	2.4 ± 0.4**	2.2 ± 0.2*	3.5 ± 1.5	4.5 ± 1.0
sICAM	1.0 ± 0.0	1.3 ± 0.2	1.5 ± 0.2**	1.2 ± 0.1*	1.3 ± 0.1	1.5 ± 0.1
C5a	1.0 ± 0.2	1.5 ± 0.2	1.4 ± 0.4	4.0 ± 0.6*	4.0 ± 0.7*	3.2 ± 0.9
TREM-1	1.0 ± 0.1	1.8 ± 1.1	3.6 ± 0.1**	12.3 ± 1.2*	10.4 ± 1.5*	14.2 ± 2.8*
IFN-γ	1.0 ± 0.2	0.9 ± 0.2	1.5 ± 0.3	2.7 ± 0.4*	2.6 ± 0.9	3.0 ± 1.0
CCL2	1.0 ± 0.1	0.8 ± 0.5	1.5 ± 0.1	8.8 ± 0.1*	8.9 ± 0.7*	7.9 ± 0.3*
CCL3	1.0 ± 0.4	1.9 ± 1.1	6.7 ± 0.2**	8.6 ± 0.8*	9.2 ± 1.0*	10.5 ± 1.5*
CCL4	ND	ND	ND	1.2 ± 0.1*	1.5 ± 0.6	1.4 ± 0.3*
CCL5	1.0 ± 0.4	2.7 ± 1.1	3.8 ± 0.4	6.8 ± 0.7*	5.1 ± 1.8	5.5 ± 1.3
CXCL1	1.0 ± 0.3	0.8 ± 0.2	1.1 ± 0.3	15.8 ± 0.3*	16.1 ± 1.0*	14.1 ± 0.6*
CXCL2	1.0 ± 0.1	1.4 ± 0.1	3.0 ± 0.8**	18.7 ± 1.0*	19.0 ± 3.2*	19.0 ± 1.4*
CXCL9	1.0 ± 0.2	1.6 ± 0.4	2.7 ± 0.1**	3.4 ± 0.4*	3.4 ± 0.9	2.7 ± 0.9
CXCL10	1.0 ± 0.5	4.7 ± 1.1	5.2 ± 1.4**	3.9 ± 0.3*	3.1 ± 1.0	3.4 ± 1.2
CXCL11	1.0 ± 0.1	2.0 ± 0.8	4.4 ± 0.9**	3.1 ± 0.6*	2.5 ± 0.9	2.6 ± 1.9
CXCL12	1.0 ± 0.1	2.2 ± 0.8	2.6 ± 0.5	1.4 ± 0.1*	1.4 ± 0.3	1.5 ± 0.3
CXCL13	1.0 ± 0.3	3.0 ± 0.3	7.5 ± 0.9**	2.5 ± 0.2*	3.2 ± 1.4	6.4 ± 1.0#

Values are means ± SE for four mice in each group. ND stands for Not Detectable. $^{**}P < 0.05$ *vs. Vehicle.* $^{*}P < 0.05$ *vs. Without ischemia/reperfusion (I/R).* $^{\#}P < 0.05$ *vs. Vehicle + I/R.*

was detected at 24 h of reperfusion in the contralateral hemisphere. Ethanol altered post-ischemic IgG leakage at 24 h of reperfusion in the ipsilateral hemisphere of the ischemic brain as indicated by a significant main effect of gavage feeding ($F_{(2,12)}$ = 16.43; p = 0.000366, n = 5). *Post hoc* analysis showed that 0.7 g/kg/day ethanol reduced post-ischemic IgG leakage compared to vehicle (p = 0.015192; **Figure 7B**). In contrast, 2.8 g/kg/day ethanol worsened post-ischemic IgG leakage compared to vehicle (p = 0.044803; **Figures 7A,B**). Ethanol also altered post-ischemic brain edema in the ipsilateral hemisphere of the ischemic brain as indicated by a significant main effect of gavage feeding ($F_{(2,15)}$ = 15.45; p = 0.000229, n = 5). *Post hoc* analysis revealed that 0.7 g/kg/day ethanol significantly alleviated post-ischemic brain edema (p = 0.036270), whereas 2.8 g/kg/day significantly worsened the post-ischemic brain edema (p = 0.018484; **Figure 7C**). Ethanol altered baseline MMP-9 activity as indicated by a significant main effect of gavage feeding ($F_{(2,12)}$ = 6.26; p = 0.013741, n = 5). *Post hoc* analysis showed that 0.7 g/kg/day ethanol significantly reduced baseline MMP-9 activity (p = 0.010701; **Figures 7D,E**). A 90-min MCAO significantly increased MMP-9 activity at 24 h of reperfusion in all three groups (Vehicle group: $F_{(1,8)}$ = 81.90; p = 0.000018, n = 5; 0.7 g/kg/day group: $F_{(1,8)}$ = 20.84; p = 0.001837, n = 5; 2.8 g/kg/day group: $F_{(1,8)}$ = 7.15; p = 0.028171, n = 5; **Figures 7D,E**). There was no significant interaction of ethanol and ischemic stroke on MMP-9 activity at 24 h of reperfusion ($F_{(5,24)}$ = 3.14; p = 0.061657, n = 5). In addition, ethanol did not significantly alter MMP-9 activity at 24 h of reperfusion ($F_{(2,12)}$ = 3.14; p < 0.079986, n = 5; **Figures 7D,E**). In contrast to MMP-9, MMP-2 activity was not altered by ethanol and at 24 h of reperfusion (data not shown).

DISCUSSION

The present study investigated the influence of chronic consumption of low to high doses of ethanol on basal and post-ischemic inflammatory profiles in the brain. There are several new findings from this study. First, 0.35–0.7 g/kg/day ethanol tends to reduce baseline expression of ICAM-1 and E-selectin, but increase baseline expression of VCAM-1. Second, post-ischemic upregulation of ICAM-1 and E-selectin were attenuated in all ethanol groups. Third, low to moderate ethanol alleviated but high-dose ethanol aggravated post-ischemic microglial activation and neutrophil infiltration. Fourth, ethanol tended to dose-dependently increase both pro- and anti-inflammatory cytokines/chemokines at basal conditions. Fifth, low-dose ethanol reduced post-ischemic pro-inflammatory cytokines/chemokines and enhanced post-ischemic anti-inflammatory cytokines/chemokines. Sixth, low-dose ethanol reduced but high-dose ethanol worsened post-ischemic BBB breakdown. Thus, ethanol may affect both basal and post-ischemic inflammatory profiles of the brain in a dose-dependent manner. Low-dose ethanol tends to induce an anti-inflammatory effect, whereas high-dose ethanol produces an inflammatory effect.

Although numerous experimental studies have investigated the effect of ethanol consumption on cardiovascular diseases, there have only been a limited amount of studies investigating the effect of ethanol consumption on ischemic brain damage.

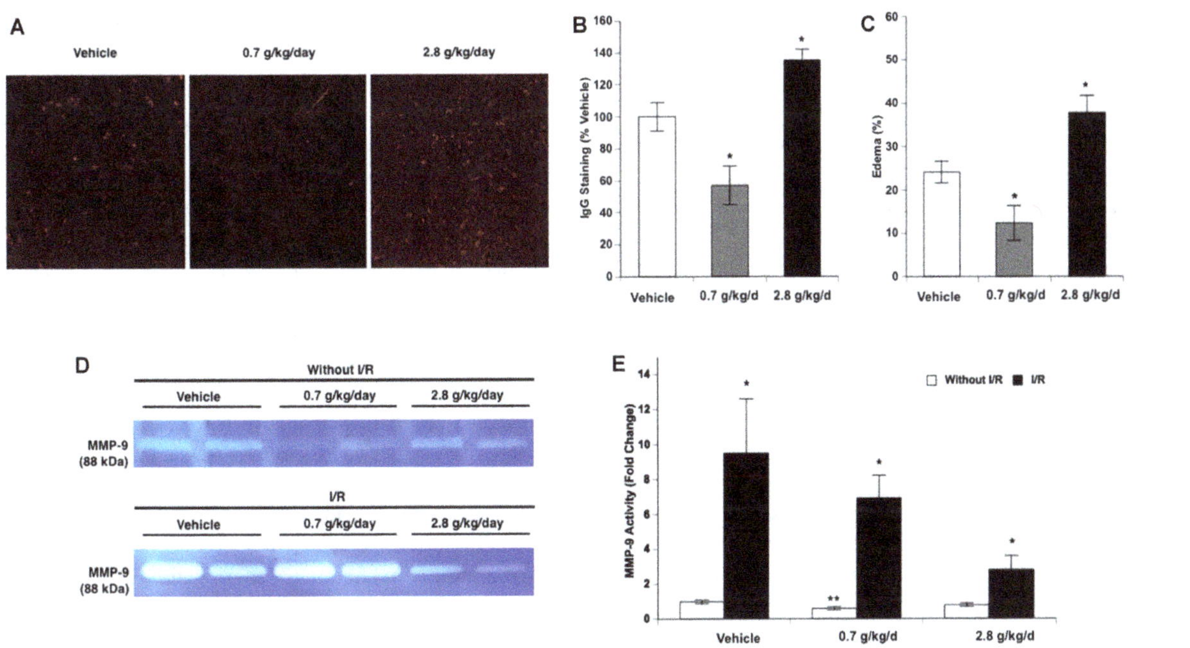

FIGURE 7 | Influence of ethanol on blood-brain barrier (BBB) permeability following a 90-min MCAO/24-h reperfusion. **(A)** Representative IgG staining. **(B)** Values are means ± SE for five mice in each group. **(C)** Values are means ± SE for six mice in each group. **(D)** Representative gelatin zymography. **(E)** Values are means ± SE for five mice in each group. *P < 0.05 vs. Vehicle. **P < 0.05 vs. Vehicle without I/R. #P < 0.05 vs. Without I/R.

In an early study, Mandybur and Mendenhall (1983) found that chronic alcoholism significantly contributes to the risk of mortality associated with ischemic brain infarction in gerbils. Later, Favalli et al. (2002) found that chronic ethanol consumption leads to an increased excitotoxicity and ischemic brain damage during early withdrawal in rats. Recently, Oliveira et al. (2014) found that heavy ethanol consumption exacerbates post-ischemic motor impairment and cortical neuronal loss in female adolescent rats. Our previous studies have shown that 2-month feeding with a liquid diet containing high-dose ethanol (6.4% v/v) worsened post-ischemic brain damage in rats (Sun et al., 2008; Zhao et al., 2010), whereas the diet containing low-dose ethanol (1% v/v) protected the brain against its I/R injury in both rats and mice (Zhao et al., 2011; Sun et al., 2012). To mimic the drinking pattern of humans, different doses of ethanol were given once a day *via* oral gavage feeding in the present study. We found that 0.7 g/kg/day ethanol significantly protected against brain I/R injury and 2.8 g/kg/day ethanol significantly exacerbated brain I/R injury. The peak blood ethanol concentration of the dose associated with a neuroprotective effect was 9.0 mM, which usually can be seen in a man with average body weight (70 kg or 154 Ibs) after ingestion of one and a half American standard drinks (14 grams of ethanol/each; Fisher et al., 1987). On the other hand, the peak blood ethanol concentration of the dose associated with a detrimental effect was 37.0 mM, which usually can be seen in a man with average body weight after ingestion of slightly more than seven American standard drinks. Therefore, the results of the present study complement and extend that which we have reported previously.

As far as we are aware, the present study is the first to systematically investigate the influence of chronic consumption of low to high doses of ethanol on early post-ischemic inflammation in the brain. We found that transient focal cerebral ischemia increased the expression of ICAM-1 and E-selectin, but not VCAM-1 and P-selectin at 24 h of reperfusion. Interestingly, the magnitude of the increase in ICAM-1 and E-selectin was significantly less in all ethanol groups when compared to the vehicle. The selectins facilitate the diapedesis of leukocytes on the endothelial surface while the immunoglobulin superfamily mediates the firm adhesion and transendothelial migration of leukocytes (Langer and Chavakis, 2009). Animals deficient in ICAM-1 or treated with strategies that block ICAM-1 have decreased ischemic damage and less brain neutrophil infiltration (Kitagawa et al., 1998). In addition, E-selectin inhibition is associated with improved neurological outcome (Huang et al., 2000). Of the various types of leukocytes, neutrophils are among the first to infiltrate the ischemic brain (Gronberg et al., 2013). Neutrophils may worsen brain I/R injury by obstructing capillaries resulting in reduced blood flow during reperfusion as well as by releasing cytotoxic products. Numerous studies have shown that inhibition of neutrophil infiltration is associated with a decrease in brain I/R injury (Egashira et al., 2013; Herz et al., 2015). In the present study, neutrophil infiltration was significantly inhibited in the 0.175–1.4 g/kg/day ethanol groups. The maximum inhibition was observed in the 0.7 g/kg/day ethanol group, in which the brain I/R injury was significantly reduced. Therefore, the neuroprotective effect of low-dose ethanol may be related to a reduction in expression of adhesion molecules and subsequent neutrophil infiltration.

Microglia are resident immune cells of the brain and are important modulators of homeostasis and immune response in the brain (Ziebell et al., 2015). Upon stimulation, microglia become activated and undergo several key morphological changes characterized by an amoeboid shape with little to no extending processes (Ziebell et al., 2015). Activated microglia may contribute to brain I/R injury *via* phagocytosis and elaboration of neuroinflammatory mediators toxic to cells (Ceulemans et al., 2010). In the present study, although post-ischemic microglia activation was significantly attenuated in the 0.175–1.4 g/kg/day ethanol groups, the maximum reduction occurred in the 0.7 g/kg/day ethanol group. Therefore, the neuroprotective effect of low-dose ethanol may be linked to a reduction in microglial activation.

Following transient focal cerebral ischemia, cytokines/chemokines are elaborated from injured neurons, infiltrated leukocytes, activated astrocytes, microglia, and endothelial cells (Kim et al., 2014). Pro-inflammatory cytokines, such as IL-1β, TNFα, and IL-6, contribute to brain I/R injury by stimulating pro-apoptotic signaling and cytotoxic proteins, activating microglia, and increasing the expression of adhesion molecules (Doll et al., 2014). In contrast, anti-inflammatory cytokines, such as IL-1ra, IL-4, and IL-10, inhibit post-ischemic inflammation by inhibiting pro-inflammatory cytokines and suppressing cytokine receptor expression and downstream signaling (Kim et al., 2014). Chemokines play a crucial role in the infiltration of leukocytes under inflammatory conditions (Kim et al., 2014). In the present study, one pro-inflammatory mediator, IL-1β, was less and one anti-inflammatory cytokine, IL-1ra, was greater in the 0.7 g/kg/day ethanol group compared to the vehicle group. IL-1 is a strong neurotoxic mediator and has two isoforms, IL-1α and IL-1β. However, IL-1β rather than IL-1α is considered to be more engaged in ischemic brain damage (Boutin et al., 2001). IL-1ra is an endogenous inhibitor of IL-1. Overexpression of IL-1ra as well as treatment with IL-1ra led to reduced ischemic brain damage (Mulcahy et al., 2003). Thus, it is conceivable that the neuroprotective effect of low-dose ethanol may also be related to an altered post-ischemic expression of cytokines/chemokines.

In the present study, post-ischemic inflammatory response produced conflicting results in the 2.8 g/kg/day ethanol group where the cerebral I/R injury was significantly exacerbated. Surprisingly, although neutrophil infiltration and microglial activation were increased, post-ischemic upregulation in adhesion molecules was reduced. Furthermore, both pro-inflammatory and anti-inflammatory cytokines/chemokines were increased after ischemic stroke. In addition to adhesion molecules, pro-inflammatory cytokines/chemokines and BBB breakdown can also influence the infiltration of neutrophils (Kim et al., 2014). In the present study, post-ischemic increase in three pro-inflammatory (IL-3, IL-23, and CCL12) was significant greater in the 2.8 g/kg/day ethanol group. Unfortunately, no studies that we are aware of have attempted to relate alterations of IL-3 and CCL12 to neutrophil infiltration following ischemic stroke. CCL12 is a potent monocyte chemokine homologous to human CCL2 (Sarafi et al., 1997). Although the role of CCL12 in ischemic brain damage has not been elucidated, overexpression of CCL2 worsens ischemic brain damage (Chen et al., 2003). A recent study report that IL-23 can aggravate neuron damage and further impair the integrity of BBB (Wang et al., 2015). In the present study, post-ischemic BBB breakdown was significantly worsened in the 2.8 g/kg/day ethanol group. On the other hand, reactive oxygen species (ROS) and extracellular ATP from dying cells have been demonstrated to promote post-ischemic microglial activation (Doll et al., 2014). We previously have found that heavy ethanol consumption exacerbates brain I/R injury by increasing NMDA-mediated excitotoxicity and NAD(P)H oxidase-mediated oxidative stress (Zhao et al., 2010, 2011). Thus, the increased neutrophil infiltration and microglia activation may be resulted from exacerbated cell death and BBB breakdown. Post-ischemic inflammation begins immediately after arterial occlusion and contributes to potential enlargement of the infarct size. In the present study, although we were not able to directly establish the correlation between post-ischemic inflammatory response and infarct volume, we evaluated the inflammatory response in the peri-infarct area at 24 h of reperfusion. Recent studies found that the healing type of activated microglia was predominated in the ischemic core while the pre-inflammatory type of activated microglia was predominated in the peri-infarct area (Denes et al., 2007; Villarreal et al., 2016). The spatial distribution of the microglia phenotypes suggests that the peri-infarct area at early stage may represent the enlargement of injured and damaged brain tissue over time.

In the present study, ethanol did not alter baseline P-selectin, but upregulated baseline VCAM-1 and downregulated baseline ICAM-1 and E-selectin at low-moderate doses. All these adhesion molecules have been extensively linked to atherosclerosis (Galkina and Ley, 2007). Thus, the net effect of low-dose ethanol on these adhesion molecules cannot be estimated. However, it has been reported that combined deficiency of E-selectin and P-selectin could produce the strongest inhibitory effects on atherosclerosis (Galkina and Ley, 2007). In the present study, although low-dose ethanol slightly increased baseline CCL-12, it significantly activated anti-inflammatory mediators, IL-27 and TIMP-1. In addition, low-dose ethanol reduced baseline activity of MMP-9. IL-27 has been previously shown to inhibit atherosclerosis (Hirase et al., 2013). MMP-9 not only contributes to atherosclerotic plaque progression but also associates with cap rupture (Vacek et al., 2015). TIMP-1 is a tissue inhibitor of metalloproteinases. Thus, low-dose ethanol consumption may induce an anti-inflammatory property rather than an inflammatory effect under basal conditions. The relationship between regular ethanol intake and incidence of atherosclerosis appears to be U-shaped (Kiechl et al., 1998). It is possible that the beneficial effect of low-dose ethanol against atherosclerosis as well as subsequent ischemic stroke is related to its anti-inflammatory propensity. In contrast to low-dose ethanol, while high-dose ethanol also activated the anti-inflammatory system, it increased most detected pro-inflammatory cytokines/chemokines, suggesting a propensity towards vascular inflammation.

CONCLUSION

The present study is the first to systematically evaluate the influence of chronic ethanol consumption on the inflammatory profile in the brain under basal conditions and after transient focal cerebral ischemia. We found that the inflammatory profile during low-moderate ethanol consumption tends to prevent ischemic stroke and reduce brain I/R injury. On the other hand, inflammation may contribute to the increased ischemic stroke and exacerbated brain I/R injury during heavy ethanol consumption. Therefore, anti-inflammatory therapeutic strategies may be able to significantly improve prognosis of ischemic stroke in heavy alcohol users but not in low-moderate alcohol users.

AUTHOR CONTRIBUTIONS

HS and WM conceived the experiments. GX, CL, AP, JL, KM and HS conducted the experiments. GX, CL, RS (Biostatistician), and HS analyzed the results. All authors reviewed the manuscript.

FUNDING

This study was supported by a National Institutes of Health Grant (AA023610) and funds from Louisiana State University Health Sciences Center-Shreveport to HS and WM, a postdoctoral fellowship to CL and a predoctoral fellowship to KM from the Center for Cardiovascular Diseases and Sciences, Louisiana State University Health Science Center-Shreveport.

REFERENCES

Ahmad, S., Elsherbiny, N. M., Haque, R., Khan, M. B., Ishrat, T., Shah, Z. A., et al. (2014). Sesamin attenuates neurotoxicity in mouse model of ischemic brain stroke. *Neurotoxicology* 45, 100–110. doi: 10.1016/j.neuro.2014.10.002

Benjamin, E. J., Blaha, M. J., Chiuve, S. E., Cushman, M., Das, S. R., Deo, R., et al. (2017). Heart disease and stroke statistics-2017 update: a report from the american heart association. *Circulation* 135, e146–e603. doi: 10.1161/CIR.0000000000000485

Bonnans, C., Chou, J., and Werb, Z. (2014). Remodelling the extracellular matrix in development and disease. *Nat. Rev. Mol. Cell Biol.* 15, 786–801. doi: 10.1038/nrm3904

Boutin, H., LeFeuvre, R. A., Horai, R., Asano, M., Iwakura, Y., and Rothwell, N. J. (2001). Role of IL-1α and IL-1β in ischemic brain damage. *J. Neurosci.* 21, 5528–5534. doi: 10.1523/JNEUROSCI.21-15-05528.2001

Bruno, A., Kent, T. A., Coull, B. M., Shankar, R. R., Saha, C., Becker, K. J., et al. (2008). Treatment of hyperglycemia in ischemic stroke (THIS): a randomized pilot trial. *Stroke* 39, 384–389. doi: 10.1161/strokeaha.107.493544

Ceulemans, A. G., Zgavc, T., Kooijman, R., Hachimi-Idrissi, S., Sarre, S., and Michotte, Y. (2010). The dual role of the neuroinflammatory response after ischemic stroke: modulatory effects of hypothermia. *J. Neuroinflammation* 7:74. doi: 10.1186/1742-2094-7-74

Chen, Y., Hallenbeck, J. M., Ruetzler, C., Bol, D., Thomas, K., Berman, N. E., et al. (2003). Overexpression of monocyte chemoattractant protein 1 in the brain exacerbates ischemic brain injury and is associated with recruitment of inflammatory cells. *J. Cereb. Blood Flow Metab.* 23, 748–755. doi: 10.1097/01.wcb.0000071885.63724.20

Chen, W., Sun, Y., Liu, K., and Sun, X. (2014). Autophagy: a double-edged sword for neuronal survival after cerebral ischemia. *Neural Regen. Res.* 9, 1210–1216. doi: 10.4103/1673-5374.135329

Choi, D. H., Kim, J. H., Lee, K. H., Kim, H. Y., Kim, Y. S., Choi, W. S., et al. (2015). Role of neuronal NADPH oxidase 1 in the peri-infarct regions after stroke. *PLoS One* 10:e0116814. doi: 10.1371/journal.pone.0116814

Denes, A., Vidyasagar, R., Feng, J., Narvainen, J., McColl, B. W., Kauppinen, R. A., et al. (2007). Proliferating resident microglia after focal cerebral ischaemia in mice. *J. Cereb. Blood Flow Metab.* 27, 1941–1953. doi: 10.1038/sj.jcbfm.9600495

Doll, D. N., Barr, T. L., and Simpkins, J. W. (2014). Cytokines: their role in stroke and potential use as biomarkers and therapeutic targets. *Aging Dis.* 5, 294–306. doi: 10.14336/ad.2014.0500294

Ducroquet, A., Leys, D., Al Saabi, A., Richard, F., Cordonnier, C., Girot, M., et al. (2013). Influence of chronic ethanol consumption on the neurological severity in patients with acute cerebral ischemia. *Stroke* 44, 2324–2326. doi: 10.1161/STROKEAHA.113.001355

Egashira, Y., Suzuki, Y., Azuma, Y., Takagi, T., Mishiro, K., Sugitani, S., et al. (2013). The growth factor progranulin attenuates neuronal injury induced by cerebral ischemia-reperfusion through the suppression of neutrophil recruitment. *J. Neuroinflammation* 10:105. doi: 10.1186/1742-2094-10-105

Favalli, L., Rozza, A., Frattini, P., Masoero, E., Scelsi, R., Pascale, A., et al. (2002). Ischemia-induced glutamate release in rat frontoparietal cortex after chronic alcohol and withdrawal. *Neurosci. Lett.* 326, 183–186. doi: 10.1016/s0304-3940(02)00352-x

Favate, A. S., and Younger, D. S. (2016). Epidemiology of ischemic stroke. *Neurol. Clin.* 34, 967–980. doi: 10.1016/j.ncl.2016.06.013

Fisher, H. R., Simpson, R. I., and Kapur, B. M. (1987). Calculation of blood alcohol concentration (BAC) by sex, weight, number of drinks and time. *Can. J. Public Health* 78, 300–304.

Galkina, E., and Ley, K. (2007). Vascular adhesion molecules in atherosclerosis. *Arterioscler. Thromb. Vasc. Biol.* 27, 2292–2301. doi: 10.1161/atvbaha.107.149179

Gronberg, N. V., Johansen, F. F., Kristiansen, U., and Hasseldam, H. (2013). Leukocyte infiltration in experimental stroke. *J. Neuroinflammation* 10:115. doi: 10.1186/1742-2094-10-115

Hansagi, H., Romelsjö, A., Gerhardsson de Verdier, M., Andréasson, S., and Leifman, A. (1995). Alcohol consumption and stroke mortality. *Stroke* 26, 1768–1773. doi: 10.1161/01.STR.26.10.1768

Herz, J., Sabellek, P., Lane, T. E., Gunzer, M., Hermann, D. M., and Doeppner, T. R. (2015). Role of neutrophils in exacerbation of brain injury after focal cerebral ischemia in hyperlipidemic mice. *Stroke* 46, 2916–2925. doi: 10.1161/strokeaha.115.010620

Hirase, T., Hara, H., Miyazaki, Y., Ide, N., Nishimoto-Hazuku, A., Fujimoto, H., et al. (2013). Interleukin 27 inhibits atherosclerosis *via* immunoregulation of macrophages in mice. *Am. J. Physiol. Heart Circ. Physiol.* 305, H420–H429. doi: 10.1152/ajpheart.00198.2013

Huang, J., Choudhri, T. F., Winfree, C. J., McTaggart, R. A., Kiss, S., Mocco, J., et al. (2000). Postischemic cerebrovascular E-selectin expression mediates tissue injury in murine stroke. *Stroke* 31, 3047–3053. doi: 10.1161/01.str.31.12.3047

Ikehara, S., Iso, H., Toyoshima, H., Date, C., Yamamoto, A., Kikuchi, S., et al. (2008). Alcohol consumption and mortality from stroke and coronary heart disease among Japanese men and women: the Japan collaborative cohort study. *Stroke* 39, 2936–2942. doi: 10.1161/strokeaha.108.520288

Jean, W. C., Spellman, S. R., Nussbaum, E. S., and Low, W. C. (1998). Reperfusion injury after focal cerebral ischemia: the role of inflammation and the therapeutic horizon. *Neurosurgery* 43, 1382–1396; discussion 1396–1387. doi: 10.1227/00006123-199812000-00077

Kalogeris, T., Baines, C. P., Krenz, M., and Korthuis, R. J. (2012). Cell biology of ischemia/reperfusion injury. *Int. Rev. Cell Mol. Biol.* 298, 229–317. doi: 10.1016/B978-0-12-394309-5.00006-7

Kiechl, S., Willeit, J., Rungger, G., Egger, G., Oberhollenzer, F., and Bonora, E. (1998). Alcohol consumption and atherosclerosis: what is the relation? Prospective results from the Bruneck Study. *Stroke* 29, 900–907. doi: 10.1161/01.str.29.5.900

Kim, J. Y., Kawabori, M., and Yenari, M. A. (2014). Innate inflammatory responses in stroke: mechanisms and potential therapeutic targets. *Curr. Med. Chem.* 21, 2076–2097. doi: 10.2174/0929867321666131228205146

Kitagawa, K., Matsumoto, M., Mabuchi, T., Yagita, Y., Ohtsuki, T., Hori, M., et al. (1998). Deficiency of intercellular adhesion molecule 1 attenuates microcirculatory disturbance and infarction size in focal cerebral ischemia. *J. Cereb. Blood Flow Metab.* 18, 1336–1345. doi: 10.1097/00004647-199812000-00008

Lakhan, S. E., Kirchgessner, A., and Hofer, M. (2009). Inflammatory mechanisms in ischemic stroke: therapeutic approaches. *J. Trans. Med.* 7:97. doi: 10.1186/1479-5876-7-97

Langer, H. F., and Chavakis, T. (2009). Leukocyte-endothelial interactions in inflammation. *J. Cell. Mol. Med.* 13, 1211–1220. doi: 10.1111/j.1582-4934.2009.00811.x

Mandybur, T. I., and Mendenhall, C. L. (1983). The effects of chronic alcoholism on development of ischemic cerebral infarcts following unilateral carotid artery ligation in gerbils. *Alcohol. Clin. Exp. Res.* 7, 357–361. doi: 10.1111/j.1530-0277.1983.tb05481.x

McCarter, K. D., Li, C., Jiang, Z., Lu, W., Smith, H. C., Xu, G., et al. (2017). Effect of low-dose alcohol consumption on inflammation following transient focal cerebral ischemia in rats. *Sci. Rep.* 7:12547. doi: 10.1038/s41598-017-12720-w

Meretoja, A., Keshtkaran, M., Saver, J. L., Tatlisumak, T., Parsons, M. W., Kaste, M., et al. (2014). Stroke thrombolysis: save a minute, save a day. *Stroke* 45, 1053–1058. doi: 10.1161/STROKEAHA.113.002910

Mulcahy, N. J., Ross, J., Rothwell, N. J., and Loddick, S. A. (2003). Delayed administration of interleukin-1 receptor antagonist protects against transient cerebral ischaemia in the rat. *Br. J. Pharmacol.* 140, 471–476. doi: 10.1038/sj.bjp.0705462

Oliveira, G. B., Fontes Ede, A. Jr., de Carvalho, S., da Silva, J. B., Fernandes, L. M., Oliveira, M. C., et al. (2014). Minocycline mitigates motor impairments and cortical neuronal loss induced by focal ischemia in rats chronically exposed to ethanol during adolescence. *Brain Res.* 1561, 23–34. doi: 10.1016/j.brainres.2014.03.005

Patra, J., Taylor, B., Irving, H., Roerecke, M., Baliunas, D., Mohapatra, S., et al. (2010). Alcohol consumption and the risk of morbidity and mortality for different stroke types—a systematic review and meta-analysis. *BMC Public Health* 10:258. doi: 10.1186/1471-2458-10-258

Ronksley, P. E., Brien, S. E., Turner, B. J., Mukamal, K. J., and Ghali, W. A. (2011). Association of alcohol consumption with selected cardiovascular disease outcomes: a systematic review and meta-analysis. *BMJ* 342:d671. doi: 10.1136/bmj.d671

Sarafi, M. N., Garcia-Zepeda, E. A., MacLean, J. A., Charo, I. F., and Luster, A. D. (1997). Murine monocyte chemoattractant protein (MCP)-5: a novel CC chemokine that is a structural and functional homologue of human MCP-1. *J. Exp. Med.* 185, 99–109. doi: 10.1084/jem.185.1.99

Shukla, V., Shakya, A. K., Perez-Pinzon, M. A., and Dave, K. R. (2017). Cerebral ischemic damage in diabetes: an inflammatory perspective. *J. Neuroinflammation* 14:21. doi: 10.1186/s12974-016-0774-5

Sun, H., Xiong, W., Arrick, D. M., and Mayhan, W. G. (2012). Low-dose alcohol consumption protects against transient focal cerebral ischemia in mice: possible role of PPARγ. *PLoS One* 7:e41716. doi: 10.1371/journal.pone.0041716

Sun, H., Zhao, H., Sharpe, G. M., Arrick, D. M., and Mayhan, W. G. (2008). Effect of chronic alcohol consumption on brain damage following transient focal ischemia. *Brain Res.* 1194, 73–80. doi: 10.1016/j.brainres.2007.11.061

Supanc, V., Biloglav, Z., Kes, V. B., and Demarin, V. (2011). Role of cell adhesion molecules in acute ischemic stroke. *Ann. Saudi Med.* 31, 365–370. doi: 10.4103/0256-4947.83217

Taylor, R. A., and Sansing, L. H. (2013). Microglial responses after ischemic stroke and intracerebral hemorrhage. *Clin. Dev. Immunol.* 2013:746068. doi: 10.1155/2013/746068

Turner, R. J., and Sharp, F. R. (2016). Implications of MMP9 for Blood Brain Barrier Disruption and Hemorrhagic Transformation Following Ischemic Stroke. *Front. Cell Neurosci.* 10: 56. doi: 10.3389/fncel.2016.00056

Vacek, T. P., Rehman, S., Neamtu, D., Yu, S., Givimani, S., and Tyagi, S. C. (2015). Matrix metalloproteinases in atherosclerosis: role of nitric oxide, hydrogen sulfide, homocysteine, and polymorphisms. *Vasc. Health Risk Manag.* 11, 173–183. doi: 10.2147/vhrm.s68415

Villarreal, A., Rosciszewski, G., Murta, V., Cadena, V., Usach, V., Dodes-Traian, M. M., et al. (2016). Isolation and characterization of ischemia-derived astrocytes (IDAs) with ability to transactivate quiescent astrocytes. *Front. Cell. Neurosci.* 10:139. doi: 10.3389/fncel.2016.00139

Wang, M., Zhong, D., Zheng, Y., Li, H., Chen, H., Ma, S., et al. (2015). Damage effect of interleukin (IL)-23 on oxygen-glucose-deprived cells of the neurovascular unit *via* IL-23 receptor. *Neuroscience* 289, 406–416. doi: 10.1016/j.neuroscience.2015.01.012

Weinstein, J. R., Koerner, I. P., and Moller, T. (2010). Microglia in ischemic brain injury. *Future Neurol.* 5, 227–246. doi: 10.2217/fnl.10.1

Yang, Y., Salayandia, V. M., Thompson, J. F., Yang, L. Y., Estrada, E. Y., and Yang, Y. (2015). Attenuation of acute stroke injury in rat brain by minocycline promotes blood-brain barrier remodeling and alternative microglia/macrophage activation during recovery. *J. Neuroinflammation* 12:26. doi: 10.1186/s12974-015-0245-4

Zhang, C., Qin, Y. Y., Chen, Q., Jiang, H., Chen, X. Z., Xu, C. L., et al. (2014). Alcohol intake and risk of stroke: a dose-response meta-analysis of prospective studies. *Int. J. Cardiol.* 174, 669–677. doi: 10.1016/j.ijcard.2014.04.225

Zhao, H., Mayhan, W. G., Arrick, D. M., Xiong, W., and Sun, H. (2010). Alcohol-induced exacerbation of ischemic brain injury: role of NAD(P)H oxidase. *Alcohol. Clin. Exp. Res.* 34, 1948–1955. doi: 10.1111/j.1530-0277.2010.01284.x

Zhao, H., Mayhan, W. G., Arrick, D. M., Xiong, W., and Sun, H. (2011). Dose-related influence of chronic alcohol consumption on cerebral ischemia/reperfusion injury. *Alcohol. Clin. Exp. Res.* 35, 1265–1269. doi: 10.1111/j.1530-0277.2011.01461.x

Ziebell, J. M., Adelson, P. D., and Lifshitz, J. (2015). Microglia: dismantling and rebuilding circuits after acute neurological injury. *Metab. Brain Dis.* 30, 393–400. doi: 10.1007/s11011-014-9539-y

18

Adapentpronitrile, a New Dipeptidyl Peptidase-IV Inhibitor, Ameliorates Diabetic Neuronal Injury Through Inhibiting Mitochondria-Related Oxidative Stress and Apoptosis

Lu Yang[1†], Wenli Han[2†], Ying Luo[1], Xiangnan Hu[3], Ying Xu[4], Huan Li[1], Congli Hu[1], Dan Huang[5], Jie Ma[1], Yang Yang[1], Qi Chen[1], Yuke Li[1], Jiahua Zhang[1], Hui Xia[1], Zhihao Chen[1], Hong Wang[1], Dongzhi Ran[1] and Junqing Yang[1]*

[1] Department of Pharmacology, The Key Laboratory of Biochemistry and Molecular Pharmacology, Chongqing Medical University, Chongqing, China, [2] Laboratory Animal Center, Chongqing Medical University, Chongqing, China, [3] Department of Pharmacology, The Laboratory of Pharmaceutical Chemistry, Chongqing Medical University, Chongqing, China, [4] Department of Pharmaceutical Sciences, School of Pharmacy and Pharmaceutical Sciences, University at Buffalo, The State University of New York (SUNY), Buffalo, NY, United States, [5] Department of Pharmacology, The Laboratory of Pharmaceutical Analysis, Chongqing Medical University, Chongqing, China

***Correspondence:**
Junqing Yang
cqyangjq@cqmu.edu.cn;
cqjqyang2004@aliyun.com

† Co-first authors

Our previous studies indicated that adapentpronitrile, a new adamantane-based dipeptidyl peptidase-IV (DPP-IV) inhibitor, has a hypoglycemic effect and ameliorates rat pancreatic β cell dysfunction in type 2 diabetes mellitus through inhibiting DPP-IV activity. However, the effect of adapentpronitrile on the neurodegenerative diseases has not been studied. In the present study, we first found that adapentpronitrile significantly ameliorated neuronal injury and decreased amyloid precursor protein (APP) and amyloid beta (Aβ) expression in the hippocampus and cortex in the high fat diet/STZ rat model of diabetes. Furthermore, adapentpronitrile significantly attenuated oxidative stress, downregulated expression of the pro-apoptotic proteins BAX, cytochrome c, caspase-9, and caspase-3, and upregulated expression of the anti-apoptotic protein Bcl-2, although there was no effect on GLP-1R expression. At 30 min post-injection of adapentpronitrile (50 mg/kg) *via* the tail vein, its concentration in normal rat brain was 0.2034 ± 0.0094 μg/g. Subsequently, we further confirmed the neuroprotective effects and mechanism of adapentpronitrile in HT22 cells treated with high glucose (HG) and aluminum maltolate [Al(mal)$_3$] overload, respectively. Our results showed significant decreases in mitochondrial membrane potential (MTP) and Bcl-2 expression, accompanied by a significant increase in apoptosis, reactive oxygen species (ROS) generation, and the expression of pro-apoptotic proteins in HT22 cells exposed to these stimuli. Adapentpronitrile treatment protected against neuronal injury, suppressed ROS generation, and reduced MTP and mitochondrial apoptosis in HT22 cells; however, DPP-IV activity was not detected. Our results suggest that adapentpronitrile protects against diabetic neuronal injury, at least partially, by inhibiting mitochondrial oxidative stress and the apoptotic pathway in a DPP-IV-independent manner.

Keywords: adapentpronitrile, DPP-IV inhibitor, neuron injury, mitochondrial apoptosis pathway, reactive oxygen species

INTRODUCTION

Diabetes is a multifactorial metabolic disease characterized by hyperglycemia and high morbidity. The incidence of diabetes has increased sharply in the last decade. Cognitive impairment induced by neuronal injury is one of the chronic complications of diabetes (Maher and Schubert, 2009; Biessels and Reagan, 2015; Baglietto-Vargas et al., 2016). Epidemiological studies show that diabetes significantly increases the risk of dementia and may finally develop into Alzheimer's disease. β-Amyloid peptide (Aβ), a neuropathological hallmark of AD, is accumulated in specific brain regions (Hardy and Selkoe, 2002). Recent research demonstrates that insulin increases extracellular Aβ levels by elevating its secretion from neurons or modulating γ-secretase activity, and decreasing Aβ degradation by inhibiting Aβ-degrading enzymes (Gasparini et al., 2002; Phiel et al., 2003; Qiu and Folstein, 2006; Dineley et al., 2014). In addition, numerous studies have demonstrated that oxidative stress and mitochondrial abnormalities are common to the etiologies of both diabetes and Alzheimer's disease (Bosco et al., 2011; Moreira, 2012). Hence, anti-diabetic agents might have important clinical and social value in the treatment of AD.

Mitochondria are essential organelles with multiple functions in energy metabolism, reactive oxygen species (ROS) generation, and apoptosis induction. Neurodegenerative diseases, which are induced by inflammation, oxidative stress, and metal and glucose toxicity, are usually accompanied by mitochondrial dysfunctions (Lin and Beal, 2006; Kumar and Gill, 2009; Verdile et al., 2015; Kandimalla et al., 2016; Koliaki and Roden, 2016). Furthermore, abnormal Aβ and tau proteins were shown to have a direct impact on mitochondrial function (Schmitt et al., 2012). Amyloid precursor proteins (APP) accumulates in mitochondrial import channels, thereby resulting in mitochondrial dysfunction (Devi et al., 2006). DuBoff et al. (2012) revealed that mitochondrial elongation was significantly increased in hippocampal neurons from tau transgenic mice. Thus, mitochondrial dysfunction is implicated as a critical step toward neuronal death.

Although ROS play a vital role in cellular survival and signaling pathways at physiological condition (cellular cycle regulation, phagocytosis, and enzyme activation), excessive ROS lead to a series of harmful effects including DNA, lipid and protein damage, mitochondrial dysfunction, or even cell death (Knock and Ward, 2011; Verbon et al., 2012; Son et al., 2013). Because mitochondria are both targets and sources of ROS, oxidant-induced mitochondrial dysfunction may lead to an increased production of superoxide anion radicals by the electron transport chain, thereby triggering a "vicious cycle" (Wallace, 2005). Oxidative stress is an important causative factor in the pathogenesis of aging, diabetes, and neurodegenerative diseases, which also cause remarkable accumulation of Aβ (Smith et al., 2007; Valko et al., 2007; Chen et al., 2012; Manoharan et al., 2016). In fact, persistent mitochondrial dysfunction and oxidative stress contribute to apoptosis *via* the mitochondria-dependent caspase cascade induced by the release of cytochrome c into the cytosol (Wallace, 2005).

The incretin hormone glucagon-like-peptide 1 (GLP-1), secreted by enteroendocrine L-cells in response to ingestion of nutrients, plays an important role in stimulating insulin secretion, ameliorating glycemic control, and repairing β-cell function. Since GLP-1 is degraded rapidly by dipeptidyl peptidase-IV (DPP-IV), the inhibitors of which have been regarded as appropriate agents to maintain blood glucose levels. Pipatpiboon et al. (2013) found that DPP-IV inhibitor vildagliptin could increase GLP-1 levels in both plasma and brain, restore neuronal insulin receptor function, and prevent brain mitochondrial dysfunction, thus ameliorating cognitive function caused by high-fat diet (HFD) consumption. Saxagliptin ameliorates Aβ, tau phosphorylation, and inflammatory markers in a streptozotocin-induced model of Alzheimer's disease by increasing GLP-1 levels in the hippocampus (Kosaraju et al., 2013). Saxagliptin is also regarded as a novel therapeutic target for Parkinson's disease *via* antioxidant, anti-inflammatory, and antiapoptotic mechanisms (Nassar et al., 2015). However, the lack of evidence demonstrating the ability of these DPP-IV inhibitors to penetrate the blood–brain barrier (Golightly et al., 2012), and the role of DPP-IV inhibitors in the neuroprotective mechanisms remain to be clarified.

Our previous study showed that adapentpronitrile (APPN, CMD-05), an adamantane-based anti-diabetic agent synthesized in our laboratory, exerted DPP-IV inhibitory activity *in vitro*, and also mediated hypoglycemic functions in diabetic rats (Ma et al., 2017). Considering the neuroprotective effects of vildagliptin and saxagliptin, we hypothesized that the new DPP-IV inhibitor adapentpronitrile represents a novel agent for the protection against neurodegenerative disease and neuronal injury. The aim of the present study was to investigate the neuroprotective effect and mechanisms of adapentpronitrile in diabetic rat from the flowing aspects: (1) the effects of adapentpronitrile on the neuronal injury were observed in diabetic rat induced by HFD/STZ and in HT22 cells induced by HG/aluminum maltolate [$Al(mal)_3$]. (2) To primarily explore the mechanism of adapentpronitrile in neuronal injury. (3) Whether the neuroprotective mechanism of adapentpronitrile was related to the classic DPP-IV-dependent pathway, the adapentpronitrile concentration, and GLP-1R expression in rat brain and the DPP-IV activity in HT22 cells were detected.

MATERIALS AND METHODS

Chemicals

Adapentpronitrile (CMD-05; 98.9% purity) was synthesized by Laboratory of pharmaceutical chemistry, Chongqing Medical University (Patent apply number: 201610818878.5), and its purity was detected by high-performance liquid chromatography (HPLC).

Animals and Protocol

Sprague-Dawley (SD) male rats were obtained from Animal Laboratory Administrative Center, Chongqing Medical University (Chongqing, China), and housed in the barrier housing facility (SPF scale), which according with national standard "Laboratory Animal-Requirements of Environment and Housing Facilities." The care and experimental operation of animal have conforming to "Chongqing Administration Rule of Laboratory Animal." The experimental procedures were approved by the animal laboratory administrative center and the institutional ethics committee of Chongqing Medical University (License number: SYXK YU 2012-0001) and also in accordance with the National Institutes of Health guidelines. All experiments reviewed and approved by the Instructional Animal Care and Use Committee (IACUC).

The experiments were performed in 70 male rats (aged 9 weeks, 80–100 g). The rats were housed in controlled conditions of temperature (22 ± 2°C), relative humidity (50 ± 10%), and 12/12-h light/dark cycle with water *ad libitum*. After a week of acclimation, 10 rats were randomly selected and fed with basal diet as the control group, 60 rats were fed a HFD (20% sugar, 10% lard, 10% egg yolk, and 60% basal feed) for 4 weeks to induce insulin resistance (Ma et al., 2017). Diabetes was induced by a single intraperitoneal injection of streptozotocin (Solarbio, China, S8050; STZ, 30 mg/kg), which is particularly toxic to pancreatic beta cells in mammals. Control rats were injected with the same volume of vehicle (citrate buffer solution). Hyperglycemia was defined as blood glucose >16.7 mmol/L, 72 h after STZ injection. Diabetic rats were maintained on the HFD for 4 weeks and randomly divided into following groups (n = 7): HFD/STZ group (0.5% CMC-Na), low dose group (adapentpronitrile 1.5 mg/kg), high dose group (adapentpronitrile 4.5 mg/kg). The dose of adapentpronitrile was based on our previous study (Ma et al., 2017). Diabetic rats in the adapentpronitrile groups were chronically administered adapentpronitrile (4.5 or 1.5 mg/kg) for 30 days *via* the intragastric route, while the control and model groups received the same amount of vehicle (0.5% CMC-Na; **Figure 1**).

After administration, three rats in each group were randomly selected and used for histopathological examination, and the remaining four rats were used for biochemical examination and Western blot.

HE Staining Observation

Three rats in each group were randomly selected and transcardially perfused with phosphate-buffered saline (PBS). Then, the brain tissues were isolated and fixed overnight in 4% paraformaldehyde. After embedded by paraffin, serial sections (5 μm) of brain tissue were obtained, which were stained by hematoxylin–eosin (HE). Proceed as follows: dewaxing in xylen, hydration in alcohols, HE staining, dehydration in alcohols, transparent in xylen and mounting with neutral resins. Ten consecutive fields were selected randomly from the hippocampal and cortical neurons, and the morphological changes were observed under an optical microscope (Olympus, Japan) at 400× magnification (Guo et al., 2016).

Measurement of SOD Activity and MDA Content

After anesthesia of another four rats in each group, the cortex and hippocampus were separated on an ice plate and washed by normal saline. Then the isolated tissues were dried and stored at −80°C until use. The superoxide dismutase (SOD) activity and malondialdehyde (MDA) content were measured using the Total Superoxide Dismutase Assay Kit (Beyotime, China, S0101) and the Lipid Peroxidation MDA Assay Kit (Beyotime, China, S0131), respectively. The protein content was determined using the BCA Protein Assay Kit (Beyotime, China, P0010S).

Measurement of Adapentpronitrile Concentration

Male SD rats (200–220 g) were injected a single dose of adapentpronitrile (50 mg/kg, n = 4) *via* tail vein after fasting 12 h. At 30 min post-injection, blood samples were collected from abdominal aorta and the brain tissues were isolated on ice (Ma et al., 2017). Plasma was obtained after centrifugation. Then the plasma and isolated brain tissues were stored at −80°C until used.

Pipette 100-μL plasma samples and 200-μL acetonitrile [containing 500-ng internal standard (IS)] into 1.5-ml eppendorf tube. After that, the mixture was centrifuged for supernatant at 12,000 × g for 15 min at 4°C.

The brain tissues were weighed and homogenized in a twofold volume of acetonitrile containing 500 ng. Briefly, acetonitrile was used to homogenize brain tissue according to a ratio of 2-mL acetonitrile to 1-g tissue sample. The homogenates were centrifuged for supernatant at 12,000 × g for 15 min at 4°C.

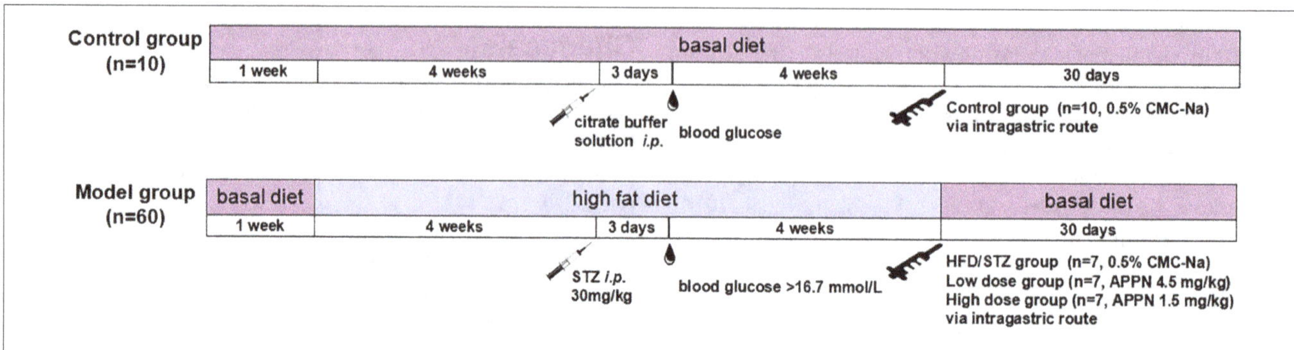

FIGURE 1 | The general procedure of this study *in vivo*.

Adapentpronitrile concentration in plasma and brain were determined using an HPLC system equipped with a UV detector. An octadecyl endcapped Phecda-C_{18} column (250 mm × 4.5 mm, 5-μm particle size) and Waters universal injector (100 μL capacity) were used. The optimum mobile phase was identified and consisted of acetonitrile and 10 mmol/L ammonium acetate (40:60, vol/vol). Samples (50 μL) were injected and a flow rate of 1 mL/min was equilibrated. The elution was monitored at 204 nm. The system was operated at the ambient temperature. Calibration curve was constructed by plotting standard peak area vs. concentration. Recoveries were calculated as the ratio of peak-area of the analyte from the fortified samples to the corresponding peak-area ratio of standard solutions.

Cell Culture

Immortalized murine hippocampal HT22 cell lines were obtained from BNCC, China. HT22 cells were cultured in DME/F12 medium (Hyclone, United States) supplemented with 10% fetal bovine serum (FBS; Hyclone, United States) and 1% 100× penicillin–streptomycin (Gibco, United States) at 37°C and 5% CO_2.

In Vitro Glucose (HG)/Al(mal)$_3$ Overload Model

HT22 cells were plated in 96-well plates (8 × 10^4 neurons/mL). The cells were divided into the control group (mannitol 100 mM) and four HG overloaded groups (glucose 25–100 mM). The cells were divided into the control group (maltol 600 μM) and four aluminum overloaded groups [Al(mal)$_3$ 50–400 μM; Ma et al., 2016]. After incubation, the relevant indicators were detected and the optimum concentrations of HG and Al(mal)$_3$ were selected in following experiments.

HT22 cells were divided into the control, HG overload and adapentpronitrile intervention groups induced by HG. HT22 cells were divided into the control group, Al(mal)$_3$ overloaded groups and adapentpronitrile intervention groups induced by Al(mal)$_3$. After incubation, the relevant indicators were detected in following experiments.

MTT Assay

HT22 cells were cultured in the 96-well plates at 8 × 10^4 cells/mL and subjected to HG or Al(mal)$_3$ as described above. After the intervention, 3-(4,5-dimethyl-thiazol-2-yl)-2,5-diphenyl-tetrazolium bromide (MTT, 20 μL, 5 mg/ml; Sigma, United States, M2128) was added per well. After 4 h of incubation, the medium was removed, and 150 μL dimethyl sulfoxide (DMSO) was added to solubilize the purple formazan. Then, the plate shook slowly on the horizontal shaking table free from light for 10 min at room temperature. Finally, optical density (OD) was detected at 490 nm using a microplate reader (BioTek, United States; Lobner, 2000).

LDH Leakage Rate Detection

Cell death was evaluated using the lactate dehydrogenase (LDH) Cytotoxicity Assay Kit (Beyotime, China, C0017). HT22 cells were cultured in 96-well plates at 5 × 10^4 cells/ml. After HG or Al(mal)$_3$ treatment for 36 h, the LDH leakage rate in the cell culture supernatant was measured according to the manufacturer's instruction.

Flow Cytometry Analysis

HT22 cells were seeded in six-well plates at 8 × 10^4 cells/mL and exposed to HG or Al(mal)$_3$ as described above. After the incubation period, cells were trypsinized without EDTA, collected and suspended in 1 ml PBS. Apoptosis was determined by flow cytometry using the Annexin V-FITC/propidium iodide (annexin V/PI) apoptosis detection kits according to the manufacturer's protocol. Three separate experiments were performed.

Transmission Electron Microscopy Observation

The changes in mitochondrial ultrastructure were confirmed by transmission electron microscopy (TEM) examination. After treatment, HT22 cells were collected and fixed in glutaraldehyde solution at 4°C. The fixed samples were sent to the electron microscope center of Chongqing Medical University for microscopic observed and photographed.

DPP-IV Activity Determination

Supernatant of HT22 cells and lysed HT22 cells were collected to measure DPP-IV activity in control group. Culture medium and equivoluminal lysis buffer were collected and regarded as blank group. DPP-IV enzyme assay was carried out according to the manufacturer's instructions. DPP-IV Activity Assay Kits (AnaSpec, United States, AS-24098) were used according the manufacturer's instructions. In this assay, DPP4 cleaves a substrate [H-Gly-Pro-7-amino-4-methyl coumarin (AMC)] to release a quenched fluorescent group, AMC, which can be easily detected using a fluorescence microplate reader at excitation and emission wavelengths of 354 and 442 nm, respectively.

TUNEL Assays

HT22 cells were cultured in cover slides and washed in ice-cold PBS. Samples were fixed with 4% paraformaldehyde for 15 min and permeabilized in PBS containing proteinase K for 3 min at room temperature. Apoptosis was determined using TUNEL FITC Apoptosis Detection Kits (Vazyme Biotech, China, A111-02) according to the manufacturer's protocol. Apoptotic cells were observed using a fluorescence microscopy. Four consecutive fields were selected randomly and the apoptosis rate was calculated as the ratio of the number of apoptotic cells to the total number of cells (expressed as a percentage).

Mitochondrial ROS Assay

Mitochondrial ROS levels were measured using ROS Assay Kits (Beyotime, China, S0033). 2′,7′-Dichloro-dihydro-fluorescein diacetate (DCFH-DA) is a non-fluorescent probe that can be oxidized to the highly fluorescent derivative DCF by intracellular

ROS. The cells were stained with 2-μM DCFH-DA and incubated at 37°C for 20 min. Four consecutive fields were selected randomly and the fluorescence intensity was measured under a fluorescence microscope after removal of the culture medium.

Mitochondrial Membrane Potential ($\Delta\psi_m$) Assay

The mitochondrial membrane potential (MMP, $\Delta\psi_m$) was measured using Mitochondrial Membrane Potential Assay Kits with JC-1 (Beyotime, China, C2006). JC-1, a cationic fluorescent dye, can be accumulated in the mitochondrial matrix to form polymer, which gives off a strong red fluorescence. At low MMP, JC-1 exists in the form of monomer in the cytoplasm and yields green fluorescence. The cells were strained with JC-1 dye at 37°C for 20 min. After washing with dilution buffer, four consecutive fields were selected randomly and the fluorescence intensity was measured under a fluorescence microscope.

Western Blot Analysis

After treatment, HT22 cells were washed in ice-cold PBS and lysed by RIPA lysis buffer containing phosphatase and protease inhibitors. The samples were collected and centrifuged at 12,000 × *g* and 4°C for 15 min, after incubated for 20 min on ice. The supernatant was collected and the total protein concentrations were measured with a BCA protein assay kit (Beyotime, China, P0010S). Loading buffer (Beyotime, China, P0015L) was added into the remaining supernatant and boiled at 100°C for 10 min. Ultimately, samples were stored at −20°C for further research.

Forty milligrams of rat cortex or hippocampus (n = 4) was added to 0.4 ml of RIPA Lysis Buffer for protein extraction and was centrifuged at 12,000 × *g* for 15 min at 4°C after homogenization. The supernatant was collected and determined with the BCA protein assay kit (Beyotime, China, P0010S) for protein concentrations. The remaining supernatant was mixed with Loading buffer (Beyotime, China, P0015L) and boiled at 100°C for 10 min. Finally, samples were stored at −20°C for further research.

According to the Cell Mitochondrial Isolation kit (Beyotime, China, C3601), the mitochondria can be separated quickly and conveniently, and the cytoplasmic protein can be obtained to study the release of mitochondrial proteins to the cytoplasm, such as cytochrome c.

Equal amounts of protein (20 mg) were separated by sodium dodecyl sulfate polyacrylamide gel electrophoresis (SDS–PAGE). The proteins were then transferred to PVDF membranes (Millipore, United States) and blocked with 5% bovine serum albumin (BSA) in Tris-buffered saline/Tween-20 (TBST) buffer for 4 h at room temperature. Membranes were probed overnight at 4°C with primary antibodies for specific detection of APP (dilution 1:500; Boster, China, BA0581), Aβ (dilution 1:1000; Abcam, United Kingdom, ab62658), GLP-1R (dilution 1:500, Bioss, China, bs-1559R), Bcl-2 (dilution 1:500; Abcam, United Kingdom, ab196495), Bax (dilution 1:400; Proteintech, China, 50599-2-Ig), cytochrome c (dilution 1:1000; Abcam, United Kingdom, ab133504), caspase-9 (dilution 1:1000; Abcam, United Kingdom, ab184786), caspase-3 (dilution 1:1000; Abcam, United Kingdom, ab184787), and β-actin (dilution 1:3000; Proteintech, United States, 60008-1-Ig; **Table 1**). The blots were incubated with HRP-conjugated secondary antibodies (dilution 1:2000; **Table 1**) at room temperature for 1 h. Finally, immunoreactive bands were visualized by ECL (Bio-Rad, United States) and quantified using Image Lab software (Bio-Rad, United States). All experiments were performed in triplicate.

Statistical Analysis

All investigators were complete randomization in the implementation process of experiments. All experiments were repeated at least four times, and representative results are shown. Data were presented as mean ± SD. Statistical analysis was carried out using SPSS 17.0 (SPSS Inc. Chicago, IL, United States). Normal distribution of data and homogeneity of variance were determined by Shapiro–Wilk test and one-way analysis of variance (ANOVA) test, respectively, followed

TABLE 1 | List of primary and secondary antibodies used in the study.

	Host	Dilution	Supply	Cat. No.	Application
Primary antibody					
APP	Rabbit	1:500	Boster	BA0581	WB
Aβ	Rabbit	1:1000	Abcam	ab62658	WB
GLP-1R	Rabbit	1:500	Bioss	bs-1559R	WB
Bcl-2	Rabbit	1:500	Abcam	ab196495	WB
Bax	Rabbit	1:400	Proteintech	50599-2-Ig	WB
Cytochrome c	Rabbit	1:1000	Abcam	ab133504	WB
Caspase-9	Rabbit	1:1000	Abcam	ab184786	WB
Caspase-3	Rabbit	1:1000	Abcam	ab184787	WB
β-Actin	Mouse	1:3000	Proteintech	60008-1-Ig	WB
Secondary antibody					
Anti-mouse HRP	Goat	1:2000	Proteintech	SA00001-1	WB
Anti-rabbit HRP	Goat	1:2000	Proteintech	SA00001-2	WB

by Dunnett-t type multiple comparison tests. $P < 0.05$ was considered to indicate statistical significance.

RESULTS

Effects of Adapentpronitrile on Pathomorphology and the Expression of APP and Aβ Proteins in Hippocampus and Cortex of Rat

Histopathological examination revealed that the neurons were in clear and intact structure, and arranged regularly in the control group. By contrast, HFD/STZ group showed severe hippocampal and cortical neurons injuries including karyopyknosis, hyperchromatic nuclei, and cell loss. Administration of adapentpronitrile (4.5 mg/kg) obviously ameliorated the pathomorphological injury in the hippocampus and cortex (**Figure 2A**).

As shown in **Figure 2B**, the expression of APP and Aβ proteins elevated significantly in HFD/STZ-treated rat, while adapentpronitrile (4.5 mg/kg) significantly blunted the changes of APP and Aβ protein expressions.

Effects of Adapentpronitrile on Oxidative Stress in the Hippocampus and Cortex of Rat

Both hippocampal and cortex SOD activity in HFD/STZ group significantly decreased compared with the control group. Adapentpronitrile treatment reversed the decrease of SOD activity (**Figure 3A**). Both hippocampal and cortex MDA content in HFD/STZ group significantly increased compared with the control group. Adapentpronitrile administration significantly blunted the increase of MDA content in HFD/STZ rats (**Figure 3B**).

Effects of Adapentpronitrile on GLP-1R and Mitochondria-Dependent Apoptosis Protein Expression Induced by HFD/STZ in the Rat Hippocampus and Cortex

Glucagon-like-peptide 1 is an incretin hormone, which plays a role in controlling synaptic plasticity and reversing memory impairment. As shown in **Figure 4**, there were no significant difference among these four groups in the protein expressions of GLP-1R. On the basis of this evidence, we deduced that the mechanism underlying the protective effects of adapentpronitrile may be GLP-1 independent.

Therefore, we also examined the impact of adapentpronitrile on the expression of the apoptosis-related proteins. The expression of the anti-apoptotic Bcl-2 was significantly decreased in HFD/STZ group, whereas the expressions of the pro-apoptotic proteins Bax, cytochrome c, caspase-9, and caspase-3 were significantly increased. However, all the alterations were significantly reversed by adapentpronitrile (4.5 mg/kg) treatment (**Figure 4**).

Concentration of Adapentpronitrile in the Rat Plasma and Brain Tissue

To confirm the ability of adapentpronitrile to permeate the BBB to protective against neuronal apoptosis, we used a HPLC method to determine the concentration of adapentpronitrile in rat plasma and brain tissue. According to HPLC methodology, the maximum ultraviolet absorption of adapentpronitrile is 204 nm, the quantitation limit and the detection limit were 0.03 μg/ml (S/N = 10) and 0.09 μg/ml (S/N = 3), respectively. The standard curve of adapentpronitrile had good linear relation in the range of 0.1–10 μg/mL in plasma, the equation was $Y = 0.5267X–0.0796$ ($r = 0.9997$, $n = 4$). The intra-day and inter-day precision RSD were 3.66–8.71 and 4.33–5.59%, respectively. The recovery of adapentpronitrile was 82.19 ± 6.57–118.21 ± 3.72%, and which has good stability in 48 h. The linear relation of adapentpronitrile was excellent within the range of 0.09–5 μg/ml in brain tissue; the equation was $Y = 0.325X–0.0125$ ($r = 0.9999$, $n = 4$). The intra-day and inter-day precision RSD were 1.71–5.69 and 3.77–4.54%, respectively. The recovery of adapentpronitrile was 106.68 ± 2.47–117.50 ± 5.10 and which has good stability in 48 h. These methods are stable, sensitive, and practicable for examination of adapentpronitrile distribution. As shown in **Figure 5**, HPLC-MS was confirmed to have good specificity to detect adapentpronitrile.

As shown in **Table 2**, the adapentpronitrile concentrations in plasma and brain were 2.8002 ± 0.5691 μg/100 μL and 0.2034 ± 0.0094 μg/g, respectively. Therefore, these data confirmed that adapentpronitrile permeates the BBB.

Establishment of HG Overload Model in HT22 Cells

To determine whether adapentpronitrile could protect neurons from HG injury, HT22 cells were treated with appropriate concentration of glucose (HG) to establish the neuronal damage model *in vitro*. As is shown in **Figure 6A**, treatment of glucose caused cytotoxicity in HT22 cells in a time- and concentration-dependent manner, showing that treatment of 200-μM glucose for 36 h resulted in a suitable neuronal injury model (66.24%).

The LDH leakage rate and apoptosis rate were elevated with the increase of glucose concentration, and treatment of 75-mM glucose led to a suitable LDH leakage rate (20.02%) and apoptosis rate (21.62%) for model establishment (**Figures 6B,C**).

As shown in **Figure 6D**, the cell number decreased with concentration of glucose from 25 to 100 mM, illustrating that cell proliferation was inhibited by HG.

Based on these results, the treatment of 75 mM glucose for 36 h was used in further experiments.

Adapentpronitrile Prevented HT22 Cells Against HG-Induced Cytotoxicity

Prior to explore the effect of adapentpronitrile on HG-induced cytotoxicity, the safety of adapentpronitrile on HT22 cells was evaluated by MTT assay. Treatment with adapentpronitrile at concentrations lower than 1×10^{-5} M did not caused significant cytotoxicity in HT22 cells (**Figure 7A**).

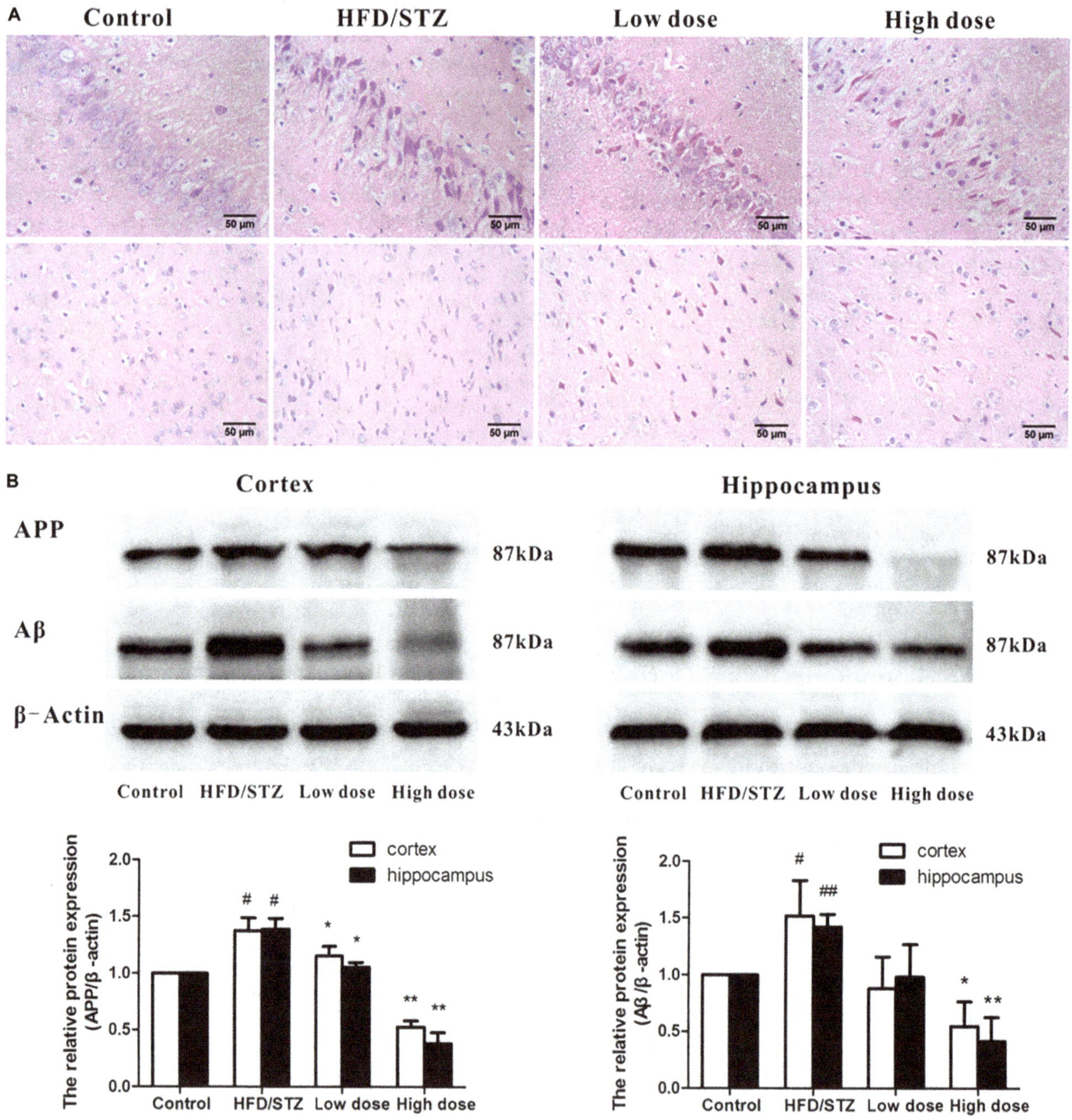

FIGURE 2 | Effects of adapentpronitrile on pathomorphology and the expression of APP and Aβ proteins in hippocampus and cortex of rat. **(A)** Representative neuronal pathomorphology in hippocampus and cortex. Sections were pictured at 400×. Scale bar = 50 μm. **(B)** The expressions of APP and Aβ proteins were measured by Western Blotting. Data were expressed as mean ± SD of four independent experiments, and were analyzed statistically using one-way ANOVA, followed by Dunnett-t type multiple comparison tests. $^{\#}P < 0.05$ and $^{\#\#}P < 0.01$ vs. Control group, respectively; $^{*}P < 0.05$ and $^{**}P < 0.01$ vs. HFD/STZ group, respectively.

The results showed that treatment with adapentpronitrile significantly increased the viability and reduced LDH leakage rate induced by HG overload in a concentration-dependent manner (**Figures 7B,C**). Treatment with adapentpronitrile (1×10^{-5} M) could ameliorate the apoptosis rate and pathomorphological change induced by 75-mM HG (**Figures 7D,E**). Therefore, these results together indicated that adapentpronitrile can inhibit neuronal apoptosis induced by HG overload *in vitro*.

DPP-IV Activity in HT22 Cells

To confirm whether dipeptidyl peptidase IV (DPP-IV) exists in HT22 cells. Supernatant from both HT22 cells incubation and the HT22 cells lysate were collected to measure DPP-IV activity

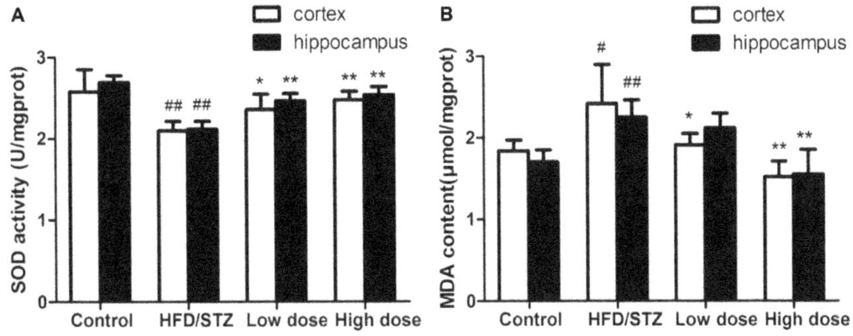

FIGURE 3 | Effects of adapentpronitrile on oxidative stress in the hippocampus and cortex of rat. **(A)** The change of SOD activity in hippocampus and cortex. **(B)** The alteration of MDA content in hippocampus and cortex. Data were expressed as mean ± SD of four independent experiments, and were analyzed statistically using one-way ANOVA, followed by Dunnett-t type multiple comparison tests. $^{\#}P < 0.05$ and $^{\#\#}P < 0.01$ vs. control group, $^{*}P < 0.05$ and $^{**}P < 0.01$ vs. HFD/STZ group, respectively.

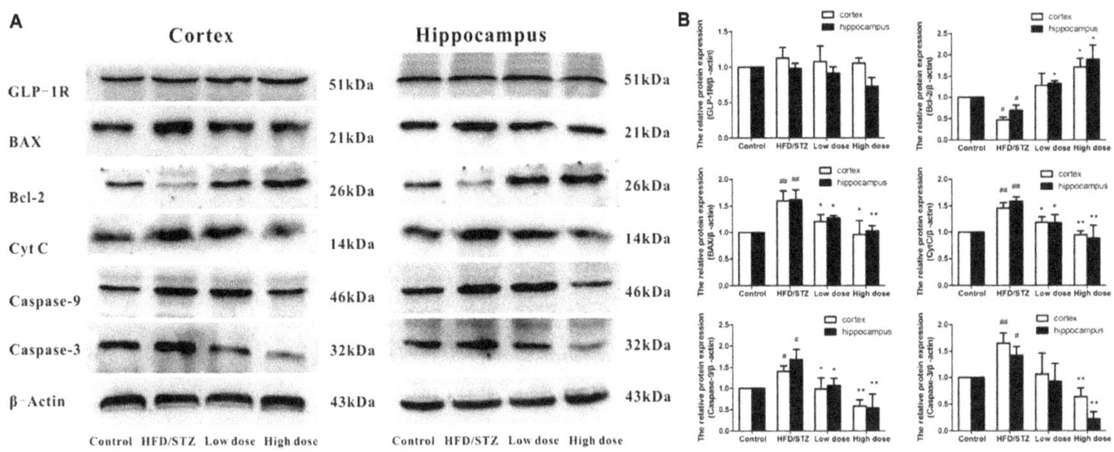

FIGURE 4 | Effects of adapentpronitrile on GLP-1R and mitochondria-dependent apoptosis protein expression induced by HFD/STZ in the rat hippocampus and cortex. **(A)** The expressions of GLP-1R and mitochondria-dependent apoptosis proteins were measured by Western Blotting. Representative images of experiments are shown. **(B)** The relative expression of GLP-1R and mitochondria-dependent apoptosis proteins were standardized to endogenous β-actin protein for each sample. Data were expressed as mean ± SD of four independent experiments, and were analyzed statistically using one-way ANOVA, followed by Dunnett-t type multiple comparison tests. $^{\#}P < 0.05$ and $^{\#\#}P < 0.01$ vs. Control group, respectively; $^{*}P < 0.05$ and $^{**}P < 0.01$ vs. HFD/STZ group, respectively.

as the control group. Equivoluminal culture medium and lysis buffer were collected and regarded as the blank group. As shown in **Figure 8**, there was no significant difference in the fluorescence intensity between the culture supernatant of HT22 cells and that of the cell-free control. There was also no significant difference in the fluorescence intensity between HT22 cell lysates and that of lysis buffer. Therefore, we concluded that DPP-IV activity was not present in HT22 cells, and indicating the protective effect of adapentpronitrile on neuronal injury *in vitro* is independent of DPP-IV.

Adapentpronitrile Protected Against HG-Induced Mitochondrial Apoptosis

As shown in **Figures 9A–C**, the numbers of TUNEL-positive cells and the ratio of green to red fluorescence of JC-1 and ROS level were significantly increased in the HG-overload group, while a reduction was noted in the adapentpronitrile-treated group.

The changes in mitochondrial ultrastructure were confirmed by TEM examination. As is shown in **Figure 9D**, in the control group, the nuclei of HT22 cells were round or oval with regular shape and evenly distributed chromatin, and the mitochondrial morphology was normal with a complete structure. In HG overload group, the chromatin was aggregated at the nuclear membrane, the mitochondrial cristae were thick and short accompanied with apoptotic bodies, thereby indicating the occurrence of mitochondrial fission; all alterations were ameliorated by adapentpronitrile treatment.

Effect of Adapentpronitrile on Mitochondria-Dependent Apoptosis-Related Protein Expression Caused by HG in HT22 Cells

As shown in **Figure 10**, exposure of HT22 cells to 75 mM HG for 36 h significantly decreased the expression of the

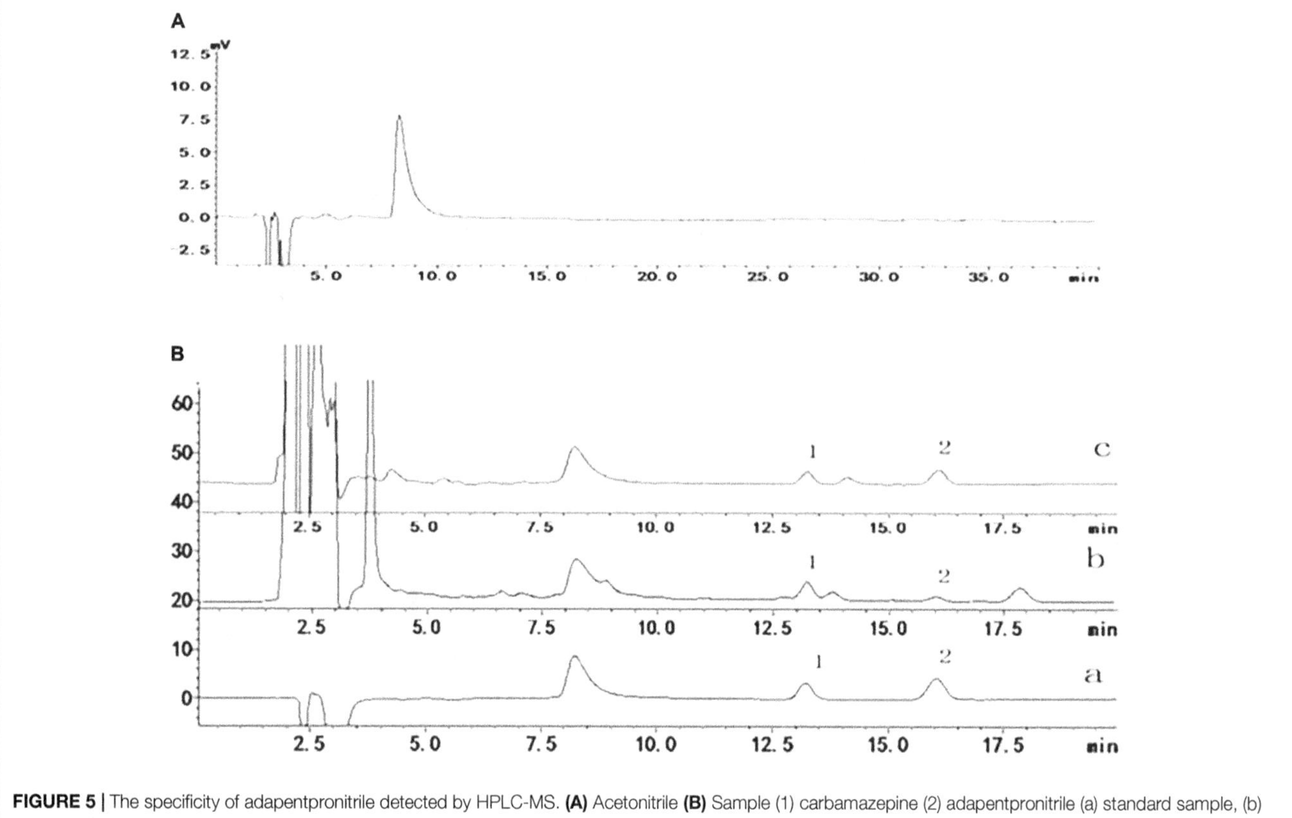

FIGURE 5 | The specificity of adapentpronitrile detected by HPLC-MS. **(A)** Acetonitrile **(B)** Sample (1) carbamazepine (2) adapentpronitrile (a) standard sample, (b) plasma, (c) brain.

anti-apoptotic protein Bcl-2 and increased the expression of the pro-apoptotic proteins Bax, cytochrome c, caspase-9, and caspase-3. All alterations in the expression of apoptosis-related proteins were reversed by adapentpronitrile treatment. Our results indicated that adapentpronitrile protects against HG-induced cell apoptosis *via* the mitochondrial apoptotic pathway.

Establishment of $Al(mal)_3$ Overload Model in HT22 Cells

To determine whether adapentpronitrile could protect neurons from non-HG injury, HT22 cells were treated with appropriate concentration of $Al(mal)_3$ to establish the neuronal damage model *in vitro*. As is shown in **Figure 11A**, treatment of $Al(mal)_3$ caused cytotoxicity in HT22 cells in a time- and concentration-dependent manner, showing that treatment of 200 μM $Al(mal)_3$ for 36 h resulted in a suitable neuronal injury model (66.24%).

The LDH leakage rate and apoptosis rates were elevated with the increase of $Al(mal)_3$ concentration, and treatment of 200 μM $Al(mal)_3$ led to a suitable LDH leakage rate (23.54%) and apoptosis rate (33.76%) for model establishment (**Figures 11B,C**).

As shown in **Figure 11D**, the cell number decreased with concentration of $Al(mal)_3$ from 50 to 400 μM, while only 400 μM $Al(mal)_3$ could contribute to a morphological change, illustrating that cell proliferation was inhibited by $Al(mal)_3$.

Based on these results, the treatment of 200 μM $Al(mal)_3$ for 36 h was used in further experiments.

TABLE 2 | Concentration of APPN in rat plasma and brain (mean ± SD, n = 4).

Sample	Unit	Concentration
Plasma	μg/ml	28.002 ± 5.691
Brain	μg/g	0.2034 ± 0.0094

Adapentpronitrile Prevented HT22 Cells Against $Al(mal)_3$-Induced Cytotoxicity

The results showed that treatment with adapentpronitrile significantly increased the viability and reduced LDH leakage rate induced by $Al(mal)_3$-overload in a concentration-dependent manner (**Figures 12A,B**). Treatment with adapentpronitrile (1×10^{-6} M) could ameliorate the apoptosis rate and pathomorphological change induced by 200 μM $Al(mal)_3$ (**Figures 12C,D**). Therefore, these results together indicated that adapentpronitrile can inhibit neuronal apoptosis induced by $Al(mal)_3$ overload *in vitro*.

Adapentpronitrile Protected Against $Al(mal)_3$-Induced Mitochondrial Apoptosis

As shown in **Figures 13A–C**, the numbers of TUNEL-positive cells, the ratio of green to red fluorescence of

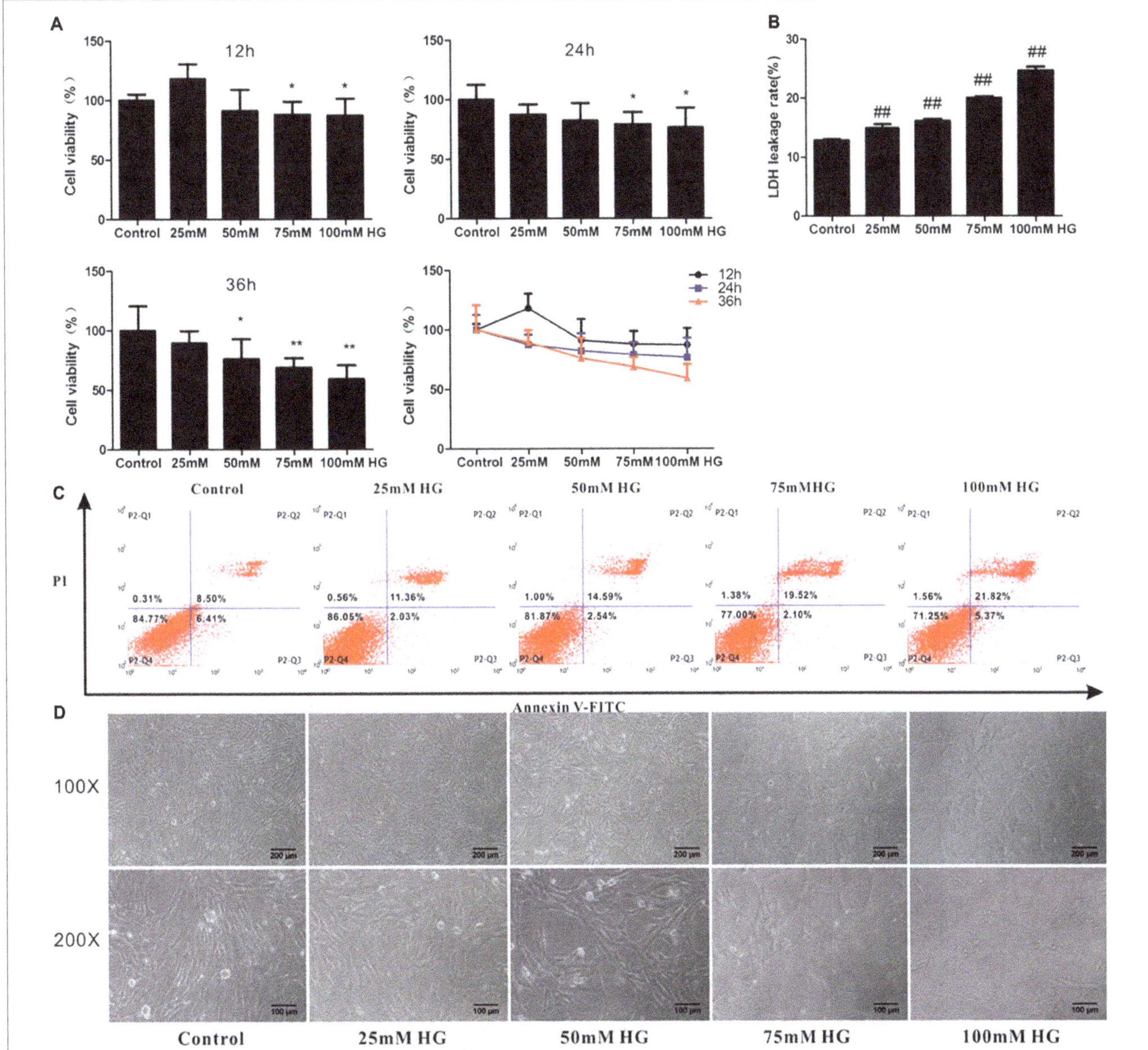

FIGURE 6 | The effects of HG overload on HT22 cells. **(A)** The viability of HT22 cells treated with different concentrations of glucose. Data were expressed as mean ± SD of six independent experiments, and were analyzed statistically using one-way ANOVA, followed by Dunnett-t type multiple comparison tests. $^{*}P < 0.05$, $^{**}P < 0.01$ vs. the control group. **(B)** The LDH leakage rate of HT22 cells treated with different concentration of glucose. Data were expressed as mean ± SD of six independent experiments, and were analyzed statistically using one-way ANOVA, followed by Dunnett-t type multiple comparison tests. $^{\#\#}P < 0.01$ vs. the control group. **(C)** The flow cytometry apoptosis analysis of HT22 cells were treated with high glucose for 36 h. The representative images of flow cytometry analysis are shown. **(D)** The cytomorphology changes in HT22 cells treated with different concentration of glucose. Representative images of experiments are shown. The magnification of images were 100× and 200×, respectively. Scale bars were 200 and 100 μm, respectively.

JC-1 and ROS level were significantly increased in the $Al(mal)_3$ overload group, while a reduction was noted in the adapentpronitrile-treated group. The photograph of TEM showed that the chromatin was aggregated at the nuclear membrane and the cristae of mitochondria was thick and short in the $Al(mal)_3$-overloaded group, which indicated that mitochondrial fission was broadly raised, while all alterations were ameliorated by adapentpronitrile treatment (**Figure 13D**).

Effect of Adapentpronitrile on Mitochondria-Dependent Apoptosis-Related Protein Expression Caused by $Al(mal)_3$ in HT22 Cells

As shown in **Figure 14**, the expression of Bcl-2 protein was significantly decreased in the $Al(mal)_3$-overload group, whereas the expressions of Bax, cytochrome c, caspase-9, and caspase-3 protein were significantly increased. All the alterations of

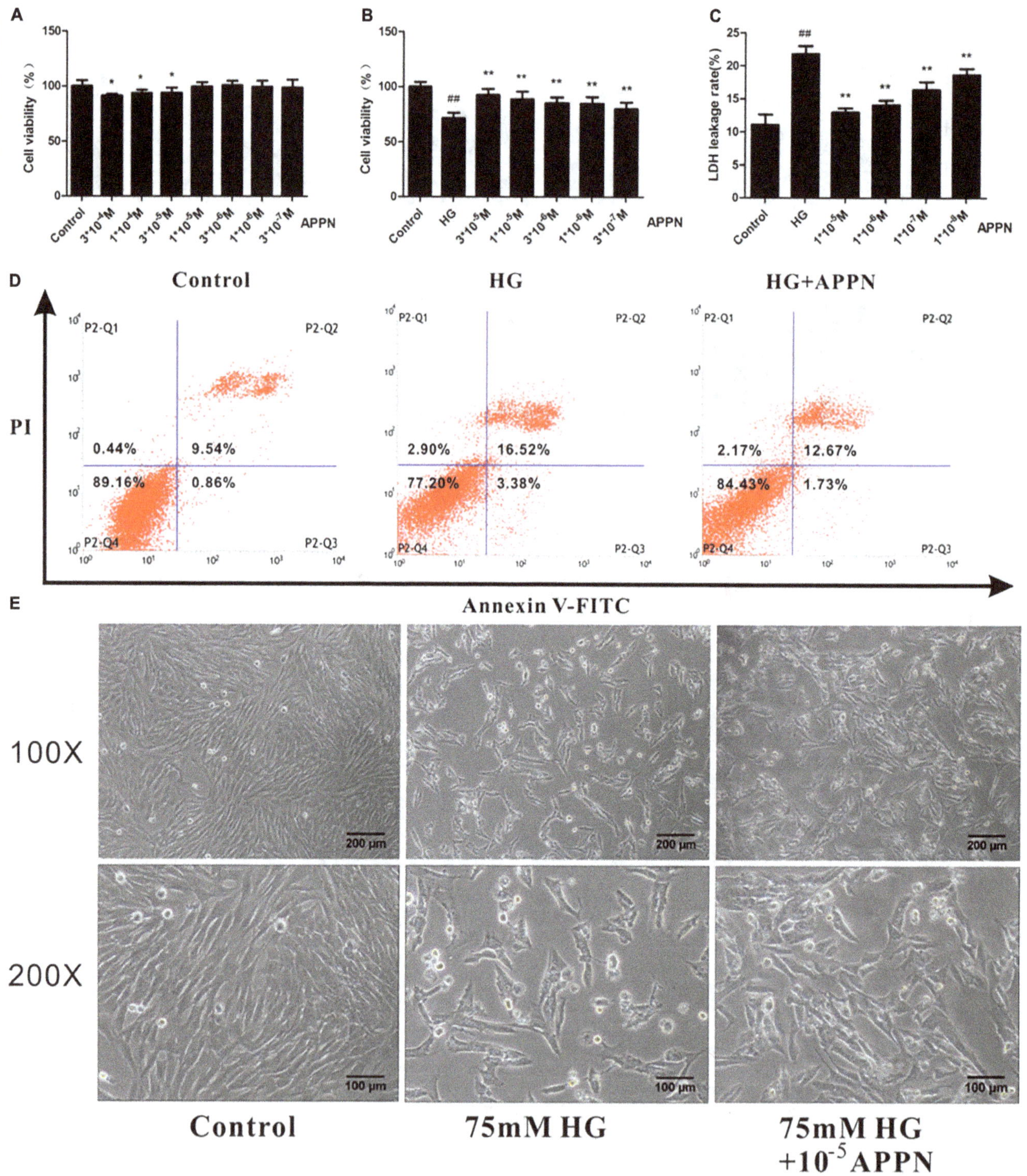

FIGURE 7 | The effect of adapentpronitrile on HG-induced cytotoxicity in HT22 cells. **(A)** The cytotoxicity of adapentpronitrile on HT22 cells. Data were expressed as mean ± SD of six independent experiments, and were analyzed statistically using one-way ANOVA, followed by Dunnett-t type multiple comparison tests. $^{*}P < 0.05$ vs. the control group. **(B)** The effect of adapentpronitrile on the viability in HT22 cells induced by HG-overload. **(C)** The effect of adapentpronitrile on the LDH leakage rate in HT22 cells induced by HG-overload. Data were expressed as mean ± SD of six independent experiments, and were analyzed statistically using one-way ANOVA, followed by Dunnett-t type multiple comparison tests. $^{\#\#}P < 0.01$ vs. the control group; $^{*}P < 0.05$ and $^{**}P < 0.01$ vs. the HG group, respectively. **(D)** The effect of adapentpronitrile on apoptosis in HT22 cells induced by HG-overload. The representative images of flow cytometry analysis are shown. **(E)** The effect of adapentpronitrile on the changes of cytomorphology in HT22 cells induced by HG overload. Representative images of experiments are shown. The magnification of images were 100× and 200×, respectively. Scale bars were 200 and 100 μm, respectively.

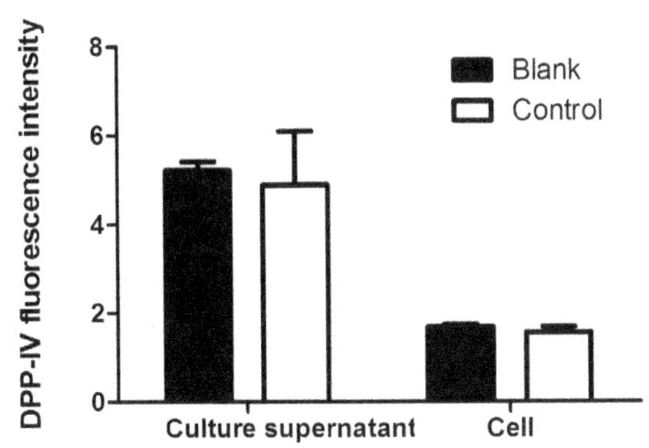

FIGURE 8 | The DPP-IV activity in HT22 cells. Data were expressed as mean ± SD of six independent experiments, and were analyzed statistically using one-way ANOVA, followed by Dunnett-t type multiple comparison tests.

apoptosis-related proteins were reversed by adapentpronitrile treatment.

DISCUSSION

Alzheimer's disease is an irreversible progressive neurodegenerative disorder characterized by cognitive deficits and memory loss. Despite various strategies have been explored, unfortunately, promising preclinical outcomes were generally disappointing (Mullard, 2016). In recent years, epidemiological studies suggest that diabetes mellitus is a risk factor for Alzheimer's disease, which may include three common pathological properties as follows, cerebrovascular inflammation, amyloid deposition, and impairment of brain insulin signaling (Takeda et al., 2010; De Felice and Ferreira, 2014). Antidiabetic agents, therefore, may have value in the treatment of AD.

In the present study, neuronal injury in rats was induced by a HFD combined with low-dose STZ (30 mg/kg). It is postulated that a persistent high-fat and high-sucrose diet contributes to an accumulation of glucolipotoxicity and β cell dysfunction, thereby leading to insulin resistance and hyperinsulinemia (Li et al., 2015). STZ is particularly toxic to islet cells in mammals and has been utilized to establish T2DM model, which accelerates β cell dysfunction and insulin deficiency (Lenzen, 2008). The pathology of HFD/STZ model reflects the progression from insulin resistance to hyperglycemia and hypoinsulinemia associated with diabetes (Reed et al., 2000; Li et al., 2015). In our previous study, we observed a reduction in β cell numbers by approximately 40% in HFD/STZ rats, which consistent with those observed in reports of patients with diabetes in the clinic (Butler et al., 2003; Ma et al., 2017). It is well known that hippocampus and cortex play an important role in the learning, cognition, and memory, and is also one of the earliest signs of neurodegenerative disorder such as Alzheimer's disease. Numerous investigations indicated that the atrophy and apoptosis of brain may occur in type 2 diabetes, especially in the hippocampus and cortex, and that may contribute to cognitive impairment (den Heijer et al., 2003; McCrimmon and Ryan, 2012; Ho and Sommers, 2013; Moran et al., 2013; Hirabayashi et al., 2016). In the present study, we observed significant pathomorphological changes and neuronal injury in the cortex and vulnerable hippocampal CA4 region following HFD/STZ insult. The protein expressions of APP and Aβ, which are a major hallmark in the pathologic progression of AD, were elevated significantly in both the hippocampus and cortex of the HFD/STZ rats. These results confirmed that the diabetic AD rat model was established successfully.

Treatment with adapentpronitrile, a new DPP-IV inhibitor, resulted in a dose-dependent amelioration of the pathological changes in the hippocampal CA4 region of T2DM rats. Furthermore, the abnormal protein expressions of APP and Aβ were reversed. These findings demonstrate the protective effects of adapentpronitrile against neuronal injury.

Glucagon-like-peptide 1, which is an incretin hormone secreted mainly by intestinal L-cells, plays a vital role in motivating insulin secretion, suppressing glucagon release, thus ameliorating glycemic control (Holst, 2007; Ma et al., 2014). In addition to the expression in peripheral tissues, the GLP-1 receptor is expressed in the brain, particularly in the hippocampus (Dunphy et al., 1998). Accumulating evidence demonstrates that GLP-1 analogs play a role in controlling synaptic plasticity and reversing memory impairment (Gault and Hölscher, 2008; McClean and Hölscher, 2014). Moreover, GLP-1 acts as a neurotropic factor by promoting proliferation and inhibiting apoptosis. The half-life of endogenous GLP-1 in the circulation is approximately 2 min due to its rapid degradation by DPP-IV (Drucker and Nauck, 2006; Ranganath, 2008). Therefore, DPP-IV inhibitors have been utilized to improve glycemic control in the treatment of T2DM since the first agent sitagliptin was approved by FDA in 2006 (Drucker and Nauck, 2006; Verspohl, 2009). DPP-IV inhibitors adapentpronitrile have been shown to stimulate insulin biosynthesis and secretion, improve glycemic control, and decrease HbA1c in diabetic rats induced by HFD/STZ (Ma et al., 2017). In the present study, adapentpronitrile significantly attenuated the neuronal injury in the hippocampus and cortex of rats caused by HFD/STZ. However, there was no significant difference among these groups in the protein expressions of the GLP-1R, indicating that the neuroprotective effects of adapentpronitrile are, at least partially, independent of the DPP-IV pathway. Therefore, the neuroprotective mechanism of adapentpronitrile remains to be fully elucidated.

The neurotoxic mechanism of HFD/STZ might be attributed to the overproduction of ROS. SOD is an important antioxidant enzyme, which functions primarily as a free radical scavenger to protect against oxidative stress. MDA, a biomarker of lipid peroxidation, is generated *via* a series of enzyme reactions (Del Rio et al., 2005). In the present study, we found that the SOD activity was significantly decreased and the MDA content was significantly increased in the brain of T2DM rat. Adapentpronitrile treatment reversed the abnormal decrease in SOD activity and increased MDA levels. These results further confirmed the involvement of oxidative stress in the rat model of diabetic neuronal injury induced by HFD/STZ, whereas adapentpronitrile treatment improved the oxidative imbalance.

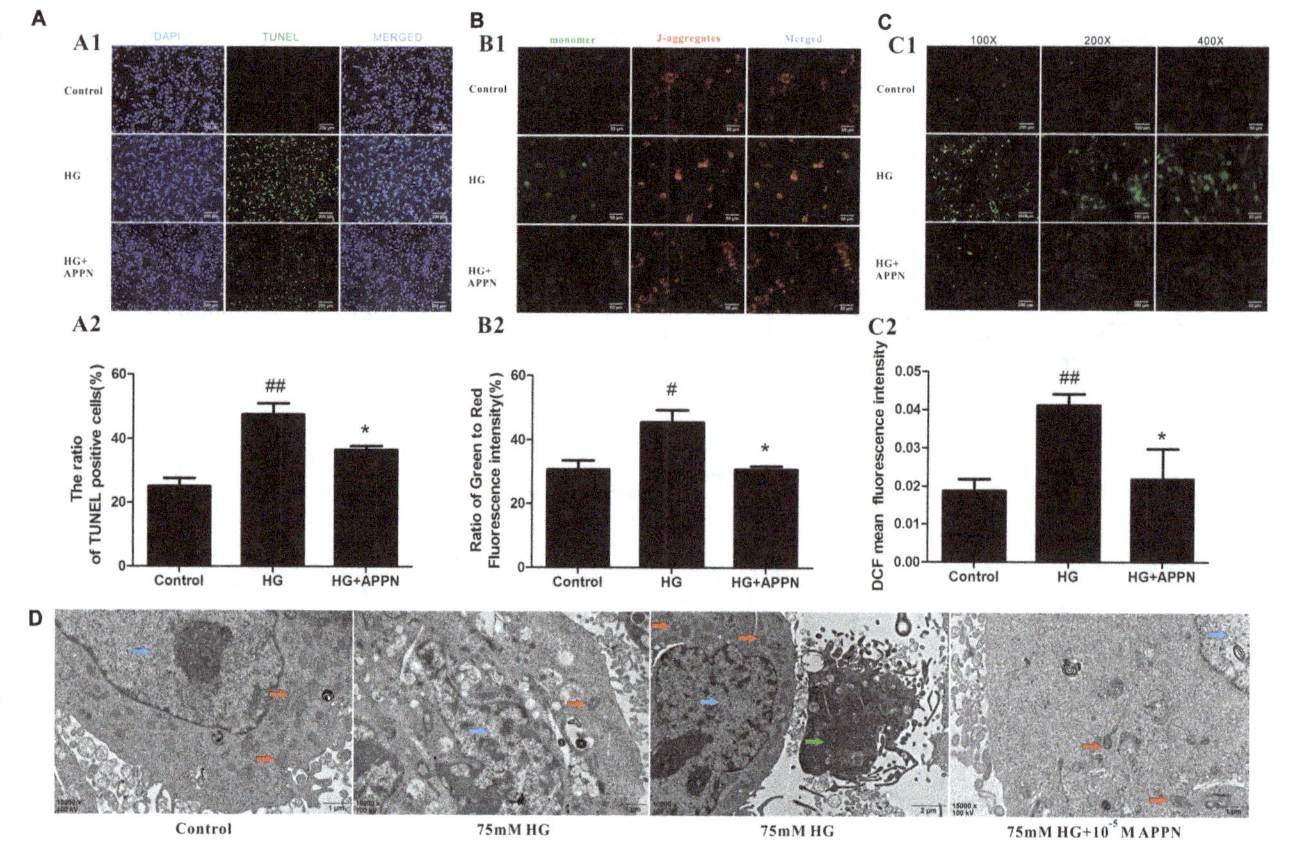

FIGURE 9 | Effects of adapentpronitrile on $\Delta\psi m$, ROS level, apoptosis, and mitochondria morphology in HT22 cells induced by HG overload. **(A)** Effects of adapentpronitrile on the TUNEL-positive cell number in HT22 cells induced by HG overload. **(B)** Effects of adapentpronitrile on mitochondrial membrane potential in HT22 cells induced by HG overload. **(C)** Effects of adapentpronitrile on ROS generation in HT22 cells induced by HG overload. Representative images of experiments are shown. Data were expressed as mean ± SD of four independent experiments, and were analyzed statistically using one-way ANOVA, followed by Dunnett-t type multiple comparison tests. $^{\#}P < 0.05$ and $^{\#\#}P < 0.01$ vs. the control group, respectively; $^{*}P < 0.05$ vs. the HG group. **(D)** The ultrastructure in HT22 cells detected by TEM. Representative images of experiments are shown. Sections were pictured at 15,000×. Scale bar = 1 μm. The blue, red, and green arrows were pointed to the nucleus, mitochondria, and apoptotic body, respectively.

Additionally, previous studies confirmed that oxidative stress promotes mitochondrial dysfunction. The mitochondrial respiratory chain can be impaired by mitochondrial dysfunction to produce excess ROS and exacerbate oxidative stress even further, forming a "vicious circle" (Vučetić-Arsić et al., 2013). Mitochondrial dysfunction initiates apoptosis by activating caspase-dependent or caspase-independent pathways (Arun et al., 2016). This process is regulated by the proteins of Bcl-2 family, including Bcl-2, Bcl-xL, Bax, and Bak. After a conformational shift, the pro-apoptotic proteins Bax and Bak insert themselves into mitochondrial membranes, where pro-apoptotic factors cytochrome c is released into the cytosol through the mitochondrial permeability transition pore (MPTP) or other channels (Tait and Green, 2010). Elevated cytosolic levels of soluble cytochrome c can lead to the increased cell mortality associated with neurodegeneration (Perier et al., 2005). In our present study, expression of the anti-apoptotic protein Bcl-2 was decreased significantly in the cortex and hippocampus of HFD/STZ rats, while the expression of mitochondria-associated pro-apoptotic proteins were increased significantly; these alterations were reversed by adapentpronitrile treatment. Thus, the current study indicates that the neuroprotective effects of adapentpronitrile are mediated *via* the mitochondrial apoptosis pathway.

Numerous studies suggest that disruption of the BBB is associated with age, obesity, and diabetes, and could contribute to early cognitive impairment (Tucsek et al., 2014; Montagne et al., 2015; van de Haar et al., 2016; Xu et al., 2016). Extensive research has revealed candidate drugs that have a better effect on CNS diseases in preclinical studies, while the clinical application has little or no effect. The main reason is that a candidate drug has to be administered directly into the cerebrospinal fluid, where it can enter the brain to mediate the neuroprotective effect (Pardridge, 2011). Therefore, it is necessary to determine whether a candidate drug can penetrate the BBB for the treatment of CNS diseases. In the present study, adapentpronitrile was detected in the brain of normal rats at 30 min after intravenous injection, indicating that adapentpronitrile can penetrate BBB. Hence, further studies are required to determine whether the neuroprotective effects of adapentpronitrile are mediated direct

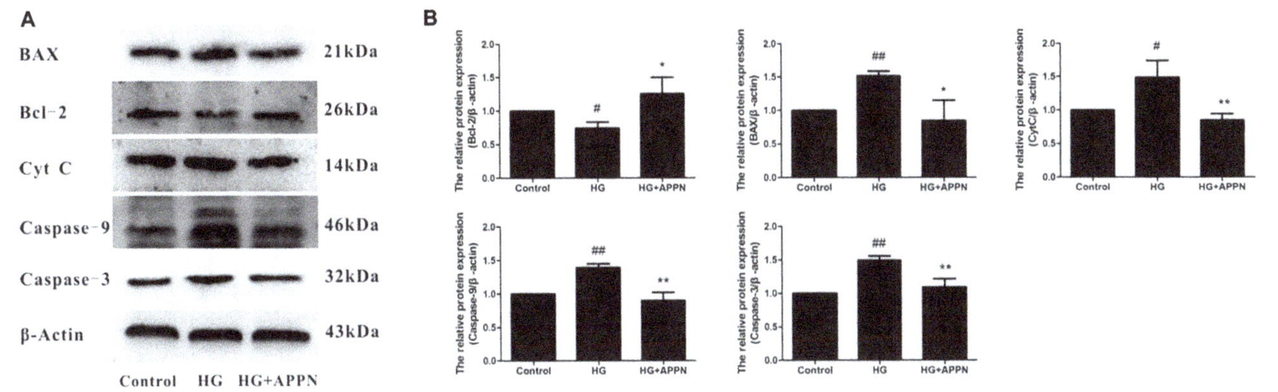

FIGURE 10 | Effect of adapentpronitrile on mitochondria-dependent apoptosis-related protein expression caused by HG in HT22 cells. **(A)** Representative blots of adapentpronitrile on the expressions of apoptosis-related proteins in HT22 cells induced by HG-overload. **(B)** The relative of protein expression were standardized to endogenous β-actin protein for each sample. Data were expressed as mean ± SD of four independent experiments, and were analyzed statistically using one-way ANOVA, followed by Dunnett-t type multiple comparison tests. $^{\#}P < 0.05$ and $^{\#\#}P < 0.01$ vs. the control group; $^{*}P < 0.05$, $^{**}P < 0.01$ vs. the HG group.

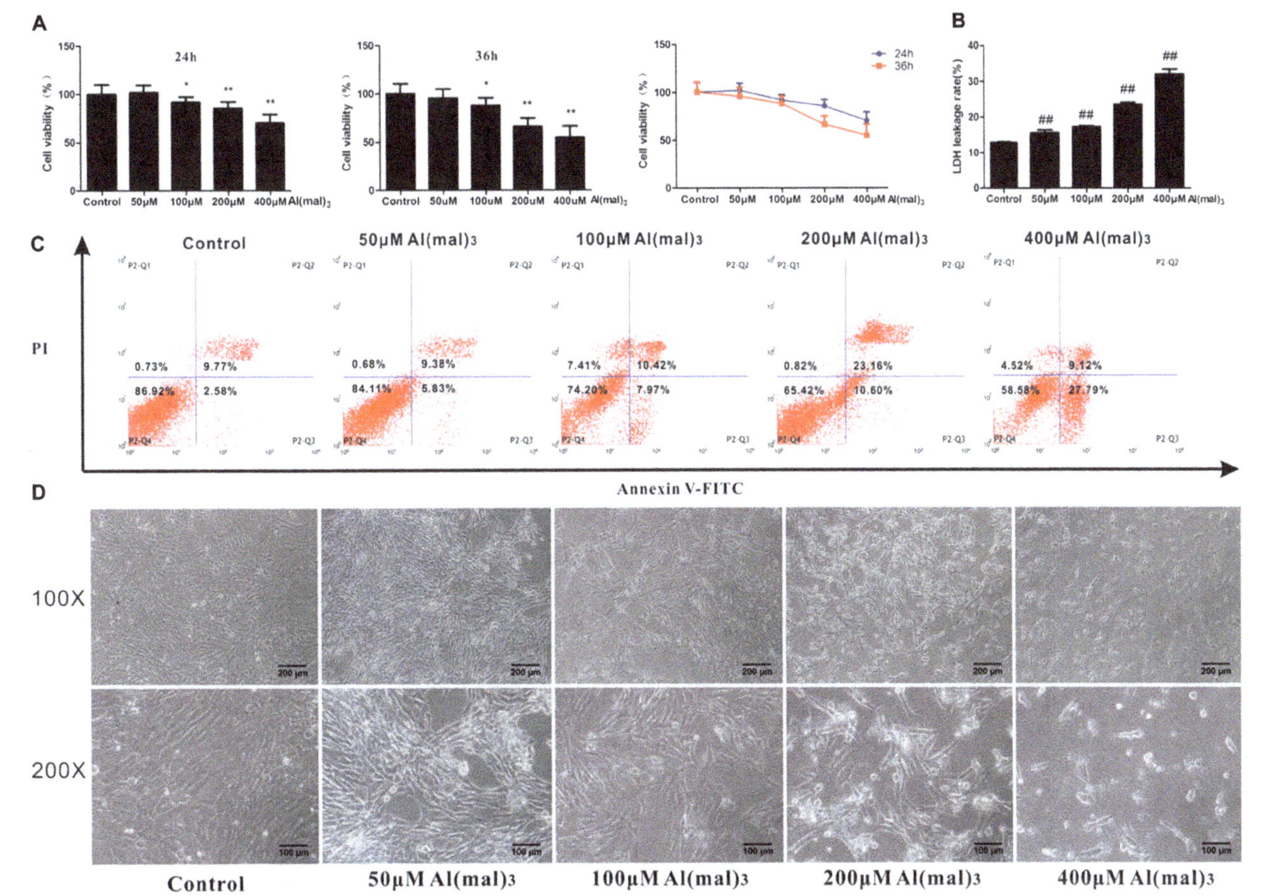

FIGURE 11 | The effects of $Al(mal)_3$ on HT22 cells. **(A)** The viability of HT22 cells treated with different concentrations of $Al(mal)_3$. Data were expressed as mean ± SD of 10 independent experiments, and were analyzed statistically using one-way ANOVA, followed by Dunnett-t type multiple comparison tests. $^{*}P < 0.05$, $^{**}P < 0.01$ vs. the control group. **(B)** The LDH leakage rate of HT22 cells treated with different concentration of $Al(mal)_3$. Data were expressed as mean ± SD of six independent experiments, and were analyzed statistically using one-way ANOVA, followed by Dunnett-t type multiple comparison tests. $^{\#\#}P < 0.01$ vs. the control group. **(C)** The flow cytometry apoptosis analysis of HT22 cells were treated with $Al(mal)_3$ for 36 h. The representative images of flow cytometry analysis are shown. **(D)** The cytomorphology changes of HT22 cells treated with different concentration of $Al(mal)_3$. Representative images of experiments are shown. The magnification of images were 100× and 200×, respectively. Scale bars were 200 and 100 μm, respectively.

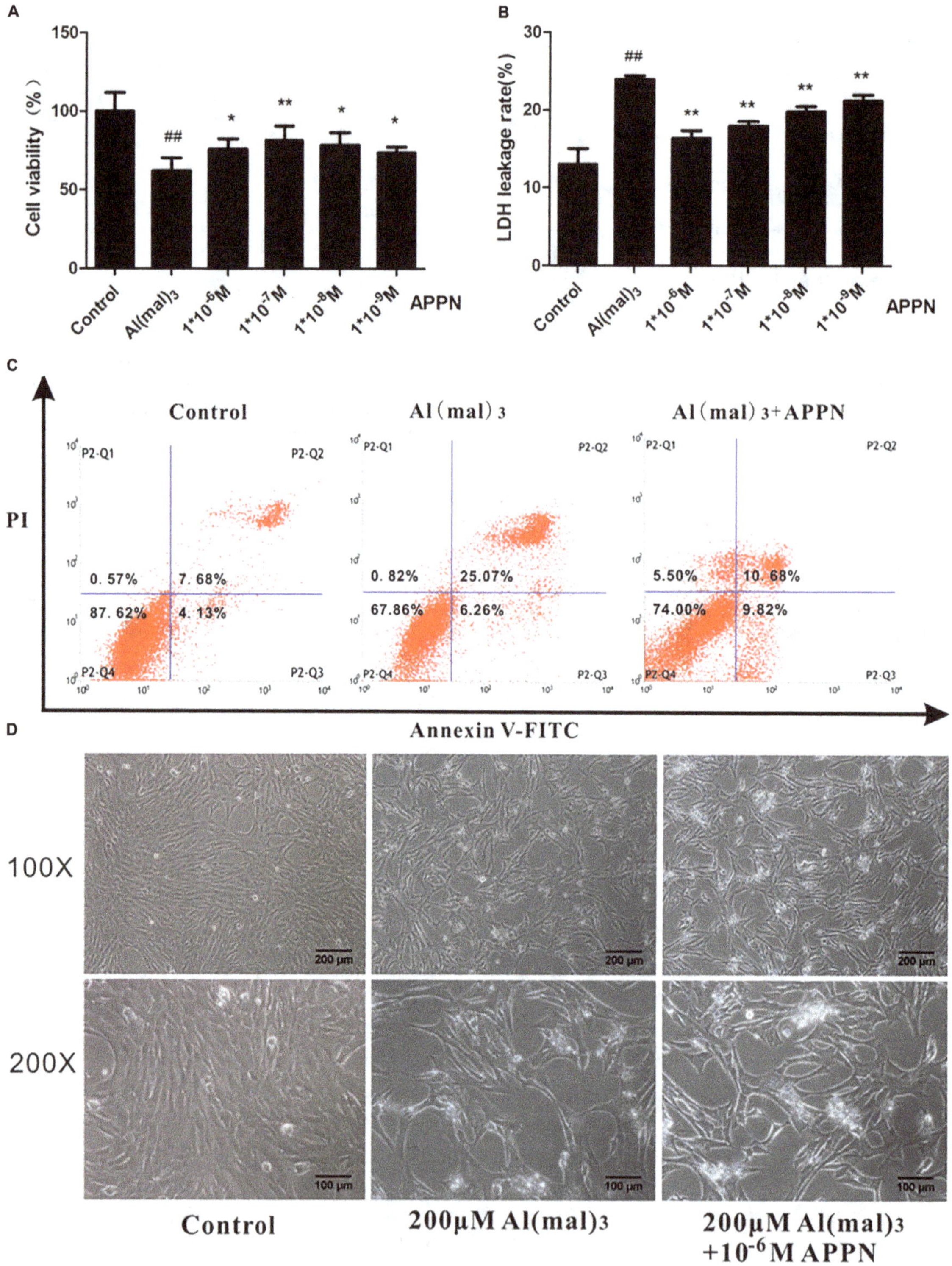

FIGURE 12 | The effect of adapentpronitrile on Al(mal)3-induced cytotoxicity in HT22 cells. **(A)** The effect of adapentpronitrile on the viability in HT22 cells induced by $Al(mal)_3$ overload. **(B)** The effect of adapentpronitrile on the LDH leakage rate in HT22 cells induced by $Al(mal)_3$ overload. Data were expressed as mean ± SD of six independent experiments, and were analyzed statistically using one-way ANOVA, followed by Dunnett-t type multiple comparison tests. $^{\#\#}P < 0.01$ vs. the control group; $^{*}P < 0.05$ and $^{**}P < 0.01$ vs. the $Al(mal)_3$ group, respectively. **(C)** The effect of adapentpronitrile on apoptosis in HT22 cells induced by $Al(mal)_3$-overload. The representative images of flow cytometry analysis are shown. **(D)** The effect of adapentpronitrile on the changes of cytomorphology in HT22 cells induced by $Al(mal)_3$-overload. Representative images of experiments are shown. The magnification of images were 100× and 200×, respectively. Scale bars were 200 and 100 μm, respectively.

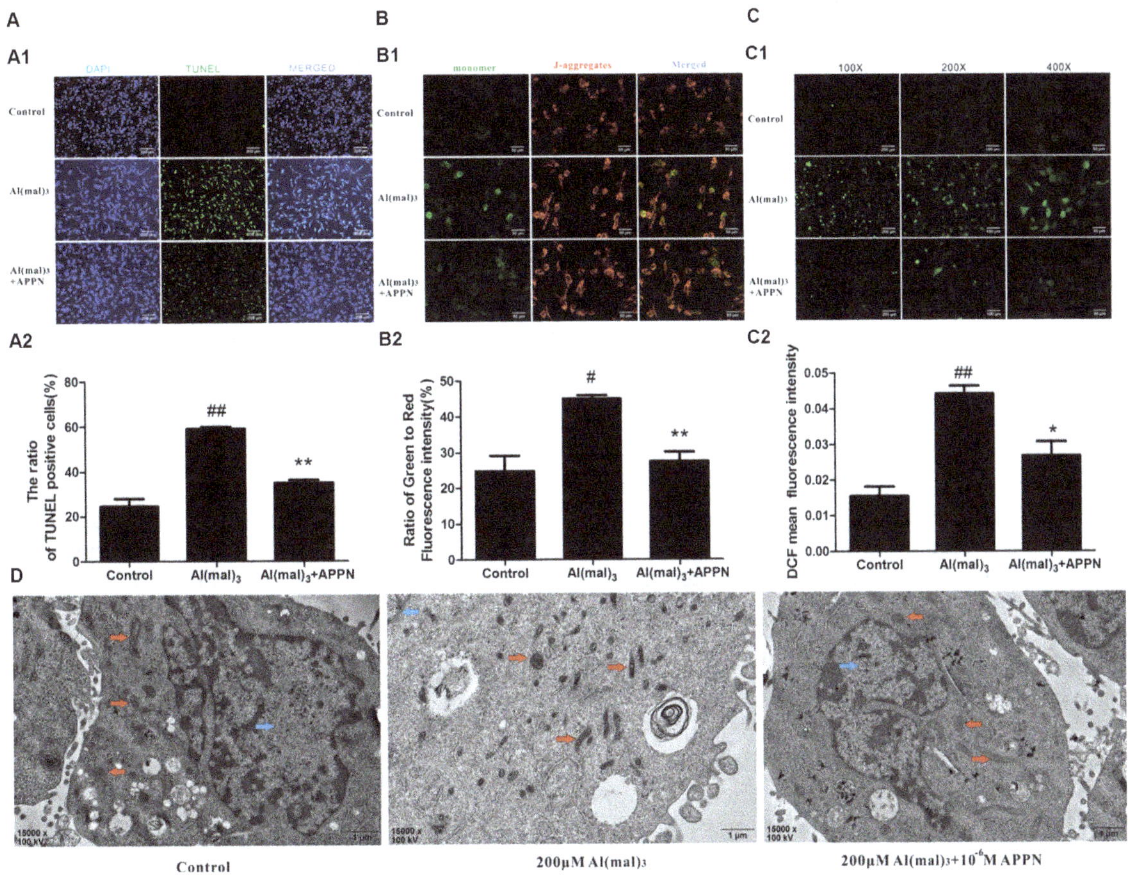

FIGURE 13 | Effects of adapentpronitrile on $\Delta\psi m$, ROS level, apoptosis, and mitochondria morphology in HT22 cells induced by $Al(mal)_3$ overload. **(A)** Effects of adapentpronitrile on the TUNEL-positive cell number in HT22 cells induced by $Al(mal)_3$ overload. **(B)** Effects of adapentpronitrile on mitochondrial membrane potential in HT22 cells induced by $Al(mal)_3$ overload. **(C)** Effects of adapentpronitrile on ROS generation in HT22 cells induced by $Al(mal)_3$ overload. Representative images of experiments are shown. Data were expressed as mean ± SD of four independent experiments, and were analyzed statistically using one-way ANOVA, followed by Dunnett-t type multiple comparison tests. $^{\#}P < 0.05$ and $^{\#\#}P < 0.01$ vs. the control group, respectively; $^{*}P < 0.05$ and $^{**}P < 0.01$ vs. the $Al(mal)_3$ group, respectively. **(D)** The ultrastructure in HT22 cells detected by TEM. Representative images of experiments are shown. Sections were pictured at 15,000×. Scale bar = 1 μm. The blue, red, and green arrows were pointed to the nucleus, mitochondria, and apoptotic body, respectively.

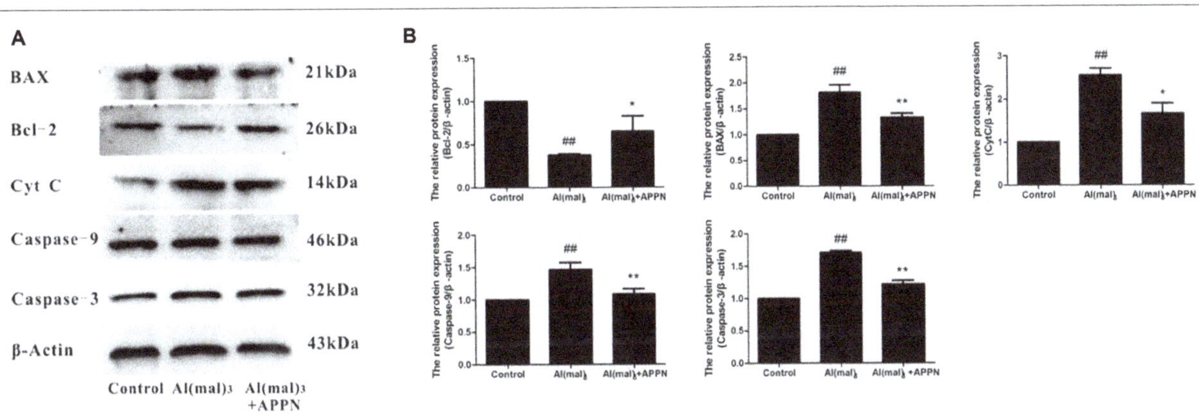

FIGURE 14 | Effect of adapentpronitrile on mitochondria-dependent apoptosis-related protein expression caused by $Al(mal)_3$ in HT22 cells. **(A)** Representative blots of adapentpronitrile on the expressions of apoptosis-related proteins in HT22 cells induced by $Al(mal)_3$. **(B)** The relative of protein expression were standardized to endogenous β-actin protein for each sample. Data were expressed as mean ± SD of four independent experiments, and were analyzed statistically using one-way ANOVA, followed by Dunnett-t type multiple comparison tests. $^{\#}P < 0.05$ and $^{\#\#}P < 0.01$ vs. the control group; $^{*}P < 0.05$, $^{**}P < 0.01$ vs. the $Al(mal)_3$ group.

or indirect action on neurons and whether the mechanism is related to DPP-IV dependent or independent.

To imitate the hyperglycemic state in the CNS of diabetic patients, we subjected HT22 cells, which are a neuronal cell line derived from murine hippocampus, to HG treatment *in vitro*. We found that neuronal injury aggravated with the HG concentration increasing, which was ameliorated by adapentpronitrile treatment.

In accordance with the results of our *in vitro* study, adapentpronitrile significantly abrogated the increase in ROS levels and neuronal apoptosis, and the decrease in MMP in HT22 cells following HG insult. Furthermore, adapentpronitrile treatment significantly increased Bcl-2 protein expression in HT22 cells, while the expression of Bax, cytochrome c, caspase 3, and caspase 9 proteins was decreased.

In order to further confirm the neuroprotection and mechanism of adapentpronitrile, the cell injury model was established by aluminum overload in HT22 cells. Metals play a risk role in AD *via* the production of free radicals, including iron, aluminum, mercury, copper, and zinc (Christen, 2000). Extensive literature illustrated that the neurotoxic effects of aluminum are beyond any doubt, and it cannot be discarded that aluminum may contribute to the development of AD (Gupta et al., 2005). Epidemiological evidence indicated that aluminum concentrations of drinking water is associated to the prevalence of AD with a dose–response relationship, and a similar link between exposure and the prevalence were also reported in elderly populations (Crapper et al., 1980; Rondeau et al., 2009). Furthermore, elevation of aluminum content were observed in the brains of patients with AD (Becaria et al., 2002), and it was also detected in *post mortem* neurofibrillary tangles and senile plaques of AD patients (Meiri et al., 1993). Both aluminum and aggregated β-amyloid stimulate free radicals production and contribute to mitochondrial dysfunction relating to the pathology of AD. $Al(mal)_3$ is a salt forms of aluminum used to imitate AD-like neuronal injury *in vivo* and *in vitro* for its stability at physiological pH (Johnson et al., 2005). Our experimental results showed that treatment of $Al(mal)_3$ decreased the viability and increase the LDH leakage rate in a concentration-dependent manner, which was ameliorated by adapentpronitrile treatment. Adapentpronitrile significantly blunted the reduction of mitochondrial membrane potential, ROS overproduction, of TUNEL-positive cell number and pro-apoptotic protein expressions triggered by $Al(mal)_3$-overload.

To explore the association of the neuroprotective effect of adapentpronitrile with DPP-IV inhibition, we determined DPP-IV activity in HT22 cells. We did not detect significant activity of DPP-IV in HT22 cells, indicating that the neuroprotective effects of adapentpronitrile are mediated *via* a DPP-IV-independent pathway *in vitro*.

CONCLUSION

The DPP-IV inhibitor adapentpronitrile effectively attenuates the neuronal injury caused by HG/$Al(mal)_3$ overload *in vitro* and ameliorates both the hippocampal and cortical neuron injury caused by HFD combined with low dose STZ *in vivo*. Pharmacokinetic studies confirmed the ability of adapentpronitrile to penetrate the blood–brain barrier *in vivo*, while no significant DPP-IV activity was detected in HT22 cells *in vitro*. These results together suggest that adapentpronitrile mediates obvious protection against diabetic neuronal injury, at least partially, by inhibiting mitochondrial oxidative stress and the apoptosis pathway *via* a DPP-IV-independent pathway. Thus, adapentpronitrile is implicated as a promising candidate for AD therapy in the clinical setting. However, the mechanism underlying the neuroprotective effects of adapentpronitrile and the potential of other whether the other DPP-IV inhibitors to mediate similar effects remain to be fully explored.

AUTHOR CONTRIBUTIONS

JY made substantial contribution to conception and design and performance of the study. LY, WH, YiL, HL, CH, DH, JM, YY, QC, YuL, JZ, HX, ZC, HW, and, DR participated in performance of all experiments and carried out the data analysis. XH provided adapentpronitrile and experimental guidance. YX participated in the grammar and writing instruction. LY participated in performance of the study and in writing the manuscript. All authors read and approved the final manuscript. JY is the guarantor of this work and, as such, had full access to all the data in the study and takes responsibility for the integrity of the data and the accuracy of the data analysis.

FUNDING

This work was supported by research grants from the Chongqing Science and Technology Commission Fund (cstc2015zdcy-ztzx120003).

REFERENCES

Arun, S., Liu, L., and Donmez, G. (2016). Mitochondrial biology and neurological diseases. *Curr. Neuropharmacol.* 14, 143–154. doi: 10.2174/1570159X13666150703154541

Baglietto-Vargas, D., Shi, J., Yaeger, D. M., Ager, R., and LaFerla, F. M. (2016). Diabetes and Alzheimer's disease crosstalk. *Neurosci. Biobehav. Rev.* 64, 272–287. doi: 10.1016/j.neubiorev.2016.03.005

Becaria, A., Campbell, A., and Bondy, S. C. (2002). Aluminum as a toxicant. *Toxicol. Ind. Health* 18, 309–320. doi: 10.1191/0748233702th157oa

Biessels, G. J., and Reagan, L. P. (2015). Hippocampal insulin resistance and cognitive dysfunction. *Nat. Rev. Neurosci.* 16, 660–671. doi: 10.1038/nrn4019

Bosco, D., Fava, A., Plastino, M., Montalcini, T., and Pujia, A. (2011). Possible implications of insulin resistance and glucose metabolism in Alzheimer's disease pathogenesis. *J. Cell. Mol. Med.* 15, 1807–1821. doi: 10.1111/j.1582-4934.2011.01318.x

Butler, A. E., Janson, J., Bonner-Weir, S., Ritzel, R., Rizza, R. A., and Butler, P. C. (2003). Beta-cell deficit and increased beta-cell apoptosis in humans with type 2 diabetes. *Diabetes Metab. Res. Rev.* 52, 102–110. doi: 10.2337/diabetes.52.1.102

Chen, X., Guo, C., and Kong, J. (2012). Oxidative stress in neurodegenerative diseases. *Neural Regen. Res.* 7, 376–385. doi: 10.3969/j.issn.1673-5374.2012.05.009

Christen, Y. (2000). Oxidative stress and Alzheimer disease. *Am. J. Clin. Nutr.* 71, 621S–629S. doi: 10.1093/ajcn/71.2.621s

Crapper, D. R., Quittkat, S., Krishnan, S. S., Dalton, A. J., and De Boni, U. (1980). Intranuclear aluminum content in Alzheimer's disease, dialysis encephalopathy, and experimental aluminum encephalopathy. *Acta Neuropathol.* 50, 19–24. doi: 10.1007/BF00688530

De Felice, F. G., and Ferreira, S. T. (2014). Inflammation, defective insulin signaling, and mitochondrial dysfunction as common molecular denominators connecting type 2 diabetes to Alzheimer disease. *Diabetes Metab. Res. Rev.* 63, 2262–2272. doi: 10.2337/db13-1954

Del Rio, D., Stewart, A. J., and Pellegrini, N. (2005). A review of recent studies on malondialdehyde as toxic molecule and biological marker of oxidative stress. *Nutr. Metab. Cardiovasc. Dis.* 15, 316–328. doi: 10.1016/j.numecd.2005.05.003

den Heijer, T., Vermeer, S. E., van Dijk, E. J., Prins, N. D., Koudstaal, P. J., Hofman, A., et al. (2003). Type 2 diabetes and atrophy of medial temporal lobe structures on brain MRI. *Diabetologia* 46, 1604–1610. doi: 10.1007/s00125-003-1235-0

Devi, L., Prabhu, B. M., Galati, D. F., Avadhani, N. G., and Anandatheerthavarada, H. K. (2006). Accumulation of amyloid precursor protein in the mitochondrial import channels of human Alzheimer's disease brain is associated with mitochondrial dysfunction. *J. Neurosci.* 26, 9057–9068. doi: 10.1523/JNEUROSCI.1469-06.2006

Dineley, K. T., Jahrling, J. B., and Denner, L. (2014). Insulin resistance in Alzheimer's disease. *Neurobiol. Dis.* 72(Pt A), 92–103. doi: 10.1016/j.nbd.2014.09.001

Drucker, D. J., and Nauck, M. A. (2006). The incretin system: glucagon-like peptide-1 receptor agonists and dipeptidyl peptidase-4 inhibitors in type 2 diabetes. *Lancet* 368, 1696–1705. doi: 10.1016/S0140-6736(06)69705-5

DuBoff, B., Götz, J., and Feany, M. B. (2012). Tau promotes neurodegeneration via DRP1 mislocalization in vivo. *Neuron* 75, 618–632. doi: 10.1016/j.neuron.2012.06.026

Dunphy, J. L., Taylor, R. G., and Fuller, P. J. (1998). Tissue distribution of rat glucagon receptor and GLP-1 receptor gene expression. *Mol. Cell. Endocrinol.* 141, 179–186. doi: 10.1016/S0303-7207(98)00096-3

Gasparini, L., Netzer, W. J., Greengard, P., and Xu, H. (2002). Does insulin dysfunction play a role in Alzheimer's disease? *Trends Pharmacol. Sci.* 23, 288–293.

Gault, V. A., and Hölscher, C. (2008). GLP-1 agonists facilitate hippocampal LTP and reverse the impairment of LTP induced by beta-amyloid. *Eur. J. Pharmacol.* 587, 112–117. doi: 10.1016/j.ejphar.2008.03.025

Golightly, L. K., Drayna, C. C., and McDermott, M. T. (2012). Comparative clinical pharmacokinetics of dipeptidyl peptidase-4 inhibitors. *Clin. Pharmacokinet.* 51, 501–514. doi: 10.2165/11632930-000000000-00000

Guo, Y., Lei, W., Wang, J., Hu, X., Wei, Y., Ji, C., et al. (2016). Misoprostol reverse hippocampal neuron cyclooxygenase-2 downstream signaling imbalance in aluminum-overload rats. *Curr. Alzheimer Res.* 13, 1006–1016. doi: 10.2174/1567205013666160401114601

Gupta, V. B., Anitha, S., Hegde, M. L., Zecca, L., Garruto, R. M., Ravid, R., et al. (2005). Aluminium in Alzheimer's disease: are we still at a crossroad? *Cell. Mol. Life Sci.* 62, 143–158. doi: 10.1007/s00018-004-4317-3

Hardy, J., and Selkoe, D. J. (2002). The amyloid hypothesis of Alzheimer's disease: progress and problems on the road to therapeutics. *Science* 297, 353–356. doi: 10.1126/science.1072994

Hirabayashi, N., Hata, J., Ohara, T., Mukai, N., Nagata, M., Shibata, M., et al. (2016). Association between diabetes and hippocampal atrophy in elderly japanese: the hisayama study. *Diabetes care* 39, 1543–1549. doi: 10.2337/dc15-2800

Ho, N., and Sommers, M. S. (2013). Effects of diabetes on hippocampal neurogenesis: links to cognition and depression. *Neurosci. Biobehav. Rev.* 37, 1346–1362. doi: 10.1016/j.neubiorev.2013.03.010

Holst, J. J. (2007). The physiology of glucagon-like peptide 1. *Physiol. Rev.* 87, 1409–1439. doi: 10.1152/physrev.00034.2006

Johnson, V. J., Kim, S. H., and Sharma, R. P. (2005). Aluminum-maltolate induces apoptosis and necrosis in neuro-2a cells: potential role for p53 signaling. *Toxicol. Sci.* 83, 329–339. doi: 10.1093/toxsci/kfi028

Kandimalla, R., Vallamkondu, J., Corgiat, E. B., and Gill, K. D. (2016). Understanding aspects of aluminum exposure in Alzheimer's disease development. *Brain Pathol.* 26, 139–154. doi: 10.1111/bpa.12333

Knock, G. A., and Ward, J. P. (2011). Redox regulation of protein kinases as a modulator of vascular function. *Antioxid. Redox Signal.* 15, 1531–1547. doi: 10.1089/ars.2010.3614

Koliaki, C., and Roden, M. (2016). Alterations of mitochondrial function and insulin sensitivity in human obesity and diabetes mellitus. *Annu. Rev. Nutr.* 36, 337–367. doi: 10.1146/annurev-nutr-071715-050656

Kosaraju, J., Gali, C. C., Khatwal, R. B., Dubala, A., Chinni, S., Holsinger, R. M., et al. (2013). Saxagliptin: a dipeptidyl peptidase-4 inhibitor ameliorates streptozotocin induced Alzheimer's disease. *Neuropharmacology* 72, 291–300. doi: 10.1016/j.neuropharm.2013.04.008

Kumar, V., and Gill, K. D. (2009). Aluminium neurotoxicity: neurobehavioural and oxidative aspects. *Arch. Toxicol.* 83, 965–978. doi: 10.1007/s00204-009-0455-6

Lenzen, S. (2008). The mechanisms of alloxan- and streptozotocin-induced diabetes. *Diabetologia* 51, 216–226. doi: 10.1007/s00125-007-0886-7

Li, L., Liao, G., Yang, G., Lu, Y., Du, X., Liu, J., et al. (2015). High-fat diet combined with low-dose streptozotocin injections induces metabolic syndrome in *Macaca mulatta*. *Endocrine* 49, 659–668. doi: 10.1007/s12020-015-0542-9

Lin, M. T., and Beal, M. F. (2006). Mitochondrial dysfunction and oxidative stress in neurodegenerative diseases. *Nature* 443, 787–795. doi: 10.1038/nature05292

Lobner, D. (2000). Comparison of the LDH and MTT assays for quantifying cell death: validity for neuronal apoptosis? *J. Neurosci. Methods* 96, 147–152. doi: 10.1016/S0165-0270 (99)00193-4

Ma, J., Li, H., Hu, X., Yang, L., Chen, Q., Hu, C., et al. (2017). CMD-05, a novel promising clinical anti-diabetic drug candidate, in vivo and vitro studies. *Sci. Rep.* 7:46628. doi: 10.1038/srep46628

Ma, J., Yang, Q., Wei, Y., Yang, Y., Ji, C., Hu, X., et al. (2016). Effect of the PGD2-DP signaling pathway on primary cultured rat hippocampal neuron injury caused by aluminum overload. *Sci. Rep.* 6:24646. doi: 10.1038/srep24646

Ma, X., Guan, Y., and Hua, X. (2014). Glucagon-like peptide 1-potentiated insulin secretion and proliferation of pancreatic β-cells. *J. Diabetes* 6, 394–402. doi: 10.1111/1753-0407.12161

Maher, P. A., and Schubert, D. R. (2009). Metabolic links between diabetes and Alzheimer's disease. *Expert Rev. Neurother.* 9, 617–630. doi: 10.1586/ern.09.18

Manoharan, S., Guillemin, G. J., Abiramasundari, R. S., Essa, M. M., Akbar, M., and Akbar, M. D. (2016). The role of reactive oxygen species in the pathogenesis of Alzheimer's disease, Parkinson's disease, and Huntington's disease: a mini review. *Oxid. Med. Cell. Longev.* 2016:8590578. doi: 10.1155/2016/8590578

McClean, P. L., and Hölscher, C. (2014). Liraglutide can reverse memory impairment, synaptic loss and reduce plaque load in aged APP/PS1 mice, a model of Alzheimer's disease. *Neuropharmacology* 76(Pt A), 57–67. doi: 10.1016/j.neuropharm.2013.08.005

McCrimmon, R. J., and Ryan, C. M. (2012). Diabetes and cognitive dysfunction. *Lancet* 379, 2291–2299. doi: 10.1016/S0140-6736(12)60360-2

Meiri, H., Banin, E., Roll, M., and Rousseau, A. (1993). Toxic effects of aluminium on nerve cells and synaptic transmission. *Prog. Neurobiol.* 40, 89–121. doi: 10.1016/0301-0082(93)90049-X

Montagne, A., Barnes, S. R., Sweeney, M. D., Halliday, M. R., Sagare, A. P., Zhao, Z., et al. (2015). Blood-brain barrier breakdown in the aging human hippocampus. *Neuron* 85, 296–302. doi: 10.1016/j.neuron.2014.12.032

Moran, C., Phan, T. G., Chen, J., Blizzard, L., Beare, R., Venn, A., et al. (2013). Brain atrophy in type 2 diabetes: regional distribution and influence on cognition. *Diabetes Care* 36, 4036–4042. doi: 10.2337/dc13-0143

Moreira, P. I. (2012). Alzheimer's disease and diabetes: an integrative view of the role of mitochondria, oxidative stress, and insulin. *J. Alzheimers Dis.* 30(Suppl. 2), S199–S215. doi: 10.3233/JAD-2011-111127

Mullard, A. (2016). Symptomatic AD treatment fails in first phase III. *Nat. Rev. Drug Discov.* 15:738. doi: 10.1038/nrd.2016.225

Nassar, N. N., Al-Shorbagy, M. Y., Arab, H. H., and Abdallah, D. M. (2015). Saxagliptin: a novel antiparkinsonian approach. *Neuropharmacology* 89, 308–317. doi: 10.1016/j.neuropharm.2014.10.007

Pardridge, W. M. (2011). Drug transport in brain via the cerebrospinal fluid. *Fluids Barriers CNS* 8:7. doi: 10.1186/2045-8118-8-7

Perier, C., Tieu, K., Guégan, C., Caspersen, C., Jackson-Lewis, V., Carelli, V., et al. (2005). Complex I deficiency primes Bax-dependent neuronal apoptosis through mitochondrial oxidative damage. *Proc. Natl. Acad. Sci. U.S.A.* 102, 19126–19131. doi: 10.1073/pnas.0508215102

Phiel, C. J., Wilson, C. A., Lee, V. M., and Klein, P. S. (2003). GSK-3alpha regulates production of Alzheimer's disease amyloid-beta peptides. *Nature* 423, 435–439. doi: 10.1038/nature01640

Pipatpiboon, N., Pintana, H., Pratchayasakul, W., Chattipakorn, N., and Chattipakorn, S. C. (2013). DPP4-inhibitor improves neuronal insulin receptor function, brain mitochondrial function and cognitive function in rats with insulin resistance induced by high-fat diet consumption. *Eur. J. Neurosci.* 37, 839–849. doi: 10.1111/ejn.12088

Qiu, W. Q., and Folstein, M. F. (2006). Insulin, insulin-degrading enzyme and amyloid-beta peptide in Alzheimer's disease: review and hypothesis. *Neurobiol. Aging* 27, 190–198. doi: 10.1016/j.neurobiolaging.2005.01.004

Ranganath, L. R. (2008). Incretins: pathophysiological and therapeutic implications of glucose-dependent insulinotropic polypeptide and glucagon-like peptide-1. *J. Clin. Pathol.* 61, 401–409. doi: 10.1136/jcp.2006.043232

Reed, M. J., Meszaros, K., Entes, L. J., Claypool, M. D., Pinkett, J. G., Gadbois, T. M., et al. (2000). A new rat model of type 2 diabetes: the fat-fed, streptozotocin-treated rat. *Metabolism* 49, 1390–1394. doi: 10.1053/meta.2000.17721

Rondeau, V., Jacqmin-Gadda, H., Commenges, D., Helmer, C., and Dartigues, J. F. (2009). Aluminum and silica in drinking water and the risk of Alzheimer's disease or cognitive decline: findings from 15-year follow-up of the PAQUID cohort. *Am. J. Epidemiol.* 169, 489–496. doi: 10.1093/aje/kwn348

Schmitt, K., Grimm, A., Kazmierczak, A., Strosznajder, J. B., Götz, J., and Eckert, A. (2012). Insights into mitochondrial dysfunction: aging, amyloid-β, and tau-A deleterious trio. *Antioxid. Redox Signal.* 16, 1456–1466. doi: 10.1089/ars.2011.4400

Smith, D. G., Cappai, R., and Barnham, K. J. (2007). The redox chemistry of the Alzheimer's disease amyloid beta peptide. *Biochim. Biophys. Acta* 1768, 1976–1990. doi: 10.1016/j.bbamem.2007.02.002

Son, Y., Kim, S., Chung, H. T., and Pae, H. O. (2013). Reactive oxygen species in the activation of MAP kinases. *Methods Enzymol.* 528, 27–48. doi: 10.1016/B978-0-12-405881-1.00002-1

Tait, S. W., and Green, D. R. (2010). Mitochondria and cell death: outer membrane permeabilization and beyond. *Nat. Rev. Mol. Cell Biol.* 11, 621–632. doi: 10.1038/nrm2952

Takeda, S., Sato, N., Uchio-Yamada, K., Sawada, K., Kunieda, T., Takeuchi, D., et al. (2010). Diabetes-accelerated memory dysfunction via cerebrovascular inflammation and abeta deposition in an Alzheimer mouse model with diabetes. *Proc. Natl. Acad. Sci. U.S.A.* 107, 7036–7041. doi: 10.1073/pnas.1000645107

Tucsek, Z., Toth, P., Sosnowska, D., Gautam, T., Mitschelen, M., Koller, A., et al. (2014). Obesity in aging exacerbates blood-brain barrier disruption, neuroinflammation, and oxidative stress in the mouse hippocampus: effects on expression of genes involved in beta-amyloid generation and Alzheimer's disease. *J. Gerontol. A Biol. Sci. Med. Sci.* 69, 1212–1226. doi: 10.1093/gerona/glt177

Valko, M., Leibfritz, D., Moncol, J., Cronin, M. T., Mazur, M., and Telser, J. (2007). Free radicals and antioxidants in normal physiological functions and human disease. *Int. J. Biochem. Cell Biol.* 39, 44–84. doi: 10.1016/j.biocel.2006.07.001

van de Haar, H. J., Burgmans, S., Jansen, J. F., van Osch, M. J., van Buchem, M. A., Muller, M., et al. (2016). Blood-Brain barrier leakage in patients with early Alzheimer Disease. *Radiology* 281, 527–535. doi: 10.1148/radiol.2016152244

Verbon, E. H., Post, J. A., and Boonstra, J. (2012). The influence of reactive oxygen species on cell cycle progression in mammalian cells. *Gene* 511, 1–6. doi: 10.1016/j.gene.2012.08.038

Verdile, G., Keane, K. N., Cruzat, V. F., Medic, S., Sabale, M., Rowles, J., et al. (2015). Inflammation and oxidative stress: the molecular connectivity between insulin resistance, Obesity, and Alzheimer's disease. *Mediators Inflamm.* 2015:105828. doi: 10.1155/2015/105828

Verspohl, E. J. (2009). Novel therapeutics for type 2 diabetes: incretin hormone mimetics (glucagon-like peptide-1 receptor agonists) and dipeptidyl peptidase-4 inhibitors. *Pharmacol. Ther.* 124, 113–138. doi: 10.1016/j.pharmthera.2009.06.002

Vučetić-Arsić, S., Radonjić, N. V., Jovanović, M., Selaković, V., Nikolić, T., Velimirović, M., et al. (2013). Oxidative stress precedes mitochondrial dysfunction in gerbil brain after aluminum ingestion. *Environ. Toxicol. Pharmacol.* 36, 1242–1252. doi: 10.1016/j.etap.2013.10.008

Wallace, D. C. (2005). A mitochondrial paradigm of metabolic and degenerative diseases, aging, and cancer: a dawn for evolutionary medicine. *Annu. Rev. Genet.* 39, 359–407. doi: 10.1146/annurev.genet.39. 110304.095751

Xu, Z., Zeng, W., Sun, J., Chen, W., Zhang, R., Yang, Z., et al. (2016). The quantification of blood-brain barrier disruption using dynamic contrast-enhanced magnetic resonance imaging in aging rhesus monkeys with spontaneous type 2 diabetes mellitus. *Neuroimage* 158, 480–487. doi: 10.1016/j.neuroimage.2016.07.017

Permissions

All chapters in this book were first published by Frontiers; hereby published with permission under the Creative Commons Attribution License or equivalent. Every chapter published in this book has been scrutinized by our experts. Their significance has been extensively debated. The topics covered herein carry significant findings which will fuel the growth of the discipline. They may even be implemented as practical applications or may be referred to as a beginning point for another development.

The contributors of this book come from diverse backgrounds, making this book a truly international effort. This book will bring forth new frontiers with its revolutionizing research information and detailed analysis of the nascent developments around the world.

We would like to thank all the contributing authors for lending their expertise to make the book truly unique. They have played a crucial role in the development of this book. Without their invaluable contributions this book wouldn't have been possible. They have made vital efforts to compile up to date information on the varied aspects of this subject to make this book a valuable addition to the collection of many professionals and students.

This book was conceptualized with the vision of imparting up-to-date information and advanced data in this field. To ensure the same, a matchless editorial board was set up. Every individual on the board went through rigorous rounds of assessment to prove their worth. After which they invested a large part of their time researching and compiling the most relevant data for our readers.

The editorial board has been involved in producing this book since its inception. They have spent rigorous hours researching and exploring the diverse topics which have resulted in the successful publishing of this book. They have passed on their knowledge of decades through this book. To expedite this challenging task, the publisher supported the team at every step. A small team of assistant editors was also appointed to further simplify the editing procedure and attain best results for the readers.

Apart from the editorial board, the designing team has also invested a significant amount of their time in understanding the subject and creating the most relevant covers. They scrutinized every image to scout for the most suitable representation of the subject and create an appropriate cover for the book.

The publishing team has been an ardent support to the editorial, designing and production team. Their endless efforts to recruit the best for this project, has resulted in the accomplishment of this book. They are a veteran in the field of academics and their pool of knowledge is as vast as their experience in printing. Their expertise and guidance has proved useful at every step. Their uncompromising quality standards have made this book an exceptional effort. Their encouragement from time to time has been an inspiration for everyone.

The publisher and the editorial board hope that this book will prove to be a valuable piece of knowledge for researchers, students, practitioners and scholars across the globe.

List of Contributors

Zsófia Hoyk, András Kincses, Fruzsina R. Walter, Szilvia Veszelka, Judit Vígh, Beáta Barabási, András Harazin and Mária A. Deli
Institute of Biophysics, Biological Research Centre, Hungarian Academy of Sciences, Szeged, Hungary

Melinda E. Tóth, Nikolett Lénárt, Dóra Nagy, Brigitta Dukay, Alexandra Csefová, Miklós Sántha and László Vígh
Institute of Biochemistry, Biological Research Centre, Hungarian Academy of Sciences, Szeged, Hungary

Ágnes Zvara and László G. Puskás
Laboratory of Functional Genomics, Core Facilities, Biological Research Centre, Hungarian Academy of Sciences, Szeged, Hungary

György Seprényi
Department of Anatomy, Histology and Embryology, Faculty of Medicine, University of Szeged, Szeged, Hungary

Ágnes Kittel
Laboratory of Molecular Pharmacology, Department of Pharmacology, Institute of Experimental Medicine, Hungarian Academy of Sciences, Budapest, Hungary

Botond Penke
Department of Medical Chemistry, Faculty of Medicine, University of Szeged, Szeged, Hungary

Jialiang Wei
Department of Neurosurgery, Xijing Hospital, Fourth Military Medical University, Xi'an, China
Department of Health Services, Fourth Military Medical University, Xi'an, China

Xiuquan Wu, Peng Luo, Kangyi Yue, Yang Yu, Jingnan Pu, Lei Zhang, Shuhui Dai and Zhou Fei
Department of Neurosurgery, Xijing Hospital, Fourth Military Medical University, Xi'an, China

Donghui Han
Department of Urology, Xijing Hospital, Fourth Military Medical University, Xi'an, China

Rudy Chang and Alexander C. Zambon
Department of Biopharmaceutical Sciences, School of Pharmacy and Health Sciences, Keck Graduate Institute, Claremont, CA, United States

Juan Castillo
Department of Neuroscience, Claremont McKenna College, Claremont, CA, United States

Tatiana B. Krasieva
Beckman Laser Institute, University of California, Irvine, Irvine, CA, United States

Mark J. Fisher
Departments of Neurology and Pathology & Laboratory Medicine, University of California, Irvine, Irvine, CA, United States

Rachita K. Sumbria
Department of Biopharmaceutical Sciences, School of Pharmacy and Health Sciences, Keck Graduate Institute, Claremont, CA, United States
Departments of Neurology and Pathology & Laboratory Medicine, University of California, Irvine, Irvine, CA, United States

Si-Hao Du, Wei Zhang, Xia Yue, Xiao-Hui Tan, Dong-Fang Qiao and Huijun Wang
School of Forensic Medicine, Southern Medical University, Guangzhou, China

Xiao-Qing Luo
School of Forensic Medicine, Southern Medical University, Guangzhou, China
Nanfang Hospital, Southern Medical University, Guangzhou, China

Chao Liu
Guangzhou Forensic Science Institute, Guangzhou Public Security Bureau, Guangzhou, China

Yaying Song
Department of Neurology, Ruijin Hospital, Shanghai Jiao Tong University School of Medicine, Shanghai, China

Peixi Liu, Yuan Shi, Sichen Li, Yingjun Liu and Wei Zhu
Department of Neurosurgery, Huashan Hospital of Fudan University, Shanghai, China

Zongwei Li, Zhijun Zhang and Yongting Wang
Neuroscience and Neuroengineering Research Center, School of Biomedical Engineering, Med-X Research Institute, Shanghai Jiao Tong University, Shanghai, China

Jun Huang
Shanghai Key Laboratory of Hypertension, Department of Hypertension, Shanghai Institute of Hypertension, Ruijin Hospital, Shanghai Jiao Tong University School of Medicine, Shanghai, China

Guo-Yuan Yang
Department of Neurology, Ruijin Hospital, Shanghai Jiao Tong University School of Medicine, Shanghai, China
Neuroscience and Neuroengineering Research Center, School of Biomedical Engineering, Med-X Research Institute, Shanghai Jiao Tong University, Shanghai, China

Haiyun Chen
Institute of Biomedical and Pharmaceutical Sciences, Guangdong University of Technology, Guangzhou, China
Institute of New Drug Research and Guangzhou Key Laboratory of Innovative Chemical Drug Research in Cardio-Cerebrovascular Diseases, Jinan University College of Pharmacy, Guangzhou, China

Jie Cao, Zeyu Zhu, Gaoxiao Zhang, Luchen Shan, Pei Yu, Yuqiang Wang, Yewei Sun and Zaijun Zhang
Institute of New Drug Research and Guangzhou Key Laboratory of Innovative Chemical Drug Research in Cardio-Cerebrovascular Diseases, Jinan University College of Pharmacy, Guangzhou, China

Yingzhu Chen, Lingling Zhang, Beilei Chen and Yuping Li
Clinical Medical College of Yangzhou University, Yangzhou, China
Department of Neurology, Northern Jiangsu People's Hospital, Yangzhou, China

Liangzhu Wang and Liu Yang
Department of Neurology, Northern Jiangsu People's Hospital, Yangzhou, China
Dalian Medical University, Dalian, China

Xiaobo Li
Clinical Medical College of Yangzhou University, Yangzhou, China
Department of Neurology, Northern Jiangsu People's Hospital, Yangzhou, China
Institute of Neuroscience, Northern Jiangsu People's Hospital, Yangzhou, China

Hailong Yu
Clinical Medical College of Yangzhou University, Yangzhou, China
Department of Neurology, Northern Jiangsu People's Hospital, Yangzhou, China
Institute of Neuroscience, Northern Jiangsu People's Hospital, Yangzhou, China
Drum Tower Hospital, Medical School of Nanjing University, Nanjing, China

Seung Eun Lee
Virus Facility, Research Animal Resource Center, Korea Institute of Science and Technology (KIST), Seoul, South Korea

Bei Zhang, Yi-Zheng Wei, Guo-Qing Wang, Dai-Di Li, Jing-Shan Shi and Feng Zhan
Key Laboratory of Basic Pharmacology of Ministry of Education, Joint International Research Laboratory of Ethnomedicine of Ministry of Education, Zunyi Medical University, Zunyi, China

Minhee Jang
Department of Convergence Medical Science, College of Korean Medicine, Kyung Hee University, Seoul, South Korea

Ik-Hyun Cho
Department of Convergence Medical Science, College of Korean Medicine, Kyung Hee University, Seoul, South Korea
Brain Korea 21 Plus Program and Institute of Korean Medicine, College of Korean Medicine, Kyung Hee University, Seoul, South Korea

Chiara D'Angelo
Department of Clinical Immunology and IdISSC, Hospital Clínico San Carlos, Madrid, Spain
Department of Immunology, Ophthalmology and ENT, Complutense University School of Medicine, Madrid, Spain
Department of Medical, Oral and Biotechnological Sciences, University "G. d'Annunzio" Chieti-Pescara, Chieti, Italy

Oriol Franch
Department of Neurology, Hospital Ruber Internacional, Madrid, Spain

Lidia Fernández-Paredes, Alejandra Comins-Boo and Silvia Sánchez-Ramón
Department of Clinical Immunology and IdISSC, Hospital Clínico San Carlos, Madrid, Spain
Department of Immunology, Ophthalmology and ENT, Complutense University School of Medicine, Madrid, Spain

Celia Oreja-Guevara
Department of Neurology, Hospital Clínico San Carlos, Madrid, Spain

María Núñez-Beltrán
Department of Clinical Immunology and IdISSC, Hospital Clínico San Carlos, Madrid, Spain

Marcella Reale
Department of Medical, Oral and Biotechnological Sciences, University "G. d'Annunzio" Chieti-Pescara, Chieti, Italy

Abdelali Agouni
Department of Pharmaceutical Sciences, College of Pharmacy, Qatar University, Doha, Qatar

Xuan He, Shuangshuang Yang, Rui Zhang, Lina Hou, Jianrong Xu, Yaer Hu, Hao Wang and Yongfang Zhang
Department of Pharmacology, Institute of Medical Sciences, Shanghai JiaoTong University School of Medicine (SJTUSM), Shanghai, China

Rang Xu
Scientific Research Center, Xinhua Hospital, Shanghai JiaoTong University School of Medicine (SJTUSM), Shanghai, China

Tânia Faustino-Mendes
Faculty of Health Sciences, University of Beira Interior, Covilhã, Portugal

Marta Machado-Pereira and Raquel Ferreira
Faculty of Health Sciences, University of Beira Interior, Covilhã, Portugal
Health Sciences Research Centre (CICS-UBI), University of Beira Interior, Covilhã, Portugal

Miguel Castelo-Branco
Faculty of Health Sciences, University of Beira Interior, Covilhã, Portugal
Health Sciences Research Centre (CICS-UBI), University of Beira Interior, Covilhã, Portugal
Hospital Center of Cova da Beira, Covilhã, Portugal

Yiwei Wang, Yinan Chen, Qin Zhou, Jiawen Xu, Qingqing Qian, Pengfei Ni and Yanning Qian
Department of Anesthesiology, The First Affiliated Hospital of Nanjing Medical University, Nanjing, China

Aijaz S. Parray, Naveed Akhtar, Paula J. Bourke, Sujata Joseph, Deborah M. Morgan, Mark D. Santos, Muhammad F. Wadiwala and Saadat Kamran
The Stroke Program, The Neuroscience Institute, Academic Health System, Hamad Medical Corporation, Doha, Qatar

Fayaz A. Mir and Siveen K. Sivaraman
Interim Translational Institute, Academic Health System, Hamad Medical Corporation, Doha, Qatar

Ashfaq Shuaib
The Stroke Program, The Neuroscience Institute, Academic Health System, Hamad Medical Corporation, Doha, Qatar
Department of Medicine (Neurology), University of Alberta, Edmonton, AB, Canada

Qian Li, Xi Lan, Xiaoning Han and Jian Wang
Department of Anesthesiology and Critical Care Medicine, The Johns Hopkins University School of Medicine, Baltimore, MD, United States

Qiang Hao, Jun-Lin Lu, Li Ma, Xiao-Lin Chen, Xun Ye, Ya-Hui Zhao, Ming-Tao Li and Yu Chen
Department of Neurosurgery, Beijing Tiantan Hospital, Capital Medical University, Beijing, China
Department of Neurosurgery, Peking University International Hospital, Peking University, Beijing, China

Hao Wang
Department of Neurosurgery, Beijing Tiantan Hospital, Capital Medical University, Beijing, China

Yuan-Li Zhao
Department of Neurosurgery, Beijing Tiantan Hospital, Capital Medical University, Beijing, China
Department of Neurosurgery, Peking University International Hospital, Peking University, Beijing, China
China National Clinical Research Center for Neurological Diseases, Beijing, China
Stroke Center, Beijing Institute for Brain Disorders, Beijing, China
Beijing Key Laboratory of Translational Medicine for Cerebrovascular Disease, Beijing, China
Basic Medical Science Department, Capital Medical University, Beijing, China

Guodong Xu
Department of Cellular Biology & Anatomy, Louisiana State University Health Sciences Center-Shreveport, Shreveport, LA, United States
Department of Neurology, Hebei General Hospital, Shijiazhuang, China

Chun Li, Anne L. Parsiola, Jiyu Li, Kimberly D. McCarter and Hong Sun
Department of Cellular Biology & Anatomy, Louisiana State University Health Sciences Center-Shreveport, Shreveport, LA, United States

Runhua Shi
Department of Medicine/Feist-Weiller Cancer Center, Louisiana State University Health Sciences Center-Shreveport, Shreveport, LA, United States

William G. Mayhan
Basic Biomedical Sciences, Sanford School of Medicine, The University of South Dakota, Vermillion, SD, United States

Lu Yang, Ying Luo, Huan Li, Congli Hu, Jie Ma, Yang Yang, Qi Chen, Yuke Li, Jiahua Zhang, Hui Xia, Zhihao Chen, Hong Wang, Dongzhi Ran and Junqing Yang
Department of Pharmacology, The Key Laboratory of Biochemistry and Molecular Pharmacology, Chongqing Medical University, Chongqing, China

Wenli Han
Laboratory Animal Center, Chongqing Medical University, Chongqing, China

Xiangnan Hu
Department of Pharmacology, The Laboratory of Pharmaceutical Chemistry, Chongqing Medical University, Chongqing, China

Ying Xu
Department of Pharmaceutical Sciences, School of Pharmacy and Pharmaceutical Sciences, University at Buffalo, The State University of New York (SUNY), Buffalo, NY, United States

Dan Huang
Department of Pharmacology, The Laboratory of Pharmaceutical Analysis, Chongqing Medical University, Chongqing, China

Yang Yang, Ying Luo, Weimin Du, Hong Wang, Huan Li, Lu Yang, Congli Hu, Jiahua Zhang, Yuke Li, Hui Xia, Zhihao Chen, Jie Ma, Xiaoyan Tian and Junqing Yang
Department of Pharmacology, Chongqing Medical University, The Key Laboratory of Biochemistry and Molecular Pharmacology, Chongqing, China

Index

M

N

O

P

R

S

T

V

W

www.ingramcontent.com/pod-product-compliance
Lightning Source LLC
LaVergne TN
LVHW060059220926
848484LV00008BA/2237